Subramania Jayaraman
Lawrence H. Lanzl

Clinical Radiotherapy Physics

Second Edition

With the Editorial Assistance of Elisabeth F. Lanzl

With 246 Figures and 62 Tables

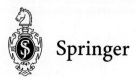

Springer

Subramania Jayaraman, Ph.D.
Chief Medical Physicist
Valley Radiation Oncology
1301 S 7th Avenue, Suite 400
Phoenix, Arizona 85007
USA

Lawrence H. Lanzl†, Ph.D.
Professor Eremitus Medical Physics
University of Chicago, Chicago Illinois
5750 S Kennwood Avenue
Chicago, Illinois 60637
USA

Title of the original edition:
Clinical Radiotherapy Physic: Volume I and II
© CRC Press, Boca Raton, New York, London, Tokyo 1996

ISBN 3-540-40284-5 Springer-Verlag Berlin Heidelberg New York

Library of Congress Cataloging-in-Publication-Data
Jayaraman, Subramania. Clinical radiotherapy physics   S. Jayaraman and L.H. Lanzl ; with the editorial assistance of
Elisabeth F. Lanzl. -- 2nd ed. p. ; cm. Includes bibliographical references and index.
ISBN 3-540-40284-5 (alk. Paper)
1. Medical physics. 2. Radiotherapy. I. Lanzl, Lawrence H. (Lawrence Herman). 1921- II. Title. [DNLM: 1. Radiotherapy.
2. Physics, 3. Radiation, Ionizing. 4. Radiometry. WN 250 J42c 2004]
R895.J39 2004   615.8'42--dc21   203054202

Springer-Verlag is a part of Springer Science+Business Media
springeronline.com

© Springer-Verlag Berlin Heidelberg 2004
Printed in Germany

Cover design: E. Kirchner, Heidelberg
Typesetter: Mitterweger & Partner, Plankstadt

Printed on acid-free paper   21/3150 hs – 5 4 3 2 1 0

Dedication

As the thoughts and ideas for this second edition were being finalized, I lost my coauthor and my senior by many years in the field, Prof. Lawrence H. Lanzl. He passed away at age 80 after making a tremendous contribution to the field of medical physics. His career had many brilliant facets. He was a researcher, developer, inventor, innovator, teacher, organizer, and leader par excellence. He commanded special respect and love from the international community of medical physicists, not only as a professional, but also as a person. He was full of noble thoughts and, together with his wife Elisabeth, lived a life with great values. It was my special privilege and honor to have known him and worked with him both as colleague and friend. Quite appropriately, this second edition of Clinical Radiotherapy Physics is dedicated to his memory.

November 2002   Subramania Jayaraman

Preface to Second Edition

The first edition of Clinical Radiotherapy Physics was published in 1996 and was received well. It consisted of two volumes and contained a total of twenty chapters. The current second edition contains the same number of chapters under the same headings, but combines them into one single volume. The scope of the text has remained the same as for the first edition. Several sections have been revised and expanded. Some new sections have been added to make the text current. All references and citations have been updated. More recent practices, recommendations, and protocols have been covered. Our purpose to outline the accepted standards of practice, rather than upcoming but as yet unproved trends, has been maintained. However, such trends are mentioned with references wherever appropriate to arouse the curiosity of research-minded readers.

Preface to First Edition

This text is an introduction to radiotherapy physics. The emphasis in much of the work is on the clinical aspects of the field; thus, the book should be especially useful for persons who are already graduate physicists and plan for a career in clinical radiotherapy physics. At present, the treatment of cancer patients with ionizing radiation is a team effort by radiation oncologists, radiation therapists, as well as clinical physicists. The book is intended to be of use to persons in each of these areas.

Historically, clinical medical physics as a profession can be dated to the year 1913, when William Duane became the first full-time hospital-employed physicist in the United States and Sydney Russ, the first in the United Kingdom. These two physicists worked on similar problems related to the use of radium and radon for the treatment of cancer and other diseases.

Although there were no full-time clinical medical physicists before 1913, the utility of physics to the practice of medicine was recognized much earlier. For example, Galileo's work on the principle of the pendulum was used by physicians of his day for measuring the heart rate of patients. In the early 1800s, the physician Neil Arnott, in England, pioneered the idea that the curriculum of physicians in training should include the study of physics. Arnott's textbooks were translated from English into several languages. He also appears to have been the first to use the term "medical physics" in his writings (1825). To this day, the study of physics is included either in medical schools (e.g., in England, Russia, and China) or in the premedical curriculum (e.g., in the United States and Canada).

In this text, we have tried to keep the treatment of a patient in perspective as much as possible, in order to keep the book clinically oriented. The sequence and depths of coverage of the different topics reflect our preference based on our own teaching experience and may be found to differ from other texts on the subject.

We have made an attempt to have the subject develop gradually from chapter to chapter, with minimum cross-references between chapters. However, we recommend that a reader do a quick read-through of all the chapters, and then do a more thorough study of each chapter. In this way, it may be possible to appreciate best how some basic aspects that are covered in the early chapters have relevance for discussions to follow in later chapters that are progressively more clinically oriented. With a desire to have a presentation that can satisfy physicists, we have used mathematical expressions as needed, but we have made an effort to add enough narrative descriptions. Non-physicist users of the book can merely browse the equations and study the text around them.

The first fourteen chapters of the text cover basic physics and principles of radiation dosimetry. The beginning chapters cover the essentials of atomic and nuclear physics, which provide the background for the later chapters. The physics of the use of photons and electrons has been emphasized because of their widespread application in radiotherapy clinics. The use of hadronic particles (such as neutrons, protons, pions), still being experimental, has been addressed only in minimum detail. A few paragraphs are devoted to leptons, quarks, and other recently identified fundamental particles for the purpose of completeness.

The sources of high-energy photons and electrons are particle accelerators, particularly linear accelerators. We believe that the principles of accelerators of charged particles are covered in sufficient detail for present-day medical physicists.

Radiation fields are quantified in terms of radiation units and measurements. Quantities used in clinical practice are defined and explained. The terms and definitions used in the text follow the recommendations of the appropriate international committees. However, where it was necessary, we felt the need to add a few new terms to improve the clarity of the presentations.

Chapters 15 to 20 are devoted to planning of radiation treatments and radiation safety. The text is written to include recent concepts and new refinements. Brachytherapy is an important area of present-day radiotherapy. Thus, radioactivity and the accompanying dosimetry considerations are included in the text. It should be realized that the largest exposure of man to ionizing radiations comes from deliberate irradiation in procedures of diagnostic and therapeutic radiology. Therefore, the later chapters are devoted to radiation safety and safety standards. The philosophy on which these standards are based has undergone a change in recent years, and the authors felt strongly that the changes should be included in the text.

Acknowledgements

When writing a book, one calls on past experiences and insights from one's teachers, associates, students, both past and present, as well as previous writers. I would like to acknowledge my debt to all of these. The authors thank Elisabeth F. Lanzl, who has helped to make the text readable by making her expertise in editing available for both the first and second editions.

Lawrence H. Lanzl

First, I wish to thank my (late) father, Ayakarambulam Rajagopalan Subramanian, and my mother, Saraswathi Subramanian, for showering their love and affection on me, as they believed in me and encouraged me since childhood toward accomplishment. So also I acknowledge the special love and affection of my wife Syamala and my daughters, Saramati and Sahana.

My career in medical physics developed largely due to the opportunities of associations with several eminent physicists in the field. Among them I wish especially to recognize and thank Professor Lawrence H. Lanzl, Professor Nagalingam Suntharalingam (Thomas Jefferson University, Philadelphia), Dr. R. Chidambaram (Chairman, Atomic Energy Commission, India), S. Somasundaram (Bhabha Atomic Research Center, India), Professor Suresh K. Agarwal (University of Virginia, Charlottesville, Virginia), Anthony Chung-Bin (Anchorage, Alaska), and Dr. Martin Rozenfeld (Chicago, Ilinois). I am indebted to their closeness and expressions of faith in me at different phases of my career.

I also find it appropriate to mention the extraordinary resilience of my coauthor, Lawrence H. Lanzl, who worked with me until his very last days amidst all his health challenges. He was an inspiration to me in many ways ever since I first met him in 1967.

I am thankful to John A. Dover, M.D., President, Valley Radiation Oncology, and his senior partner, Herbert Hitchon, D.O., for their especial interest and support for completion of this second edition. So also, I thank the Springer-Verlag, Heidelberg, Germany, for publishing this second edition.

Subramania Jayaraman

The Authors

The two authors were associated with each other professionally for more than 34 years. They first met in 1967, when they took on assignments in the Dosimetry Section of the International Atomic Energy Agency, Vienna, Austria. S. Jayaraman was on leave of absence from the Bhabha Atomic Research Center, Bombay, India, and Lawrence H. Lanzl was on leave from the Argonne Cancer Research Hospital of the University of Chicago, Chicago, Illinois. Also, for a few months in the 1970s, Lanzl spent some time at the Bhabha Atomic Research Center. Next, in the 1980s, both Jayaraman and Lanzl worked in the Departments of Medical Physics and Therapeutic Radiology at Rush-Presbyterian-St. Luke's Medical Center, Chicago. It was then that the idea of writing a book crystallized and resulted in the publication of the first edition in 1996.

At present, S. Jayaraman is Chief Medical Physicist at Valley Radiation Oncology, Phoenix, Arizona. L.H. Lanzl, who retired as Professor of Medical Physics, Department of Medical Physics, Rush University, Chicago, unfortunately passed away as the preparation of this second edition was in its final stages.

Contents

Part I   Basic Physics and Radioactivity Decay

1	**Scope of Clinical Radiotherapy Physics**	3
1.1	A Physicist in a Clinic?	3
1.2	Physical Concepts and Radiotherapy	3
1.3	Cooperation between Physicist and Physician	4
1.4	Scope of this Book	5
	References	6
2	**Atoms, Molecules, and Matter**	7
2.1	Historical Origin of Atomic Physics	7
2.2	Formation of Atoms and Elements	8
2.3	Atomic Electron Configuration	11
2.3.1	Electron Orbits and Energy Levels	11
2.3.2	Ionization and Excitation of Atoms	14
2.3.3	Characteristic X-Rays and Auger Electrons	14
2.4	Definition of an Electron Volt (eV)	15
2.5	Atomic Mass, Molecular Mass, and Atomic Mass Unit	15
2.6	Avogadro's Number (N_{Av})	16
2.7	Periodic Table of Elements	17
2.8	Molecular Bonds	17
2.8.1	Ionic Bonds	17
2.8.2	Covalent Bonds	17
2.8.3	Hydrogen Bonds	19
2.9	Elementary Particles	20
2.10	Outer Space and Particle Research	24
	References	25
3	**Propagation of Energy by Electromagnetic Waves**	26
3.1	Radio Waves, Heat Waves, and Light Waves	26
3.2	Wave Propagation	26
3.3	Photons, Quanta, and the Electromagnetic Spectrum	28
3.4	Louis de Broglie's Matter Waves	29

4   **Nuclear Transitions and Radioactive Decay** 31
4.1   Discovery of Natural Radioactivity 31
4.2   Nuclear Forces and Energy Levels 32
4.3   Nuclear Decay Schemes 33
4.4   Alpha Decay 33
4.5   Beta Decay 34
4.5.1   Neutron-Proton Imbalance 34
4.5.2   Beta-Minus (β^-) Decay 35
4.5.3   Beta-Plus (β^+) Decay 37
4.5.4   Electron Capture (EC) 37
4.6   Internal Conversion (IC) 38
4.7   Isomeric Transition 40
4.8   Nuclear Fission 40
4.9   Nuclear Fusion 41
4.10   Induced Nuclear Transformations 42

5   **Radioactive Decay Calculations** 43
5.1   Introduction 43
5.2   Decay of a Single Isotope 43
5.2.1   Observing an Instant 43
5.2.2   Observing Decay Over Lengthy Periods 44
5.2.3   Half Life (T_h) 45
5.2.4   Mean Life (T_M) 46
5.3   Radioactive Decay Chains 48
5.3.1   Daughter Product Buildup and Decay 48
5.3.2   Secular Equilibrium 49
5.3.3   Transient Equilibrium 50
5.4   Neutron Activation 52

Part II   **Interaction of Radiation with Matter**

6   **Collision and Radiation Loss in Charged-Particle Interactions** 59
6.1   Slowing Down of Charged Particles 59
6.2   Collision Loss 60
6.2.1   Collision Energy Loss Formula 60
6.2.2   Bragg Ionization Curve 62
6.3   Radiative Loss 63
6.3.1   Bremsstrahlung 63
6.3.2   Radiative Stopping Power 63
6.3.3   Angular Distribution of Bremsstrahlung X-Rays 64
6.3.4   Energy Distribution of Bremsstrahlung Radiation 65
6.3.5   Linear Energy Transfer 67
       References 68

7	**Photon Interactions**	69
7.1	Nature of the Interactions	69
7.2	Attenuation Coefficient	70
7.2.1	Diminution of Photon Flux	70
7.2.2	Linear Attenuation Coefficient	71
7.2.3	Mass Attenuation Coefficient	71
7.2.4	Atomic Attenuation Coefficient	72
7.2.5	Electronic Attenuation Coefficient	72
7.3	Coherent Thompson Scattering	72
7.4	Photoelectric Absorption	73
7.4.1	Early Photoelectron Experiment	73
7.4.2	Photon Energy and Photoelectric Interaction	75
7.4.3	Atomic Number and Photoelectric Interaction	76
7.4.4	Local Energy Absorption in Photoelectric Interaction	76
7.4.5	Angular Emission of Photoelectrons	76
7.4.6	Photoelectric Cross Section	77
7.5	Incoherent Compton Scattering	77
7.5.1	Kinematics of Compton Scattering	77
7.5.2	Angular Distribution of Scattered Photons	79
7.5.3	Scattered Energy at Specific Angles	80
7.5.4	Compton Cross Section	80
7.5.5	Energy and Atomic Numbers vs. Compton Cross Section	81
7.6	Negatron-Positron Pair Production	82
7.6.1	Threshold Energy for Pair Production	82
7.6.2	Electron-Positron Annihilation	83
7.6.3	Pair Production Cross Section	84
7.6.4	Photon Energy and Atomic Number vs. π	84
7.6.5	Local Energy Absorption and Pair Production	84
7.7	Summing up the Local Energy Absorbed	85
7.8	Components of μ at Different Energies	85
7.9	Attenuation Coefficients for Mixtures and Compounds	87
7.9.1	Weighted Addition of μ/ρ Values	87
7.9.2	Effective Z for Mixtures and Compounds	87
7.10	Broad- and Narrow-Beam Attenuation Geometries	88
7.10.1	Primary and Scatter Fluence	88
7.10.2	Scatter Build-Up Factor	89
7.11	Photonuclear Reactions	90
Part III	**Radiation Beam Therapy Equipment**	
8	**Conventional X-Ray Machines**	95
8.1	Discovery of X-Rays	95
8.2	Gas-Discharge X-Ray Tube	96
8.3	Features of Modern X-Ray Tubes	96
8.3.1	Coolidge's X-Ray Tube	96
8.3.2	Heat Generation	97

8.3.3   Line Focus Principle 97
8.3.4   Heel Effect 98
8.3.5   Rotating Anode 99
8.3.6   Avoidance of Overheating 99
8.4   High-Voltage Supply and Rectification 100
8.4.1   Stepping up the AC Supply 100
8.4.2   Self-Rectified X-Ray Tube 101
8.4.3   Half-Wave Rectification 101
8.4.4   Full-Wave Rectification 102
8.4.5   Three-Phase Power Supply and Full-Wave Rectification 103
8.5   A Typical X-Ray Circuit 104
8.6   X-Ray Spectra and Quality 105
8.6.1   X-Ray Spectra in Practicle 105
8.6.2   Beam Quality and Half-Value Thickness 106
8.6.3   Homogeneity Index 106

9   **Equipment for Radioisotope Teletherapy** 107
9.1   Concept of Teletherapy 107
9.2   Radioisotope Sources 107
9.2.1   Requirements for the Source 107
9.2.2   Some Radioisotopes to be Considered for Teletherapy 108
9.3 ^{60}Co Teletherapy Machines 109
9.3.1   The Source Head 109
9.3.2   Light Beam Localizer 110
9.3.3   Source on-off Mechanism 110
9.3.4   Source Capsule 111
9.3.5   Geometric Penumbra 111
9.3.6   Transmission Penumbra 113
9.3.7   Designs of Adjustable Diaphragms 113
9.4   Miscellaneous Features and Accessories 114
9.4.1   Movement of Treatment Head and Patient Support 114
9.4.2   Optical Distance Indicator 114
9.4.3   Back-Pointing Device 116
9.5   Closing Remarks 117

10   **Particle Accelerators** 118
10.1   Three Categories of Accelerators 118
10.2   Direct-Voltage, Electrostatic Accelerators 119
10.2.1   Tube for Acceleration 119
10.2.2   Cockcroft-Walton Voltage Multiplier 119
10.2.3   Van de Graaff Electrostatic Generator 120
10.3   Linear Accelerators 121
10.3.1   Principle of Linacs 121
10.3.2   Phase Stability in Linacs 122
10.3.3   Wave Guides 123
10.3.4   Standing Wave and Traveling Wave 124
10.3.5   Clinical Linear Accelerator 124

10.4   Betatron 127
10.5   Cyclotron 129
10.6   Microtron 130

Part IV   Radiation Quantities, Units, and Detectors

11   Quantification of Radiation Field: Radiation Units and Measurements 135
11.1   Radiation Field 135
11.2   Some Theoretical Concepts 135
11.2.1   Fluence 135
11.2.2   Energy Fluence 136
11.2.3   Fluence Rate 136
11.2.4   Energy Fluence Rate 137
11.2.5   Energy Transferred and Kerma (k_{med}) 137
11.2.6   Energy Absorbed and Dose (D_{med}) 138
11.2.7   Charged-Particle Equilibrium 138
11.2.8   Relationship between Kerma and Dose 139
11.3   Dose and Kerma Profiles – An Interface Example 140
11.4   Air Kerma (k_{air}) and Water Kerma (k_{water}) 142
11.5   Exposure 142
11.5.1   Concept of Exposure 142
11.5.2   Relationship Among Exposure, Air Kerma, and Dose to Air 143
11.5.3   Relationship of Dose in Medium to Air Kerma and Exposure 144
11.6   Measurement of Exposure 146
11.6.1   Free-Air Ionization Chamber 146
11.6.2   Cavity Chambers 147
11.6.3   Exposure Calibration Factor 149
11.7   Use of Calibrated Ion Chamber in Therapy Beams 150
11.7.1   Need for Calibration of Beams 150
11.7.2   ”Dose to Tissue in Air“ for a Cobalt-60 Beam 151
11.7.3   Dose in Water for a Cobalt-60 Beam 152
11.7.4   Ideal Bragg-Gray Cavity 152
11.7.5   Less than Ideal (Larger) Cavity 154
11.7.6   Walled Chamber in a Medium 154
11.7.7   Determining N_{gas} from $N_{X,Co}$ 155
11.7.8   Dose Delivered by Electron Beams 156
11.7.9   Converting Dose to Plastic to Dose to Water 157
11.8   Calorimetry and Protocols Based on Absorbed Dose to Water 157
11.9   Air-Kerma Rate Constant for Radionuclide Sources 159
11.10   Reference Air-Kerma Rate
         for Specifying Brachytherapy Source Strength 162
11.10.1   Reference Air-kerma Rate (S_{ak}) 162
11.10.2   Dose-Rate Constant (Λ) 163
         References 165

12	**Instruments for Radiation Detection**	168
12.1	Introduction	168
12.2	Ionization Detectors	168
12.2.1	Role of Applied Potential	168
12.2.2	Condenser Chamber	169
12.2.3	Cylindrical (Thimble) Chamber	171
12.2.4	Parallel-Plate (Pancake) Chamber	171
12.2.5	Extrapolation Chamber	172
12.3	Photographic Film Detector	173
12.3.1	Photographic Process	173
12.3.2	Optical Density	173
12.3.3	Calibration of a Film	174
12.3.4	Film Response Curves	174
12.3.5	Intensifying Screens and Grids	175
12.3.6	High-Energy Port Films	176
12.4	Scintillation Detector	176
12.5	Solid-State Electrical Conductivity Detectors	177
12.6	Thermoluminescent Dosimeters (TLDS)	178
12.6.1	Thermoluminescence	178
12.6.2	TLD Instrumentation	179
12.6.3	Measuring an Unknown Dose by TLD	179
12.7	Chemical Dosimeters	180
12.8	Optically Stimulated Luminescence (OSL) Dosimetry	181
12.9	Nuclear Magnetic Resonance (NMR) Dosimetry	182
12.10	Radiochromic Film Dosimetry	182
12.11	Concluding Remarks	183
	References	183

Part V   Dosimetry of Radiation Beams

13	**Basic Ratios and Factors for the Dosimetry of External Beam**	189
13.1	Introduction	189
13.2	Defining the Beam Geometry	189
13.3	Quality of Beams	191
13.4	Central-Axis Dose Profile	192
13.5	Calculation of Dose in the Depth: General Approach	193
13.6	Dose to Tissue in Air	194
13.7	Inverse-Square Fall-Off	195
13.8	Irradiation Parameters	196
13.9	Tissue-Air Ratio (TAR)	197
13.10	Peak Scatter Factor (PSF)	198
13.11	Normalized PSF (NPSF)	200
13.12	Percent Depth Dose (PDD)	200
13.13	Tissue Maximum Ratio (TMR)	205
13.14	Tissue-Phantom Ratio	206
13.15	Dose Output Factors	206

13.15.1   Calibrated Dose Output 206
13.15.2   In-Air Output and Peak Output 210
13.16   Methods of Deriving the Dose Rate $\dot{D}_P$ at Point P 212
13.17   Calculation of Treatment Duration 214
13.18   Equivalent Squares and Circles 214
13.19   Relationship of TAR and TMR to PDD 217
13.20   Converting PDD for One SSD to that for Another 217
13.21   Concluding Remarks 227
          References 229

14   **Beam Dosimetry: Additional Corrections – Special Situations** 230
14.1   Introduction 230
14.2   Scatter Considerations 230
14.2.1   Scatter in Blocked Fields 230
14.2.2   Effective Rectangular Field 231
14.2.3   Scatter-Air Ratio, SAR(d, A_d) 234
14.2.4   Scatter-Radius Integration 235
14.2.5   Day's Method 237
14.3   General Approach for Off-Central Axis Points 238
14.3.1   Surface Curvature, Distance, and Depth 238
14.3.2   Off-Center Ratios in Air, OCR_{air} 239
14.3.3   Dose Rate at Off-Center Point Q 240
14.4   Correction for Body Inhomogeneities 240
14.4.1   Inhomogeneities 240
14.4.2   Inhomogeneity Correction Factor (ICF) 241
14.4.3   Lung and Bone 241
14.4.4   Lung Phantom Geometry 242
14.4.5   Effective Depth (d_{eff}) 243
14.4.6   ICF Based on Accounting for d_{eff} 243
14.4.7   Effective Field Size (A_{eff}) 243
14.4.8   ICF Based on Equivalent TAR, with d_{eff} and A_{eff} 244
14.4.9   ICF by Batho's Method 244
14.4.10   Comparison of ICF Obtained by Different Methods 245
14.4.11   Lung Density and Lateral Electronic Equilibrium 248
14.5   Bone Attenuation and Absorption 248
14.6   Beams of Non-Uniform Intensity 251
14.7   Concluding Remarks 252
          References 253

Part VI   **Radiation Treatment Planning**

15   **Treatment Dose Distribution Planning: Photon Beams** 259
15.1   Introduction 259
15.2   Isodose Surfaces and Curves 259
15.3   Single-Beam Isodose Curves 260
15.3.1   General Features 260

15.3.2   Low-Energy Kilovoltage X-Ray Beam 261
15.3.3 ^{60}Co Beam 262
15.3.4   Megavoltage X-Rays 262
15.4   Concept of Combining Beams 264
15.5   Derivation of Dose Distribution 265
15.5.1   General Approach.. 265
15.5.2   Dose at P_I for Fixed-SSD Technique 265
15.5.3   Dose at P_i for Isocentric Technique 267
15.5.4   Correction for Contour Shape 267
15.5.5   Influence of Obliquity on Dose Build-Up 270
15.6   Planning of Dose Distributions 271
15.6.1   Zones to be Considered 271
15.6.2   Examining a Dose Distribution 272
15.7   Principles of the Use of Wedge Filters 273
15.7.1   Wedge Angle 273
15.7.2   Wedged Oblique Pair 276
15.7.3   Three-Field Techniques with Wedges 277
15.8   Irradiations with Parallel Opposed Beams................... 279
15.8.1   On a Body Section of Medium Thickness.................... 279
15.8.2   On a Thin Body Section.................................... 280
15.8.3   On a Thick Body Section 284
15.8.4   In a Four-Field Box Geometry 284
15.8.5   On a Section of Uneven Body Thickness 287
15.9   Other Common Techniques 288
15.10   Treatment Planning: A Practical Case...................... 294
15.10.1   Therapy Simulator 294
15.10.2   Localization for Treatment of the Esophagus 296
15.10.3   Case-Specific Isodose Planning 298
15.10.4   Comparative Evaluation of the Plans 300
15.10.5   Use of Dose-Volume Plots 300
15.10.6   Integral Dose (Σ) 301
15.10.7   Simulating the Accepted Plan 303
15.11   Use of CT Data 306
15.11.1   CT Transverse Cuts.. 306
15.11.2   CT for Field Shaping 306
15.12   Treatment of Adjacent Sites 309
15.12.1   Problem of Concern 309
15.12.2   Both Sites Treated from One Direction 309
15.12.3   Adjacent Parallel Opposed Fields.......................... 311
15.12.4   Matching Opposed Beams with a Single Beam 314
15.12.5   Angle Match Between Orthogonal Beams 314
15.13   3D-CRT, SRT, IMRT 315
15.14   Concluding Remarks 318
          References 318

16	**Physical Aspects of Electron Beam Therapy**	323
16.1	Electron Transport	323
16.2	Electron Beam from Machine to Patient	323
16.3	Electron Beam After Entering the Patient	325
16.4	Electron Beam Depth Dose Date	329
16.5	Planning a Simple Electron Beam Treatment	330
16.6	Electron Beam Depth Dose and Field Size	331
16.7	Electron Pencil Beam	333
16.8	Oblique Incidence and Depth Dose	333
16.9	Electron Beams: Some Practical Consideration	335
16.9.1	Electron Beam Output Factors	335
16.9.2	Output Factors for Non-Square Fields	337
16.9.3	Field Shaping and Selective Shielding	337
16.9.4	Effective SSD	340
16.9.5	Agreement of Light Field and Radiation Field	341
16.10	Influence of Inhomogeneities	342
16.11	Comparison of Kilovoltage X-Ray and Electron Beams	345
16.12	Total-Skin Electron Treatment	346
16.13	Intraoperative Electron Therapy	347
16.14	Electron Arc Therapy	348
16.15	Adjacent Electron Fields	350
	References	352
17	**Physics of the Use of Small Sealed Sources in Brachytherapy**	357
17.1	Brachytherapy	357
17.2	Categories of Applications	359
17.3	Source Strength of Brachytherapy Sources	361
17.3.1	Need for Specification of Source Strength	361
17.3.2	Specification by Radium-Equivalent Mass	362
17.3.3	Specification by Activity	363
17.3.4	Specification by Air-Kerma Rate Yield	364
17.3.5	Specification by Water-Kerma Rate Yield	364
17.4	Source Strength and Time Product	365
17.4.1	Significance	365
17.4.2	Milligram Hours of Treatment	365
17.4.3	Air-Kerma Yield of Treatment	365
17.5	Dosimetry of a Point Source in Water	366
17.5.1	Theoretical Approach	366
17.5.2	AAPM and ICWG Empirical Approach for Dosimetry of Radioactive Seeds	369
17.6	Dosimetry of a Linear Source	371
17.6.1	Encapsulated Source in Air	371
17.6.2	Unencapsulated Source in Air	373
17.6.3	Linear Source in Water	375
17.6.4	Dose Distribution for Linear Sources	375
17.6.5	AAPM and ICWG Approach for Linear Source Dosimetry	376
17.7	A Simple Line Source Treatment	377

17.8	Forming Multiple Source Arrays	379
17.8.1	Sources as Dose Building Blocks	379
17.8.2	Uniform vs. Differentially Distributed Arrays	379
17.9	Systems for Brachytherapy	384
17.9.1	What are Systems or Approaches?	384
17.9.2	Quimby Approach	385
17.9.3	Paris Approach	387
17.9.4	Approach of Memorial Hospital in New York	389
17.9.5	Manchester Approach of Paterson and Parker	390
17.9.6	Pitfalls of Mixing Systems or Approaches	394
17.10	Manchester (Paterson and Parker) Distribution Rules	394
17.10.1	Surface Applications	394
17.10.2	Single-Plane Implants	397
17.10.3	Two-Plane Implants	397
17.10.4	Volume Implants	398
17.11	Planning and Implementing a Practical Case	399
17.11.1	A Sample Target Volume	399
17.11.2	Planning the Geometry of the Array	399
17.11.3	Determining the Source Strengths	400
17.11.4	Procuring the Sources	400
17.11.5	Implanting the Sources	401
17.11.6	Radiographic Localization of Sources	401
17.11.7	Orthogonal Reconstruction – A Practical Case	404
17.11.8	Dosimetry Using Computer and Interpretation	405
17.12	Permanent Implants	408
17.13	Intracavitary Irradiation	409
17.13.1	Vaginal Cylinder	409
17.13.2	Pairs of Colpostats	410
17.13.3	Irradiations of Uterine Cervix	411
	References	414

Part VII   Radiation Safety

18	Radiation Safety Standards	421
18.1	Introduction	421
18.2	Harmful Effects of Radiation	422
18.2.1	Acute Radiation Syndrome	422
18.2.2	Stochastic Effects and Deterministic Effects	422
18.2.3	Somatic and Genetic Effects	423
18.3	Evaluation of Dose for Radiation Protection	423
18.3.1	Inadequacy of Dose as an Index of Harm	423
18.3.2	Microscopic Energy Deposition	424
18.3.3	Relative Biological Effectiveness (RBE)	425
18.3.4	Quality Factor and Dose Equivalent	425
18.3.5	Weighting Factors for Different Radiations	426
18.3.6	Equivalent Dose	427

18.3.7   Weighting Factors for Different Body Tissues 428
18.3.8   Effective Dose 428
18.4   Uncertainties in Radiation Risk Assessment 430
18.4.1   Problem of Sample Size 430
18.4.2   Imperfect Knowledge of Radiation Dose 431
18.4.3   Dose-Response Projection 431
18.4.4   Lifetime Risk Projection 432
18.4.5   Dose and Dose Rate Effectiveness Factor (DDREF) 433
18.4.6   Assessed Radiation Risk 434
18.5   Radiation Safety Philosophy 434
18.5.1   Natural Background Radiation 434
18.5.2   Medical Exposures 435
18.5.3   Risk vs. Benefit Philosophy 435
18.6   Safety of Radiation Workers 436
18.6.1   Limits for Adult Workers 436
18.6.2   Limits for Embryo or Fetus 438
18.6.3   Limits for Workers Under Age 18 438
18.6.4   Personnel Monitoring 438
18.7   Safety of the General Public 439
          References 440

19   **Radiation Safety in External-Beam Therapy** 443
19.1   Introduction 443
19.2   Time, Distance, and Shielding 444
19.3   Approach to Shielding Design of a Beam-Therapy Facility 444
19.3.1   Selection of Acceptable Weekly Equivalent Dose Limits (P) 444
19.3.2   Radiation Components 445
19.3.3   Recommended Leakage Levels 445
19.3.4   Shielding Data 447
19.3.5   Architectural and Equipment Data 449
19.3.6   Workload (W) 449
19.3.7   Use Factor (U) 450
19.3.8   Occupancy Factor (T) 450
19.4   Estimating the Allowable Barrier Transmission 451
19.4.1   Primary Shielding Barrier 451
19.4.2   Secondary Protective Barrier 452
19.4.3   Entrance Door Barrier 454
19.4.4   Roof Protection and Skyshine 456
19.5   High-Energy X-Rays and Neutron Production 457
19.5.1   Neutron Shielding at the Door 457
19.5.2   Neutron Capture Gamma Rays 459
19.5.3   Induced Radioactivity 460
19.6   An Example of Shielding Calculations for a Facility 460
19.6.1   Basic Data and Assumptions 460
19.6.2   Side Walls 461
19.6.3   Entrance Door Shield 462
19.6.4   Skyshine Shielding 463

19.7   Ozone Production... 467
19.8   Miscellaneous Aspects of Planning a Facility 467
          References 474

20   **Radiation Safety in Brachytherapy** 478
20.1   Introduction 478
20.2   Role of Time and Afterloading 479
20.3   Role of Distance 479
20.4   Role of Shielding.. 480
20.5   Monitoring Instruments 480
20.6   Source Storage and Preparation 480
20.7   Source Inventory.. 482
20.8   Source Wipe Tests... 482
20.9   Source Transport 483
20.10   Safety of Nurses and Visitors During Treatment 484
20.11   Procedure After Treatment 484
20.12   Permanent Implants.. 486
20.13   Personnel Monitoring 486
20.14   Conclusion 487
          References 487

Appendix A and B

Appendix A. Electron Mass Stopping Powers (in MeV cm^2 g^{-1}) for Various
Materials 491

Appendix B. Mass Attenuation Coefficients, Mass Energy Transfer Coefficients,
and Mass Energy Absorption Coefficients (in cm^2 g^{-1}) for Various Materials 499

Subject Index 507

Basic Physics and Radioactivity Decay

CHAPTER 1

Scope of Clinical Radiotherapy Physics

1.1
A Physicist in a Clinic?

The word "physician," rather than "physicist," is commonly associated with the word "clinic." It is natural that the term "clinical physicist" may provoke a reaction among lay people. They may ask whether indeed "physicist" and not "physician" was meant. Next could come the query, what role does a physicist play in a clinic? The reply is that medical physicists function in those clinics that need their expertise to ensure proper patient care. In general, medical physics includes all applications of physics to medicine, being concerned with the use of physical principles and techniques in any aspect of the prevention, diagnosis, and treatment of human diseases, and in medical research for the promotion of human health. Although medical physics encompasses this wider territory, rather than merely radiation therapy, radiation therapy remains one area in which the physicist has some influence on every individual patient treated. It is an area in which the physicist can interact with the physician and contribute to the better management of specific patients. For an understanding of this, it is necessary to discuss briefly what radiation therapy involves.

1.2
Physical Concepts and Radiotherapy

Radiation therapy is the treatment of neoplastic diseases with ionizing radiation. The radiation can be electromagnetic (X-rays, gamma rays) or corpuscular (electrons, protons, neutrons, alpha particles, mesons, heavy ions, etc.). The radiation effect is produced by the energy absorbed in living tissues through the processes of ionization and excitation of the atoms and molecules that form these tissues. Thus, the radiation energy delivered is the medicine that is administered. The "radiation dose" is the amount of energy absorbed by the tissues. In practical radiotherapy, the radiation dose needs to be controlled within an accuracy of a few percent, i.e., with a very narrow margin for error. This need to accomplish such a high level of accuracy in the amount of "medicine" delivered distinguishes radiation therapy from other disciplines of clinical care. A pain-killing medicine like ibuprofen may be prescribed in steps of 200 mg, 400 mg, or 800 mg for different clinical effects. Compared to this, a change in the radiation dose of ± 5 to 10% can make the difference between acceptable and adverse clinical outcomes.

Radiotherapy clinics are equipped with specially designed, expensive radiation-producing machines. A physician who sets out to treat a patient with radiation aims to deliver a preplanned radiation dose within acceptable margins of uncertainty to

Fig. 1.1. Resolution of a tumor in the esophagus after radiation beam treatment. Radiographic appearance of esophagus (**a**) before treatment, and (**b**) after treatment. (Picture adapted and reproduced with permission from [1])

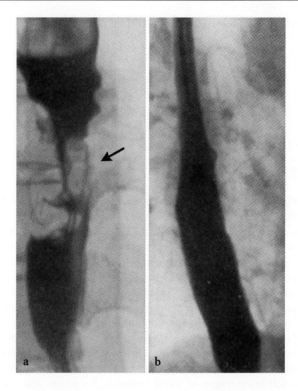

selected sites in the patient's body. The method of administration of a radiation dose is complicated. It is inevitable that some radiation dose will be delivered to tissues in the body that are not the intended main targets of treatment. However, the methods of irradiation can be optimized so that the damage to such incidentally irradiated tissues is minimal. The production of the radiation, the techniques of tumor localization, the planning of the irradiation, the implementation of the treatment, and the estimation of the radiation doses received by different sites in the body are based on principles of physics. Figures 1.1 and 1.2, respectively, show examples of tumor regression accomplished by the two well known modes of radiation therapy, viz. external-beam therapy and brachytherapy.

1.3
Cooperation between Physicist and Physician

Only a close collaboration between the physicist and the physician can ensure optimum management of patients. In a sense, this resembles the cooperation between surgeons and anesthetists. The wide range of radiotherapy machines available to modern clinics, the complexity of the dose calculation procedures, and the high degree of patient-specific individualization of treatment approaches have made clinical radiotherapy physics a specialty in itself. A trained medical physicist can provide his or her input and influence the course of the radiation treatment of any individual patient. The

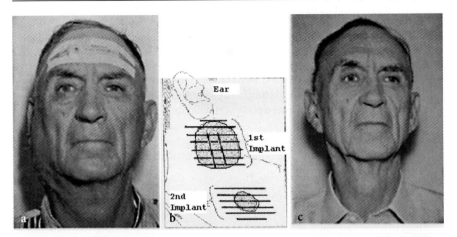

Fig. 1.2. Resolution of a tumor on the right neck of a patient after treatment by implanted radioactive needles. (a) Appearance of patient before treatment, (b) schematic diagram of the implanted needles, and (c) patient several years after treatment. (Picture adapted and reproduced with permission from [2])

type of reasoning that a physicist employs is of enormous value for superior patient management in a radiotherapy clinic. There may be instances when the radiation therapy physician has to rely on a physicist's interpretation and judgment about a particular treatment. To what extent a physicist can contribute depends on (a) the radiotherapy physician's interest in using the physicist's input and (b) the physicist's interest in raising issues and discussing with the physician the possible ramifications and improvements of the treatment. The overall emphasis should be on producing the best clinical outcome for the patients being treated.

1.4
Scope of this Book

This book is directed toward providing a basic course in clinical radiotherapy physics. The book aims to serve more than one category of users. First, it is intended to help those who have a well-established physics background and want to become clinical physicists. Second, it should help resident physicians entering the specialty of radiation therapy to become familiar with the physics involved. A clinical physicist is a physicist who has added to his or her experience radiotherapy physics in a clinical environment. The training in a clinical setting with physicians, patients, and machines is vital for a physicist to become clinically oriented.

In turn, a radiation therapy physician should add physics knowledge to his or her clinical background, so that his or her insight will be adequate for managing patients who undergo radiation treatment. Without the necessary physics background, it will be difficult for him or her (a) to understand the technical advantages and limitations of the equipment available in a particular clinic, (b) to know to what degree and when to seek the physicist's help, and (c) to comprehend what he or she can do or not do in a particular patient context.

In addition to clinical physicists and physicians, radiation therapy technologists form an integral part of the radiation therapy team. The accuracy of the treatment delivery rests not only on the quality and sophistication of the equipment used, but also on the caliber of the members of the technical staff who set up the machines for the treatment of patients on a daily basis. Hence, this book is written also to satisfy the needs of physics instructors who train radiotherapy technologists. In short, it is intended to be of help to anyone who is seriously interested in learning or teaching the physics aspects of radiotherapy. It is not to be regarded as a data book or atlas for obtaining numerical information for clinical use. It should be used only as a pedagogic and descriptive text. Users of the book will judge to what extent we succeeded in this endeavor.

References

1. Lanzl, L.H., and Carpender, W.J., Moving Field Radiation Therapy, p. 211, Fig. 147, University of Chicago Press, Chicago, 1962.
2. Martin, C.L., and Martin, J.A., Low Intensity Radium Therapy, Plate 20, Little Brown, and Co., Boston, 1959.

CHAPTER 2

Atoms, Molecules, and Matter

2.1
Historical Origin of Atomic Physics

One aspect of scientific inquiry is to try to perceive all materials as being made up of smaller components. Chemical experiments showed that compounds could be split into components, each of which has its own distinct chemical behavior. These individual components were given the name "elements." Groups of elements have been identified as alkali, halogens, and inert gases, with elements in each group behaving alike chemically. In 1816, Prout suggested that all of the heavier elements might have been built from the lightest element, hydrogen. Soon afterwards, Dalton stated that samples of different sizes of any particular chemical compound contained the constituent elements in the same proportions. He referred to the smallest entity of any compound as a molecule of that compound, and to the smallest entity of any element as an atom of that element. A molecule and an atom are the smallest samples that display a characteristic chemical behavior.

Since the beginning of the 19th century, our understanding of what constitutes matter has grown by leaps and bounds. Matter and energy, the two quantities with which physics is concerned, have been found to be mutually convertible. From Einstein's special theory of relativity, the energy, E_0, of a free body at rest is given by the relation

$$E_0 = mc^2$$

where m is the mass of the free body and c is the velocity of light in a vacuum. E_0 is called the rest energy. Thus, the mass of a particle at rest is (E_0/c^2). The energy, E, of the same free body when it moves with a velocity $\bar{v}$ is given by

$$E^2 = p^2c^2 + m^2c^4 \quad \text{and} \quad \bar{p} = \bar{v}\frac{E}{c^2}$$

where $\bar{p}$ is the momentum of the free body.

Atoms are made up of three different particles, electrons, protons, and neutrons, the characteristics of which are summarized in Table 2.1. Protons are positively charged and electrons are negatively charged. Neutrons were discovered in the early 1930s. They were found to have a mass slightly larger than that of the proton and to have no electric charge. For many years, these three particles were believed to be indivisible and fundamental particles. In more recent times, our understanding has changed, as presented in the last two sections of this chapter.

Table 2.1. Some Physical Characteristics of Electrons, Protons, and Neutrons

Name	Symbol	Charge[a]	Mass[b]		
Electron	e^-	-1	9.109×10^{-31} kg	5.5×10^{-4} amu	0.511 MeV
Proton	p	$+1$	1.672×10^{-27} kg	1.007 amu	938 MeV
Neutron	n	0	1.676×10^{-27} kg	1.009 amu	940 MeV

[a] Charge expressed in units of 1.602×10^{-19} C, which is the charge of the positron (e^+), a positively charged electron.

[b] Stated in kilograms, atomic mass units (amu), and rest energy in million electron volts (MeV). See Sections 2.1, 2.5, and 2.6 in text.

2.2
Formation of Atoms and Elements

The word "atom" is derived from the Greek word atomos, meaning "indivisible." The assumption that atoms are indivisible has been disproved. Every atom has a nucleus composed of protons and neutrons. The charge of a particular nucleus depends upon the number of protons in the nucleus, and the mass of the nucleus is governed by the sum of the protons and neutrons that it contains. Neutrons and protons are jointly referred to as nucleons. Electrons are attracted to the nucleus and move in orbits around it like the planets around the sun in the solar system. The electrons, being negatively charged particles, are held in their orbits by the attraction of the positive charges of the protons in the nucleus. This attractive force provides the binding energy that keeps the electrons bound to the nucleus. An external supply of energy equivalent to or greater than the binding energy is needed to free the electron from its bound state within the atom. In addition, there is a binding energy that ties the nucleons to one another within the nucleus. Any change or transition within the nucleus or within the atom as a whole, including the orbital electrons, represents a change in the energy contained in the atomic system. If the energy in the system is reduced due to any transition, the energy conservation law requires that this energy lost by the system be emitted in some form. The form can be either electromagnetic radiation, such as light, or a fast-moving particle, or both.

To be electrically neutral, an atom must have as many electrons in the atomic orbits as there are protons in the nucleus. The hydrogen atom is the simplest atom, and thus hydrogen is the simplest element. A hydrogen atom consists of one proton that forms the nucleus and one electron in the orbit (Figure 2.1a). The next element in the periodic table, which has two protons in the nucleus and two orbital electrons, is helium (Figure 2.1b). A few other elements are also illustrated schematically in Figure 2.1c, d, and e. Each has a specific number of electrons and protons.

Chemical binding and chemical reactions between different elements occur because of interaction among orbital electrons. Thus, what governs the chemical behavior of an element is the number of electrons in the atom. This number is referred to as the atomic number, designated by the symbol Z. Table 2.2 lists 106 elements ranging from hydrogen ($Z = 1$) to Seaborgium ($Z = 106$). The atoms of these different elements with their distinct chemical behavior can be thought of as being formed by a gradual increase in the number of orbital electrons from 1 to 106 and being matched by an

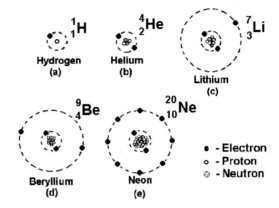

Fig. 2.1. Diagrams showing electrons in the orbits of hydrogen, helium, lithium, beryllium, and neon atoms

equal number of protons in the nucleus. The number of neutrons in the nucleus does not relate to Z or to the chemical behavior of the element. Hence, a difference in the number of neutrons in the nucleus can contribute to the formation of a heavier or lighter nuclide of one and the same element having the same Z. For example, Figure 2.2 illustrates three forms of hydrogen atoms. Figure 2.2a (also Figure 2.1a) shows a light hydrogen atom, which is abundantly present in our universe. Figure 2.2b shows a rarer and heavier hydrogen atom which has one neutron added to the proton in the nucleus. Adding a further neutron to the nucleus results in the still rarer, and heavier, hydrogen atom of Figure 2.2c. The nuclei of the two heavy hydrogens are called deuteron and triton. Their atomic names are deuterium and tritium, respectively. Deuterium and tritium behave chemically the same way as hydrogen because they, too, have Z = 1, with one orbital electron. We call them isotopes of hydrogen.

Isotopes are formed by a change in the number, N, of neutrons in a nucleus that contains a given number, Z, of protons. The total number, M, of nucleons is given by M = Z + N. M is called the mass number. Isotopes of the same element have a common value of Z, but different N and hence different M values. Each element is identified by a symbol, such as H for hydrogen, He for helium, Li for lithium, etc. An isotope of an element X is identified by Z appended as a subscript and M as a superscript:

$$^{M}_{Z}X$$

According to this convention, the three isotopes of hydrogen are

$$^{1}_{1}H \qquad ^{2}_{1}H \qquad ^{3}_{1}H$$

Fig. 2.2. Three isotopes of hydrogen

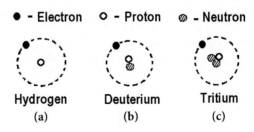

Table 2.2. List of Elements

Atomic Number	Symbol	Name	Atomic Number	Symbol	Name
1	H	Hydrogen	54	Xe	Xenon
2	He	Helium	55	Cs	Cesium
3	Li	Lithium	56	Ba	Barium
4	Be	Beryllium	57	La	Lanthanum
5	B	Boron	58	Ce	Cerium
6	C	Carbon	59	Pr	Praseodymium
7	N	Nitrogen	60	Nd	Neodymium
8	O	Oxygen	61	Pm	Promethium
9	F	Fluorine	62	Sm	Samarium
10	Ne	Neon	63	Eu	Europium
11	Na	Sodium	64	Gd	Gadolinium
12	Mg	Magnesium	65	Tb	Terbium
13	Al	Aluminum	66	Dy	Dysprosium
14	Si	Silicon	67	Ho	Holmium
15	P	Phosphorus	68	Er	Erbium
16	S	Sulfur	69	Tm	Thulium
17	Cl	Chlorine	70	Yb	Ytterbium
18	Ar	Argon	71	Lu	Lutetium
19	K	Potassium	72	Hf	Hafnium
20	Ca	Calcium	73	Ta	Tantalum
21	Sc	Scandium	74	W	Tungsten
22	Ti	Titanium	75	Re	Rhenium
23	V	Vanadium	76	Os	Osmium
24	Cr	Chromium	77	Ir	Iridium
25	Mn	Manganese	78	Pt	Platinum
26	Fe	Iron	79	Au	Gold
27	Co	Cobalt	80	Hg	Mercury
28	Ni	Nickel	81	Tl	Thallium
29	Cu	Copper	82	Pb	Lead
30	Zn	Zinc	83	Bi	Bismuth
31	Ga	Gallium	84	Po	Pollonium
32	Ge	Germanium	85	At	Astatine
33	As	Arsenic	86	Rn	Radon
34	Se	Selenium	87	Fr	Francium
35	Br	Bromine	88	Ra	Radium
36	Kr	Krypton	89	Ac	Actinium
37	Rb	Rubidium	90	Th	Thorium
38	Sr	Strontium	91	Pa	Protactinium
39	Y	Yttrium	92	U	Uranium
40	Zr	Zirconium	93	Np	Neptunium
41	Nb	Niobium	94	Pu	Plutonium
42	Mo	Molybdenum	95	Am	Americium
43	Tc	Technetium	96	Cm	Curium
44	Ru	Ruthenium	97	Bk	Berkelium
45	Rh	Rhodium	98	Cf	Californium
46	Pd	Palladium	99	Es	Einsteinium
47	Ag	Silver	100	Fm	Fermium
48	Cd	Cadmium	101	Md	Mendelevium
49	In	Indium	102	No	Nobelium
50	Sn	Tin	103	Lw	Lawrencium
51	Sb	Antimony	104	Rf	Rutherfordium
52	Te	Tellurium	105	Ha	Hahnium
53	I	Iodine	106	Sg	Seaborgium

The isotopes of helium are

$$^2_2\text{He} \qquad ^3_2\text{He} \qquad ^4_2\text{He}$$

The common isotopes of nitrogen and oxygen are

$$^{14}_7\text{N} \qquad ^{15}_7\text{N}$$

$$^{15}_8\text{O} \qquad ^{16}_8\text{O} \qquad ^{17}_8\text{O}$$

Not all isotopes that one could conceive of by arbitrarily adding neutrons to the nucleus can actually exist. This is because the nuclear kinetics may not permit a stable binding of the nucleons. In fact, nuclei that are heavily loaded with neutrons become unstable, and this instability may result in radioactive disintegration of the nucleus. For example, tritium undergoes radioactive decay to ^3_2He, a stable isotope of helium.

The isotopes can be classified as either naturally occurring or artificially produced. Bombardment of a naturally occurring atom with neutrons in a nuclear reactor or with fast-moving protons or helium ions from a high-energy accelerator can result in the formation of an artificial isotope. All of the elements with Z values higher than 92 (uranium) are artificially produced. They are called transuranic elements.

Atoms that have a common M but a different Z value are called isobars, and atoms that have the same N but a different M are called isotones. It is possible for a nuclide (with a given Z, M, and N) to remain for a significant period in an excited energy state above its normal stable state. It can, in the course of time, deexcite to the normal state by emission of radiation energy. Such a transition of a nuclide between its two energy states is referred to as an isomeric transition. The nuclides in the two states are called isomers of the same nuclide.

2.3
Atomic Electron Configuration

2.3.1
Electron Orbits and Energy Levels

The positive charge of the nucleus exerts an attractive electrical force on the electrons, just as the earth's gravitational force attracts any mass. The electrons in an atom are distributed in different orbits. Depending upon their orbits, electrons are in different energy states. Although one might think that the electron orbits could have any arbitrary radius and energy, the rules of quantum mechanics, which govern the physics of atomic levels, forbid this. In quantum mechanics, not all continuous energy values are possible. Instead, the momentum of the motion of the electrons changes from one permissible level to another, and so do the allowable energies. Figure 2.3a schematically represents the atomic structure in the form of an orbital diagram. It can be seen that the orbits cluster close to one another and appear to belong to different groups. The groups of orbits are designated as K, L, M, etc. in an alphabetical sequence. It is usual to refer to them as K shell, L shell, M shell, etc. The innermost allowable shell is the K shell.

In quantum mechanics, any particular electron's "orbital" state is specified by the assignment of particular values to the so-called quantum numbers n, ℓ, m_ℓ, and m_s. In addition, Pauli's exclusion principle, which is known to apply to the configuration of

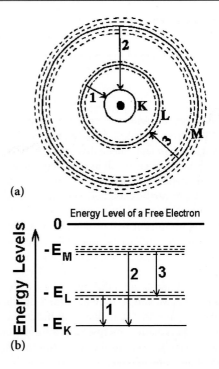

Fig. 2.3. (a) Electron-orbital
diagram showing K, L, and
M shells. (b) Energy level
diagram. The dashed lines
represent the allowed minor
variations around K, L, and M
shells.

the atomic electrons, stipulates that only one electron can occupy any one state defined by a particular combination of the four quantum numbers. The value of n, called the principal quantum number, can be any positive integer value 1, 2, 3, . . ., and each shell corresponds to a particular value of n. The K shell corresponds to n = 1, the L shell to n = 2, the M shell to n = 3, etc. In any shell, the azimuthal quantum number ℓ, can have a positive integer value from 0 to n − 1. For a given ℓ, the quantum number m_ℓ, called the magnetic quantum number, can assume any positive or negative integer value up to a maximum of ℓ, thereby giving $2\ell + 1$ different possible values of m_ℓ. The value of m_s, called spin quantum number, can be either −1/2 or +1/2, implying a positive or negative spin orientation. Each combination of quantum numbers defines a particular energy state possible for an electron. According to a rule called Pauli's exclusion principle, any particular state can be occupied by only one electron. Thus, a shell for quantum number n can accommodate a maximum of $2n^2$ electrons. Hence the K, L, M, and N shells can contain not more than 2, 8, 18, and 32 electrons, respectively.

Figure 2.3b is a schematic diagram showing the potential energy levels applicable to electrons bound to an atomic nucleus. In physics, the potential energy of an object is the work done to bring that object to its current state from its reference state. The reference state, which, by the above definition, is also the zero energy state, can be chosen arbitrarily. In the convention used for measuring the energy of atomic electrons, a free electron, unbound to any atom, is assigned zero energy. Thus, the bound electrons are in negative energy states. As an analogy, imagine that three stones are at the bottom of a well. Let us assume that they are lifted up from the bottom of the well to three different heights, and that only one of them is lifted all the way to the

Table 2.3. Binding Energies of Atomic Orbital Electrons (from Orbit K to M_5) in keV.

Z	Element	E_K	E_{L1}	E_{L2}	E_{L3}	E_{M1}	E_{M2}	E_{M3}	E_{M4}	E_{M5}
1	Hydrogen	0.014								
2	Helium	0.025	0.001							
6	Carbon	0.284	0.013	0.005	0.005					
7	Nitrogen	0.400	0.018	0.007	0.007					
8	Oxygen	0.533	0.024	0.009	0.009					
13	Aluminum	1.560	0.118	0.073	0.073	0.005				
15	Phosphorus	2.144	0.188	0.130	0.130	0.010	0.002	0.002		
19	Potassium	3.607	0.377	0.296	0.294	0.034	0.018	0.018		
20	Calcium	4.037	0.438	0.350	0.346	0.044	0.025	0.025		
22	Titanium	4.966	0.563	0.462	0.456	0.060	0.035	0.035		
26	Iron	7.112	0.846	0.721	0.708	0.093	0.053	0.053	0.003	0.003
29	Copper	8.981	1.096	0.953	0.933	0.122	0.074	0.074	0.007	0.007
42	Molybdenum	20.00	2.867	2.625	2.521	0.505	0.410	0.392	0.230	0.238
46	Palladium	24.35	3.605	3.330	3.174	0.670	0.559	0.532	0.340	0.335
47	Silver	25.51	3.806	3.524	3.351	0.718	0.602	0.571	0.373	0.367
50	Tin	29.20	4.465	4.156	3.929	0.884	0.756	0.714	0.493	0.485
53	Iodine	33.17	5.188	4.852	4.557	1.072	0.931	0.876	0.633	0.619
56	Barium	37.44	5.987	5.623	5.247	1.291	1.135	1.061	0.794	0.780
74	Tungsten	69.53	12.10	11.54	10.20	2.820	2.575	2.281	1.871	1.809
77	Iridium	76.11	13.42	12.82	11.22	3.173	2.908	2.551	2.116	2.040
78	Platinum	78.40	13.88	13.27	11.56	3.297	3.027	2.645	2.202	2.122
79	Gold	80.73	14.35	13.73	11.92	3.425	3.150	2.743	2.291	2.206
82	Lead	88.00	15.86	15.20	13.04	3.851	3.554	3.066	2.586	2.484

Data extracted from Reference 1. With permission.

ground level. The stone lifted to the ground required more work than did the other two stones, which are below the ground state. If this stone is assumed to be in the reference (or zero) energy state, the two other stones inside the well are in negative energy states with respect to it. Of the two stones inside the well, the one closer to the bottom of the well is at a lower energy. The stone on the ground is analogous to a free electron that is unbound to any atom. The two stones trapped inside the well are comparable to L and K electrons bound to the nucleus. Table 2.3 lists the binding energies of electrons in the low-energy orbits for several elements. A given shell can contain electrons of differing (and discrete) energies. However, here, for the sake of simplicity, we will refer to the K-, L-, and M-shell electrons as being at energies $-E_K$, $-E_L$, and $-E_M$, respectively. We say that a K-shell electron is bound to the nucleus by the binding energy E_K, and an amount of energy E_K is needed to free the K electron from its orbit. L-, M-, and N-shell electrons have binding energies E_L, E_M, and E_N, respectively.

In the sequence of elements, electrons are accommodated in orbits of increasing energy. An increase in the number of protons in the nucleus results in elements of progressively increasing Z, as has been illustrated in Figure 2.1. The first element, hydrogen (H), has only one orbital electron occupying the K shell. The next element, helium (He), has two orbital electrons, both of which are accommodated in the K shell. The next element, lithium (Li), has Z = 3 and three orbital electrons. For quantum-mechanical reasons, the K shell can have no more than two electrons. Therefore, the third electron in the Li atom is located in the next shell, the L shell. The L shell can hold a maximum of eight electrons. Thus, for neon (Ne), with Z = 10, the L orbit is completely filled. In the next element, sodium (Z = 11), the last electron occupies the next higher energy orbit, in the M shell. This process continues for increasing Z values. As we move to higher-order shells, it is possible that the energy levels in the adjacent shells overlap, that is, the energy of some of the orbits of a lower shell can exceed that of some orbits of a higher shell.

The foregoing discussion shows that both He and Ne have completed outer orbits with full complements of electrons. These elements are known to be chemically inert. On the other hand, hydrogen, lithium, and sodium each have only one electron in their outer orbits. They are chemically alike and very active. The role of the electronic configuration of the atom of any element in influencing its chemical behavior is discussed with examples later (Sections 2.7 and 2.8).

2.3.2
Ionization and Excitation of Atoms

A normal atom is electrically neutral, with all of its electrons in their proper orbits. An abnormal situation results if, for example, a K electron receives just enough energy from an external source to be lifted to the L or M orbit. Then the atom is said to be in an excited state. It is also possible that the K electron receives a large enough energy to be removed from the atom. The atom then is a positive ion with a vacancy in the K shell. The atom can be said to be in an ionized state. Any bound electron in an atom can be released if it is supplied with the energy needed to free it from its bond. The energy can be supplied by interaction with electromagnetic radiation (photons), or a moving electron, or even heat. Accordingly, the liberated electron may be called a photo-electron, a secondary electron, or thermionic emission.

2.3.3
Characteristic X-Rays and Auger Electrons

A vacancy in the K shell is an invitation to a higher-orbital electron to come closer to the nucleus. An L electron may transfer into the K-shell vacancy. The L electron is bound less tightly than the K electron in an atom. Also, the energy of the L electron is higher than that of the K electron. The transition of the L electron to fill a K vacancy will result in an energy loss by the system (atom) that is given by

$$E_{ph} = E_K - E_L$$

The energy E_{ph} will be in the form of electromagnetic radiation i.e., a photon (see Chapter 3). If a loosely bound outer orbital electron or a free electron fills the K vacancy, the energy of the photon released will be

$$E_{ph} = E_K$$

Sometimes a K vacancy may be filled by an L electron, an L vacancy by an M electron, and so on, resulting in a cascade of photons.

Because E_K, E_L, E_M, etc. are characteristic for each type of atom and E_{ph} depends on them, the photons emitted are also characteristic of the atom. Hence they are called characteristic photons or characteristic X-rays. In Figures 2.3a and b, the arrows marked 1, 2, and 3 are possible electronic orbital transitions that can result in emission of characteristic X-rays.

Another process that is known to occur in an ionized atom is Auger electron emission. As an alternative to emission of the characteristic photon, the excess energy, e. g., E_K, in an atom with a K-shell vacancy, might be transferred to another existing orbital electron, say, an L electron. Then a part of the excess energy E_K will be needed to strip the bound L electron. The stripped L electron, called an Auger electron, will be emitted with an energy E_{el} given by

$$E_{el} = E_K - E_L$$

After the emission of the Auger electron, the atom will be in a doubly ionized state, with two electron vacancies.

In general, an atom that is ionized by an interaction will lose its excess energy by emission of either characteristic photons or Auger electrons.

2.4
Definition of an Electron Volt (eV)

As energy is measured in work units, the energy of K, L, and M electrons can be expressed in the common unit of work, the joule (J). A different, but somewhat arbitrary and convenient unit for measuring the energy of particles is the electron volt (eV), defined as the energy gained by an electron when it is accelerated by an electrical potential difference of one volt. (Continuing the analogy with the gravitational field, this is like defining an energy unit in terms of the energy gained by a brick as it falls through 1 cm. However, the selection of the electron in the definition of the electron volt is much more specific in terms of the charge and mass.) Any particle of charge q will reach an energy E given by

$$E = qV$$

when accelerated by a potential V. The greater the charge q, the higher the energy reached will be. Also, for a given charge q, increasing V will increase the energy E attained. If q is measured in coulombs (C) and V in volts (V), then E will be in joules. If q is given in multiples of the electronic charge e and V is in volts, E will be in electron volts.

Because an electron has a charge of 1.602×10^{-19} C, acceleration by 1 V will give an energy of

$$1.602 \times 10^{-19}\,C \times 1\,V = 1.602 \times 10^{-19}\,J$$

That is,

$$1\,eV = 1.602 \times 10^{-9}\,J.$$

For many practical purposes, the units of kiloelectron volts (keV) and million electron volts (MeV) are also used.

2.5
Atomic Mass, Molecular Mass, and Atomic Mass Unit

It is often useful to compare the mass of one atom or isotope to that of another. For this purpose, in 1961 the International Union of Pure and Applied Physics and the International Union of Pure and Applied Chemistry selected carbon-12 as the official standard for atomic masses. (Before that time, oxygen was used as standard by both

Unions, but in two different ways. Thus, there were two standards for the atomic mass unit.) The following is the definition of the atomic mass unit (amu):

$$\text{One amu} = \frac{\substack{\text{Mass of a neutral atom of the most abundant} \\ \text{isotope of carbon in its ground state}}}{12}$$

The most abundant form of carbon is the isotope The isotopes of carbon are

Artificially produced	$^{10}_{6}C$	$^{11}_{6}C$	
Naturally occurring	$^{12}_{6}C$	$^{13}_{6}C$	
Artificially produced	$^{14}_{6}C$	$^{15}_{6}C$	$^{16}_{6}C$

The two stable isotopes, $^{12}_{6}C$ and $^{13}_{6}C$, occur in nature in relative abundances of 98.89% and 1.11%, respectively. In a simplistic sense, each amu can be thought of as approximating the mass of one nucleon, which is close to the mass of the hydrogen atom.

The atomic mass, A, of any element is the average mass of an atom of that element stated in amu. A sample of any element may be a mixture of many isotopes of that element in any proportion, and thus the average mass of an atom may not be an integral multiple of the amu. The atomic mass of chlorine is 35.5 amu, which is almost half-way between 35 and 36. The presence of heavier isotopes of hydrogen results in an atomic mass of hydrogen of 1.0078256 amu.

In a similar definition, the molecular mass of any compound is the average mass of one molecule in amu.

2.6
Avogadro's Number (N_{Av})

If we take a sample of any element and its mass is exactly one"kilogram atomic mass" (that is, A kg), it will contain 6.022×10^{26} atoms. This quantity is known as Avogadro's number (N_{Av}). A sample of any compound with a one "kilogram molecular mass" (i. e., M kg) will also contain N_{Av} molecules. The number N_{Av} is a universal constant. It is the same for all elements and molecules, under all circumstances, regardless of whether they are in gaseous, liquid, or solid form. For example, molecular mass of carbon is 12, and that of water is (almost) 18. Therefore, 12 kg of carbon and 18 kg of water contain 6.022×10^{26} carbon atoms and water molecules, respectively. (An amount of material has a certain mass that is the same in any gravitational field. However, the weight of a given amount of material changes with the gravitational field. The weight will depend on the altitude at which a material is located and whether it is on the earth or, for example, on the moon. The weight of a substance is equal to mass times the acceleration due to gravity.) From the definition of amu we derive the following:

$$1\ \text{amu} = (1/12)\ \text{mass of}\ ^{12}C\ \text{atom}$$
$$= (1/12)(12\ \text{kg}/N_{Av}) = 1.66056 \times 10^{-27}\ \text{kg}$$

2.7
Periodic Table of Elements

We know that the value of Z determines the possible electronic structure. We also know that there are groups of elements that have similar affinities or chemical behaviors. These groups were identified long before we had any insight into the electronic structure. The elements can be arranged in tabular form, from $Z = 1$ to 106, in such a way that the elements showing the same chemical behavior lie in the same column. Such a table is the Periodic Table of Elements (Table 2.4), first conceived of in 1869 by Dimitri Mendeleev. In this table, the elements in the last column are known to be chemically inert. All of these elements are known to have just the right number of electrons to have a completed outer shell. Adding one electron to the inert gas elements results in the elements of column 1 that form the chemical group called alkali. All of these elements have only one electron in their outermost shell. They all behave chemically alike and are highly reactive substances. The second to the last column contains elements that have one less electron than needed to complete their outer electron shell. These also behave alike and are highly reactive in forming molecules. We will briefly describe how the orbital electrons play a role in the formation of molecules.

2.8
Molecular Bonds

There are three important types of chemical bonds: ionic bonds, covalent bonds, and hydrogen bonds.

2.8.1
Ionic Bonds

Chemical bonds between atoms exhibit a tendency for any atom to have eight electrons in its outermost orbit. In an ionic bond, one atom combines with just one other atom. For example, the lithium (Li) atom, with $Z = 3$, has a completed K shell and one electron (called the valence electron) in its outermost L shell. It seeks to give away the single electron of the L shell in chemical reactions. The fluorine (F) atom, with $Z = 9$, has a completed K shell, but an L shell with seven rather than eight electrons. The compound lithium fluoride (LiF) is formed (Figure 2.4) by the combination of Li and F atoms. F takes away the extra electron of Li and becomes a negative ion, and the Li atom becomes a positive ion. The molecule LiF as a whole is electrically neutral.

2.8.2
Covalent Bonds

In covalent bonds, several atoms come together and share their outer orbital valence electrons. The water molecule H_2O combines two atoms of hydrogen with one atom of oxygen in a covalent bond. Oxygen ($Z = 8$) has a completed K shell and an incomplete L shell with 6 electrons. The hydrogen atom has an incomplete K shell with only one

Table 2.4. Periodic Table of Elements

	Alkali		METALS (Transition Metals)										Metalloids and Nonmetals				Halogens	Inert Gases
	I	II											III	IV	V	VI	VII	VIII
	1H																	2He
	3Li	4Be											5B	6C	7N	8O	9F	10Ne
	11Na	12Mg											13Al	14Si	15P	16S	17Cl	18Ar
	19K	20Ca	21Sc	22Ti	23V	24Cr	25Mn	26Fe	27Co	28Ni	29Cu	30Zn	31Ga	32Ge	33As	34Se	35Br	36Kr
	37Rb	38Sr	39Y	40Zr	41Nb	42Mo	43Tc	44Ru	45Rh	46Pd	47Ag	48Cd	49In	50Sn	51Sb	52Te	53I	54Xe
	55Cs	56Ba	57La	72Hf	73Ta	74W	75Re	76Os	77Ir	78Pt	79Au	80Hg	81Tl	82Pb	83Bi	84Po	85At	86Rn
	87Fr	88Ra	89Ac															
Lanthanides		58Ce	59Pr	60Nd	61Pm	62Sm	63Eu	64Gd	65Tb	66Dy	67Ho	68Er	59Tm	70Yb	71Lu			
Actinides		90Th	91Pa	92U	93Np	94Pu	95Am	96Cm	97Bk	98Cf	99Cs	100Fm	101Md	102No	103Lw	104Rf	105Ha	106Sg

Fig. 2.4a,b. A molecule of lithium fluoride (LiF) combines one atom of lithium with one atom of fluorine

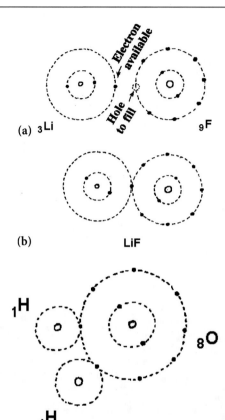

(a) $_3$Li

$_9$F

(b)

LiF

Fig. 2.5. A water (H_2O) molecule is formed by two hydrogen atoms and one oxygen atom

$_1$H

$_8$O

$_1$H

H_2O

electron in it. In H_2O (Figure 2.5), two hydrogen atoms come together and donate their two electrons to oxygen to make its L shell complete with eight electrons.

Ammonia (NH_3) is made up of one nitrogen (N) atom (with $Z = 7$, a completed K shell and an incomplete L shell with only five electrons) combined with three hydrogen (H) atoms in a covalent bond (Figure 2.6).

Aluminum oxide (Al_2O_3) combines two atoms of aluminum ($Z = 13$) with three oxygen atoms ($Z = 8$), because each oxygen atom requires two additional electrons to complete its L shell (Figure 2.7).

2.8.3
Hydrogen Bonds

The hydrogen bond refers to the attraction between two molecules containing hydrogen atoms. An example is the bond between two water (H_2O) molecules. In a water molecule, the hydrogen atoms give up their electrons and oxygen receives them. As a result, there is a concentration of electrons on the oxygen side of the molecule. This

Fig. 2.6. A molecule of ammonia (NH_3) combines one nitrogen atom and three hydrogen atoms

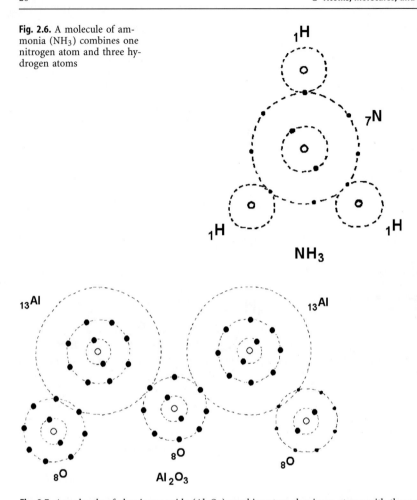

NH_3

Al_2O_3

Fig. 2.7. A molecule of aluminum oxide (Al_2O_3) combines two aluminum atoms with three oxygen atoms

causes a charge imbalance by which the hydrogen side could appear to be positively charged and the oxygen side negatively charged. If there are two water molecules, there is an attractive force between the oxygen atom of one and a hydrogen atom of the other. The two molecules will be held together in a bond referred to as a hydrogen bond.

2.9
Elementary Particles

We have discussed atoms and molecules by considering electrons, protons, and neutrons as the building blocks of matter. For completeness, in this section we present a brief summary of the modern trends in the understanding of the substructure of matter.

All materials around us are made up of fundamental particles. These particles are characterized by their mass, charge, spin, and other characteristics which have been established. Some of the particles are more stable than others. Their stability is characterized by their mean life. Particles that are unstable have a certain probability of disappearing. When this occurs, their mass may be split into smaller masses. Either their entire mass or a part of the mass may be converted into energy, in accordance with the laws of modern physics. The particles interact with each other, exerting mutually attractive or repulsive forces. These forces function like invisible strings holding them in a relationship to one another. Sometimes this mutual interaction can result in the transformation of one fundamental particle into another.

The physical theories (such as quantum electrodynamics, quantum chromodynamics) that deal with particles and their behavior are fascinating. The elementary particles may be grouped into three main categories: vector bosons, leptons, and quarks. Vector bosons are responsible for the forces between particles. We know that the four known forces of interactions between particles are electromagnetic, weak, strong, and gravitational. Among these, the electromagnetic forces and gravitational forces have been well known for a long time. Gravitational forces are about 10^{36} times weaker than the electromagnetic forces, and hence they play no known role of consequence in particle physics. Electromagnetic interaction occurs between particles that carry electric charge. The mediating particle in an electromagnetic interaction is the vector boson called a photon (hv). Any charged particle interacts with a photon field. Electromagnetic forces are long-range forces.

There are two other forces, weak and strong, that particles mutually exert in the nucleus. These forces are rather short-range forces, extending over nuclear dimensions of 10^{-13} to 10^{-16} cm. The strong force is known to be an attractive force that acts between neutron and neutron, neutron and proton, and proton and proton, and holds them together in the nucleus. The strong force vanishes at 4×10^{-13} cm or more, but is much stronger than the coulomb force (i. e., the force between electric charges) at 2×10^{-13} cm or less. Weak forces are about 10^{14} times weaker than the strong forces. In the modern theory, the weak and electromagnetic interactions are separate manifestations of one common electroweak force, just as electricity and magnetism are different manifestations of the same phenomenon. In the same manner that the electromagnetic interactions are mediated by photons, the weak interactions are mediated by vector bosons, $W^{\pm}$ and Z^0. The strong forces are known to be mediated by gluons (g).

Leptons are weakly interacting particles with no known internal structure and hence are considered to be truly fundamental. There are three known families of leptons: electron (e^-) and electron-neutrino (ν_e), negative muon (μ^-) and muon-neutrino(ν_μ), and negative tau (τ^-) and tau-neutrino (ν_τ) (see Figure 2.8). Each of these particles has a corresponding antiparticle having the same mass. The antiparticles of the lepton families are positron (e^+) and electron-antineutrino $(\bar{\nu}_e)$, the positive muon (μ^+) and muon-antineutrino, and tau plus (τ^+) and tau-antineutrino. Thus, there are 12 known leptons. Electrons are the best known among them. Neutrinos (an Italian word meaning tiny neutral ones) are chargeless, weakly interacting particles. They can penetrate the earth as if it were transparent. They travel the vast interstellar spaces with minimum interactions.

The characteristics of the three lepton particle families are given in Table 2.5. The lepton count (given by the number of leptons minus the number of antileptons) before

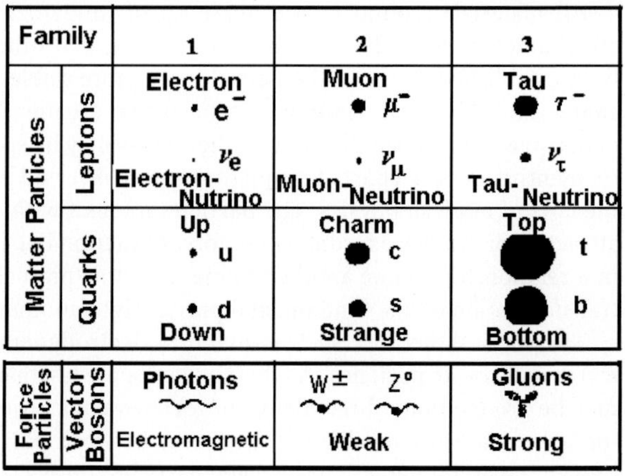

Fig. 2.8. Chart of leptons, quarks, and vector bosons

Family	1	2	3
Leptons (Matter Particles)	Electron • e^-	Muon • μ^-	Tau • τ^-
	ν_e Electron-Nutrino	ν_μ Muon-Neutrino	ν_τ Tau-Neutrino
Quarks (Matter Particles)	Up • u	Charm • c	Top • t
	• d Down	• s Strange	• b Bottom
Vector Bosons (Force Particles)	Photons 〜 Electromagnetic	$W^\pm$ Z^0 〜 〜 Weak	Gluons 丫 Strong

and after any particle transition is known to be conserved. The electron, positron, and all neutrinos and antineutrinos are stable, that is, they do not decay. The muon and tau are not stable. The leptons have dimensions of less than 10^{-16} cm. The name lepton, meaning light in Greek, was coined when the heaviest known lepton was the muon. However, tau, discovered in 1975, is heavier than many other particles that are not classified as leptons.

The name baryons (meaning heavy ones) refers to particles of large mass that take part in strong interactions. Before 1950, there was evidence of only two known baryons, which were the neutron and proton. There was also evidence for three particles, called mesons (meaning medium-heavy ones). These consisted of pions of positive charge (π^+), negative charge (π^-), and no charge (π^0). The strong force between baryons was considered to result from exchange of mesons between the baryons. By 1960, many more baryons and mesons had been discovered. At present, more than 100 such particles are known to exist. These are collectively called hadrons. Scientists wondered whether so many particles could be fundamental. Presently, it is understood

Table 2.5. Leptons

Family	Name of particle	Charge	Symbol	Rest Energy (Mass $\times c^2$)	Mean Life (sec)
(1)	Electron	−1	e^-	0.51 MeV	Stable
	Electron-neutrino	0	ν_e	<18 eV	Stable
(2)	Muon	−1	μ^-	105 MeV	2.197×10^{-6}
	Muon-neutrino	0	ν_μ	<0.25 MeV	Stable
(3)	Tau	−1	τ^-	1785 MeV	3.0×10^{-13}
	Tau-neutrino	0	ν_τ	<35 MeV	Stable

All particles have their corresponding antiparticles. The ν_τ has only been established as missing momentum and spin in the decay of tau lepton. Charges are in units of the charge of positron (e^+), which is 1.602×10^{-19} C.

Data based on Reference 2, p626.

Table 2.6. Quarks

Family	Name of Particle	Charge	Symbol	Rest Energy (Mass $\times$ c^2)
(1)	Up	2/3	u	5 MeV
	Down	−1/3	d	10 MeV
(2)	Charm	2/3	c	1.4 GeV
	Strange	−1/3	s	200 MeV
(3)	Top	2/3	t	80–200 GeV
	Bottom	−1/3	b	5 GeV

All quarks are of three kinds, called "colors": "red," "yellow," and "blue." All have their corresponding antiquarks. Charges are in units of the charge of positron (e$^+$), which is 1.602×10^{-19} C. Only recently (in 1994 at Fermilab, Illinois) has there been experimental evidence for the presence of the top quark. (Data based on Reference 2, p329).

that mesons and hadrons, in contrast to leptons, are not fundamental particles. They are composite structures of more fundamental constituents, called quarks.

There are now three known families of quarks. These are (up, down), (strange, charm), and (top, bottom) (see Figure 2.8). The characteristics of quarks are listed in Table 2.6. The six quarks listed are referred to as having u, d, s, c, t, and b "flavors." There is evidence for the presence of all quarks. Each of the six flavors of quarks can have three different "colors," viz., "red," "yellow," or "blue." For example, there are u-red, u-yellow, and u-blue quarks. Hence, there are 18 quarks and their corresponding antiquarks (which are shown by an overbar), making up a total of 36 quarks. (The flavors and colors of quarks are symbolic and have nothing to do with the human sensory perceptions.)

Mesons are combinations of a quark and an antiquark. Baryons are a combination of three quarks. A proton is the combination uud; a neutron is ddu; π^+ is u$\bar{\text{d}}$, π^- is $\bar{\text{u}}$d, and π^0 can be either u$\bar{\text{u}}$ or d$\bar{\text{d}}$. The quarks in the hadrons are held together by the strong force mediated by gluons. The strength of the gluon field is almost independent of distance. This independence of the strong force from distance of separation between the two quarks makes the quarks inseparable. Hence, we do not expect to see a free quark or a free gluon.

Hadrons have sizes of the order of 10^{-13} cm. The quarks and gluons have dimensions of less than 10^{-16} cm. Thus, a hadron volume contains quarks, gluons, and much empty space. We already mentioned that there are two types of hadrons: mesons and baryons. Among baryons, there are very heavy ones called hyperons. Table 2.7 lists the characteristics of several hadrons.

The mass of the quarks in the three quark families increases progressively from that of (u, d), (c, s) to (t, b). Likewise, the mass of the charged lepton increases in the three lepton families, with electron, muon, and tau having masses $\times$ c^2 of 0.51 MeV, 105 MeV, and 1785 MeV, respectively. The three sets of quarks and leptons are believed to be conjoined in three quark-lepton families: (u, d, e$^-$, ν_e), (c, s, μ^-, ν_μ), and (t, b, τ^-, ν_τ).

In the context of radiotherapy, it is worthwhile to mention that beams of protons, neutrons, electrons, and pions have all been used for treatment of cancer.

Table 2.7. Hadrons

Subcategory	Name of Particle	Symbol	Charge	Rest Energy (Mass $\times$ c^2) (MeV)	Mean Life (sec)	Quark Content
Mesons	pi$^+$ meson	π^+	1	140	2.6×10^{-8}	u$\bar{\text{d}}$
	pi^0 meson	π^0	0	140	8.7×10^{-17}	u$\bar{\text{u}}$ or d$\bar{\text{d}}$
	pi$^-$ meson	π^-	-1	140	2.6×10^{-8}	$\bar{\text{u}}$d
	K$^+$ meson	K$^+$	1	490	1.2×10^{-8}	$\bar{\text{s}}$u
	K^0 meson	K^0	0	490	5.2×10^{-8}	$\bar{\text{s}}$d
	K$^-$ meson	K$^-$	-1	490	1.2×10^{-8}	s$\bar{\text{u}}$
	D$^+$ meson	D$^+$	$+1$	1869	9×10^{-13}	c$\bar{\text{d}}$
	D^0 meson	D^0	0	1865	4×10^{-13}	c$\bar{\text{u}}$
	D$^-$ meson	D$^-$	-1	1869	9×10^{-13}	$\bar{\text{c}}$d
Baryons	Proton	p	$+1$	938	Stable	uud
	Neutron	n	0	940	898	udd
	Lambda	Λ^0	0	1115	2.6×10^{-10}	uds
H						
Y	Sigma$^+$	Σ^+	$+1$	1189	8×10^{-11}	uus
P	Sigma^0	Σ^0	0	1193	7×10^{-20}	uds
E	Sigma$^-$	Σ^-	-1	1197	1.5×10^{-10}	dds
R						
O	Xi^0	Ξ^0	0	1315	2.9×10^{-10}	uss
N	Xi$^-$	Ξ^-	-1	1321	1.6×10^{-10}	dss
S						
	Omega$^-$	Ω^-	-1	1672	0.8×10^{-10}	sss

There are more than 100 hadrons; only a few are listed here. Charges are in units of the charge of positron (e$^+$), which is 1.602×10^{-19} C. Antiquarks are marked by an overbar above the symbol. (Data based on Reference 2, p335 and 469).

2.10
Outer Space and Particle Research

Many laws of physics are based on symmetry. Developments in particle physics have repeatedly indicated that particles indeed exist in pairs. For every particle there is an antiparticle, such as, for example, electron and positron, proton and antiproton, which have the same mass, but opposite charge. As matter is mostly made up of protons, neutrons, and electrons, antimatter should be composed of antiprotons, antineutrons, and positrons. When matter and antimatter come together, a total disappearance or annihilation of both occurs. Hence, antimatter cannot exist amid matter in our surroundings on earth. The evidence for the existence of antimatter has to come from the cosmos. Cosmic rays that bring the dust of exploding stars (supernovae) can bring antimatter if it exists in outer space. Secondary antiprotons produced by cosmic rays colliding with interstellar matter have been detected, but the search for the presence of any heavier antimatter species, such as antihelium, continues. Cosmologists and theoretical particle physicists share a common interest in exploring for antimatter in distant galaxies.

References

1. Storm, E., and Israel, H.I., Photon cross sections from 1 keV to 100 MeV for elements $Z = 1$ to $Z = 100$, Nuclear Data Tables, A7, U.S. Atomic Energy Commission (and Academic Press). p565–681, 1970.
2. Lerner, R.G., and Trigg, G.L., (Eds.) Encyclopedia of Physics, VCH Publishers, New York, 2nd Edition, 1991.

CHAPTER 3

Propagation of Energy by Electromagnetic Waves

3.1
Radio Waves, Heat Waves, and Light Waves

If a stone is thrown, travels, and hits a target, the damage caused is readily attributed to the energy of the stone. That the moving stone is a carrier of energy is easily understood. It is less easy to understand how the energy coming from a radio transmitter is sensed by a radio receiver. The propagation of energy, in this case, is through electromagnetic waves that are invisible. The heat we feel when we place our hand near a hot oven is due to the infrared waves from the oven, which are also electromagnetic waves. The visible light from an electric lamp also consists of electromagnetic waves. In this chapter, we discuss electromagnetic waves and what causes the difference among radio waves, infrared waves, visible light, and any other manifestation of these waves. After presenting the classical description based on wave theory that applies to their macroscopic behavior, we briefly introduce the quantum-mechanical concepts that operate on atomic and microscopic scales, as needed for the purposes of this book.

3.2
Wave Propagation

First of all, we should understand wave propagation. A wave is a disturbance that travels through an extended medium. If a stone is thrown into the calm water of a pond (Figure 3.1), the waves (or disturbances) travel in all directions around the point where the stone fell. One can see the motion of the waves and get the erroneous impression that the water itself is moving outward from the spot where the stone fell. In reality, the water does not move outward; only the level of the water in a given location changes with time and creates the impression of motion. In other words, the disturbance (i. e., the wave) and not the water itself moves outward. Figure 3.2 shows the instantaneous ripple at some distance away (along a radial direction) from the point where the stone fell. The horizontal line indicates the level of the water before it was disturbed. The continuous wavy line represents the disturbance as it looks at one instant. It has peaks or "crests" at regular intervals, with valleys or "troughs" between them. The distance between two adjacent crests is the wavelength, denoted by λ. The dashed wavy line in Figure 3.2 represents the disturbance as it would appear a little later, as the wave moves. The dashed curve and the continuous curve are called different phases of the same wave. As the wave moves continuously, a time (or phase) will soon come when, once again, the disturbance looks exactly like the continuous curve. When the original phase first repeats, one cycle has passed. The number of wave crests that pass a fixed

Fig. 3.1. Waves formed in water
by a falling stone

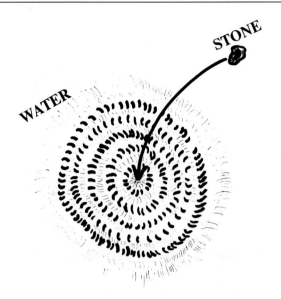

point in one second is called the frequency, denoted by ν. The wave velocity **v** is the distance a crest (or trough) travels in one second. The above definitions of wavelength, frequency, and wave velocity imply the following relationship among them for any wave propagation:

$$\mathbf{v} = \nu\lambda$$

The term "electromagnetic waves" implies that an electric wave and a magnetic wave are propagated in conjunction. From discoveries in the early nineteenth century, it was well known that moving electric charges produce a magnetic field, and that a changing magnetic flux produces an electric field. Maxwell formulated the relationship between electricity and magnetism into a set of laws. According to these laws, electromagnetic

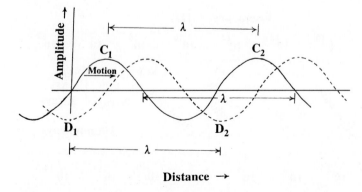

Fig. 3.2. Illustration of wavelength and wave motion. A wave moves from the position indicated by the continuous curve to that of the dashed curve over time. C_1 and C_2 are successive crests, and D_1 and D_2 are successive troughs

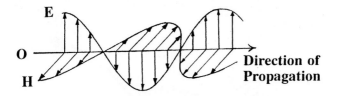

Fig. 3.3. Electric (E) and magnetic (H) fields associated with an electromagnetic wave, and their direction of propagation

waves consist of a varying electric field (**E**) and a varying magnetic field (**H**), in mutually perpendicular planes, sustaining each other as they are propagated through space (Figure 3.3).

3.3
Photons, Quanta, and the Electromagnetic Spectrum

Electromagnetic waves can have any wavelength. If the wavelength changes (for example, from 10^6 m to 10^{-10} m), the type of interaction of the waves with the surroundings also changes. Because of the manifestation of the behavior of the waves, different names have been given to them for different wavelengths. The electromagnetic spectrum spanning wavelengths from 10^2 m to 10^{-14} m, which covers radio waves, microwaves, infrared rays, visible light, ultraviolet rays, X-rays, and gamma rays, is presented in Figure 3.4.

A century ago, scientists believed that a medium was needed for any wave to travel. The question arose as to the medium in which electromagnetic waves travel. With the assumption that a medium was necessary, a mythical medium called "ether" was proposed. The "ether" was hypothesized to be so fine and all-pervading that it filled not only the spaces between stars and planets, but also the microspaces in atoms. However, scientific experiments very carefully designed to detect any "ether wind"

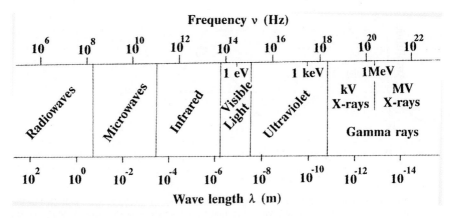

Fig. 3.4. The electromagnetic spectrum from radio waves to gamma rays

gave negative results. After Einstein developed his special theory of relativity, it could be inferred that electromagnetic waves traveled even through empty, "etherless" space. Visible light, which is a part of the electromagnetic spectrum, is known to travel even through a vacuum. Furthermore, electromagnetic waves of all wavelengths were found to travel in empty space with the same constant velocity, $c = 2.9979 \times 10^8$ m sec^{-1}. Thus, frequency ν, wavelength λ and velocity c are connected by relation

$$c = \nu\lambda$$

The value **c** is a universal constant. In media other than a vacuum, the velocity depends on both the medium and the wavelength. The velocity in air for any λ is almost equal to **c**.

Experimental studies of light, including the photoelectric effect (to be discussed in Section 7.4), revealed another aspect of electromagnetic waves, that the electromagnetic energy flows as discrete packets of energy, or quanta. Each quantum is called a photon. The energy E_ν of a photon is related to the frequency and wavelength as follows:

$$E_\nu = h\nu = h\frac{c}{\lambda}$$

where **h** ($= 6.625 \times 10^{-34}$ J sec) is a universal constant called Planck's constant. The greater the frequency ν, the larger the energy of the quantum will be, and the greater the wavelength λ, the smaller the quantum energy will be. For example, a photon of infrared radiation has very little energy compared to that of blue light, and a photon of X-rays will have more energy than does a photon of blue light. Hence, blue light with its low-energy quanta may not be able to perform a task (such as freeing electrons bound to a metal) that X-rays can do. Increasing the brightness of the blue light will only increase the number of photons, but each photon will remain as weak as before. (You may have learned that, in a darkroom where silver bromide emulsions are processed, red illumination may be used because it does not affect the photographic image.)

Photons also behave like particles. The mass-energy conversion relation, $E_0 = mc^2$, suggests that the mass of a particle is given by energy divided by c^2. This, in turn, suggests that a photon has an "associated" mass of $h\nu/c^2$. The corresponding momentum (given by mass multiplied by velocity) is $h\nu/c$. This means that photons can act like projectiles. We will show later (in Section 7.5) that, during incoherent photon scattering, known as the Compton effect, the photons do behave like particulate projectiles.

3.4
Louis de Broglie's Matter Waves

In modern quantum physics, this wave-particle duality is not reserved exclusively for electromagnetic energy. Louis de Broglie speculated in 1924 that particles with a mass, such as electrons, could exhibit wave properties. According to this suggestion, a particle of mass **m** and velocity **v** will have an equivalent wavelength of **h/mv**. This also implies that particles are not well localized, but are diffused and spread out like waves. Furthermore, interference and diffraction are features of the wave-like behavior. Such features of the wave-like behavior of matter were also soon verified by the demonstration of diffraction patterns produced by electrons. The wavelength of electrons was found to limit the resolution of electron microscopes in the same way as does the wavelength of visible light in optical microscopes.

CHAPTER 4

Nuclear Transitions and Radioactive Decay

4.1
Discovery of Natural Radioactivity

In 1896, Henri Becquerel in Paris identified a fluorescent compound of uranium which emitted penetrating radiation that produced a photographic image. In 1898, G.C. Schmidt in Germany and Marie Curie in Paris found another element, thorium, with a similar emission. Soon afterwards, Marie and Pierre Curie identified two additional radiation-producing elements, polonium and radium. An unusual characteristic of these elements was that all of them emitted radiation.

In an early experiment, Rutherford placed a sample of radium in a cavity shielded on all sides except in one direction, as is illustrated in Figure 4.1. A magnetic field was applied perpendicular to the plane of the diagram. A photographic plate was placed above the aperture and exposed to the radiation emerging from the sample. The image on the film revealed the emission of three radiation components. The three types of radiation were called alpha (α), beta (β), and gamma (γ) rays. The alpha radiation was found to be intensely ionizing and was bent slightly in the magnetic field. The beta radiation was lightly ionizing and was bent much more, though in the direction opposite to that of the alphas. These behaviors indicated that the alpha particles were heavy particles that carried a positive electric charge and beta particles were light particles that carried a negative electric charge. The gamma component was not bent by the magnetic field, indicating that it carried no charge. In other experiments, the gamma radiation was found to be the least ionizing among the three. Alpha particles were later identified to be helium atoms without their two orbital electrons; thus, they are doubly charged, positive ions. Beta particles are known to be

Fig. 4.1. Illustration of an early experiment on radioactivity. The magnetic field is directed perpendicular to the plane of the paper, as is a photographic film

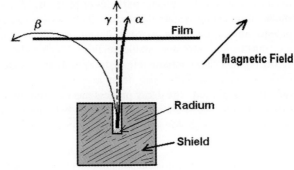

negatively charged electrons, and gamma rays consist of photons. All three originate in the nucleus.

Scientific research with particle accelerators and nuclear reactors has made it possible to obtain a number of artificially produced radioisotopes (in addition to the naturally occurring radioactive elements such as radium) for medical uses. The various known nuclear radioactive decay transitions are the subject of this chapter.

4.2
Nuclear Forces and Energy Levels

In Chapter 2, we addressed atomic energy levels and transitions. Radioactive decay is concerned in a similar way with nuclear transitions. The nucleus is composed of protons and neutrons, which together are referred to as nucleons. Nucleons are known to have a substructure made up of more fundamental particles, called quarks. The nucleons tend to be bound to each other by nuclear exchange forces of strong interaction. These strong forces are attractive in nature and have a rather short range. The relative scale of these short-range forces can be imagined from the fact that the atomic electron orbits have radii of the order of 10^{-8} cm, whereas the nuclear radii are of the order of 10^{-12} cm. The nucleons are still smaller. In an enlarged view, if the nucleus has the size of a peanut, the atom will be spread over an entire house. The protons have positive charges and, because the electromagnetic force between like charges is one of repulsion, they should tend to come apart. However, the attractive strong forces keep the nucleons bound. Another known nuclear exchange force is a so-called "weak force" that is known to be associated with beta decay.

It is known that the total mass of a nucleus is less than the sum of the masses of its constituent nucleons. The difference between the two is referred to as a mass defect. The mass defect converted into its energy equivalent is the energy that binds the nucleons together to form the nucleus and hence is called the binding energy. The binding energy is the energy required to split a nuclide* with mass number M into Z protons and N neutrons.

We described (in Chapter 2) that the atomic electrons have different quantized energy levels in the atom. The nucleons also have specific energy levels in the nucleus. Nuclear transitions occur when the nucleons change from one energy level to another. Furthermore, a neutron may be converted into a proton, and vice versa. Nuclear transitions can occur spontaneously, or they can be induced artificially by striking of the nuclei of atoms with energetic particles or photons. Whereas some nuclides are highly stable, others show instability because they possess excess energy that results in turbulence among the nucleons. Such unstable nuclides undergo radioactive decay and are transformed into more stable nuclides. (Each radioactive decay process happens according to a characteristic rate of decay with an associated half-life, T_h. Such mathematical details of radioactive decay are discussed in Chapter 5.) During the decay, radiation is emitted. The decay process has different names, depending upon the nature of the emitted radiation. Alpha decay, beta decay, internal conversion, isomeric transition, nuclear fission, and nuclear fusion are the processes that are covered in this chapter.

---

* A nuclide is any nuclear structure that exists long enough to be identified.

4.3
Nuclear Decay Schemes

During a nuclear transformation, the energy levels and the atomic number of the nucleus undergo changes. This can be depicted in diagrams called decay schemes. Figures 4.2 and 4.4 to 4.8 are decay schemes for various radionuclides. In these diagrams, the vertical positions represent the energy levels and the horizontal axis the atomic number. A line going from an upper to a lower level represents a loss of energy of the nucleus. A line going toward the right indicates an increase, and a line going toward the left, a decrease in atomic number. Each line and level are labeled to give information about the decay path they represent and the nucleus that results. There can be more than one route of decay, and the probabilities for competing routes are indicated in percent.

It is common to present a nuclear transition in the form of an equation showing the nuclide that existed before and the nuclide that results after a transition, connected by an arrow indicating the direction of the change. The equations have a balance that conserves the following before and after the transition:

(i) The total charge (given by positive charge minus negative charge)
(ii) The number of nucleons (given by the sum of protons and neutrons)
(iii) The number of leptons (given by the sum of leptons minus antileptons)

The above conservation laws are effective in addition to the physical laws of conservation of mass-energy and momentum. The equations use the following notation for the different particles:

$^1_0 n$ Neutron

$^1_1 p$ Proton

$^0_{-1} e^-$ Electron (also called β^- particle)

$^0_1 e^+$ Positron (also called β^+ particle)

$^0_0 \nu_e$ Electron-neutrino

$^0_0 \bar{\nu}_e$ Electron-antineutrino

$^4_2 He$ Doubly ionized helium atom (also called α particle)

$^0_0 \gamma$ Gamma photon

$^M_Z X$ A nuclide X with M nucleons that include Z protons

In all of the above, the subscript gives the charge of the particle (in units of the charge of the positron), and the superscript gives the mass number of the particle (in units of the mass of a nucleon).

4.4
Alpha Decay

When a helium atom is stripped of its electrons and is in a doubly ionized state, it is called an alpha (α) particle. Helium has the mass number 4, with two protons and two neutrons in its nucleus. In a nonionized state, the helium atom has two orbiting electrons. When any nucleus $^M_Z X$, with atomic number Z and mass number M, decays by alpha emission, it changes to a radioactive daughter nuclide Y with atomic number $(Z - 2)$ and mass number $(M - 4)$. This nuclear decay can be expressed in the form of the equation

$$_Z^M X \rightarrow \, _{Z-2}^{M-4} Y + _2^4 He$$

where $_2^4 He$ is the helium ion (i.e., alpha particle). It is to be noted that the total mass number is the same before and after the decay, and so is the sum of the charges as represented by the Z values, thus balancing the equation.

A classic example of alpha decay is the decay of radium to radon, which occurs as follows:

$$_{88}^{226} Ra \rightarrow \, _{86}^{222} Rn + _2^4 He \ (4.78 \, MeV)$$

In the above example, the alpha particles have an energy of 4.78 MeV. An unstable nuclide may decay in more than one way. This is the case for $_{88}^{226} Ra$, as is shown in the decay scheme of Figure 4.2. Whereas 95% of the $_{88}^{226} Ra$ nuclides decay as above, the residual 5% decay by emission of alpha particles of a lower energy, 4.60 MeV. In that scheme, the resulting radon nuclide is in an interim excited state and subsequently decays to a more stable state, shedding the excess energy of $(4.78 \, MeV - 4.60 \, MeV) = 0.18 \, MeV$ by emitting a gamma photon. $_{86}^{222} Rn$ undergoes a further series of decays with alpha, beta, and gamma emissions until it is transmuted to stable lead, $_{82}^{206} Pb$.

Fig. 4.2. Alpha decay scheme of radium-226 to radon-222

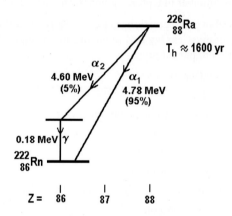

4.5
Beta Decay

4.5.1
Neutron-Proton Imbalance

Nuclear stability is influenced by the neutron-proton balance. An unstable nucleus can improve its neutron-proton ratio and become more stable through three different decay processes. These processes are β^- decay, β^+ decay, and electron capture (EC). In β^- decay, a neutron converts to a proton. In both β^+ decay and EC, a proton converts to a neutron. After β decay, the mass number M of the nuclide undergoing the transition remains unchanged, but the atomic number Z either increases or decreases by one. All of these processes result in the emission of a neutrino (v_e) or antineutrino ($\bar{v}_e$) associated with the electron (see Section 2.9). The electrons emitted in the decay process are called beta particles. Beta-minus (β^-) particles are negatively charged electrons (also called negatrons). Beta-plus (β^+) particles are positively charged electrons (also called positrons).

4.5.2
Beta-Minus (β^-) Decay

A nuclide that is unstable because it contains an excess neutron can change to a more stable state by a transition of one of its neutrons to a proton. A neutron (n), which has a net charge of zero, can decay into a proton (p), an electron (e^-), and an electron-antineutrino ($\bar{v}_e$):

$$_0^1 n \rightarrow {}_1^1 p + {}_{-1}^0 e^- + {}_0^0 \bar{v}_e$$

The antineutrino is a particle of negligible mass, but carries with it enough energy to maintain conservation of energy and momentum.

Both the antineutrino and the beta particle are emitted from the nucleus. They share between them the excess energy of the nucleus in a continuum of all possible combinations, so that the sum of the energies of the two particles has the same value for a given beta transition. Thus, unlike alpha particles, which have well-defined, discrete energies, beta particles can have continuous energies up to a maximum value. The maximum occurs in the extreme situation in which all of the available excess energy is given to the beta particle, with none going to the antineutrino. At the other extreme, the antineutrino may carry all of the energy, leaving none for the beta particle.

A typical beta-particle energy spectrum (i.e., the observed spread of beta-particle energies over many disintegrations) is shown in Figure 4.3. The diagram shows the maximum energy, E_{max}, the most probable energy, E_f, and the average energy, E_a.

In β^- decay, a neutron is converted into a proton; therefore, the atomic number of the residual nuclide increases by 1, but the mass number remains unchanged. The equation representing the transition of a nuclide X to a nuclide Y by β^- decay is of the form

$$_Z^M X \rightarrow {}_{Z+1}^M Y + {}_{-1}^0 e^- + {}_0^0 \bar{v}_e$$

Fig. 4.3. Energy spectrum of $_{83}^{210}$Bi beta particles, showing their maximum energy, E_{max}, the average energy, E_a, and the most probable energy, E_f

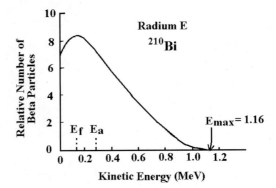

Fig. 4.4. Decay scheme of cobalt-60

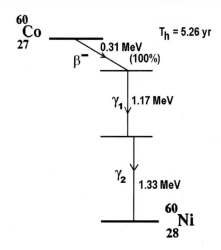

For example, $^{60}_{27}$Co decays as follows:

$$^{60}_{27}\text{Co} \rightarrow \ ^{60}_{28}\text{Ni} + \ ^{0}_{-1}e^- + \ ^{0}_{0}\bar{\nu}_e + \ ^{0}_{0}\gamma$$

The decay scheme of ^{60}Co shown in Figure 4.4 is rather simple. The beta particles have a maximum energy of 0.31 MeV, and the resulting nickel (Ni) nuclide is in an excited state. This leads to emission of two photons, of energies 1.17 and 1.33 MeV, in a cascade before the stable state of nickel is reached.

A more complicated decay is that of $^{131}_{53}$I, shown in Figure 4.5. In this case, there are five different beta spectra having E_{max} values of 0.808, 0.608, 0.469, 0.335, and 0.249 MeV, with relative abundances of 0.6%, 90.4%, 0.5%, 6.9%, and 1.6%, respectively. After the emission of beta particles by any of these branches, the balance of the energy necessary to reach the stable nuclide of $^{131}_{54}$Xe is emitted in the form of gamma rays.

Fig. 4.5. Decay scheme of iodine-131. Only major pathways are shown

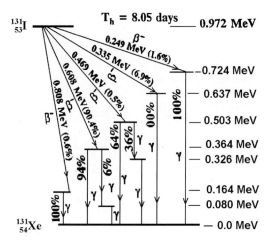

4.5.3
Beta-Plus (β^+) Decay

In β^+ decay (which is positron decay), a nucleus that is unstable because of an excess proton will tend to convert one of its protons into a neutron. Electrons and positrons have the same mass of 0.51 MeV, but have opposite charge. Thus, in theory, if a nucleus has an excess energy of $(2 \times 0.51 =) 1.02$ MeV, an electron-positron pair can be formed by mass-energy conversion. (See discussion on pair production in Section 7.6.) Then the following transition that converts a proton to a neutron is possible:

$$\,^1_1p + \left(\,^0_{-1}e^- + \,^0_1e^+\right) \rightarrow \,^1_0n + \,^0_1e^+ + \,^0_0\nu_e$$

In the above transition, the negative charge of the electron combines with the positive charge of the proton to annul the charge, and the proton becomes a neutron. The positron, which is the β^+ particle, is emitted with a neutrino. β^+ particles have a continuous energy spectrum similar to that of β^- particles. β^+ decay results in a daughter nuclide that has an atomic number lower by one than that of the parent, but having the same mass number as the parent. This can be expressed as

$$\,^M_Z X \rightarrow \,^M_{Z-1}Y + \,^0_1e^+ \,^0_0\nu_e$$

An example is

$$\,^{13}_7N \rightarrow \,^{13}_6C + \,^0_1e^+ + \,^0_0\nu_e$$

4.5.4
Electron Capture (EC)

We noted that an energy of 1.02 MeV is needed for β^+ decay to be possible. A nuclide may not possess this amount of excess energy, but may be unstable because it has an excess proton. Decay by electron capture is another option available to such a nuclide. In electron capture, an atomic orbital electron is drawn into the nucleus to neutralize the positive charge of a proton. This results in the following transition, in which the proton becomes a neutron with a neutrino being emitted:

$$\,^1_1p + \,^0_{-1}e^- \rightarrow \,^1_0n + \,^0_0\nu_e$$

The captured electron can come from any one of the electron shells, K, L, M, etc. Accordingly, the capture is called K capture, L capture, etc. The probability for K capture is higher than that for L capture, which, in turn, is higher than that for M capture, and so on for shells farther from the nucleus. After an electron capture occurs, the atom goes to an ionized state with an orbital-electron vacancy. This leads to the emission of characteristic X-rays and Auger electrons (see Section 2.3.3).

Some nuclides may decay entirely by electron capture. Some others may decay entirely by positron emission. For some, electron capture and β^+ decay can become competing processes. For example, the decay scheme of $\,^{22}_{11}Na$ is shown in Figure 4.6. The vertical line on the right shows, first, the loss of 1.02 MeV in electron-positron pair production (which is a requirement for the conservation of mass and energy). The oblique line below from the right toward the left represents the emission of the positron with an E_{max} of 0.91 MeV and a reduction in the atomic number by 1. The slanting line on the left indicates decay by electron capture. The figures in parentheses

Fig. 4.6. Decay scheme
of sodium-22. Only major
pathways are shown

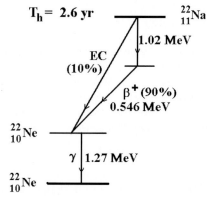

Fig. 4.7. Decay scheme
of iodine-125. Only major
pathways are shown

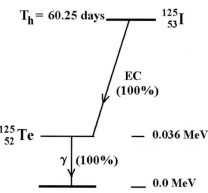

(10% and 90%) next to the decay paths indicate the relative probabilities of decay along
these paths.

$^{125}_{53}I$ is an example of a nuclide that decays only by electron capture. Its decay scheme
is shown in Figure 4.7.

4.6
Internal Conversion (IC)

The daughter nuclide formed after a radioactive transition may have excess energy
to give away. This excess energy (say, E_{ph}) is often released in the form of a photon.
Photons, which are electromagnetic radiations of nuclear origin, are given the name
gamma rays. Gamma rays have clearly defined, discrete energies.

Sometimes the gamma ray energy, E_{ph}, is transferred to an orbital electron, resulting in the emission of that electron. This process is called internal conversion, and
the released orbital electron is called an internal conversion electron. The internal
conversion can occur from any electron shell. Accordingly, there can be K-conversion
electrons, L-conversion electrons, etc. The probability for conversion decreases from
the K shell to the outer shells. The K-conversion electron has an energy $E_{K,c}$ given by

$$E_{K,c} = E_{ph} - E_K$$

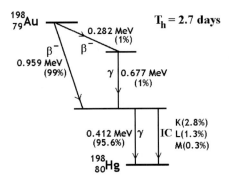

Fig. 4.8. Decay scheme of gold-198. Only major pathways are shown

where E_{ph} is the excitation energy available and E_K is the K-electron binding energy. Likewise, the L-conversion electron will have energy $E_{L,c}$, given by

$$E_{L,c} = E_{ph} - E_L$$

where E_L is the binding energy of an L electron.

Gamma ray emission and internal conversion can be competing processes. For example, the decay scheme of $^{198}_{79}\text{Au}$ is shown in Figure 4.8. In the initial state, $^{198}_{79}\text{Au}$ can emit a β^- particle belonging to one of two spectra, with E_{max} of 0.959 or 0.282 MeV. The numbers in parentheses (99% and 1%) indicate the branching ratio for these two possibilities, with the total adding up to 100%. The 1% branch also results in the emission of a gamma ray of energy (0.959 MeV $-$ 0.282 MeV) $= 0.677$ MeV. The nuclide now is still in an excited state. To reach its stable state of $^{198}_{80}\text{Hg}$, it needs to shed an excess energy of 0.412 MeV. It does this by gamma emission with a probability of 95.6%. The remaining 4.4% results in internal conversion, with K, L, and M conversions having 2.8%, 1.3%, and 0.3% probabilities, respectively.

Internal conversion electrons can be distinguished by their discrete energies. They can be seen as peaks superimposed on the continuous nuclear beta-particle spectrum. Such a spectrum (showing a plot of the relative number of beta particles versus momentum) is shown in Figure 4.9.

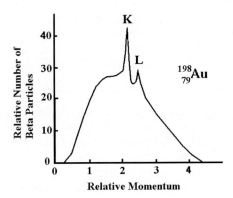

Fig. 4.9. Beta-particle spectrum of gold-198, showing the discrete peaks for K and L internal conversion electrons

4.7
Isomeric Transition

Generally, the gamma rays accompanying radioactive transitions are emitted instantly along with alpha or beta rays; there is no decay that results in the emission of gamma rays only. However, there are instances in which the daughter nuclide that is formed remains in an excited state for a significant period before becoming deexcited by a gamma emission. Such a "temporary" or "metastable" excited state is called an isomeric state. The radioactive isotope $^{99m}_{43}$Tc, which is widely used in medicine, is an example of such a state. $^{99}_{42}$Mo emits a β^- particle (Figure 4.10) and becomes $^{99m}_{43}$Tc (where the letter m appended to the mass number implies a metastable condition). $^{99m}_{43}$Tc subsequently becomes stable $^{99}_{43}$Tc on emission of a 140-keV gamma photon. The $^{99m}_{43}$Tc is stable for a sufficiently long duration so that it can be separated chemically from Mo if needed. ^{99m}Tc-labeled pharmaceuticals are used as pure gamma emitters in nuclear medicine (see Section 5.3.2).

Fig. 4.10. Decay scheme of molybdenum-99. The isomeric state of technetium-99m is shown. Only major pathways are shown

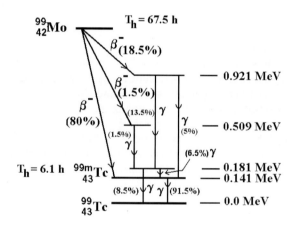

4.8
Nuclear Fission

In alpha or beta decay, the emitted particle has a small size and low mass compared to those of the nuclide. Nuclear fission is a type of decay in which a heavy nuclide becomes fragmented into two smaller heavy nuclides. For example, $^{235}_{92}$U can split into two fragments, $^{137}_{55}$Cs and $^{96}_{37}$Rb, and two neutrons; that is,

$$^{235}_{92}\text{U} \rightarrow {}^{137}_{55}\text{Cs} + {}^{96}_{37}\text{Rb} + 2\,{}^{1}_{0}\text{n}$$

The mass distribution of the fission fragments is random, but within the constraints of the mass-energy conservation law. Figure 4.11 illustrates the mass spectrum of fragments of U^{235} fission, which shows a double-peaked distribution. The two daughter nuclides formed in a nuclear fission reaction are often radioactive themselves. The nuclear fission reaction transfers a large amount of energy to the recoiling fission fragments. This is the source of energy in nuclear power stations.

Fig. 4.11. Mass spectrum of fission products of uranium-235. The peaks correspond to the most abundant fission fragments

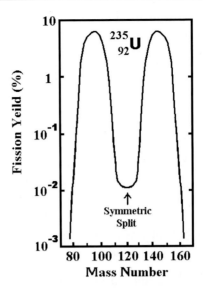

A fission reaction either can be spontaneous or can be induced by addition of a neutron from an external source. In most fission reactions, neutrons are released in addition to the main fission fragments. Sometimes two and sometimes three neutrons are released. These neutrons can be reabsorbed in other fissionable nuclides and further fission reactions can result. This can cause the release of more energy and more neutrons. This process can continue on and on. It is such a neutron chain reaction used in a controlled manner that produces energy at a steady rate in a nuclear reactor. A chain reaction that is uncontrolled and that releases the energy in a sudden burst is the basis of nuclear explosives and weapons.

4.9
Nuclear Fusion

Nuclear fusion implies combining of two nuclides. Fusion is the opposite of fission. At high temperatures, matter evaporates and becomes ionized plasma. Plasma is a state of matter in which the gaseous constituents (for example, hydrogen and helium) are highly ionized. A fusion reaction occurs in such a plasma. In many fusion reactions, as in fission, a large amount of energy is released. Like fission chain reactions, fusion chain reactions are possible. The energy of the sun and stars consists entirely of fusion energy. Uncontrolled release of energy in fusion chain reactions is the basis of the thermonuclear bomb or hydrogen bomb. In such a bomb, for the fusion to happen, a fission device is first exploded, creating the plasma. An example of a fusion cycle involves hydrogen ions (protons) and helium ions. This cycle starts with two hydrogen ions and ends by producing two hydrogen ions as follows:

$$^1_1H + {}^1_1H \rightarrow {}^2_1H + {}^0_1e^+ + {}^0_0\nu_e$$
$$^2_1H + {}^1_1H \rightarrow {}^3_2He + {}^0_0\gamma$$
$$^3_2He + {}^3_2He \rightarrow {}^4_2He + 2\,{}^1_1H$$

Here, several hydrogen ions have undergone fusion to form helium. Achieving a controlled nuclear fusion chain reaction at low temperatures is still a difficult challenge that is awaiting a research breakthrough. (When this is accomplished, society will have solved its major problems of energy shortage. The abundance of hydrogen in the world can then be exploited fully.)

4.10
Induced Nuclear Transformations

When a target nuclide **X** is hit by a particle **a**, this can result in the absorption of that particle by the nucleus, and formation of a compound nucleus. The compound nucleus may subsequently emit a particle **b** and become a nuclide **Y**. Such a reaction, called an (**a**, **b**) reaction, is written as

$$X(a, b)Y$$

It can also be written as an equation of the form

$$a + X \rightarrow Y + b + Q$$

In the above equation, Q signifies a mass-energy term given by $[(Y+b)-(a+X)]$. The laws of conservation of momentum, mass-energy, and lepton number (see Section 4.3) are applicable to all nuclear reactions. A positive Q value is indicative of a release of energy in the reaction. A reaction with a negative Q value cannot take place unless the incident particle **a** is accelerated to have a minimum energy of Q. This indicates that the incoming particle **a** should have a minimum threshold energy for the reaction to take place.

Nuclear reactions provide much insight into the nucleus and nuclear structure. Accelerators that produce energetic particles have become major tools for fundamental physics research. Many new radionuclides have been produced by bombardment of nuclides of naturally occurring elements with neutrons, protons, deuterons, or alpha particles. Various examples of nuclear reactions are

(n, p) reaction $\quad {}_0^1 n + {}_7^{14} N \rightarrow {}_6^{14} C + {}_1^1 p + 0.63 \text{ MeV}$

(p, n) reaction $\quad {}_1^1 p + {}_1^3 H \rightarrow {}_2^3 He + {}_0^1 n - 0.76 \text{ MeV}$

(α, n) reaction $\quad {}_2^4 He + {}_4^9 Be \rightarrow {}_6^{12} C + {}_0^1 n + 5.6 \text{ MeV}$

(n, α) reaction $\quad {}_0^1 n + {}_3^6 Li \rightarrow {}_1^3 H + {}_2^4 He + 4.78 \text{ MeV}$

(d, n) reaction* $\quad {}_1^2 H + {}_1^2 H \rightarrow {}_2^3 He + {}_0^1 n + 3.265 \text{ MeV}$

(d, p) reaction $\quad {}_1^2 H + {}_{15}^{31} P \rightarrow {}_{15}^{32} P + {}_1^1 p$

(n, γ) reaction $\quad {}_0^1 n + {}_1^1 H \rightarrow {}_1^2 H + {}_0^0 \gamma + 2.2 \text{ MeV}$

(γ, n) reaction $\quad {}_0^0 \gamma + {}_{82}^{204} Pb \rightarrow {}_{82}^{203} Pb + {}_0^1 n - 8.2 \text{ MeV}$

(p, γ) reaction $\quad {}_1^1 p + {}_3^7 Li \rightarrow {}_4^8 Be + {}_0^0 \gamma + 17.2 \text{ MeV}$

---

* The symbol d refers to the deuteron, which is the heavy-hydrogen ion ${}_1^2 H$. This reaction is also called (d, d) reaction.

CHAPTER 5

Radioactive Decay Calculations

5.1
Introduction

A sample of a radioactive material is a collection of unstable radionuclides. It is not possible to pinpoint or predict exactly which ones among them will decay and when. This is because radioactive decay is a random process. Any radionuclide may decay in any given time interval with a certain probability, but not with any certainty. We can only predict the averages for a whole group, without being specific about a particular nuclide. Furthermore, in decay calculations, we do not consider situations in which the number of radionuclides is too small or the observation time is too short for the average to be meaningful. In this chapter, we present the mathematical approaches used for calculating the decay and buildup of radioactivity in a sample in typical situations of interest in medical physics.

5.2
Decay of a Single Isotope

We first address the simple situation of a sample of a single radioactive substance that decays to a stable daughter product.

5.2.1
Observing an Instant

Assume that there are N radioactive nuclides. Because these nuclides tend to undergo radioactive disintegration, a fraction ΔN of them will decay during a time interval Δt. The number of transitions ΔN can be expected to increase in proportion to the total number of nuclides N observed and to the observation time Δt. Hence,

$$\Delta N = -\lambda N \Delta t \tag{5-1}$$

where λ is a constant of proportionality. The negative sign on the right-hand side of the equation is included to make ΔN negative and indicates a reduction of N with the passage of time. The constant λ, called the radioactive decay constant or decay probability, is the probability per unit time that any of the N radionuclides will decay.

We define the activity of a radioactive sample as the number of disintegrations per unit time, i.e., the rate of disintegration. Because ΔN atoms decay in a time interval

Δt, the activity, A, is given by

$$A = -\Delta N / \Delta T = \lambda N \tag{5-2}$$

Thus, the decay constant λ, multiplied by the number N of radioactive atoms present, gives the activity at any instant. Activity can be expressed in units of sec^{-1}. This unit has been given the name becquerel (Bq); 1 Bq is one disintegration per second. The curie (Ci) is another unit of activity; 1 Ci is 3.7×10^{10} Bq. The size of the curie is somewhat arbitrary; it was chosen because it closely matches the disintegration rate of 1 g of radium.

5.2.2
Observing Decay Over Lengthy Periods

It is clear that, if a radioactive sample is observed over an extended period, the number of radionuclides available in it that are yet to disintegrate will gradually decline. Equations (5-1) and (5-2) address the particular instant when the number of available radionuclides is N. At any instant, the number disintegrating depends on the quantity of radionuclides present at that instant. The disintegration rate should decrease as the number of radionuclides available for decay decreases. Such a phenomenon, in which the change in a value (at any moment) is proportional to the existing value (at that same moment,) is expressed mathematically as an exponential function. The exponential function (see equations (5-4) and (5-5)) uses the universal constant e called Eyler's exponential constant. Like the universal constant **e** that has a value of 3.1416, e has a constant value of 2.7183. Most modern scientific calculators provide for an easy entering of values π and **e**.

To derive the exponential function mathematically, we transpose and rewrite Equation (5-2) as a differential equation by replacing ΔN by dN and Δt by dt:

$$\frac{dN}{dt} = -\lambda N \tag{5-3}$$

Let us say that, at the beginning of the observation, N_o radionuclides are available. As the time increases from 0 to T, the number of radionuclides changes from N_o to N. Hence, we can write

$$\int_{N_o}^{N} \frac{dN}{N} = -\lambda \int_{0}^{T} dt$$

The mathematical solution of the above integral equation gives exponential function

$$N = N_o e^{-\lambda T} \tag{5-4}$$

which employs the value e.

Similarly, if A_o is the intial activity and A is the activity after a time interval T:

$$A = A_o e^{-\lambda T} \tag{5-5}$$

The fall-off of N and A is thus exponential. In Figure 5.1a and b, the decrease of activity with time is plotted in two types of graphs. In Figure 5.1a, linear scales are used for both time and activity. Figure 5.1b is a semilogarithmic graph in which a linear scale is

Fig. 5.1. Radioactive decay of an initial activity of A_o with time, presented in a linear-linear graph (left side) and a linear-logarithmic graph (right side). T_h and T_m are half life and mean life, respectively. The activity reaches $0.5\,A_o$ and $0.37\,A_o$, respectively, at these two times

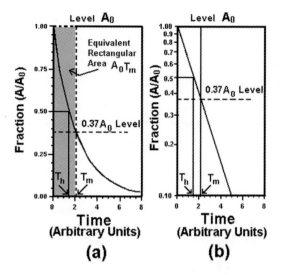

used for time and a logarithmic scale for activity. As is apparent from Equation (5-5), the fall-off of A becomes a straight line in a semilog graph.

5.2.3
Half Life (T_h)

The half life (T_h) of a radionuclide is defined as the time in which the activity A reaches half of the initial value A_o. In other words, if $T = T_h$, $A = A_o/2$. Mathematically,*

$$A_o/2 = A_o e^{-\lambda T_h}$$

or

$$e^{-\lambda T_h} = 1/2$$

$$\lambda T_h = \ln(2) = 0.693$$

and

$$T_h = 0.693/\lambda \qquad (5\text{-}6)$$

Thus, given λ, T_h can be derived, and vice versa. The exponential decay of the activity can also be written in terms of T_h as follows:

$$A = A_o e^{-0.693T/T_h} \qquad (5\text{-}7)$$

or, alternatively, as

$$A = A_o 2^{-T/T_h} \qquad (5\text{-}8)$$

---

* In general, if $y = e^x$, $\ln(y) = x$, where ln refers to the natural logarithm with base e. Because $e^{0.693} \approx 2$, $\ln(2) \approx 0.693$. Thus, the number 0.693 has a special significance. If $y = 10^x$ then $\log(y) = x$, where log refers to common logarithm with base 10.

...ause $e^{-0.693} = 2$. If T is n half lives, $T/T_h = n$, and

$$A = A_o 2^{-n} \qquad (5\text{-}9)$$

EXAMPLE 5.1

Cobalt-60 decays with a half life of 5.26 years. A source has an initial activity of 1000 Ci. What will be its activity after (i) 18 months, (ii) 10.52 years, and (iii) 10 half lives?

(i) $A_o = 1000$ Ci, $T_h = 5.26$ years, $T = 18$ months.
      T and T_h must be expressed in the same unit; thus, we express T in years.
      $T = 18$ months/(12 months/year) = 1.5 years.
      Substituting these values in the relation (5-7), we obtain

$$A = A_o e^{-0.693 T/T_h} = 1000 \text{ Ci} \times e^{(-0.693 \times 1.5/5.26)}$$
$$= 1000 \times 0.821 \text{ Ci} = 8.21 \text{ Ci}.$$

(ii) $T = 10.52$ years

$$A = A_o e^{-0.693 T/T_h} = 1000 \text{ Ci} \times e^{(-0.693 \times 10.52/5.26)}$$
$$= 1000 \times e^{(-0.693 \times 2)} = 250 \text{ Ci}.$$

   Notice that 10.52 years is twice the half life of 5.26 years. Over the first half life, the activity of 1000 Ci would be reduced by one half to 500 Ci. Over the second half life, it would again be reduced by half to 250 Ci.

(iii) $T = 10$ half lives.
      For n half lives, $A = A_o 2^{-n}$.
      $A = 1000$ Ci $\times 2^{-10} = 1000$ Ci $\times 0.00098 = 0.98$ Ci.

5.2.4
Mean Life (T_M)

We already mentioned that the radioactive decay of a nuclide is a random process. In a given radioactive sample, some of the nuclides will decay early and have short lives, whereas others may not decay for a long time. We can ask what is the average life or mean life (T_m) for the total population of N_o nuclides. To answer this question, we need to imagine that all of the N_o radionuclides live for the identical period T_m and have an abrupt demise. Such a situation is illustrated by the step-like dashed line in Figure 5.1a, which shows that the activity remains steady at its initial value A_o for a period T_m. The area under the radioactivity decay curve gives the total number of possible disintegrations. It is evident that only N_o disintegrations in all are possible. The mean life T_m is such that the area under the step curve is N_o. Thus,

$$A_o T_m = N_o$$

or

$$\lambda N_o T_m = N_o$$
$$\lambda T_m = 1 \qquad (5\text{-}10)$$

and

$$T_m = 1/\lambda$$

Because $T_h = 0.693/\lambda$, $T_m = 1.443\, T_h$.

The mean life can also be derived from the following mathematical formula for the mean or average time:

$$T_m = \frac{\int_0^\infty t A_0 e^{-\lambda t}\, dt}{\int_0^\infty A_0 e^{-\lambda t}\, dt} = \frac{1}{\lambda} \tag{5.10a}$$

The concept of mean life is useful for carrying out calculations in situations in which there is complete decay of activity.

EXAMPLE 5.2

I^{125} decays with a half life of 60.25 days. (i) What is its mean life? (ii) If 400 MBq of initial activity of I^{125} is implanted in a patient, how many disintegrations would take place before decay is complete?

(i) Half life $T_h = 60.25$ days

$$\text{Decay constant } \lambda = 0.693/T_h = 0.693/60.25 \text{ days}^{-1}$$
$$= 0.0115 \text{ days}^{-1}$$

Mean life $T_m = 1/\lambda = 86.94$ days.

(ii) Because $1 \text{ MBq} = 1 \times 10^6$ disintegrations sec^{-1},

$400 \text{ MBq} = 400 \times 10^6$ disintegrations $\text{sec}^{-1} = 4 \times 10^8$ disintegrations sec^{-1}.

Total disintegrations for complete decay are given by

(initial disintegration rate) × (mean life)

$= (4 \times 10^8 \text{ disintegrations sec}^{-1}) \times (86.94 \text{ days} \times 24 \text{ hours/day} \times 3600 \text{ sec/hour})$

$= (4 \times 10^8 \text{ disintegrations sec}^{-1}) \times (7.512 \times 10^6 \text{ sec})$

$= 3.005 \times 10^{15}$ disintegrations .

EXAMPLE 5.3

In the above example, if the initial activity were 10 millicuries (mCi), how many disintegrations would result in complete decay?

$$1 \text{ Ci} = 3.7 \times 10^{10} \text{ disintegrations sec}^{-1}$$

$$10 \text{ mCi} = 10 \times 10^{-3} \times 3.7 \times 10^{10} \text{ disintegrations sec}^{-1}$$
$$= 3.7 \times 10^8 \text{ disintegrations/sec} .$$

Total disintegrations for full decay = (initial disintegration rate) × (mean life)

$$= (3.7 \times 10^8 \text{ sec}^{-1}) \times (7.512 \times 10^6 \text{ sec})$$
$$= 2.779 \times 10^{15} \text{ disintegrations} .$$

The above two examples illustrate the relative magnitudes of the activity units MBq and mCi.

5.3
Radioactive Decay Chains

5.3.1
Daughter Product Buildup and Decay

It is possible that a parent nuclide **1** decays to its daughter nuclide **2**, which, in turn, decays to its daughter nuclide **3**, and so on. Such a process is called a decay chain. An example is that of the decay of radium-226 to radon-222, which, in turn, decays to radium A (an isotope of polonium). The decay continues until Ra G (which is a stable isotope of lead) is formed (Figure 5.2).

Let us say that the parent nuclides **1** have half life T_1 and a decay constant λ_1, and that the daughter nuclides **2** result from the decay of **1**. Let us assume that we start with a pure sample of **1** amounting to $(N_1)_0$ nuclides. At any instant, there are N_1 nuclides of **1** and N_2 nuclides of **2**. With the passage of time, the number N_1 will dwindle and N_2

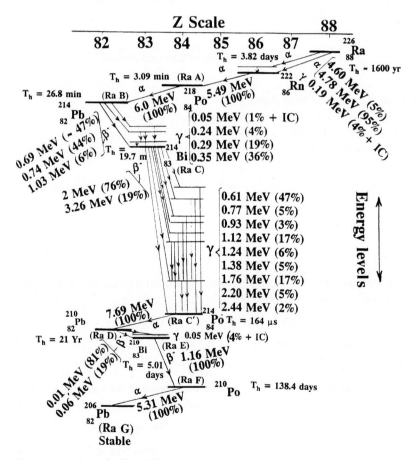

Fig. 5.2. Decay chain of radium-226

will grow. A part of **2** will decay, as these nuclides, too, are radioactive, with a half life T_2 and decay constant λ_2. We can derive a mathematical relation for the rate of change of N_2 at any time t as follows:

$$\text{Rate of change of } N_2 = \begin{bmatrix} \text{Rate for formation} \\ \text{of } N_2 \end{bmatrix} - \begin{bmatrix} \text{Rate of decay} \\ \text{of existing } N_2 \end{bmatrix}$$

$$= \begin{bmatrix} \text{Rate of decay} \\ \text{of } N_1 \end{bmatrix} - \begin{bmatrix} \text{Rate of decay} \\ \text{of } N_2 \end{bmatrix}$$

that is,

$$\frac{dN_2}{dt} = \lambda_1 N_1 - \lambda_2 N_2 \tag{5-11}$$

One can solve this differential equation by substituting

$$N_1 = (N_1)_o e^{-\lambda_1 t}$$

The solution gives the following expression:

$$\lambda_2 N_2 = (\lambda_1 N_1) \frac{\lambda_2}{\lambda_2 - \lambda_1} \left[1 - e^{-(\lambda_2 - \lambda_1)t} \right] \tag{5-12}$$

Note that $\lambda_1 N_1$ and $\lambda_2 N_2$ are, respectively, the activities A_1 and A_2 of nuclides **1** and **2**. Hence, we can rewrite the above as

$$A_2 = A_1 \frac{\lambda_2}{\lambda_2 - \lambda_1} \left[1 - e^{-(\lambda_2 - \lambda_1)t} \right] \tag{5.13a}$$

In terms of half lives,

$$A_2 = A_1 \frac{T_1}{T_1 - T_2} \left[1 - e^{-0.693[(T_1 - T_2)/(T_1 T_2)]t} \right] \tag{5.13b}$$

Equation (5-13) can be simplified for certain practical situations, depending on the relative magnitudes of the half lives of parent and daughter.

5.3.2
Secular Equilibrium

Let us assume that the parent nuclide has a very long half life and the daughter a very short half life. Under these conditions, $\lambda_1 \ll \lambda_2$ and the activity A_1 $(= \lambda_1 N_1)$ of the parent nuclide remains steady, because its decay can be considered negligible. If so, Equation (5.13a) is simplified to

$$A_2 = A_1 \left[1 - e^{-\lambda_2 t} \right] \tag{5.13c}$$

A_2 rises initially and reaches a constant equilibrium value, as shown in Figure 5.3. This is called secular equilibrium. At secular equilibrium, the number of daughter nuclides decaying is replenished exactly by the number generated by the decay of the parent. This equilibrium condition is given by

$$\lambda_1 N_1 = \lambda_2 N_2$$

that is, the activities of parent and daughter are equal.

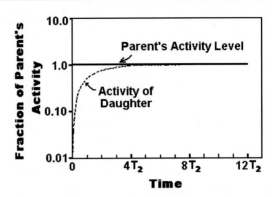

Fig. 5.3. Secular equilibrium reached by the activity of a short-lived daughter product with half life T_2 when the half life T_1 of its parent is very large (i. e., $T_2 \ll T_1$)

An example of secular equilibrium is the decay of radium into radon and its daughter products. The decay scheme of radium is shown in Figure 5.2. Radium has a very long half life of about 1600 years, but its daughter, radon, decays with a half life of 3.82 days. The several nuclides that follow radon have even shorter half lives. If one starts with a pure sample of radium nuclides in an enclosure, radon (which is a gas) will build up gradually, and so will the decay products of radon. The activity of radon and its daughter products reaches a saturation value equaling the activity of radium after about ten half lives of radon.

The equilibrium condition can be stated as follows for several nuclides in a chain:

$$\lambda_1 N_1 = \lambda_2 N_2 = \lambda_3 N_3 = \lambda_4 N_4 = \text{etc.}$$

Radium was recognized as being useful for treatment of cancer shortly after its discovery by Marie Curie in the 1890s. During the use of encapsulated radium sources in radiotherapy (see Chapter 17), most of the radiation comes from radon and its short-lived daughter products. Because, within the sealed source, radon and its daughter nuclides are in secular equilibrium with the long-lived radium, no decay corrections are needed during the use of these sources. The radon activity can be assumed to be identical to the activity of radium with its half life of 1602 years. However, if a radium capsule is damaged and radon escapes, the equilibrium condition no longer holds. If this happens, the escaping radon can diffuse into the surroundings, and, as it decays further, will deposit the decay products on surfaces and cause widespread radioactive contamination. That is why sealed radium sources should be tested frequently for radon leakage and discarded if they are damaged. It is necessary to test the integrity of the encapsulation of all sealed sources used in radiotherapy to ensure that the radioactive material is contained well and that any leakage and undesirable spread of radioactive contamination are avoided.

5.3.3
Transient Equilibrium

Let us consider a situation in which the half life of the parent, T_1, is much larger than that of the daughter, T_2. Then $T_1 > T_2$ and $\lambda_1 < \lambda_2$. The exponential term in Equations (5.13a) and (5.13b) can now be simplified as follows:

$$A_2 = A_1 \frac{\lambda_2}{\lambda_2 - \lambda_1} \left[1 - e^{-\lambda_2 t} \right] \tag{5.14a}$$

and

$$A_2 = A_1 \frac{T_1}{T_1 - T_2} \left[1 - e^{-0.693t/T_2} \right] \tag{5.14b}$$

When the time t is very large compared to T_2 (i. e., $t \gg T_2$), the above can be reduced further to

$$A_2 = A_1 \frac{T_1}{(T_1 - T_2)} \tag{5-15}$$

In such a case, the activity of the daughter increases initially (Figure 5.4) and a transient equilibrium is established, after which the activity of the daughter follows that of the parent. The ratio A_2/A_1 becomes a constant at $t \gg T_2$ and is determined by Equation (5-15). Transient equilibrium is taken advantage of for the generation of short-lived radionuclides in nuclear medicine departments.

An example is the use of the decay of molybdenum-99 (^{99}Mo) for generation of metastable technetium (^{99m}Tc) for use in diagnostic nuclear medicine studies. ^{99}Mo decays with a half life of 67 hours by beta emission. About 88% of the decay results in an isomeric state, ^{99m}Tc. This radionuclide, in turn, decays in an isomeric transition with a half life of 6 hours, emitting a 140-keV photon.

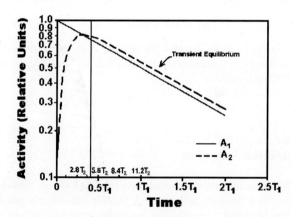

Fig. 5.4. Transient equilibrium reached by the activity of a daughter product with half life T_2 when the half life T_1 of the parent is such that $T_1 > T_2$

EXAMPLE 5.4

A nuclear medicine department receives a technetium generator that initially has a clean sample of 500 MBq of ^{99}Mo. After 18 hours, (i) what is the residual activity of ^{99}Mo, and (ii) how much ^{99m}Tc activity will be available to be chemically separated for a patient application?

(i) Decay factor for ^{99}Mo for 18 hours $= e^{-(0.693 \times 18/67)} = 0.830$.
    Activity of Mo then $= 500$ MBq $\times 0.830 = 415$ MBq.
(ii) We temporarily ignore the information that only 88% of ^{99}Mo decays to the metastable state, ^{99m}Tc. In Equation (5.14b), we substitute the following to derive

., the activity of ^{99m}Tc):

$$A_1 = 415\,\text{MBq}; \; T_1 = 67\,\text{hours}; \; T_2 = 6\,\text{hours}; \; t = 18\,\text{hours}$$

$$A_2 = 415\,[67/(67-6)]\left[1 - e^{-(0.693 \times 18/6)}\right]\,\text{MBq}$$

$$= 415 \times 1.098 \times [1 - 0.125] = 399\,\text{MBq}\,.$$

Note that 18 hours is three times the half life of 6 hours of ^{99m}Tc. During this time, the activity A_2 has become 96% of A_1.

We now recall that only 88% of ^{99}Mo results in formation of ^{99m}Tc. This means that the activity of 399 MBq should be reduced to $399 \times 0.88 = 351$ MBq to give the actual amount of ^{99m}Tc available for chemical separation for patient use.

EXAMPLE 5.5

In the previous example, what would be the available ^{99m}Tc activity after 60 hours?

Using Equation (5-7), activity of ^{99}Mo after 60 hours is $=\,500\,\text{MBq}\,e^{-(0.693 \times 60/67)} = 269\,\text{MBq}$. Sixty hours is a rather long period compared to the half life of 6 hours. Therefore, we can use Equation (5-15). With $A_1 = 269\,\text{MBq}$, $T_1 = 67\,\text{hours}$, $T_2 = 6\,\text{hours}$,

$$A_2 = A_1 T_1/(T_1 - T_2)$$

or

$$A_2 = 269 \times 67/(67-6) = 269 \times 1.098 = 295\,\text{MBq}\,.$$

The factor 1.098 denotes the ratio of daughter activity to parent activity. Of course, we must again remember that only 88% of ^{99}Mo decays to ^{99m}Tc. Therefore, the actual ^{99m}Tc available is

$$295 \times 0.88 = 260\,\text{MBq}\,.$$

5.4
Neutron Activation

Many radioisotopes are made by absorption of neutrons in stable nuclides. This process is called neutron activation. A nuclear reactor is a good source of neutrons. Let us consider that a sample of a (nonradioactive) nuclide of type 1 is placed in a nuclear reactor at a position where the neutron flux is ϕ_n neutrons cm^{-2} sec^{-1} (i. e., ϕ_n neutrons pass through a 1-cm^2 area per second). A fraction of these neutrons will be absorbed in the sample, resulting in the production of type 2 nuclides. The rate of yield of type 2 can be expected to be proportional to the number N_1 of type 1 nuclides irradiated and the neutron flux ϕ_n. This rate is given by

$$N_1 \phi_n \sigma$$

where σ (cm^2) is a proportionality constant with a value specific to the type 1 nuclide for neutron absorption (also called neutron capture). It is also referred to as the cross section for neutron absorption. The type 2 nuclides formed may themselves decay with a decay constant λ_2. The overall rate of growth of the number N_2 of nuclides of type 2 will be

$$\frac{dN_2}{dt} = \text{rate for formation} - \text{rate of decay}$$

$$= N_1\phi_n\sigma - \lambda_2 N_2 \qquad (5\text{-}16)$$

The above equation resembles Equation (5-11), with the difference that $(\phi_n\sigma)$ has now been substituted for λ_1. Thus, modifying Equation (5-12), the activity A_2 of type 2 after time t of irradiation is given by

$$A_2 = \frac{\lambda_2 N_1\phi_n\sigma}{\lambda_2 - \phi_n\sigma}\left[1 - e^{-(\lambda_2-\phi_n\sigma)t}\right] \qquad (5\text{-}17)$$

Often, in practical situations, $\lambda_2 \gg \phi_n\sigma$, so that the following approximation is possible:

$$A_2 = N_1\phi_n\sigma\left[1 - e^{-\lambda_2 t}\right] \qquad (5\text{-}18)$$

If the activation is continued for a fairly long time, i.e., $t \gg T_2$, a stage is reached where the amount of type 2 nuclide produced matches the amount of it that decays; that is, a saturation activity level is attained. The saturation activity $(A_2)_S$ is related to the available neutron flux by the expression

$$(A_2)_S = N_1\phi_n\sigma \qquad (5\text{-}19)$$

Figure 5.5 illustrates how the activity builds up to reach the saturation value. In one half life, only 50% of the maximum possible activity is attained. In about three half lives, approximately 88% is reached. It takes more than six half lives to reach the saturation limit. This applies for activation of any element.

Fig. 5.5. Buildup of activity in a sample subjected to neutron activation

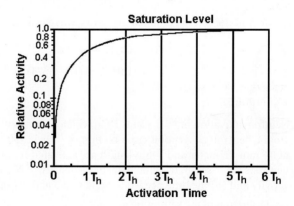

EXAMPLE 5.6

A ^{59}Co pellet of 1 g is irradiated in a nuclear reactor having a neutron flux density of 10^{11} neutrons cm^{-2} sec^{-1}. ^{59}Co has an atomic neutron activation cross section of 38×10^{-24} cm^2. The activation product, ^{60}Co, decays with a half life of 5.26 years. Calculate (i) the saturation activity and (ii) the activity after 3 years of irradiation.

1 mol of ^{59}Co is approximately 59 g $= 59 \times 10^{-3}$ kg.

59 g of ^{59}Co contains Avogadro's number, $N_{Av} = 6.02 \times 10^{23}$ atoms. (See Section 2.6)

$$\text{The number } N_1 \text{ of target atoms per gram} = (6.02 \times 10^{23}/59) \text{ target atoms g}^{-1}$$
$$= 1.02 \times 10^{22} \text{ target atoms g}^{-1}.$$

The decay constant of the product nuclide, ^{60}Co, is

$$\lambda_2 = 0.693/(5.26 \text{ years} \times 365 \text{ days/year} \times 24 \text{ hours/day} \times 3600 \text{ sec/hour})$$
$$= 4.18 \times 10^{-9} \text{ sec}^{-1}.$$

The atomic neutron absorption cross section for ^{59}Co is

$$\sigma = 38 \times 10^{-24} \text{ cm}^2$$

$$\text{Neutron flux} \quad \phi_n = 10^{11} \text{ neutron cm}^{-2} \text{ sec}^{-1}$$

$$\sigma\phi_n = 3.8 \times 10^{-12} \text{ sec}^{-1}$$

Because $\lambda_2 \gg \sigma\phi_n$, we can use the approximate expressions (5-18) and (5-19).

(i) The saturation activity $(A_2)_S$ is

$$(A_2)_S = N_1\phi_n\sigma$$
$$= (1.02 \times 10^{22})(10^{11})(38 \times 10^{-24})$$
$$= 38.76 \times 10^9 \text{ disintegrations sec}^{-1} \text{ g}^{-1}$$
$$= 38.76 \text{ giga-Becquerel (GBq) g}^{-1}$$

Because $1 \text{ Ci} = 3.7 \times 10^{10} \text{ Bq}$,

$$(A_2)_S = 1.05 \text{ Ci g}^{-1}$$

(ii) To find the activity attained in 3 years, we rewrite Equation (5-18) as

$$A_2 = (A_2)_S \times \left[1 - e^{-0.693(3/5.26)}\right]$$
$$= 1.05 \text{ Ci} \times (1 - 0.674) = 0.342 \text{ Ci}$$

EXAMPLE 5.7

Neutron activation of ^{191}Ir yields ^{192}Ir, which decays with a half life of 74.4 days. The atomic neutron absorption cross section of ^{191}Ir is 750×10^{-24} cm^2. Iridium pellets of 0.8 mm diameter and 3 mm length are activated in a reactor that has a flux of 109 neutrons cm^{-2} sec^{-1}. Iridium metal has a density of 20 g cm^{-3}. Find (i) the saturation activity and (ii) the time needed to build up an activity of 1 mCi.

(i) Evaluation of the saturation activity:
     Radius of pellet (r) $= 0.08/2 = 0.04$ cm
     Height of pellet (h) $= 0.3$ cm

$$\text{Volume of pellet} \quad (\pi r^2 h) = 3.1416 (0.04)^2 0.3 \text{ cm}^3$$
$$= 1.5 \times 10^{-3} \text{ cm}^3$$
$$\text{Mass of pellet} = (1.5 \times 10^{-3}) \times 20$$
$$= 0.03 \text{ g}.$$

One gram-atom of ^{192}Ir is approximately 192 g.

$$\text{Number } (N_1) \text{ of target nuclides} = (0.03)(\text{Avogadro's number})/(192)$$
$$= 0.03 \times 6.02 \times 10^{23}/192$$
$$= 9.4 \times 10^{-19} \text{ nuclides}$$

It is given: $\phi_n = 10^9$ neutrons $\text{cm}^{-2}\,\text{sec}^{-1}$; and $\sigma = 750 \times 10^{-24}\,\text{cm}^2$
Expected saturation activity

$$(A_2)_S = N_1\phi_n\sigma$$
$$= 9.4 \times 10^{19} \times 10^9 \times 750 \times 10^{-24}$$
$$= 7.05 \times 10^7 \text{ disintegrations sec}^{-1} = 70.5\,\text{MBq}$$

Because $1\,\text{Ci} = 3.7 \times 10^{10}\,\text{Bq}$,

$$(A_2)_S = 1.91 \times 10^{-3}\,\text{Ci} = 1.91\,\text{mCi}$$

(ii) Time needed to develop an activity of 1 mCi:
   We note that 1 mCi is 52% of the saturation activity of 1.91 mCi. According to
   Equation (5-18),

$$\left[1 - e^{-(0.693t/T_2)}\right] = 0.52$$

i. e.,

$$e^{-(0.693t/74.4)} = 0.48$$

Thus, solving for t, the time of irradiation is

$$t = \ln(0.48) \times 74.4/0.693 = 78.8\,\text{days}$$

If high specific activities of ^{60}Co are to be obtained for radiation therapy, a reactor that can provide high neutron flux densities is required. In addition, it is necessary to consider the burn-up of ^{60}Co, i. e., the absorption of a neutron by ^{60}Co by which it becomes ^{61}Co. ^{61}Co has a rather short half life of 48 days and is not of use in radiotherapy.

Interaction of Radiation with Matter

Collision and Radiation Loss in Charged-Particle Interactions

6.1
Slowing Down of Charged Particles

Energetic charged particles such as alpha particles and electrons lose their energies and slow down as they pass through matter. The rate of slowing depends on the stopping power of the medium. A light particle such as an electron may follow a zig-zag, tortuous path, changing directions during several energy-diminishing encounters, as illustrated in Figure 6.1. The thickness of the medium needed for the entire energy of a particle to be absorbed is called the range. The range must be distinguished from the path length, which is the length of the entire zig-zag distance traveled. Alpha particles, which are very heavy, do not acquire high velocities even at high energies. Also, because they are doubly charged, they produce intense ionization and have very short ranges. Electrons, on the other hand, being light particles, have high velocities even at low energies. Electrons play a key role in radiation energy absorption processes that are exploited in routine radiotherapy. In this chapter, we focus attention mainly on moving electrons.

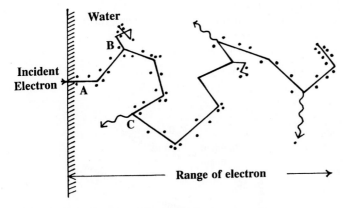

Fig. 6.1. A typical zig-zag path of an electron passing through a medium. Dots represent ionizing events. The events near *A* result in small energy losses. At *B*, a high-energy secondary electron (delta ray) is produced. At *C*, a bremsstrahlung photon is produced

6.2
Collision Loss

6.2.1
Collision Energy Loss Formula

When an electron passes near the electric field of another electron or that of a nucleus, it undergoes scattering and changes its direction. Depending upon the exact details of a collision, the energy loss and the change of direction undergone by the traveling electron may be small or large. The energy loss can be significant in the coulomb field of electrons in atoms because it involves a collision with a light particle. Such a collision can lead to the removal of a bound electron from the atom (i. e., to ionization) or to lifting of an atomic electron to a higher-energy orbit (i. e., to excitation). If the collision takes place with the strong electric field of the heavy nucleus, less energy may be lost, but the change in direction can be significant.

When a 15.7-MeV electron beam of small cross section (less than 1 mm) is directed on a thin carbon foil (the target), and the electrons are observed from a 30° angle with respect to the incident direction, an energy spread as shown in Figure 6.2 is obtained [1]. The horizontal and vertical axes represent measures of the energy of the scattered electrons and the number of electrons observed (as measured by a magnetic spectrometer and detector), respectively. The graph is a double-peaked curve. The first peak, at low energy, is due to the incident electrons and orbital electrons that suffered electron-electron scattering in the carbon foil. The second peak, at the higher energy, is attributable to electron-nuclear collisions. Any electron penetrating a thick target will undergo many electron-electron and electron-nuclear collisions. Electron-nuclear scattering has been used for spreading out thin pencil beams of electrons to make them useful clinically (see Chapter 16, Section 16.2).

If an electron loses energy dE over a distance dx in a medium, the linear stopping power, S, of that medium is defined as the ratio dE/dx. If ρ is the density of the medium, the mass stopping power of the medium, S_m, is given by

$$S_m = S/\rho = dE/(\rho dx) = (1/\rho)/(dE/dx)$$

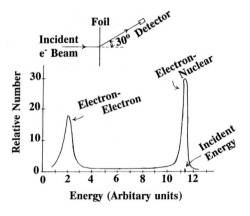

Fig. 6.2. Energy spectrum of electrons scattered by a thin carbon foil as observed at a 30° angle with respect to the incident beam by a magnetic spectrometer coupled to an electron counter

The stopping power dE/dx can be divided into a collision component, $S_c = (dE/dx)_c$, and a radiation component, $S_r = (dE/dx)_r$. Thus,

$$dE/dx = (dE/dx)_c + (dE/dx)_r$$

i. e.,

$$S = S_c + S_r$$

The collision component is that part of the energy loss occurring due to the ionization and excitation events. The radiation component, which is discussed later (in Section 6.3 of this chapter), is due to the emission of electromagnetic radiation. Stopping powers for some materials of interest in radiotherapy physics are given in Appendix A.

For the collision component, Bethe and Ashkin derived the relation [2]

$$-\left(\frac{dE}{dx}\right)_c = \frac{2\pi e^4 NZ}{m_0 v^2}\left[\ln\frac{m_0 v^2 E}{2I^2(1-\beta^2)} - \ln 2\left(2\sqrt{1-\beta^2}-1+\beta^2\right)\right.$$
$$\left. +\left(1-\beta^2\right)+\frac{1}{8}\left(1-\sqrt{1-\beta^2}\right)^2\right]$$

where

N = the number of atoms in the medium per unit volume
Z = the atomic number of the medium
v = the velocity of the electron
m_0 = the mass of the electron at rest
E = the kinetic energy of the electron
I = the mean excitation energy of the medium
e = the charge of an electron
β = v/c, where c is the velocity of light in a vacuum

The term NZ in the above equation for $(dE/dx)_c$ gives the number of electrons per unit volume of the medium. Because the collision losses occur in interactions with orbital electrons, the proportionality of $(dE/dx)_c$ to N and Z can be expected. The equation shows that collision energy loss is directly proportional to the electron density of the medium. In high-Z materials, partial screening of the inner orbital electrons occurs consequent to the presence of the outer orbital electrons. This makes the dependence of collision loss not exactly proportional to Z.

Figure 6.3 shows the dependence of the collision stopping power on energy for electrons and protons in water. $(dE/dx)_c$ is high at low electron energies and decreases rapidly to a minimum value as the electron energy increases. At very high energies, it gradually increases. At extremely low energies (not shown in the figure), the collision losses are known to be negligible because the electron does not have sufficient energy to cause ionization or excitation. The curve for protons is similar to that for electrons, but is shifted along the energy axis. The shift is caused by the higher mass of protons compared to electrons.

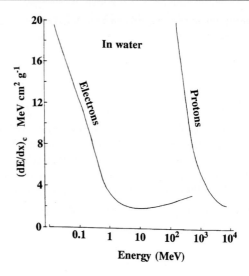

Fig. 6.3. Dependence of collision stopping power on energy for electrons and protons in water. (Based on data from Bichsel, H., Charged particle interactions, Chapter 4, in Radiation Dosimetry, Vol I, Fundamentals, Eds: Attix, F.H. and Roesch, W.C., Academic Press, New York, 1968.)

6.2.2
Bragg Ionization Curve

The Bragg curve is a plot of the ionization density (i. e., specific ionization) vs. distance as a particle slows down. Figure 6.4 shows the Bragg curve for protons as an example for heavier particles. For protons and still heavier particles, the increase in $(dE/dx)_c$ with a reduction in energy is very steep. This implies that, when a heavy particle slows down in a medium, the rate of energy loss will reach a peak toward the end of the track. As the particle slows down, it captures an electron, which reduces its charge and hence reduces its $(dE/dx)_c$.

Curve (a) in Figure 6.4 illustrates the increase in stopping power for a 100-MeV proton beam with depth in water. Curve (b) shows the associated variation of dose delivered with depth. This peak ionization is given the name "Bragg peak." In external-beam therapy, this phenomenon can be exploited for delivery of a high dose to a deep-

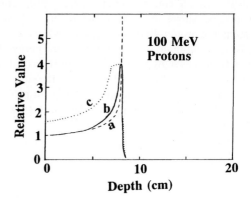

Fig. 6.4. Depth-ionization curve for 100-MeV protons. Curves (a) and (b) show the variation of collision stopping power and the dose, respectively, for a monoenergetic beam of 100 MeV. Curve (c) represents the dose profile for a beam modified by a filter to give a spread in the incident energy. (Based on data from Physical characteristics of particle beams, by W.C. Roesch, p39–43, in Particle Accelerators in Radiotherapy, Proceedings of a Conference, U.S. Atomic Energy Commission, Report LA5180-C, Washington, D.C., 1973.)

seated tumor while the overlying tissues are spared. Unfortunately, heavy particles lose energy rapidly and do not penetrate deeply enough for use in radiation therapy unless accelerated to high energies of several hundred MeV. An additional problem is that the Bragg peak for a monoenergetic beam is too narrow to cover an extended tumor. A clinically useful beam having a wider peak results only if the energy of the beam is spread out (by use of special filters). However, this will also reduce the peak-to-surface dose ratio, as illustrated by curve (c) in Figure 6.4. The cost of producing heavy charged particles of high energies at the levels of intensity needed for treatment of patients is very high. Some pilot studies have been done for exploration of such methods. These methods are far from becoming routine or practical for large-scale use in radiotherapy clinics. A peak like the Bragg peak does not occur with electrons because electrons undergo extensive lateral dispersions with respect to the incident direction.

6.3
Radiative Loss

6.3.1
Bremsstrahlung

A moving electric charge subjected to an acceleration or deceleration radiates electromagnetic energy in accordance with the electromagnetic theory. This results in an additional phenomenon that is different from the electron-nuclear scattering discussed before. When an electron passes close to the coulomb field of a nucleus of an atom, the electron loses energy by releasing electromagnetic radiation in the form of X-rays. These X-rays can have a continuum of energies and hence are called "continuous X-rays," "white X-rays," or "bremsstrahlung" (meaning braking radiation). This phenomenon of radiation emission during an electron's deceleration in a nuclear field is used in X-ray machines. The influence of the nuclear coulomb field falls off rapidly with distance from the nucleus. The fraction of the electron energy lost in a radiative process depends upon how close the electron comes to the nucleus. An electron may come so close that it loses its entire energy in the emission of a photon of the maximum possible energy. Partial energy losses by the electron result in a continuum of all possible photon energies up to this maximum. The radiation emission spectrum is discussed in greater detail in Section 6.3.4.

6.3.2
Radiative Stopping Power

The radiative component of the stopping power, as derived by Bethe and Ashkin [2], is given by

$$-\left(\frac{dE}{dx}\right)_r = \frac{NEZ(Z+1)e^4}{137m_0^2c^4}\left(4\ln\frac{2E}{m_0c^2} - \frac{4}{3}\right)$$

It can be seen that $(dE/dx)_r$ is nearly proportional to E and Z^2 (because $Z(Z+1) \approx Z^2$ for large Z). Furthermore, the path length increases with E, but decreases with Z. Thus, overall, the total bremsstrahlung yield will be nearly proportional to $(EZ^2)(E/Z) = E^2Z$.

ative Energy Loss of Electrons in Collision and Radiative Processes in Water and Lead

	Water				Lead			
	Electron energy				Electron energy			
	100 keV	1 MeV	10 MeV		100 keV	1 MeV	10 MeV	25 MeV
Collision	99.9%	99%	92%	Collision	97%	86%	49%	25%
Radiation	0.1%	1%	8%	Radiation	3%	14%	51%	75%

For low-energy electrons, the energy loss is dominated entirely by collision processes, whereas, in high-Z materials and at high electron energies, the radiative loss becomes significant (see Table 6.1).

6.3.3
Angular Distribution of Bremsstrahlung X-Rays

Bremsstrahlung X-rays have an angular distribution of intensity with respect to the direction of incidence of the electrons, as shown in Figure 6.5. The distribution at low electron energies differs markedly from that at high energies. At low energies, the maximum intensity occurs at an angle of 50° to 60° with respect to the incident direction, and the intensity in the backward direction is negligible. The forward intensity is considerably lower than the maximum intensity. At very high energies, on the other hand, the intensity has a peak in the forward direction. The practical difficulty that this causes in the production of high-energy beams of uniform intensity over a

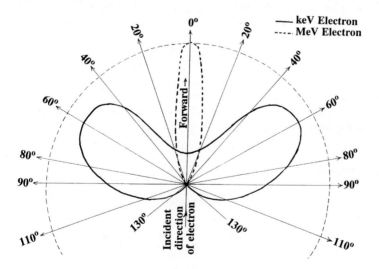

Fig. 6.5. Polar diagram showing the intensity of bremsstrahlung emission in different directions with respect to the direction of the incident electrons. The radial distance in the diagram is proportional to the relative intensity. Curves are shown for keV and MeV electrons. (Based on data from Figure 2.16, p67, Johns, H.E., and Cunningham, J.R., Physics of Radiology, 4th Edition, 1983, Charles C Thomas, Springfield, Illinois.)

therapeutically usable wide angle is discussed in Section 10.3.5. The diagram in Figure 6.5 is strictly true only for a medium that is very thin and in which the assumption that the electrons travel in a single incident direction can be valid. In a thick target, electrons diffuse in successive layers and move in various directions. X-ray machines operating at low energies (60 to 100 keV) use the intensity emerging at almost 90° from the incident electron beam; at high energies, the forward emission is used.

6.3.4
Energy Distribution of Bremsstrahlung Radiation

In Chapters 8 and 10, we discuss the machines that accelerate electrons for production of bremsstrahlung X-rays for use in radiotherapy. In these machines, energized electrons are made to impinge on high-Z target materials to produce X-rays. Because the electrons lose energy by collision events, a progressive reduction in their energies occurs as they pass through the target material. The spectrum of the slowed-down electrons is a function of the thickness of the target material. Hence, the distribution of X-ray energies (i. e., the X-ray spectrum) differs for thick and thin targets [3–9].

We define the energy intensity I(E) at photon energy E as given by

$$I(E)dE = N(E)E\,dE$$

where N(E) refers to the number of photons per unit energy interval at the energy E, and dE is a small energy interval. The intensity distribution shown in Figure 6.6a is for a simplified model for an ideally thin target. This spectrum has a maximum photon energy E_{max}, which equals the energy of the electrons incident on the target. Photons of energy E_{max} result when an incoming electron loses its entire energy in a single radiative interaction. The constant level of I(E) in Figure 6.6a means that N(E) varies as $1/E$ when a large number of electrons are incident on the target. For example, for

Fig. 6.6. (a) A theoretical low-energy thin-target bremsstrahlung X-ray spectrum for an unfiltered beam. (b) Summed- up thick-target spectrum for both unfiltered and filtered emission

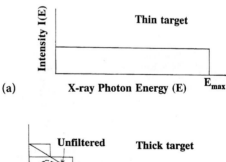

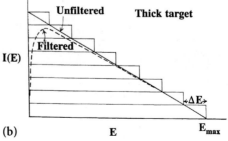

every photon of energy Emax that is observed, there would be 2 photons of energy $E_{max}/2$ and three photons of energy $E_{max}/3$.

In a thick target, electrons will be slowed down in successive layers of the target material. The maximum possible energy will decrease from layer to layer, and the X-ray intensities from each of these layers will be added together. In Figure 6.6b, this is shown in distinct steps, with the electron losing ΔE at each step. The total intensity from all layers will add up to the values given by the inclined straight line. Mathematically, this line is described by

$$I(E) = CZ(E_{max} - E)$$

where C is a constant of proportionality. An integration of the intensity, $I(E)dE$, from $E = 0$ to $E = E_{max}$, gives the total intensity, I_{total}:

$$I_{total} = CZ(E_{max})^2/2$$

The above relationships apply to a hypothetical situation in which the bremsstrahlung emerges unfiltered. In practice, there will be some inevitable filtration of photons within the target itself, and other filters may be placed in the path of emergence of the X-rays. The reduction in intensity due to filtration can be particularly significant for low-energy photons. The filtered spectrum will tend to resemble the dashed curve in Figure 6.6b.

Figure 6.7 shows the shape of the X-ray spectra for thick and thin targets (with no added filtration) at relativistic electron energies ($> m_0c^2$). The thin-target spectrum in Figure 6.7 (curve 1) applies to megavoltage X-ray beams from radiotherapy accelerators [9].

Fig. 6.7. Typical unfiltered bremsstrahlung spectra at relativistic megavoltage energies. Curve 1 is for thin-target emission and curve 2 is for thick-target emission. (Figure is adapted from Figure 3.10, p55, Anderson, D.W., Absorption of Ionizing Radiation, University Park Press, Baltimore, 1984.)

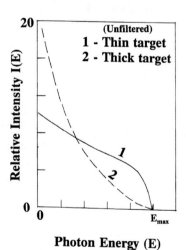

6.3.5
Linear Energy Transfer

As a charged particle traverses a medium, it leaves a trail of ions along its own track and along the tracks of the secondary electrons that it sets in motion in the collision events. The specific ionization, I_s, is the linear density of ionization. It is a measure of the number of ions produced per unit path length of the particle track. If W is the average energy expended per ionization event, I_s is given by

$$I_s = \frac{S_c}{W}$$

I_s is a function of the type of charged particle and its energy. Some particles, such as alpha particles, can be densely ionizing. Others, such as electrons, are sparsely ionizing. Figure 6.8 is a schematic diagram of the tracks of two different particles. In both tracks, some of the secondary electrons have sufficient energies to travel up to a significant distance away from the path of the primary particle. Such secondary electrons of high energies are referred to as delta rays. Thus, not all energy loss accounted for in the stopping power S_c results in ionizations close to the primary particle track. Hence, S_c is called the "total" or "unrestricted" collision stopping power.

In radiobiology, there is a need to distinguish the ionization events that occur in the immediate vicinity of the track from those that occur remotely. For this purpose, the concept of linear energy transfer (LET) is defined [10]. LET_Δ is the part of S_c attributable to collision events that transfer less than a specified energy Δ to the secondary particles. The smaller the size of Δ, the stricter the applicability of LET_Δ to the track of the primary particle. The higher the value chosen for the limit Δ, the closer is the value of LET_Δ to S_c. This upper limit of LET is also designated as LET_∞; that is,

$$LET_\infty = S_c$$

In the above discussion, we referred to an upper limit of Δ for the energy transferred to the secondary electrons. A different demand for specification of a lower limit of Δ is encountered in the radiation dosimetry problems discussed in Chapter 11. It is customary to use the symbol L_Δ for the part of the collision stopping power S_c that restricts the events to those that result in losses of more than a specified energy Δ. L_Δ is called the restricted stopping power.

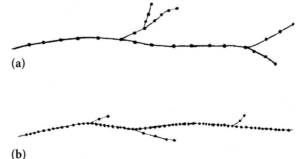

Fig. 6.8. Dots represent ionizing events along particle tracks shown as lines. (a) Track of a sparsely ionizing particle with a low specific ionization; (b) track of a densely ionizing particle. Secondary electron tracks are also shown

(a)

(b)

References

1. Lyman, E.M., Hanson, A.O., and Scott, M.B., Scattering of 15.7 MeV electrons by nuclei, Phys. Rev., Vol 84, p626, 1951.
2. Bethe, H.A. and Ashkin, J., Passage of radiation through matter, in Experimental Nuclear Physics, Vol. I, Ed: E. Segre, John Wiley & Sons, New York, p166–379, 1953.
3. Kulenkampff, H., Uber das kontinuierliche Roentgen Spektrum, Ann. Phys. Leipzig, Vol 69, p548–596, 1922.
4. Kramers, H.A., On the theory of X-ray absorption and of the continuous X-ray spectrum, Philos. Mag., Vol 46, p836–871, 1923.
5. Schiff, L.I., Energy angle distribution of thin target bremsstrahlung, Phys. Rev., Vol 83, p252–253, 1951.
6. Soole, B.W., The effect of target absorption on the attenuation characteristics of bremsstrahlung generated at constant medium potentials, J. Phys., Vol B5, p1583–1595, 1972.
7. Storm, E., Calculated bremsstrahlung spectra from thick tungsten targets, Phys. Rev., Vol A5, p2328–2338, 1972.
8. Desobry, G.E. and Boyer, A.L., Bremsstrahlung review: An analysis of the Schiff spectrum, Med. Phys., Vol 18, p497–505, 1991.
9. Anderson, D.W., Figure 3.10, p54–57, Absorption of Ionizing Radiation, University Park Press, Baltimore, 1984.
10. ICRU, Report 16, Linear Energy Transfer, International Commission on Radiation Units and Measurements, Washington, D.C., 1970.

Additional Reading

1. Evans, R.E., Atomic Nucleus, McGraw-Hill, New York, 1972.
2. Anderson, D.W., Absorption of Ionizing Radiation, University Park Press, Baltimore, 1984.
3. Fermi, E., Nuclear Physics, Course Notes, Eds: Orear, J., Rozenfeld, A.H., and Schluter, R.A., University of Chicago Press, Chicago, 1950.
4. Attix, F.H., Charged particle interactions in matter, Chapter 8, p160–195, and X-ray production and quality, Chapter 9, p203–221, in Introduction to Radiological Physics and Radiation Dosimetry, John Wiley & Sons, New York, 1986.

CHAPTER 7

Photon Interactions

7.1
Nature of the Interactions

As photons pass through matter, such as a patient's soft tissue, bone, or any other structure, various interactions (i. e., events that cause changes) may take place. These different interactions become competing processes. The relative prevalence of any particular type of interaction depends on two major factors, the photon energy and the atomic composition of the medium. In some interactions, a part of the energy of the photon is transferred to the electrons belonging to the atoms or molecules in the tissue. These electrons, because of their short range (compared to photons), dissipate their energy locally around the sites of the interactions. Such locally absorbed energy becomes the cause of radiation effects or damage. If a photon enters and leaves the medium with its entire energy intact, or if it merely changes its direction in an interaction, no radiation dose is delivered.

In this chapter, we discuss the principal modes of interaction of photons with matter and their relative dependence on E_ν (the photon energy at frequency ν) and the atomic number Z of the medium. The interactions to be discussed are

(i)   Coherent Thompson scattering
(ii) Photoelectric absorption
(iii) Incoherent Compton scattering
(iv) Pair production
(v)   Photonuclear reaction

In general, the above interactions should be regarded as mutually competing processes at all energies. The above sequence ranks them as to their predominance and importance with increasing photon energy. At very low energies, only (i) is important. At the energies commonly used in radiotherapy, (ii), (iii), and (iv) play the major roles. Because (v) becomes important only at very high energies, only a short discussion of it has been included at the end of this chapter.

There is a difference in emphasis in our approach to photons and charged particles. For charged particles, we emphasize their energy loss in their slowing-down process until they come to a stop. Accordingly, for these particles we talk about the stopping power of the medium (see Chapter 4). On the other hand, we consider photons as undergoing a reduction in number or a diminution in intensity. We account for them as being either present and available for interactions or lost in an encounter. Such loss or diminution of the photon intensity in any medium is governed by the photon attenuation coefficient of that medium.

7.2
Attenuation Coefficient

7.2.1
Diminution of Photon Flux

In Figure 7.1a, a narrow parallel pencil beam of photons strikes a thin plane slab of an absorbing medium perpendicularly. Let the incident surface receive N_0 photons per unit area. Let us consider a thin slice of thickness d, within the slab. If N photons per unit area are falling on the entrance side of this slice, we can expect that a lesser number, $(N - dN)$ per unit area, will emerge on its exit side. The diminution by dN is attributed to the photons that interact within the slice and are either absorbed or scattered out of the beam. The loss dN is directly proportional to (1) the incident number N and (2) the thickness $d\ell$. We can also write this as

$$dN = -\mu N \, d\ell \qquad (7\text{-}1)$$

where μ is a proportionality constant. The negative sign of μ makes dN a negative number, indicating a reduction in N.

Fig. 7.1. (a) N, photons exit after passing through a slab of thickness, on which N_0 photons forming a thin beam are incident. The variation of N_ℓ/N_0 with ℓ, is shown in a linear-linear graph in (b) and a semi-logarithmic graph in (c). HVT refers to half-value thickness

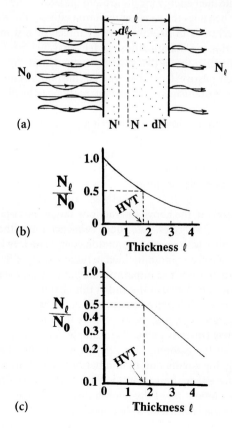

7.2.2
Linear Attenuation Coefficient

The constant μ is called the linear attenuation coefficient and has the dimension of the reciprocal of length. Sometimes, the term "cross section" rather than "coefficient" is used. μ is a characteristic of both the medium and the photon energy. Equation (7-1) holds true only for the situation in which both the thickness $d\ell$ and the loss dN are infinitesimally small. To find the photon flux, N_ℓ, at the exit side of a slab of a significant thickness ℓ, we can rewrite Equation (7-1) and integrate over the thickness ℓ.

$$\int_{N_0}^{N_\ell} \frac{dN}{N} = \int_0^\ell -\mu \, d\ell \qquad (7\text{-}2)$$

Solving the above gives the expression

$$N_\ell = N_0 \, e^{-\mu \ell} \qquad (7\text{-}3)$$

In practice, the thickness ℓ, can be in centimeters, and the value of μ would, accordingly, be cm^{-1}. Hence,

$$\left[N_\ell \text{ photons/cm}^2 \right] = \left[N_0 \text{ photons/cm}^2 \right] e^{-[\mu \, \mathrm{cm}^{-1}][\ell \, \mathrm{cm}]} \qquad (7\text{-}3\mathrm{a})$$

The thickness of the material that reduces the beam intensity to one half of the incident intensity is called half-value thickness (HVT), i. e.,

$$e^{-\mu(\mathrm{HVT})} = 1/2$$

or

$$\mathrm{HVT} = \frac{\ln(2)}{\mu} = \frac{0.693}{\mu} \qquad (7\text{-}4\mathrm{a})$$

and

$$\mu = \frac{0.693}{\mathrm{HVT}} \qquad (7\text{-}4\mathrm{b})$$

The exponential photon attenuation bears resemblance to radioactive decay (discussed in Sections 5.2.2 and 5.2.3.) It can be noticed that μ and HVT have a relationship similar to that between the decay constant λ and the half life T_h in radioactive decay. The distance $1/\mu$ is the statistical average distance between successive photon interactions and is called the mean free path. (This is analogous to mean life $T_m = 1/\lambda$ in radioactive decay). Figure 7.1b shows the exponential curve of the change of the ratio (N_ℓ/N_0) with ℓ in a linear-linear graph. The same graph becomes a straight line in a semi-log graph, as shown in Figure 7.1c.

7.2.3
Mass Attenuation Coefficient

The thickness of the slab can also be specified in terms of the mass of the slab per unit area. The mass-equivalent thickness ℓ_m is related to ℓ by the density ρ of the medium, as follows:

$$\ell_m = \rho \ell \qquad (7\text{-}5)$$

Typically, with ℓ stated in cm and ρ in $g\,cm^{-3}$, ℓ_m will be in $g\,cm^{-2}$. We can rewrite (7-3) as

$$N_\ell = N_0\,e^{-(\mu/\rho)(\rho\ell)} = N_0\,e^{-(\mu/\rho)\ell_m} \qquad (7\text{-}6)$$

The quantity (μ/ρ) is the mass attenuation coefficient, which is evaluable in units of $cm^2\,g^{-1}$. The linear attenuation coefficient μ can vary for a given medium if the density of the medium changes. The mass attenuation coefficient is a better index of the attenuation capacity of a medium, because it eliminates the role of density. For example, water and steam will have different μ, but identical (μ/ρ) values. In general, whenever we refer to a coefficient or cross section, without specifically qualifying it as "linear," "atomic," or "electronic," it should be taken to mean the mass attenuation coefficient.

7.2.4
Atomic Attenuation Coefficient

The attenuation capacity per atom in the medium is given by the atomic attenuation coefficient, μ_{atom}, which is related to μ/ρ. We know that, if A is the atomic mass, the mass of one atom is A/N_{Av}, where N_{Av} is Avogadro's number (see Section 2.6). Thus, the fraction of (μ/ρ) attributable to one atom is

$$\mu_{atom} = (\mu/\rho)(A/N_{Av})\,cm^2\,atom^{-1} \qquad (7\text{-}7)$$

If the atomic attenuation coefficient is to be used in an expression like that of (7.3a), the thickness of the slab should be expressed in number of atoms/cm^2 to ensure consistency.

7.2.5
Electronic Attenuation Coefficient

The attenuation capacity per electron in the medium is the electronic attenuation coefficient, $\mu_{electron}$. Each (neutral) atom has Z electrons. Hence, this coefficient is given by

$$\mu_{electron} = \mu_{atom}/Z = (\mu/\rho)(A/N_{Av})(1/Z)\,cm^2/electron \qquad (7\text{-}8)$$

An expression like (7.3a) can employ the electronic coefficient along with the thickness measured in number of electrons/cm^2.

7.3
Coherent Thompson Scattering

Thompson scattering occurs at very low photon energies. This phenomenon can be explained in terms of the wave nature of electromagnetic radiation. In this interaction, the electromagnetic field of the incoming photon induces an oscillation of an atomic electron by classical electromagnetic action (Figure 7.2). In the process, the incident photon loses its energy. However, the photon energy is not large enough to free the electron from its atomic bond. In Thompson scattering, the oscillating bound electron itself becomes a source of electromagnetic emission that is of a frequency, and hence energy, identical to that of the incident photon. The angle of photon emission can be

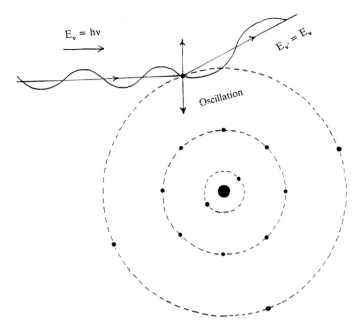

$E_v = h\nu$

Oscillation

$E_v = E_v$

Fig. 7.2. Schematic diagram of coherent scattering of a photon of energy E_v that sets an electron into oscillation, which, in turn, causes the emission of a scattered photon of the same energy E_v

different from the incident angle. The apparent result of this interaction is merely to change the direction of the incident photon, without any change in energy. Hence, this is given the name "coherent scattering." No energy absorption or transfer takes place in coherent scattering.

7.4
Photoelectric Absorption

7.4.1
Early Photoelectron Experiment

To understand the photoelectric effect, we have to treat electromagnetic radiation as quantized. The quantum aspect of radiation became evident when the photoelectric effect was first observed and needed an explanation. Figure 7.3 shows an evacuated glass tube enclosing a metallic cathode and anode. When light is incident on the cathode, electrons are ejected from the metal and are drawn to the anode, producing a current. The electrons ejected are called photoelectrons. In this experiment was noticed that no photoelectron emission occurred unless the frequency of the incident light was greater than a certain minimum value. At less than this critical frequency, there was no photoelectron emission, no matter how great the brightness of the light happened to be. Above the critical frequency, the emission occurred even at minimal brightness. For example, with an aluminum cathode, no photoelectrons could be seen

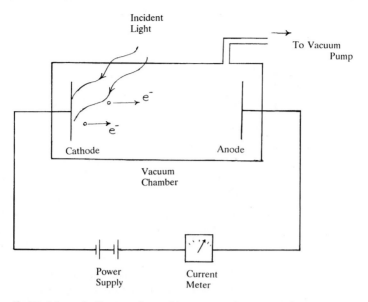

Fig. 7.3. Schematic diagram of an early experimental setup used for observation of the photoelectric effect

with green light ($\lambda = 500$ nm, $\nu = 600$ terrahertz [THz]). If the color changed to violet ($\lambda = 400$ nm, $\nu = 750$ THz), a photoelectron current was detectable. In 1921, Albert Einstein explained the photoelectric effect on the basis of photon quanta (see Section 3.3). For example, green photons are not as energetic as violet photons in liberating the electrons bound to the metallic surface.

In the photoelectric effect, the incident photon energy E_ν ($= h\nu$) is transferred to an orbital electron, say, a K-shell electron, as shown in Figure 7.4a. The K electron has a binding energy E_K. Only if $E_\nu > E_K$, can the electron be separated from its atom. The requirement for a minimum value of E_ν also means that, unless the frequency of the incident photon is sufficiently large, no K electron can be ejected. The kinetic energy T of the K photoelectron is given by

$$T = E_\nu - E_K \tag{7-9}$$

If the interaction results in an L photoelectron, T will change to

$$T = E_\nu - E_L \tag{7-10}$$

where E_L is the binding energy of an L-shell electron.

After an electron is ejected (Figure 7.4b), the electron vacancy in the atom can result in the emission of characteristic X-rays or Auger electrons (see Section 2.3.3). That is, any K-shell vacancy can give rise to either K characteristic X-rays or Auger electrons, or both, with a total energy of emission amounting to E_K. Thus, in a photoelectric interaction, the entire energy E_ν of the incident photon is converted into the energy of the characteristic X-rays, or the Auger electrons, and into the kinetic energy T of the photoelectron.

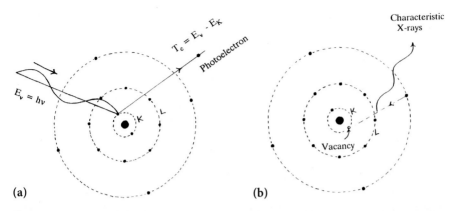

Fig. 7.4. (a) Photoelectric absorption of a photon of energy E_ν resulting in the emission of a K-shell electron. (b) The K-shell vacancy is filled by an outer-shell electron, resulting in the emission of a characteristic X-ray photon

7.4.2
Photon Energy and Photoelectric Interaction

Figure 7.5 shows the change in the photoelectric attenuation coefficient with photon energy for water and lead, in order to represent low-Z and high-Z substances. The curve for lead demonstrates sharp increases at energies just above the binding energies E_K and E_L. This is because, as the photon energy exceeds the threshold E_K for lead, its K electrons can be removed and can participate in the photoelectric process. The same effect occurs at energy E_L with L electrons. Such sharp increases in the cross section are called photoelectric absorption edges. Just past the edges at E_K and E_L, the increase in

Fig. 7.5. Variation of mass photoelectric attenuation co-efficient (τ/ρ) and mass pair production coefficient (π/ρ) with photon energy for water ($Z_{eff} = 7.4$) and lead (Z = 82)

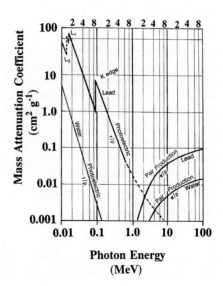

the photon energy reduces the cross section. (A photoelectric interaction is somewhat analogous to the game of golf. A golf ball can be hit successfully into a hole only if the right amount of force is applied. Weak hits will not enable the ball to go near the hole, and too forceful a hit will cause the ball to jump across the hole.) Except for the sharp rises at the absorption edges, the photoelectric cross section decreases rapidly with energy as $(1/E_v)^3$. The values of E_K and E_L for water are much lower than the lowest energy shown in Figure 7.5. Hence, the curve for water does not reveal the absorption edges.

7.4.3
Atomic Number and Photoelectric Interaction

Figure 7.5 shows that the photoelectric cross section (or mass attenuation coefficient) for lead is much higher than that for water. Lead has a Z value of 82, whereas the constituents of water, hydrogen and oxygen, have Z values of only 1 and 8. The photoelectric effect is strongly dependent on Z. Its cross section increases approximately as Z^3. Bone, which contains calcium $(Z = 20)$ and phosphorus $(Z = 15)$, has more photoelectric absorption than do the surrounding soft tissues. Diagnostic radiographs taken with 60- to 100-kV X-rays show high bone absorption, and hence contrast, with respect to that of the surroundings.

7.4.4
Local Energy Absorption in Photoelectric Interaction

In the photoelectric effect, the energy of the incident photons is divided into the following three components of secondary emissions:

(i)   The kinetic energy T of the photoelectron
(ii) The characteristic X-rays
(iii) Auger electrons

   When the secondary electrons and photons released in a photon interaction are of short range, we can regard their energies as being absorbed locally (i. e., within a few millimeters). The photoelectrons and Auger electrons have a short range and hence can be deemed to be absorbed locally. The characteristic X-rays can have a maximum energy E_K. Except in those situations that involve very high-Z materials such as lead, with a correspondingly high E_K, the characteristic X-rays, also, can be considered as being absorbed locally. Thus, in low-Z materials, the entire incident energy E_v is absorbed locally in photoelectric interactions.

7.4.5
Angular Emission of Photoelectrons

At low photon energies (50 to 100 keV), photoelectrons are emitted mostly in a direction perpendicular to that of the incident photons. With increases in photon energy, the photoelectron emission becomes peaked in the forward direction.

7.4.6
Photoelectric Cross Section

The part of the diminution in the photon intensity caused by the photoelectr alone can be calculated from an equation similar to (7-1):

$$dN = -\tau N \, d\ell \qquad (7\text{-}11)$$

where τ is the photoelectric component of the overall attenuation cross section. τ/ρ will be the corresponding mass photoelectric attenuation cross section.

7.5
Incoherent Compton Scattering

7.5.1
Kinematics of Compton Scattering

The photoelectric process involves a bound atomic electron. Whether an electron behaves like a bound or a free electron is determined by the relative magnitudes of the photon energy and the binding energy of the electron. For example, up to a photon energy of 100 keV, the K electrons of lead, with $E_K = 88$ keV, behave like bound electrons, but those of oxygen in water, with $E_K = 0.53$ keV, are like free (or quasi-free) electrons. Compton scattering is an elastic collision between a photon and a "free" electron. The collision of photon of energy E_v $(= h\nu)$, produces a scattered photon of degraded energy $E_{v'}$ $(= h\nu')$ and a recoil electron of energy T (Figure 7.6). Because the energy of the scattered photon differs from that of the incident photon, this is called an incoherent scattering process. The scattered photon and the recoil electron may travel at angles θ and ϕ with respect to the direction of the incident photon. The energies $E_{v'}$ and T can be derived based on the laws of conservation of momentum and energy. The equations conserving the momentum components along the directions parallel and perpendicular to the incident photon are

$$E_v/c = (E_{v'}/c) \cos\theta + p \cos\phi \qquad (7.12a)$$
$$0 = (E_{v'}/c) \sin\theta - p \sin\phi \qquad (7.12b)$$

where p is the momentum of the recoil electron. Energy conservation requires that

$$E_v = E_{v'} + T \qquad (7\text{-}13)$$

An electron, being a light particle, even at moderately low energies reaches velocities comparable to the velocity of light, c. At such high velocities, classical mechanics does not apply. Expressions for energy and momentum based on the theory of relativity must be used for solving the above equations. Such solutions lead to various expressions relating $E_{v'}$ and T to E_v, θ, and ϕ. An interesting outcome is that, if λ and λ' are the wavelenngths of the incident and scattered photons, the increase in the wavelength, $d\lambda = \lambda' - \lambda$, turns out to be unique for any particular value of the emission angle θ of the scattered photon. The shift in wavelength, $d\lambda$, can be calculated from the relation

$$d\lambda = \lambda' - \lambda = \frac{c}{v'} - \frac{c}{v} = \frac{h}{m_0 c}(1 - \cos\theta) \qquad (7\text{-}14)$$

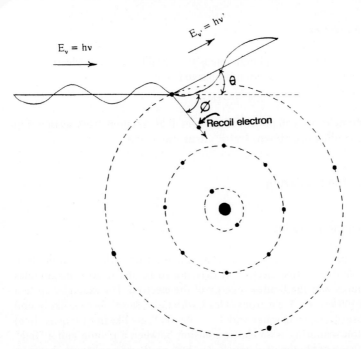

Fig. 7.6. A photon of energy E_v is Compton-scattered by an electron, resulting in a scattered photon of energy $E_{v'}$, and a recoil electron of kinetic energy T

The constant factor $[h/(m_0c)]$ has the dimension of length and is called the Compton wavelength. It is numerically equal to the wavelength of a photon with an energy identical to that of the rest energy m_0c^2 ($= 0.51$ MeV) of an electron.

The ratio $E_{v'}/E_v$ depends on the angle of scatter and is given by

$$\frac{E_{v'}}{E_v} = \frac{hv'}{hv} = \frac{1}{[1 + \alpha(1 - \cos\theta)]} \tag{7-15}$$

where $\alpha = hv/(m_0c^2)$ is the energy of the incoming photon, expressed in multiples of m_0c^2.

The kinetic energy of the Compton recoil electron is given by

$$T = E_v \frac{\alpha(1 - \cos\theta)}{1 + \alpha(1 - \cos\theta)} \tag{7-16}$$

or, in terms of the angle θ, by

$$T = E_v \frac{2\alpha \cos^2\phi}{(1 + \alpha)^2 - (\alpha^2 \cos^2\phi)} \tag{7-17}$$

For a given angle θ, ϕ is unique, and vice versa. The two angles are related to each other by

$$\cos\phi = (1 + \alpha)\tan(\theta/2) \tag{7-18}$$

In general, θ can vary from 0° to 180°, i. e., from forward scatter to backw
The value θ = 90° corresponds to perpendicular scatter. The electron angle
from 0° to 90°.

7.5.2
Angular Distribution of Scattered Photons

Compton-scattered photons have an angular distribution that depends on the incident photon energy, with the probability of scatter varying for different scattering angles. At low incident photon energies, the scatter is distributed somewhat more evenly in all directions as compared to the mainly forward scattering observed at high energies (Figure 7.7).

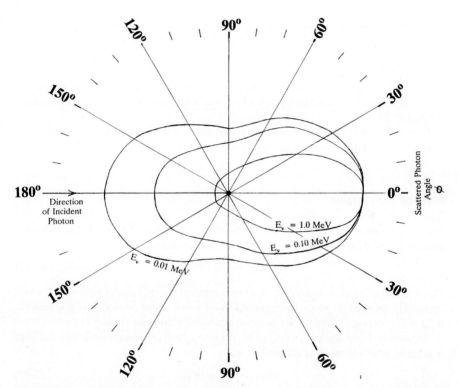

Fig. 7.7. Angular distribution of Compton-scattered photons at three energies, 0.01, 0.10, and 1.0 MeV. The radial distance in any direction is proportional to the relative Compton cross section per unit solid angle in that direction

7.5.3
Scattered Energy at Specific Angles

Direct collision and back scatter $(\theta = 180°, \phi = 0°)$ – In this case, the photon is back scattered and maximum energy is transferred to the recoil electron. If we substitute $\cos\theta = -1.0$ in (7-16),

$$T_{max} = \frac{2\alpha E_v}{2\alpha + 1} \qquad (7\text{-}19)$$

The scattered photon has the minimum possible energy and a maximum wavelength change. The electron will travel forward (i. e., $\phi = 0$).

Perpendicular scatter $(\theta = 90°)$ – In this case, $\cos\theta = 0$ and hence,

$$E_{v'} = \frac{E_v}{(1 + \alpha)} \qquad (7\text{-}20)$$

At very high energies, where $\alpha \gg 1$,

$$E_{v'} = E_v/\alpha = m_0c^2 = 0.51\,\text{MeV} \qquad (7\text{-}21)$$

This means that the 90° scatter energy gradually assumes a constant value of 0.51 MeV as the photon energy increases. This has interesting implications for shielding of radiotherapy rooms in directions perpendicular to a therapy beam (as will be discussed in Chapter 19).

Forward scatter $(\theta = 0°)$ – This is a grazing scatter. Because $\cos\theta = 1.0$, $E_{v'}$ is identical to E_v. The recoil electron receives no energy.

7.5.4
Compton Cross Section

The partial loss of the photon intensity due to the Compton effect alone can be calculated from the following relation, which resembles Equation (7-1):

$$dN = -\sigma_t N \, d\ell \qquad (7\text{-}22)$$

where σ_t is the "total" Compton scatter component of the overall attenuation cross section μ. The reason for the qualifying term "total" will become clear in later discussions. σ_t/ρ is the corresponding mass Compton attenuation cross section.

Because each photon has an energy E_v, the energy lost in a thickness $d\ell$ of a medium is given by multiplication of dN by E_v; i. e.,

$$dNE_v = -\sigma_t N \, d\ell E_v \qquad (7\text{-}23)$$

or

$$dNE_v = -[NE_{v'}][\sigma_t \, d\ell] \qquad (7.23a)$$

or

$$\text{Energy removed} = [\text{energy incident}] \times [\sigma_t \, d\ell] \qquad (7.23b)$$

In the above evaluation, the energy removed includes not only the energy given to the recoil electrons, but also the part carried away by the scattered photons. However, if we want to concentrate our attention on the energy absorbed locally, we need make a distinction between energy given to the recoil electrons and that given to scattered photons. The energy T given to the electrons can be considered as being locally absorbed because of their short range. However, the energy carried away by the highly penetrating scattered photons cannot be regarded as being absorbed locally. For dosimetric purposes, it is necessary to distinguish between local energy absorption and the energy carried away. Thus, we divide the total Compton cross section as follows:

$$\sigma_t = \sigma_s + \sigma_a \tag{7.24a}$$

$$\sigma_t/\rho = \sigma_s/\rho + \sigma_a/\rho \tag{7.24b}$$

where σ_s and σ_a, respectively, are the scatter and the absorption component of the cross section. Accordingly,

$$\text{Energy converted into scatterd photons} = \sigma_s N\, d\ell E_v \tag{7.25a}$$

and

$$\text{Energy transferred to recoil electrons and locally absorbed} = \sigma_a N\, d\ell E_v \tag{7.25b}$$

7.5.5
Energy and Atomic Numbers vs. Compton Cross Section

The Compton cross section decreases with energy, but not as rapidly as we saw it happen with the photoelectric component. The Compton cross section depends on the number of electrons available for interacting. The electron density (i. e., the concentration) in any element of atomic mass A and atomic number Z is given by

$$(N_{Av}/A)Z = N_{Av}(Z/A) \tag{7-26}$$

where N_{Av} is Avogadro's number. The electron density does not vary much for different substances. This is because, as a fortuitous natural phenomenon, the ratio Z/A remains close to 2 for element after element, except for hydrogen at the beginning of the periodic table. Hydrogen has a Z/A ratio of 1. However, in practical contexts of medical physics, hydrogen is encountered only as a compound with other, heavier elements. Because the latter make up the bulk of the source of electrons, the role of hydrogen becomes insignificant overall. Hence, the Compton cross section, with its dependence on electron density, shows very little dependence on Z. This is quite unlike the photoelectric cross section which, as we observed, shows a great dependence on Z.

The Compton interaction is the major mode of interaction for most photon energies used in radiotherapy. In diagnostic radiology, the Compton effect plays both positive and negative roles. Positively, it provides for some contrast between air, bone, and soft tissue through the differences in their linear attenuations caused by the differences in their mass densities. A negative effect results because the Compton-scattered photons travel in all directions to smear and blur the image. Special measures for cutting off the scatter, such as the use of a grid, are needed so that this undesirable blurring is reduced (See Section 12.3.5).

7.6
Negatron-Positron Pair Production

7.6.1
Threshold Energy for Pair Production

In the field of a nucleus, a photon may lose its entire energy and produce a negatron (i. e., a normal negatively charged electron) and positron (i. e., a positively charged electron) pair (Figure 7.8). This is known as pair production. The energy equivalent of the combined mass of the two electrons is

$$2 \times m_0 c^2 = 2 \times 0.51\,\text{MeV} = 1.02\,\text{MeV}$$

Thus, the minimum photon energy at which pair production can occur (in a nuclear field) is 1.02 MeV. According to Dirac's theory of the electron, the positron is a "hole" in a sea of electrons. Figure 7.9 shows the energy level diagram which Dirac used to explain the pair production phenomenon. Two horizontal lines are drawn at energy levels of $-m_0 c^2$ and $+m_0 c^2$. All continuous energies below and above these lines are allowed levels which the electrons can occupy. Between these lines, there is a band of energies which the electrons are forbidden to occupy. Dirac contended that all commonly occurring electrons are observed to be at energy levels above $+m_0 c^2$. He hypothesized that the levels below $-m_0 c^2$ are filled to saturation with electrons, creating a sea of negative charge. If it happens that a photon having an energy E_v greater than $2m_0 c^2$ is absorbed by one of the electrons (in the sea) with energy below $-m_0 c^2$, it can be lifted to a positive energy level above $+m_0 c^2$. Then it appears as a normal electron for observation. The missing electron in the negative energy region is the "hole," which behaves like a particle with a positive charge, that is, a positron. The energy excess of the photon above 1.02 MeV is divided between the positron and the

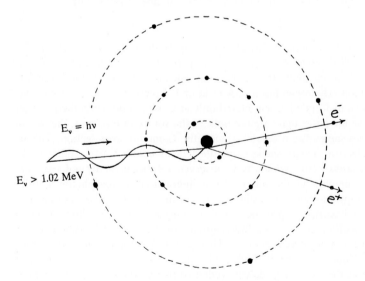

Fig. 7.8. A photon of energy E_v produces an electron-positron pair in a nuclear field

Fig. 7.9. Dirac's diagram for electron-positron pair production

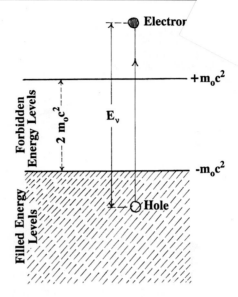

negatron. The energy conservation equation is

$$E_v = T_{e^+} + T_{e^-} + 1.02\,\text{MeV} \qquad (7\text{-}27)$$

where T_{e^+} and T_{e^-} are the kinetic energies of the positron and negatron. T_{e^+} and T_{e^-} need not be equal, although equality is highly probable. The direction of emission of the pair of particles is predominantly forward, and this characteristic becomes especially striking at high photon energies.

Pair production requires an electric field, such as that of the nucleus. Pair production occurs near the nucleus, in its electric field, and not inside it. Pair production can also occur in the field of an electron, but with a lower probability. In such an event, the electron creating the field is also set in motion, and thus three moving electrons result. This is called "triplet" production. The laws of physics require a minimum photon energy of 2.04 MeV for triplet production.

7.6.2
Electron-Positron Annihilation

The two particles, negatron and positron, travel their own separate paths and lose their energy through ionization, excitation, and bremsstrahlung production. On slowing down to near-zero energy, the positron is annihilated by recombining with a stationary electron. In terms of Dirac's theory, at this stage the "hole" reaches the energy level $-m_0c^2$ and is filled by an electron at the energy level m_0c^2. The filling should result in emission of an energy of $2m_0c^2 = 1.02\,\text{MeV}$. This indeed happens; two photons of 0.51 MeV are emitted during annihilation of a positron (Figure 7.10). The two photons travel in opposite directions to maintain the conservation of momentum.

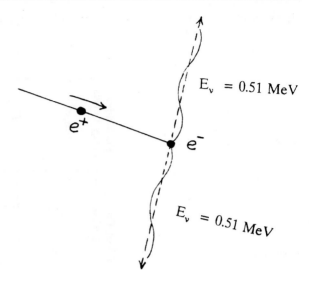

Fig. 7.10. A slowed-down positron is annihilated on meeting an electron and produces two photons, each of 0.51 MeV, that travel in opposite directions

$E_v = 0.51$ MeV

e^+

e^-

$E_v = 0.51$ MeV

7.6.3
Pair Production Cross Section

The reduction in the photon intensity caused by pair production alone can be calculated from a relation that resembles Equation (7-1):

$$dN = -\pi N\, d\ell \tag{7-28}$$

where π is the pair production component of the overall attenuation cross section μ. π/ρ is the corresponding mass pair production attenuation cross section.

7.6.4
Photon Energy and Atomic Number vs. π

The pair production yield (like the bremsstrahlung yield) increases with the nuclear field strength and hence depends on Z. The pair production atomic coefficient π_{atom} varies in proportion to Z^2. Because there are Z electrons per atom, the electronic cross section $\pi_{electron}$ is proportional to Z. We know that the number of electrons per gram remains nearly the same amount for most materials. This means that the coefficient π/ρ will also be proportional to Z. Beyond the threshold of 1.02 MeV for pair production, π/ρ increases with the photon energy E_v. Figure 7.5 compares π/ρ for lead and water, which represent high-Z and low-Z materials, respectively.

7.6.5
Local Energy Absorption and Pair Production

During pair production, the photon of energy E_v completely disappears. However, the eventual annihilation of the positron results in emission of two penetrating photons of 0.51 MeV each. This total energy of 1.02 MeV given out as annihilation radiation cannot be regarded as being absorbed locally. Thus, the net local energy absorption in pair production is the sum of the kinetic energies given to the pair of electrons. Interestingly, however, the pair production cross section is high only when E_v is much larger than 1.02 MeV. At increasing values of E_v, the assumption that almost the entire photon energy is absorbed locally becomes a possible approximation.

7.7
Summing up the Local Energy Absorbed

The value of μ and that of μ/ρ can be expressed as a sum of their components as follows:

$$\mu = \tau + \sigma_t + \pi \tag{7.29a}$$

$$\mu/\rho = \tau/\rho + \sigma_t/\rho + \pi/\rho \tag{7.29b}$$

The values μ and μ/ρ are referred to as total linear and total mass attenuation co-efficients, because they account for the attenuation of the incident beam under the assumption that the entire incident photon energy is dissipated in all interactions. However, radiation effects are due to the local energy absorption and, thus, it becomes necessary to distinguish between the part of the energy of the incident photon that is converted to the energy of the electrons and weak characteristic X-rays on the one hand, and the part that is reemitted as penetrating photons on the other. The latter part carries energy away and does not contribute to the local absorption of radiation energy. The coefficient μ/ρ can be divided into two parts, namely, μ_{tr}/ρ, the energy transfer coefficient, which applies to the energy transferred as kinetic energy to the short-range radiations of electrons and characteristic X-rays; and μ_s/ρ, the energy scatter coefficient, which applies to the energy converted into scattered photons. Hence,

$$\mu/\rho = \mu_{tr}/\rho + \mu_s/\rho \tag{7-30}$$

The value of μ_{tr}/ρ is given by

$$\mu_{tr}/\rho = \tau/\rho + \sigma_a/\rho + \pi/\rho \left[1 - (2m_0c^2/hv)\right] \tag{7-31}$$

It can happen that a part of the energy transferred to the electrons is lost by emission of bremsstrahlung photons. If g refers to the fractional energy of the electrons that is lost as bremsstrahlung, the true energy absorption coefficient, μ_{en}/ρ, is given by

$$\mu_{en}/\rho = \mu_{tr}/\rho(1 - g) \tag{7-32}$$

Appendix B gives the values of μ/ρ, μ_{tr}/ρ, and μ_{en}/ρ for a few materials of interest in radiotherapy physics.

7.8
Components of μ at Different Energies

The overall picture of the dependence of the relative magnitude of the different interaction processes on both E_v and Z is shown in Figure 7.11. The curve on the left side, in the low-energy region, marks the (E_v, Z) combinations at which photoelectric events and

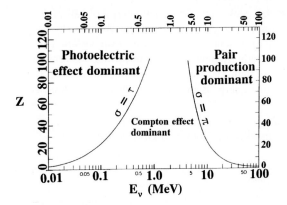

Compton events become equally likely. The curve on the right side defines the (E_v, Z) combination for which Compton and pair production events occur with the same probability. The two curves together divide the diagram into three distinct regions, in which the photoelectric, Compton, and pair production events become dominant. The middle region, with dominance of the Compton effect, has special importance for high-energy radiotherapy.

The data in Table 7.1 give the relative preponderance of different interactions at different photon energies for both water and lead. Again, water and lead are used to serve as examples of low-Z and high-Z materials. The values in the table show that, as the photon energy increases, the dominance gradually shifts from photoelectric through Compton to pair production events. At low energies, photoelectric events dominate for both water and lead. As the energy increases, the Compton effect begins to take over very significantly for water, but less significantly for lead. Photoelectric events decrease less rapidly for lead than for water. The Compton effect dominates from 100 keV to 5 MeV for water. Up to the threshold energy of 1.02 MeV, there are no pair production events. Pair production is only a small part of the overall absorption process

Table 7.1. Relative Percentages of Number of Interactions of Different Types for Water and Lead at Different Photon Energies

E_v	Coherent Scattering		Photoelectric Absorption		Incoherent (Compton) Scattering		Pair Production		Total (μ/ρ cm^2 g^{-1})	
(MeV)	H_2O	Pb	H_2O	Pb	H_2O	Pb	H_2O	Pb	H_2O	Pb
0.01	5	4	92	96	3	–	–	–	0.512	43,900
0.05	9	8	11	91	80	1	–	–	0.224	2,710
0.10	3	3	2	95	95	2	–	–	0.171	1,900
0.50	–	5	–	52	100	43	–	–	0.0969	54.7
1.00	–	3	–	26	100	71	–	–	0.0707	24.2
5.00	–	–	–	3	92	46	8	51	0.0303	14.6
10.0	–	–	–	–	77	25	23	75	0.0221	16.7
50.0	–	–	–	–	30	4	70	96	0.0166	27.6
100.0	–	–	–	–	16	2	84	98	0.0171	32.1

Note: All values are in percent. Based on data in Reference 7 (Additional Reading).

for water even at 5 MeV. However, at this energy for lead, pair production accounts for more than 50% of the total interactions because of the high Z. The photoelectric effect at low energies and pair production at high energies contribute to a significant difference between the μ/ρ values for lead and water. This is a direct consequence of the dependence on Z.

7.9
Attenuation Coefficients for Mixtures and Compounds

7.9.1
Weighted Addition of μ/ρ Values

In general, any material can be thought of as made up of fractions, by mass, of $w_1, w_2, w_3, \ldots, w_n$, of elements $1, 2, 3, \ldots, n$. The overall attenuation coefficient for the material is then

$$\mu/\rho = w_1(\mu_1/\rho) + w_2(\mu_2/\rho) + w_3(\mu_3/\rho) + \ldots + w_n(\mu_n/\rho) \qquad (7\text{-}33)$$

The same process of weighted addition can be used for the three individual components τ/ρ, σ/ρ, and π/ρ of μ/ρ.

7.9.2
Effective Z for Mixtures and Compounds

It has been emphasized throughout this chapter that the probabilities of occurrence of the different photon interactions depend both on the energy of the photon and on the atomic number of the material. To carry out experimental studies simulating the use of radiation in biomedical contexts, we need to make use of tissue substitute materials (also called phantom materials). Mixtures or compounds that are similar in their radiation interaction characteristics to soft tissue, bone, or other body constituents can be identified for this purpose. The ideal comparison between competing substitutes should be made in terms of comparing all of their attenuation coefficients at all energies; however, this is neither easy nor practical. The effective atomic number, Z_{eff}, of any mixture has been defined to serve as a single index that is useful for such comparisons. If the cross section depends on Z as Z^m, we can derive a mathematical expression for Z_{eff} for any mixture:

$$Z_{eff} = \left[w_1 Z_1^m + w_2 Z_2^m + \ldots + w_n Z_n^m \right]^{1/m} \qquad (7\text{-}34)$$

From our discussion on Z dependence in this chapter, the appropriate values of m are 3, 0, and 1 for photoelectric, Compton, and pair production events, respectively. Thus, the photoelectric effect is the most sensitive to Z. The value of m recommended for practical purposes is 2.94 (i. e., almost 3). Thus,

$$Z_{eff} = \left(w_1 Z_1^{2.94} + w_2 Z_2^{2.94} + \ldots + w_n Z_n^{2.94} \right)^{1/2.94} \qquad (7\text{-}35)$$

The number 2.94 was arrived at empirically and is a reasonable approximation for purposes of comparing radiation absorbers.

7.10
Broad- and Narrow-Beam Attenuation Geometries

7.10.1
Primary and Scatter Fluence

The attenuation curve that we discussed in Section 7.2.2 depends on the geometric relationship among the radiation beam, the attenuating medium, and the detector. Two different geometries are illustrated in Figure 7.12. In the top diagram (Figure 7.12a), the beam is just large enough to cover the size of a small detector. In this situation, any scattered photon that originates from the attenuating medium and travels at even a small angle with respect to the incident direction will not strike the detector. Thus, the detector's signal will be almost entirely due to the primary photons that travel through the medium without any interaction. Such a situation, in which a narrow beam is used and only the transmitted primary component is measured, is referred to as narrow-beam geometry. The attenuation coefficient obtained by measurement in this geometry will correspond to the total attenuation μ. This is a unique value.

The uniqueness can be lost if some amount of scattered photons can also reach the detector. This is shown in Figure 7.12b, in which a broad beam is used. Two detectors are shown, one of which is placed close to the attenuating medium and the other at a large distance. The detector located close by can be struck by scattered photons emerging at an angle with respect to the incident beam. This does not occur with the detector placed far away. Whereas one detector measures the primary photons only, the

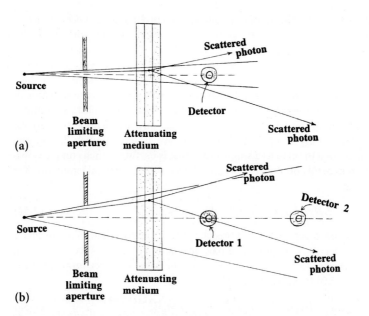

Fig. 7.12. Geometries for measurement of photon attenuation through a medium. (a) Narrow-beam geometry, in which any scattered photon from the medium will miss the detector. (b) Broad-beam geometry, in which detector 1 sees scattered photons, but detector 2 does not

Fig. 7.13. Typical broad-beam and narrow-beam transmission curves

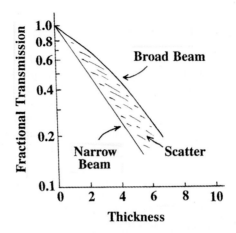

other measures scatter also. The former measures the attenuation for an approximately narrow beam, and the latter measures that for a broad beam including scatter.

Figure 7.13 illustrates the difference between broad-beam and narrow-beam attenuation curves. The attenuation coefficient of the broad beam is smaller than that of the narrow beam. The broad-beam attenuation is not unique, because of its dependence on the details of the actual geometry. However, a minimum limiting value of the broad-beam attenuation coefficient will be reached when the scatter build-up is complete, with all possible scatter reaching the detector. Sometimes, narrow-beam and broad-beam measurement geometries are referred to as "good" and "bad" geometries, respectively.

7.10.2
Scatter Build-Up Factor

If I_0 is the intensity measured at a point without an attenuator in the beam, introduction of an attenuator of thickness ℓ reduces the intensity to I. Then, under scatter-free (i. e., narrow-beam) conditions,

$$I = I_0\, e^{-\mu\ell} \qquad (7\text{-}36)$$

The addition of scatter, or "build-up of scatter," in the broad-beam situation may result in a different intensity, I', given by

$$I' = IB(\mu\ell) = I_0 B(\mu\ell) e^{-\mu\ell} \qquad (7\text{-}37)$$

where $B(\mu\ell)$ is a factor with a value > 1.0, called the "build-up factor." It is a function of the attenuation path length $\mu\ell$. The general definition of the build-up factor is

$$\text{Build-up factor} = \frac{\text{total intensity}}{\text{primary intensity}} = \frac{(\text{primary} + \text{scatter})\text{intensity}}{\text{primary intensity}}$$

In many practical calculations, it is convenient first to calculate the primary intensity I of a narrow beam by using Equation (7-36). In the next step, the actual intensity I', including the scatter, can be evaluated from Equation (7-37), using an already derived table of $B(\mu\ell)$ values applicable for specific scattering geometries and photon spectra.

7.11
Photonuclear Reactions

Photonuclear reactions occur when the energy E_v of a photon is absorbed by the nucleus of an atom. After the absorption, one or more neutrons or photons may be emitted, and the nucleus is transformed as a result of the reaction. Photonuclear reactions require a minimum or threshold photon energy. The threshold depends on the nuclide and the particular reaction. Table 7.2 gives different photonuclear reactions and their thresholds. Photonuclear reactions occur with a much smaller probability than do other photon interactions. In megavoltage radiotherapy treatment rooms, some of the photoneutrons produced in the accelerator, collimating system, and the patient reach the entrance door through the access pathways. Shielding for these neutrons should be provided with special doors incorporating hydrogenous materials to keep the radiation levels for operating personnel acceptable. High-energy electrons are also known to trigger nuclear reactions that result in the emission of neutrons and protons, although the probabilities for electron-nuclear reactions are smaller than those for photonuclear reactions.

Table 7.2. Some Photonuclear Reactions and Their Photon Energy Thresholds

Target	Photonuclear Threshold (MeV)	Reaction Product	Product Half Life
^{12}C	18.7	^{11}C	20.5 min
^{14}N	10.5	^{13}N	10 min
^{16}O	15.7	^{15}O	124 sec
^{27}Al	13.1	^{26}Al	6.5 sec
^{54}Fe	13.6	^{53}Fe	8.5 min
^{65}Cu	9.9	^{64}Cu	12.9 h
^{64}Zn	11.8	^{63}Zn	38 min
^{70}Zn	9.2	^{69}Zn	52 min
^{82}Se	9.8	^{81}Se	17 min
^{107}Ag	9.5	^{106}Ag	24 min/8.3 d
^{181}Ta	7.6	^{180}Ta	8.1 h
^{182}W	8.0	^{181}W	130 d
^{197}Au	8.1	^{196}Au	6.2 d/9.7 h
^{204}Pb	8.2	^{203}Pb	6.1 sec/52 h
^{208}Pb	7.4	^{207}Pb	Stable
^{2}H	2.20	^{1}H	Stable
^{9}Be	1.67	^{8}Be $\rightarrow$ 2 ^{4}He	Stable

Note: Most of the data are from Reference 10 (Additional Readings)

Additional Reading

1. Anderson, D.W., Absorption of Ionizing Radiation, University Park Press, Baltimore, 1984.
2. Evans, R.D., Atomic Nucleus, McGraw Hill, New York, 1955; republished by Krieger, 1986.
3. Attix, F.H. and Tochilin, E., Radiation Dosimetry, Vol 1, Academic Press, New York, 1969.
4. Hubbell, J.H., Review of photon interaction cross section data in the medical and biological context, Phys. Med. Biol., Vol. 44, pp R1–20, 1999.
5. Hubbell, J.H., Seltzer, S.M., Tables of x-ray mass attenuation coefficients and mass energy-absorption coefficients from 1 keV to 20 MeV for elements Z = 1 to 92 and 48 additional substances of dosimetric interest, Report NISTIR 5632, National Institute of Standards and Technology, Gaithersburg, MD, USA, 1996.

6. Hubbell, J.H., Photon mass attenuation and energy-absorption coefficients from 1 keV to 20 MeV, Int. J. Appl. Radiat. Isot., Vol 33, p1269–1290, 1982.
7. Storm, E. and Israel, H.I., Photon cross sections from 1 keV to 100 MeV for elements Z = 1 to Z = 100, Nuclear Data Tables, Vol A7, p641–689, 1970.
8. International Commission on Radiation Units and Measurements, Tissue Substitutes in Radiation Dosimetry and Measurement, ICRU Report 45, International Commission on Radiation Units and Measurements, Bethesda, Maryland, 1989.
9. White, D.R. and Constantinou, C., Anthropomorphic phantom materials, Chapter 3, in Progress in Medical Radiation Physics (Ed: Orton, C.G.), Plenum Press, New York, 1982.
10. National Council on Radiation Protection and Measurements, Report No. 79, Neutron Contamination from Medical Electron Accelerators, National Council on Radiation Protection and Measurements, Bethesda, Maryland, 1987.

PART III

Radiation Beam Therapy Equipment

CHAPTER 8

Conventional X-Ray Machines

8.1
Discovery of X-Rays

At the beginning of the 20th century, there was much interest among experimental physicists in the study of atomic phenomena in rarefied gases subjected to high electric potentials. They used glass discharge tubes (Figure 8.1) which contained an anode and a cathode, and in which gas was maintained at very low pressures, of the order of 0.001 mmHg. Crookes found that, when very high voltages were applied between the electrodes, the gas turned dark and the walls glowed. The glow was attributed to fast-moving, negatively charged particles, later identified as electrons. In 1895, Wilhelm Conrad Roentgen reported the emission of a mysterious and penetrating radiation from evacuated tubes that affected the photographic plates stored in light-tight containers. He was, in fact, observing the bremsstrahlung produced by electron interactions. He called the radiation "X-rays," using the letter "X" to designate something unknown. Nowadays, these rays are also called Roentgen rays. Roentgen's radiographing of his own and his wife's hands marked the beginning of the use of X-rays in the healing arts.

To produce X-rays, one first needs to have an ample supply of electrons. Next, the electrons must be accelerated to become energetic. They are then made to strike a target composed of a high-Z material, where they produce bremsstrahlung photons. In this chapter, we discuss the characteristics of conventional X-ray machines operating at kilovolt potentials and the radiation beams they produce. Acceleration of electrons to very high energies for production of megavoltage X-rays will be discussed in Chapter 10.

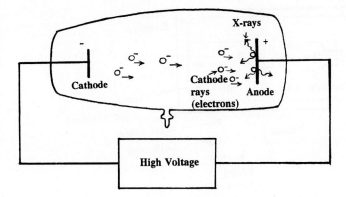

Fig. 8.1. Schematic diagram of a cold-cathode gas discharge X-ray tube

8.2
Gas-Discharge X-Ray Tube

The schematic diagram in Figure 8.1 shows an early gas discharge X-ray tube. In such a tube, gas molecules were split into electrons and positive ions by the potential difference between the electrodes. The potential also accelerated the electrons, which gained energy and struck the anode, producing X-rays. The air in the tube was continuously pumped out, and the residual pressure was controlled so that sufficient gas was in the tube to provide a constant supply of ions. These were also called Crookes' tubes or cold cathode tubes. The tubes were inexpensive and simple, but were not satisfactory for the practice of radiography. In modern times, Crookes' tubes have been superseded by hot-cathode tubes, called Coolidge tubes.

8.3
Features of Modern X-Ray Tubes

8.3.1
Coolidge's X-Ray Tube

William Coolidge, at the General Electric Company, used a heated filament as the source of electrons. The phenomenon of emission of electrons by a heated filament is called thermionic emission. The heat energy helps to liberate the electrons bound to the filament material. In Coolidge's tube (Figure 8.2), a filament, which can be a thin tungsten wire, is heated to 2000–4000°C by passage of an electric current of 2 to 5 A. The amount of electron emission depends on the temperature of the filament, which, in turn, is controlled by the current through the filament. The filament also acts as the cathode. The stream of electrons emerging from the filament is accelerated by a

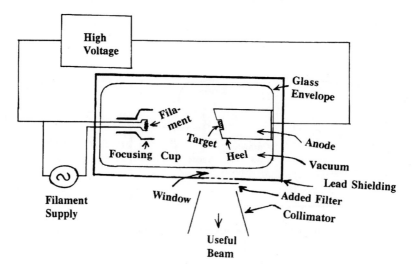

Fig. 8.2. Schematic diagram of a Coolidge X-ray tube

potential of several kilovolts (kV) which is applied between the anode and the filament. An electrical focusing cup surrounds the filament to produce a narrow pencil beam of electrons. The anode is usually made of a metal such as copper, which is capable of good electrical and heat conduction. A small piece of a high-Z metal, such as tungsten, is embedded in the anode and functions as the target for the electron impact and for production of bremsstrahlung. The entire assembly of the filament, focusing cup, and anode is covered by an evacuated glass envelope. Because the bremsstrahlung is emitted in all directions, the envelope needs to be entirely surrounded by lead shielding, except in one direction that has a window through which the useful beam emerges. The beam is usually made to pass through a metallic filter and a variable collimating aperture before it strikes a patient or object.

8.3.2
Heat Generation

The efficiency of bremsstrahlung production is less than 1% at low electron energies, where most of the energy of the electrons is dissipated in collision events. This, in turn, results in high local energy absorption and in heating of the target-anode assembly. The anode therefore should have a high heat capacity.

An irradiation for which a constant potential V is used at a tube current I, and which lasts for time t, dissipates an amount of energy E, given by

$$E = VIt \qquad (8\text{-}1)$$

This will, in turn, generate heat H, given by

$$H = E/J = VIt/J \qquad (8\text{-}2)$$

where J is Joule's mechanical equivalent of heat. The value of J is 4.18 joules/calorie. If V, I, and t are given in units of kV, mA, and seconds, respectively, E in Equation (8-2) will be in joules. The heat generated, H, can be evaluated in calories.

Managing the enormous amount of heat generated and avoiding a target meltdown is a practical problem that can be solved by various methods, which we discuss next.

8.3.3
Line Focus Principle

The area struck by the electrons, called the focal spot of X-ray emission, is heated instantly. Although the heat subsequently can be dissipated over time, the instant overheating of the focal spot can contribute to a meltdown. A large focal spot can reduce this possibility. However, this is not desirable, as it will increase the size of the X-ray source and hence reduce the resolution of the radiographic image obtained; that is, the sharpness of the image produced can suffer. The "line focus principle," illustrated in Figure 8.3a and b, provides a wide focal spot without compromising the resolution. In this approach, the face of the target presents an angle of $90° + \theta$ with respect to the direction of the incident electrons (see Figure 8.3b). The width of the target struck by the electrons is AB, but, when seen from the direction of the useful

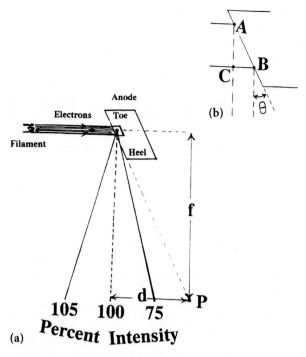

Fig. 8.3. Line focus principle. (a) Diagram showing an angled target and the resulting nonuniformity of intensity due to heel attenuation. (b) Effective focal spot size CB, the actual focal spot size AB, and angle of inclination θ

beam, its apparent width is CB, given by

$$CB = AB \sin \theta \tag{8-3}$$

The smaller the angle θ, the smaller the size of the apparent focal spot. However, one cannot use very small angles without reducing the area of coverage of the useful beam, as the discussion that follows will reveal.

8.3.4
Heel Effect

Some of the intensity of the X-rays emerging from the target is lost as the rays travel within the target-anode assembly (Figure 8.3a). The heel (see Figure 8.2 for location of the heel) of the angled anode makes the attenuation smaller for the rays on the cathode side compared to those toward the anode side. Because of this "heel effect," the intensity of the useful X-ray beam shows a fall-off in the cathode-to-anode direction. The X-ray intensity will be shielded by the full thickness of the anode assembly at point P (Figure 8.3a). In a plane at a distance f from the focal spot, the off-center distance of P is given by (f tan θ). At f = 100 cm, 7° and 15° target angles will limit the maximum possible coverage of the beam up to about 12 cm and 27 cm in the direction of P, respectively.

8.3.5
Rotating Anode

In another type of anode that is designed to reduce the possibility for overheating, a fly-wheel (Figure 8.4) is connected to a motor and is set in rotation prior to irradiation. The rotation causes successively different faces of the anode to be presented to the electrons and dissipates the heat over a large ring-shaped area. The instantaneous focal spot used for imaging is always small, and thus the sharpness of the image is not compromised.

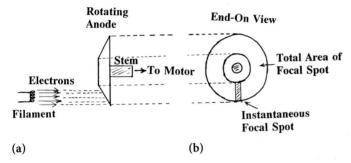

(a)   (b)

Fig. 8.4. (a) Electrons incident on a rotating anode. (b) The instantaneous focal spot and the total usable focal spot area in an end-on view of the anode

8.3.6
Avoidance of Overheating

The user of an X-ray tube constantly has to be aware of the thermal tolerance of the anode of the tube in use to avoid overload. The four important parameters to be considered in any X-ray use are (i) the tube potential, (ii) the tube current, (iii) the duration of the exposure, and (iv) the filter inserted in the path of the beam for removal of the useless soft X-ray components (see Section 8.6.2). The units commonly used for the tube potential, tube current, and duration of irradiation are kilovolts (kV), milliamperes (mA), and seconds (sec), respectively. The filter is specified in terms of its thickness and material, such as "1 mm Cu." For any chosen tube potential and filter combination, the product of the tube current and the duration of irradiation determines the total X-ray output. The product of the units mA and sec gives the unit of milliampere-seconds (mAs). For a satisfactory radiograph with X-rays, one uses a proper selection of kilovolts and milliampere-seconds, together with a filter incorporated in the beam.

The X-ray tubes used in diagnostic radiology and those used in therapeutic radiology have differing requirements. In radiography, images are formed on films, and it is necessary for the images to be sharp. It is ideal to use a small focal spot and a short exposure time (to eliminate any unsharpness due to motion of the patient or body tissues). It is usual to employ an exposure lasting only a fraction of a second with a tube current of several hundred milliamperes. In such usage, it is imperative to keep in mind the need to allow the tube to cool down between exposures as recommended by the manufacturer. Modern X-ray equipment includes circuits that have warning lights to indicate overload. Many tubes have two filaments of different sizes to give the user a choice of either a large or a small focal spot.

In diagnostic fluoroscopy, the X-ray image is seen by an image intensifier camera with a fluorescent screen. The image is amplified and projected on a TV screen to be observed at frequent intervals, or continuously, if needed, by the physician. For fluoroscopy, low tube currents of a few milliamperes are used, and this does not involve instantaneous generation of a large amount of heat.

The therapeutic use of X-rays calls for operation at moderately high currents, 10 to 20 mA, over an extended period of several minutes for delivery of an adequate dose to the patient. Hence, therapy X-ray tubes need to be provided continuously with circulating coolants around the anode assembly for removal of heat. Because therapy tubes deliver high radiation doses, they need heavy lead shielding on all sides for radiation protection. Thus, the tube assembly becomes bulky and heavy.

8.4
High-Voltage Supply and Rectification

8.4.1
Stepping up the AC Supply

The operation of an X-ray tube requires a very high applied voltage between the anode and the cathode. The normal electrical supply is an alternating current (AC) of 50 to 60 Hz, with a root mean square potential of either 110 or 220 V. This potential is too low to accelerate the electrons to sufficient energies for the production of X-rays. To be applied across an X-ray tube, this low voltage should be (i) amplified to kilovolt levels, (ii) rectified so that, at all times, it provides a positive potential between the anode and the filament, and (iii) kept constant at a chosen voltage level.

The principle of a transformer (Figure 8.5) can be employed for stepping up the normal 110- or 220-V AC supply. A transformer consists of two insulated coils of wire wound around a laminated iron core. One of these coils is the primary one, to which the input supply line is connected. The other is the secondary coil, across which an output voltage is produced through the magnetic induction of the core by the alternating current in the primary coil. The secondary output voltage, V_s, is proportional to the

Fig. 8.5. Illustration of the principle of the transformer, showing a laminated core with its (input) primary and (output) secondary windings

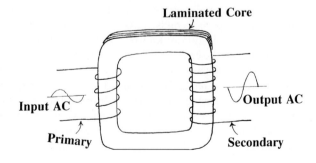

primary input, V_p, according to the relation

$$V_s/V_p = N_s/N_p \qquad (8\text{-}4)$$

where N_p and N_s are the numbers of turns in the primary and secondary coils, respectively. For an N_s/N_p ratio of 500, a 110-V input AC will be amplified to give $110\,V \times 500 = 55\,kV$. The output voltage is also an alternating one, with the same frequency as that of the primary.

8.4.2
Self-Rectified X-Ray Tube

If the transformer output is applied to an X-ray tube (Figure 8.6a), the tube current can flow only during the half-cycle of the AC for which the anode potential is positive with respect to the filament so that it draws the electrons emitted. During the negative half of the cycle, in principle, the tube current should be zero, as shown in Figure 8.6b. However, the reverse bias formed by the negative voltage between the anode and filament can draw some electrons back to strike the filament and thereby become a cause of damage to the filament. The probability for this can be reduced by incorporation of devices such as a dummy load in the secondary circuit of the transformer during the reverse cycle. Many dental and portable X-ray machines use self-rectification.

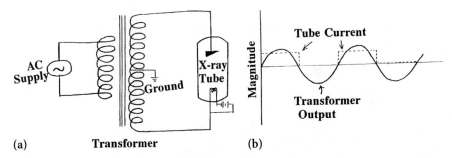

(a)   Transformer   (b)

Fig. 8.6. (a) A self-rectified X-ray circuit. (b) Time variation of the transformer output and the X-ray tube current

8.4.3
Half-Wave Rectification

Vacuum tube or semiconductor diodes can be used which allow only a positive potential to be applied to the anode of the tube. A diode (such as D1 or D2 in Figure 8.7), which has two terminals (shown as a thick arrow and a thin line), is a unidirectional conductor. It can conduct only when the potential of the arrow is positive with respect to the line. In the circuit of Figure 8.7, diodes D1 and D2 can conduct only during the half-cycle when terminal A of the transformer is positive and terminal B negative. The resulting X-ray tube potential and current will be as shown in Figure 8.7b. It can be seen that such half-wave rectification wastes one half of each cycle. The overall time of exposure can be shortened with the use of full-wave rectification.

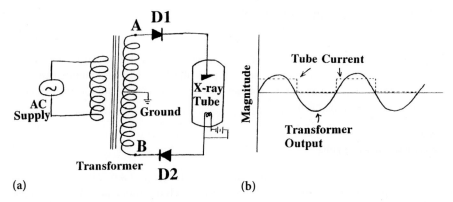

Fig. 8.7. (a) A half-wave rectification circuit connected to an X-ray tube. (b) Variation of the transformer output and tube current with time

8.4.4
Full-Wave Rectification

A four-diode bridge rectifier is shown in Figure 8.8a. If the transformer terminal A is positive and B negative, connections PQ and RS result. If B is positive and A negative, connections PS and RQ result. Thus, the anode and filament are connected to positive and negative terminals of the transformer, respectively, throughout the wave cycle (see Figure 8.8b).

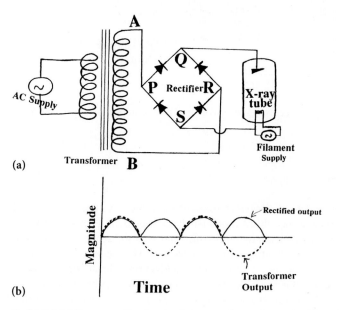

Fig. 8.8. (a) A full-wave rectification circuit connected to an X-ray tube. (b) Variation of the transformer output and tube potential

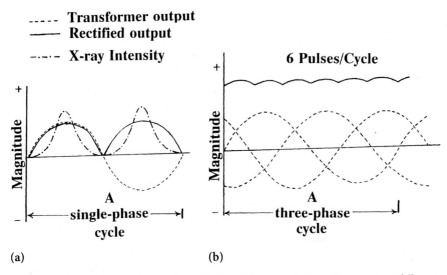

Fig. 8.9. (a) Diagram showing the variation with time of the unrectified transformer output, full-wave-rectified waveform, and X-ray intensity for a single-phase alternating-current input. (b) Same variation shown for a three-phase input

The X-ray output of the tube strongly depends on the energy of the electrons, which, in turn, is proportional to the tube potential. X-ray output is a power function of tube potential and increases rapidly with kV (see Sections 6.3.2 and 8.6.1). A single-phase (i. e., only one wave; see Figure 8.9a) AC supply after full-wave rectification provides a high X-ray intensity only at the peak of the wave in a cycle. This, once again, is not a very efficient use of a full AC cycle for production of X-rays. Ideally, there should be a constant rectified positive potential throughout each cycle. This ideal can nearly be achieved by use of a three-phase AC input.

8.4.5
Three-Phase Power Supply and Full-Wave Rectification

Three-phase transformers use specially configured coil windings to provide a simultaneous output of three wave forms with a mutual phase difference (Figure 8.9b). The sum of the three waves after full-wave rectification results in a near-constant potential with six pulses per cycle. This can be improved further (by more complex circuitry) to produce a near-ideal constant potential.

It is common practice to state the tube operating voltage in terms of the maximum (or peak) potential of the waveform, for example, 80 kVp, 100 kVp, etc., where kVp means the kilovoltage peak. Use of appropriate circuitry can enable the X-ray tube to operate at a steady potential. Only then can 80 kVp mean an 80 kV constant potential.

8.5
A Typical X-Ray Circuit

Figure 8.10 depicts a typical X-ray circuit with various meters and controls. The AC supply is varied by selection of the tap in an autotransformer. Different taps are selected for the tube and for the filament. The kilovolt meter is in the primary supply circuit, but, with proper calibration, should reflect the tube potential. The filament current is controlled by a variable resistor. There is a step-up transformer for increasing the supply voltage. The stepped-up potential is rectified and applied to the tube. A timer is incorporated which controls the exposure time. A step-down transformer provides the low voltage needed for heating of the filament. The tube current is monitored by an ammeter which (for safety reasons) is connected at a grounded point to the middle of the secondary coil of the transformer. The tube kilovoltage can be adjusted and read before the tube is energized. The tube current is related to the filament current and is determined by the selection of the latter. The time of irradiation can also be chosen in advance. Some diagnostic X-ray consoles allow selection of the total X-ray output (mAs) directly after initial selection of either the tube current or the duration of irradiation. For some special procedures, such as angiography, multiple sequential radiographs at preprogrammed intervals are needed.

Therapeutic use of X-rays requires a more exact and reproducible selection of tube potential and current than is needed for diagnostic purposes. In addition, X-ray tubes for therapy have changeable filters. By changes in the applied kilovoltage or filter, or both, beams of different penetration can be produced. For added safety, switches are usually included on the console of the machine for selection of a needed filter. These switches are wired into an electrical interlock circuit that ensures that the chosen filter is in the path of the beam before the beam can be turned on. Ideally, the consoles of therapy machines should have a press-the-button type of selection of tube potential, current, and filter, rather than a continuously adjustable selection, so that the values of the parameters can be reproduced exactly.

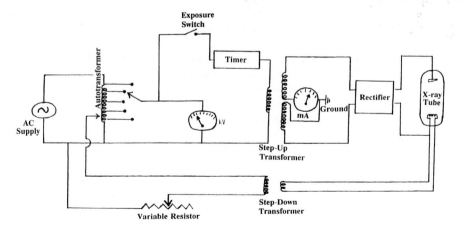

Fig. 8.10. Schematic diagram of the components of an X-ray circuit

8.6
X-Ray Spectra and Quality

8.6.1
X-Ray Spectra in Practicle

We have discussed (in Section 6.3) the production of continuous X-rays or brems-strahlung when electrons slow down in a target material. Because the electrons gain an energy of V keV when the tube potential is V kV, the value of E_{max} (representing the loss of the entire electron energy) is given by

$$E_{max} = V \ keV \qquad (8\text{-}5)$$

The low-energy photons do not penetrate deeply enough to be of any practical utility. X-ray beams for practical use need to have added filters of aluminum or copper to cut off the soft components. In the absence of prefiltering, the soft X-rays would strike the patient to be absorbed in the superficial layers, merely contributing to the skin dose. Cutting out the soft components is referred to as beam hardening. An X-ray spectrum obtained in practice (Figure 8.11) also has superimposed spikes of characteristic X-ray energies of the target element. The characteristic X-rays are due to the electron transitions within the atomic energy levels of the target atoms, and thus they have energies specific to the target material. The ionization and excitation events within the target are responsible for the characteristic X-rays that are emitted. The transitions to fill K, L, and M electron vacancies, respectively, produce K, L, and M characteristic X-rays. The K X-rays themselves can be grouped into $K_{\alpha 1}$, $K_{\alpha 2}$, $K_{\beta 1}$, $K_{\beta 2}$, etc., depending upon which outer orbital electron fills the K-shell vacancy.

Characteristic X-rays are also produced in any filter material interposed in the path of the emerging beam. For example, aluminum filters in the beam will add characteristic X-rays of aluminum. A composite filter having a layer of tin (Z = 50), followed by a layer of copper (Z = 29), followed by a layer of aluminum (Z = 13) was designed by Thoreaus for use in 200- to 240-kV therapy beams. In the Thoreaus filter, the beam

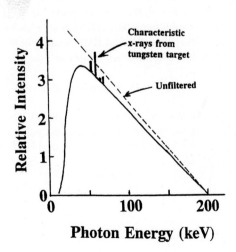

Fig. 8.11. Typical X-ray spectra including the characteristic X-ray peaks from a tungsten target at 200 kV with (——) and without (– – –) filters added in the beam

first falls on tin, which effectively filters out the low-energy components. However, it also generates its own undesirable soft characteristic X-rays. These are absorbed in the copper layer, but copper contributes its own weak characteristic X-rays. These are absorbed by the subsequent layer of aluminum. Thus, Thoreaus filters produce a well-hardened beam.

8.6.2
Beam Quality and Half-Value Thickness

The word "quality," when applied to X-ray spectra, has a broader meaning than merely energy, although it is often used in the latter sense in radiation physics. Also, X-ray beams are not monoenergetic and cannot be characterized by stating of a single energy. There is a need to have a single parameter that can be used for comparing X-ray spectra. An accepted method is to specify the beam quality in terms of the "half value thickness" (HVT), which is the thickness of a material that reduces the intensity of a beam to one half of its initial value. The HVT can be stated in thickness of aluminum or copper. We discussed in Section 7.10 the difference between narrow-beam and broad-beam conditions for attenuation measurements. Because the narrow-beam HVT values are unique, they are used as indicators of the beam quality for typical X-ray beams. Usually, the HVT is given in millimeters of aluminum for X-rays up to 120 kV and in millimeters of copper for X-rays of higher energies. Information on the waveform, kVp, added filtration, and HVT gives a comprehensive description of the beam quality for practical purposes.

8.6.3
Homogeneity Index

The HVT defined above is called the first HVT. An inhomogeneous (i. e., having a wide spectrum) X-ray beam (such as that shown in Figure 8.11) is hardened after its passage through a filter. Let us say that an X-ray beam passes through a filter of one HVT. It will emerge hardened, i. e., it will have a higher average energy, at the exit side. By addition of more filter material, the beam intensity can be reduced by another half (i. e., to one fourth of the unfiltered intensity). Such an added thickness is the second HVT, which would be thicker than the first HVT because of the hardening of the inhomogeneous beam. We define a homogeneity index as

$$\text{Homogeneity index} = \frac{\text{first HVT}}{\text{second HVT}}$$

This index is a measure of the inhomogeneity of the beam. A homogeneous monochromatic beam is not hardened or changed in quality upon filtration. It can be expected to have identical values for the first and second HVT, with a homogeneity index of unity.

CHAPTER 9

Equipment for Radioisotope Teletherapy

9.1
Concept of Teletherapy

In external-beam therapy (or teletherapy), a radiation beam coming from a source located at a distance from the patient is directed toward the patient. The source of the radiation emitted is enclosed in a heavily shielded source head. The prefix "tele" (meaning far or distant) in teletherapy (in contrast to the prefix brachy, meaning near or short, in brachytherapy) signifies the use of a large source-to-patient distance. In most practical cases, this distance is in the range of 30 to 150 cm.

The designs of individual teletherapy machines vary widely. There are two broad categories of teletherapy machines: those that make use of the nuclear gamma rays from a radioisotope source, and accelerators, in which electrons are first subjected to forces from which they gain enough energy. (The conventional X-ray machines discussed in the previous chapter are low-energy electron accelerators.) The energetic electrons can be spread out to produce an electron beam, or they can be directed to strike a target and generate an X-ray beam, for irradiating the patient. Some of the modern therapy accelerators are so versatile that they can produce electron beams of several energies and photon beams of one or two energies.

Accelerators have also been used for production of beams of neutrons, protons, helium ions, and other heavy charged particles for radiotherapy. However, it is expensive to produce these beams, and they are currently being used at research facilities for clinical trials only. Discussion of these beams is not within the scope of this book. The aim in this chapter is to discuss radioisotope teletherapy equipment and to describe, in addition, certain features and accessories that are needed for positioning and directing the beam in external-beam therapy.

9.2
Radioisotope Sources

9.2.1
Requirements for the Source

Radiation intensity falls off as the inverse square of the distance from the source. The fall-off is very rapid at short distances from the source. Improved uniformity of the dose delivered within the tumor volume results when the treatment distance is large. This large treatment distance, in turn, demands that the radioactive source used for teletherapy have a very high rate of radiation emission, so that the treatment times will be reasonably short. A typical radiation treatment (delivering a dose of 2 to 3 Gy) should require a delivery period of not more than 2 to 4 minutes to be practical. Source activities of the order of 10^{14} disintegrations/sec (i. e., 100 TBq) are needed, so that the dose rate at the patient distance will be adequate to meet this criterion. Furthermore, as will be shown later, a radiation source having a small size produces a beam with a sharp edge and an acceptable penumbra (see Section 9.3.5). Providing a large source strength in a source of less than 2.0 cm diameter requires a very high concentration of activity (specific activity). Another practical requirement is that the source isotope should have a long half life, so that there will be no need to make daily decay corrections for dose calculations, or to make frequent replacements of decayed sources.

9.2.2
Some Radioisotopes to be Considered for Teletherapy

Table 9.1 lists some radioisotope sources that have been used for teletherapy. Among these, ^{60}Co has proved to be the most viable. ^{60}Co is produced by neutron activation in a reactor. The technical advances of activation in high-neutron-flux reactors have made it possible to produce ^{60}Co sources of 0.5 to 2.0 cm diameter which have sufficient activity for use in teletherapy. ^{60}Co also has a fairly long half life of 5.26 years. It emits photons of megavoltage energies, 1.17 and 1.33 MeV, and hence not only yields sufficient photon energy per disintegration, but also gives a beam of high penetration. The phenomenon of secondary electron build-up at the air-tissue interface with such high-energy beams also provides the major advantage of a reduced skin dose and thus skin sparing (see Section 11.3).

^{137}Cs is extracted chemically from fission product wastes of nuclear reactors. During the extraction process, another isotope, ^{134}Cs, becomes a contaminant. Compared to the 30-year half life of ^{137}Cs, ^{134}Cs has a half life of only 2 years. Whereas ^{137}Cs (after first becoming metastable ^{137}Ba by beta decay) emits monoenergetic photons of 660 keV, ^{134}Cs emits several low-energy photons. The main problem with ^{137}Cs is its low specific

Table 9.1. Characteristics of Radioisotopes for Use in Teletherapy

Radioisotope	Method of Production	Useful Emission	Half Life	Activity* Needed for 1 Gy/min at 1 m
^{60}Co	Neutron activation of ^{59}Co	Photons 1.17 MeV 1.33 MeV	5.26 years	1.7×10^{14} Bq (4.6 kCi)
^{137}Cs	Fission product Extraction	Photons 0.66 MeV	30 years	6.7×10^{14} Bq (18.1 kCi)
^{192}Ir	Neutron activation of ^{191}Ir	11 photons from 0.136–0.613 MeV	74.5 d	3.76×10^{14} Bq (10.2 kCi)
^{226}Ra	Naturally occurring	Many photons up to 2.2 MeV (mean, 0.87 MeV)	1602 years	2.67×10^{14} Bq (7.22 kCi)

* These are typical estimates. Because of self-attenuation within the source, this activity can vary depending on the source diameter and design.

activity, which requires sources that are large (3 to 5 cm in diameter), and yet they have a low radiation output. ^{137}Cs teletherapy machines have been used at short treatment distances and with extended collimating cones that reduce the penumbra. Although some ^{137}Cs units are still in operation around the world, it is likely that they will gradually be phased out.

^{226}Ra is a decay product of the naturally occurring uranium isotope ^{238}U. In the past, radium in equilibrium with its daughter products has been used extensively for radiotherapy, especially for brachytherapy. Although radium became the first radioelement used for therapy after its discovery by Marie Curie in 1898, it has many disadvantages as a radioactive source. Its very long half life of about 1600 years is an advantage. However, radium is scarce and expensive, and it is difficult to make sources of high specific activity. Radium (in secular equilibrium with radon and its daughter products) emits photons with a wide range of energies. Its low-energy photons not only are partly absorbed within the source, but also do not penetrate deeply through tissue. Its high-energy photons, on the other hand, are too penetrating and demand heavy shielding around the source head so that leakage levels become acceptable.

Radium, which reigned supreme in brachytherapy for many years, never became a serious contender as a teletherapy source. Nowadays, even for brachytherapy, ^{137}Cs, ^{192}Ir, and ^{60}Co have superseded radium. Table 9.1 also lists ^{192}Ir, purely for academic interest. Some consideration had been given to adopting ^{192}Ir as a teletherapy source, but it has too short a half life and too low an average photon energy to be useful.

The discussion in the next sections focuses on ^{60}Co machines because of their remarkable worldwide acceptance and success.

9.3
^{60}Co Teletherapy Machines

9.3.1
The Source Head

The source head (or treatment head) is the heavily shielded section of the machine that contains the radioactive source. Radiation from the source is emitted in all directions. If whole-body irradiation of the patient is to be avoided, the source needs to be shielded on all sides, except for an aperture through which the beam can emerge, as shown in Figure 9.1a. This aperture, which is referred to as the primary collimator, determines the largest available cross section of the beam to be produced by the machine. For treatment of smaller cross sections, an adjustable secondary collimator is attached to the primary one. Additional shaping of the beam cross section is accomplished by placement of shaped lead blocks on a tray inserted in the beam. Heavy metals such as lead, tungsten, or uranium can be used for source shielding and collimation. Tungsten and uranium are more expensive than lead, but have higher densities. Using them can keep the shielding more compact, as the thickness needed can be 1.4 to 1.8 times less than that required for lead. Some source heads and collimation systems combine these different materials in a cost-effective way.

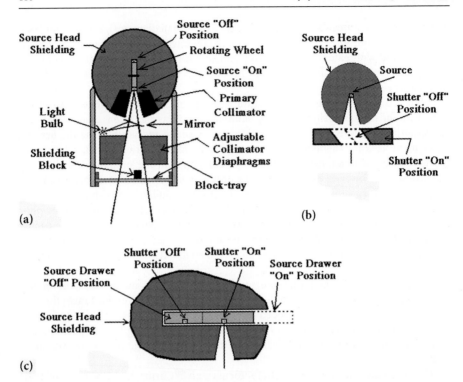

Fig. 9.1. (a) A source head of a teletherapy machine with a radioactive source on a rotating wheel as the beam on-off mechanism. The associated beam delivery system is also shown. (b) A source head having a fixed source and a shutter as the on-off mechanism. (c) A source head with a source affixed to a movable drawer as the on-off mechanism

9.3.2
Light Beam Localizer

For the purpose of visualizing the area to be irradiated on the patient's skin during treatment set-up, the radiation beam is usually simulated by a light beam. This is achieved by a light source and mirror arrangement, as shown in Figure 9.1a. The light appears to diverge from the position of the radioactive source and thus helps to show the location of the radiation beam. A cross hair made of opaque wires can be positioned in the light beam so that it casts its shadow to indicate the central ray of the beam. (Light beam localizers are also used in conventional X-ray machines and accelerators.)

9.3.3
Source on-off Mechanism

To control the dose delivered to the patient, it is necessary to control the time during which the beam emerges through the aperture. For this purpose, the source head includes a mechanism for turning the beam on and off. The source is said to be in the "off" position when it is completely shielded. In the "on" position, the radiation from the source can irradiate the patient through the primary collimator. After a precalculated treatment time, the source is to be restored to its "off" position.

The beam "off" to "on" and "on" to "off" functions are achieved by different mechanisms in different designs. In Figure 9.1a, a rotating wheel moves the source from the shielded "off" position to the "on" position, in which it is aligned with the axis of the collimating aperture. In Figure 9.1b, the "on-off" mechanism uses a shutter that opens and closes. In Figure 9.1c, the source is mounted in a rectangular drawer that moves it from the "off" to the "on" position, and vice versa. In the "off" position, a light bulb mounted in the drawer can provide the field simulation. Some early designs of ^{60}Co machines used an "on-off" shutter system in which mercury flowed into or was pumped out of the primary collimating aperture.

The specific details of the source "on-off" mechanism can have a bearing on the procedure to be used for replacement of a decayed source. ^{60}Co sources need to be replaced at intervals of 3 to 5 years. The source replacement procedure must be carried out with the utmost care. It involves, first, the transfer of the old source from the source head to a shielded transport container. This is followed by loading of the new source into the source head. Both old and new sources have high activity and hence can deliver lethal doses if handled carelessly.

9.3.4
Source Capsule

The source capsule is a double-walled, sealed container that envelops the radioactive ^{60}Co. The contents of the capsule can be made up of several metal pellets or of disks of radioactive ^{60}Co. The external dimensions of sources are made to satisfy the international standards for a source capsule agreed upon by the atomic energy control authorities of the various source-manufacturing countries. This standardization makes it possible for sources from different suppliers to be used interchangeably. The shape of the sources is generally a cylinder, and the source is used with the axis of the cylinder coinciding with the central ray of the beam. The radioactive part within the capsule may be up to 3 cm in diameter and 3 cm in height. A small source, with 1.0 to 2.0 cm diameter, is preferred because it can provide a beam of good clinical quality with sharp edges.

9.3.5
Geometric Penumbra

We can construct some geometric projections to examine the edge of the beam for a source that is not an ideal point source, but has a finite size. The right side of the top part of Figure 9.2 shows solid lines that connect the lateral edges of the source with the distal edge of the beam-limiting diaphragm (or collimator). The geometric edge of the beam is the dashed line between the continuous lines that connects the center of the source (which would be the position of an ideal point source) with the distal edge of the diaphragm. This dashed line also corresponds to the field edge projected by the light beam localizer. At the level of the patient's skin, the point P_g at the geometric edge will see one half of the source, whereas the point P_c at the central ray will see the full

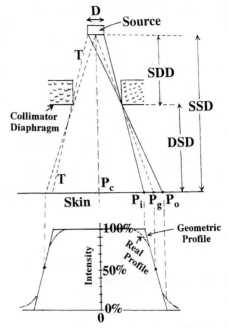

op) Geometric pro- the rays from the rough a collimating m. (Bottom) Shapes diation intensity profiles as interpreted geometrically (solid line) and as observed in reality (dashed-dotted line)

source. Thus, the intensity at P_g can be expected to be half of that at P_c. From P_i, the full source is visible. At P_o, the source just becomes invisible.

The lower part of Figure 9.2 shows the geometrically inferred radiation intensity profile, with a straight line connecting the intensities at P_i, P_g, and P_o. The points P_i and P_o mark the inner and outer edges of the penumbra. The distance P_iP_o is called the geometric penumbra width and is given by

$$P_iP_o = \frac{D(SSD - SDD)}{SDD}$$

where D, SSD, and SDD are (see Figure 9.2) the source diameter, the source-to-skin distance, and the distance from the source to the distal end of the diaphragm, respectively. It is desirable to minimize the width of the penumbra by optimizing the values of D, SDD, and SSD. P_iP_o can be reduced if D is decreased or SDD is increased. However, it is not practical to reduce the source diameter D beyond a certain limit, as the source activity will be diminished. On the other hand, reducing the DSD to very short distances causes a different problem. Ideally, we would like to produce a beam that consists of photons only, without any electrons. However, the photons interacting with the surface of the diaphragm release secondary electrons. These electrons travel to the skin and enhance the skin dose, thus spoiling the dose build-up and skin sparing possible with high-energy photon beams (see Section 11.3). Such "electron contamination" cannot be eliminated altogether, but can increase to unacceptable levels if the diaphragm is too close to the skin.

As a practical compromise between the need to keep the penumbra small and the electron contamination low, a gap of at least 20 cm between the diaphragm and skin during any treatment is recommended. Because the electron contamination is influenced by the area of the diaphragm that is exposed to the beam, it increases with the beam cross section. A sheet of plastic of a low-Z material can be used to cover the diaphragm's distal end and thus reduce the electron contamination. The plastic sheet absorbs the many electrons coming from the diaphragm; however, in turn, it releases a few secondary electrons that arise due to photon interactions taking place within it. Because more electrons are absorbed by the plastic material than are released by it, the skin dose is reduced. (X-ray machines and particle accelerators used in the X-ray mode also have a geometric penumbra. However, in general, the geometric penumbras are narrow, because of the smaller focal spots of radiation emission compared to those of radioisotope sources.)

9.3.6
Transmission Penumbra

In the foregoing discussion, we only dealt with geometric projections of the bottom edge of the diaphragm and ignored the fact that, in practice, the diaphragm is rather thick. About 6 to 7 cm of lead is commonly needed to reduce the radiation transmitted through the diaphragm to below 5%. Significant transmission can occur for the oblique rays such as the rays labeled T in Figure 9.2. These rays add a transmission penumbra and smear the geometric penumbra. The real radiation intensity profile, combining the geometric and transmission effects, is also illustrated in the lower part of Figure 9.2. The transmission penumbra can be reduced (but not eliminated) by improved design of the beam-collimating diaphragm, which we discuss next.

9.3.7
Designs of Adjustable Diaphragms

Figures 9.3a, b, and c show different diaphragm designs. In all of these figures, the dark blocks control the beam width in the plane of the paper, and the gray blocks control the beam width in the perpendicular direction. In the design shown in Figure 9.3a, the straight-edged lead blocks can be moved closer together or farther apart. In this design, the penumbra in the two perpendicular directions can be different because of their different distances from the source. In Figure 9.3b, a convergent multilayered collimator is shown, with the layers in the perpendicular directions alternating with those in the plane of the figure. The edges of the layers are aligned with the geometric edge of the beam. Figure 9.3c shows a nonconvergent multilayered collimator, and Figure 9.3d illustrates the appearance of the aperture (for all three types) as seen from the skin.

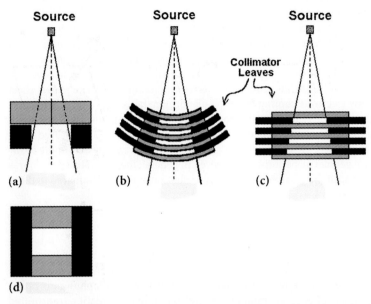

Fig. 9.3. Different diaphragm designs. The dark blocks and the gray blocks are in the plane of the paper and perpendicular to it, respectively. (**a**) Diaphragm made of thick blocks. (**b**) Multi-layered diaphragm that moves in an arc. (**c**) Multilayered diaphragm that moves in a straight line. (**d**) Axial view of the above three types of diaphragms from the position of the patient

9.4
Miscellaneous Features and Accessories

9.4.1
Movement of Treatment Head and Patient Support

Every teletherapy machine has a treatment head that encloses the source of radiation (Figure 9.4). The treatment head is mounted in such a way that it can be moved and the beam can be oriented in any desired way toward the patient. The patient is positioned for treatment on a couch (or treatment table) that is capable of controlled movement. The controllable movement and the reproducible positioning of the treatment head and of the patient support couch are very important features of any treatment machine. The total radiation dose in a typical external-beam treatment is accumulated in small daily fractions, and the treatment is carried out over several weeks. Therefore, it is imperative that the positional set up for any patient be reproduced from day to day.

9.4.2
Optical Distance Indicator

The optical distance indicator (ODI) is an accessory incorporated in the treatment head to help measure the distance of the patient surface from the source position along the central ray of the beam. The principle of its operation is illustrated in Figure 9.5.

Fig. 9.4. A view of the patient cross section, the couch and its support, and the source head and its gantry for a teletherapy set-up

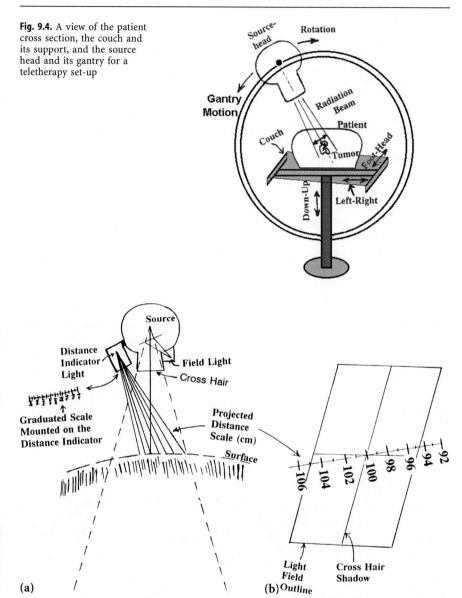

(a)

(b) Outline

Fig. 9.5. Principle of operation of an optical distance indicator. (a) The optical projection of a graduated ruler at an angle with respect to the central ray of the beam. (b) The projected scale as seen on the patient's surface within the light beam

As shown in Figure 9.5a, the distance indicator consists of a light bulb coupled to an optical device that projects the graduations of an opaque scale at an angle with respect to the central axis of the beam. The rays of the fan beam emerging from the device meet the central axis of the radiation beam at different distances from the source. The graduations indicate the distance at which the different rays meet the central ray of the fan beam. The scale as projected on the patient surface can be seen together with the light beam from the field localizer, as shown in Figure 9.5b. The reading at the central ray of the beam (which is indicated by a cross-hair shadow in the light beam) is the source-to-surface distance, which is 100 cm in the figure.

9.4.3
Back-Pointing Device

Directing a beam to cover the intended target site of irradiation is a required feature of external-beam treatments. Improperly directed beams can miss the treatment site and can damage the normal tissues that are not to be irradiated. Details of treatment planning are discussed in later chapters. A back pointer attached to the treatment head, as shown in Figure 9.6, is useful for obtaining the beam direction in situations where the skin entrance point A and the exit point B of the central ray of the treatment beam are known. This device has an arm that goes around the patient's body. It has a sliding back-pointer pin that has been aligned to move along the central ray of the beam. There is another sliding pin that acts as a front pointer, which also is aligned to coincide with the central ray of the beam. The required orientation of the beam is obtained when the patient is positioned with respect to the beam in such a way that the tips of the front-pointing pin and back-pointing pin can be adjusted to touch points A and B in the figure, respectively. The front-pointing pin carries a scale that indicates the distance from the source to the tip. Alternatively, the optical distance indicator together with the cross-hair shadow of the light beam localizer can function like a front pointer.

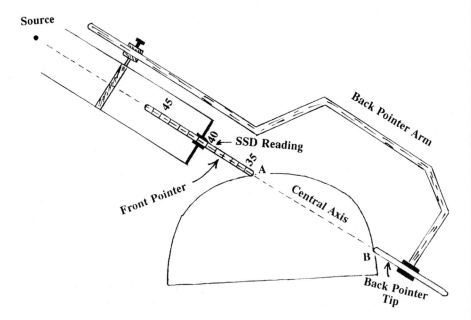

Fig. 9.6. Principle of use of a back pointer

9.5
Closing Remarks

Choosing a treatment machine among various makes and models of commercially marketed radioisotope machines or accelerators is the first important task faced by any radiotherapy clinic. Individual needs and specific situations may vary. Although medical linear accelerators offer more advanced technology compared to ^{60}Co machines, the simplicity and the cost-effectiveness of the latter continues to be proved around the world. Hence, no general recommendations as to an optimal choice of a teletherapy machine can be made. In general, the energy of the radiation emitted and the treatment distance are major considerations in the selection of a teletherapy machine for purchase. Machines having treatment distances of 80 cm or more are preferable to those with shorter distances, because they offer better depth-dose characteristics for treatment of patients (see Chapters 13 and 15). In addition, the features of the treatment head and couch motion, the ease of daily patient set-up, the beam collimation, the "on" and "off" control, and safety interlocks for avoiding catastrophic incidents (such as collision of the machine with the patient or overdosing) should all be taken into account during the selection. Purchase cost, space needed for installation, levels of radiation leakage from the source head, room shielding costs, possible down time, and ease of servicing and maintenance are all important aspects to be considered in the choice of a machine.

CHAPTER 10

Particle Accelerators

10.1
Three Categories of Accelerators

Particle or high-energy accelerators owe their development to the interest of scientists in doing physics research at high energies. Charged particles accelerated to energies of several million electron volts can be used for bombardment of target nuclides and study of their transmutations. Because electrons accelerated to high energies can be made to strike targets and produce X-rays, accelerators became useful for radiotherapy. The transformer principle used (in Chapter 8) for stepping up voltage reaches a limit at about 400 kV, where the insulation between the transformer coils breaks down. Air-core transformers extend the kilovolt range, although not significantly. Different techniques are needed for acceleration of particles to megavoltage energies. The various accelerators differ in the techniques they employ for imparting energy. Any particle of charge q is subject to a Lorentz force $\vec{F}_L$ in an electromagnetic field, given by

$$\vec{F}_L = q(\vec{E} + \vec{v} \times \vec{B})$$

where $\vec{E}$, $\vec{B}$, and $\vec{v}$ are vectors representing the magnitude and direction of the electric field, magnetic field, and particle velocity, respectively. The accelerators can be classified into three categories, according to the acceleration technique employed, as follows:

1. Direct-voltage accelerators, in which the charged particles gain energy as they travel through an applied potential difference. The electric field does not change with time during the transit of the particle. Conventional accelerators belong to this class.
2. Induction accelerators, in which the electric field is induced by a monotonically increasing magnetic flux. Betatrons belong to this type.
3. Resonance accelerators, which make use of the electric field component of a radiofrequency electromagnetic wave. The particles move along either a circular or a linear trajectory. The particles can undergo acceleration steadily if they are "in phase" with the electric field and there is a resonance between the accelerated particle and the wave pattern. The linear accelerator (linac), cyclotron, and microtron belong to this class.

10.2
Direct-Voltage, Electrostatic Accelerators

10.2.1
Tube for Acceleration

Direct-voltage electrostatic accelerators have two parts: a tube for acceleration and a high-voltage generator connected to the tube. Different types of generators can be used to produce the high voltage, but the accelerating tubes used with different generators can be of the same design.

Figure 10.1 shows an accelerating tube. The tube is maintained at a high vacuum. The high-voltage potential is divided by a series of very high resistors, and the resulting split voltages are applied to metallic electrodes inside the tube. The electric lines of force (i. e., the electric field) between successive electrodes (which are at different potentials) accelerate the particles. The fields also act to bring back to focus any particle that strays away, as is shown by a particle's track in the figure.

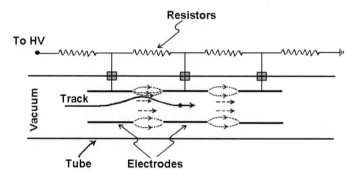

Fig. 10.1. High voltage applied to electrodes in a particle accelerating tube. The focusing effect on a particle track and the electric field lines at the gaps between electrodes are shown

10.2.2
Cockcroft-Walton Voltage Multiplier

The voltage multiplier, in principle, charges capacitors in parallel and discharges them in series. Cockcroft and Walton used two columns of capacitors for this purpose (Figure 10.2). These two columns are cross-connected through diodes (indicated as circles marked 1 and 2), which allow conduction in one direction (marked by arrows). A transformer T that produces an alternating current of peak voltage U is connected to the generator. After an initial start-up phase, voltages of 2U, 4U, and 6U are available across C_1, $(C_1 + C_2)$, and $(C_1 + C_2 + C_3)$. The voltage multiplier has been used successfully as a high-voltage supply for energies in the neighborhood of 1 MeV. Some giant accelerators, such as the one at Fermilab near Chicago and another at Los Alamos, New Mexico, employ voltage multipliers for the starting point of acceleration.

Fig. 10.2. Cockcroft-Walton
voltage multiplier circuit

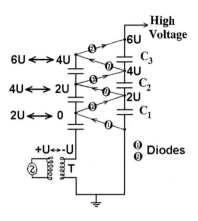

10.2.3
Van de Graaff Electrostatic Generator

The electrostatic machine, called a Van de Graaff generator (Figure 10.3), consists of a spherical high-voltage terminal supported on electrically insulated columns. A moving belt (made of a material similar to neoprene, used for electrical insulation) functions as a carrier to move electric charges. Charges of one polarity, say, negative charges (i. e., electrons), are sprayed on the belt at the grounded end from a row of sharp corona points. (Phonograph needles have been used for this purpose.) A corona discharge between these tips and ground produces ionization in the air, and charge is deposited on the moving belt. If the belt carries negative charges, the points must have a negative potential relative to ground. For accumulation of positive charges, the corona points

Fig. 10.3. Schematic diagram of
the essential parts of a Van de
Graaff generator

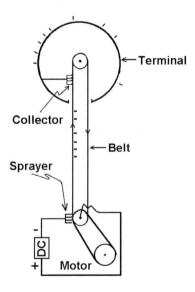

are made positive. The belt carries the charges upward. A collector screen connected to the high-voltage terminal rubs against the belt and removes the charges to store them on the terminal. With the accumulation of sufficient charge, the voltage between the high-voltage terminal and ground can reach 1 to 3 MV. (With increases in voltage, the probability of insulation breakdown increases.)

Electron, proton, and deuteron Van de Graaff generators were used for physics and biomedical research in the 1940s and 1950s. The electron machines were used for radiotherapy, but have now been retired.

10.3
Linear Accelerators

10.3.1
Principle of Linacs

In a linear accelerator (LINAC), particles travel along a straight line; hence the adjective "linear" is used. A radio frequency (RF) oscillator sends RF power to a wave guide and generates electric potential differences that accelerate a particle. The particle and the wave both move. The particle energy gradually increases, if the RF wave and the particle move in synchrony and the RF wave continues to provide a forward acceleration. This happens if there is a resonance between the RF wave and the particle.

Figure 10.4 is a schematic diagram of an early linear accelerator. An RF oscillator generates electromagnetic waves, and an electric potential results between successive tubular electrodes arranged in a cylindrical vacuum chamber. The ion source releases the ionized particles which will undergo acceleration. The RF potential changes with time in a sinusoidal manner from being positively to negatively oriented. Accordingly, the direction of the electric field at the gap betwen the elecrodes also changes. For example, if the RF frequency is 3000 MHz, the cycle will repeat every (1/3000) sec, and at intervals of (1/6000) sec the field will reverse. Thus, the direction of the electric field between the gaps will alternate, as shown by the continuous and dashed arrows. Each time a particle crosses a gap, it should find an accelerating field (and not a decelerating field), so that it will gain energy. This can be achieved by designing the separation between successive acceleration gaps to equal the distance traversed by the particle

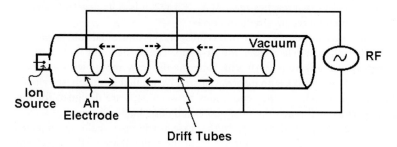

Fig. 10.4. Simplified schematic diagram of an early linear accelerator, with increasing distance between successive accelerating gaps

during one half cycle. This length is given by

$$L = \frac{1}{2} \frac{v}{f} \qquad (10\text{-}1)$$

where v is the particle velocity and f the frequency of the electric field. The separation between gaps becomes progressively larger as the particle gains more velocity and hence energy. If V_g is the voltage across the gap and q is the charge carried by the particle, the energy E gained at each gap will be

$$E = qV_g \qquad (10\text{-}2)$$

For a particle of mass m, under nonrelativistic conditions, this should be equal to the kinetic energy added. It can be shown that the length L_n of the nth electrode (which should corrrespond to a total kinetic energy of $\frac{1}{2}mv^2 = nqV_g$) will be given by

$$L_n = \frac{1}{2f} \left[2nq(V_g/m) \right]^{1/2} \qquad (10\text{-}3)$$

This expression gives the resonance condition. At relativistic energies, particles reach velocities comparable to the velocity of light c, which is also that of the RF wave, and the gap spacings become constant. This is particularly true for a particle of low mass, such as an electron, for which

$$L_n = \frac{c}{2f} = \frac{\lambda}{2} \qquad (10\text{-}4)$$

where λ is the wavelength of the applied RF.

10.3.2
Phase Stability in Linacs

In general, it is possible that a particle will cross a gap at any time during the positive cycle of the RF sine wave. Then V_g is related to the peak potential V_p (Figure 10.5) by

$$V_g = V_p \sin \phi_g \qquad (10\text{-}5)$$

where ϕ_g is the phase difference. We can understand the sine wave potential as follows: the phase ϕ_g of the wave depends on both time and location. At any location, for $\phi_g = 0$, the potential is zero. As ϕ_g increases (with time), the positive peak occurs at $\phi_g = \pi/2$. At $\phi_g = \pi$, the potential again reaches zero. At $\phi_g = 3\pi/2$, it is at its negative peak. At $\phi_g = 2\pi$, the zero potential recurs after a full cycle.

Figure 10.5 shows a continuous curve that represents the sinusoidal voltage pattern at the instant when the particle crosses the first gap. The dashed and dotted curves show the progress of the wave pattern with time. As the wave moves with its phase velocity, the particle also moves with its own velocity. We would like the phase velocity to equal the particle velocity. If the separations between gaps are designed for this condition, the particle will reach the next gap exactly one half-cycle later, at a wave phase represented by the dash-dot curve. In that case, it will once again be subjected to an acceleration by a voltage of magnitude V_g at the same phase of the wave. The same phenomenon will occur at the next gap, and so on. It is as if the particle rode on a fixed point on the wave, like a surfer. However, imagine the gap coming a little too

Fig. 10.5. Four different phases of the electric potential of an RF wave, and a charged particle riding in phase with the wave in a linear accelerator

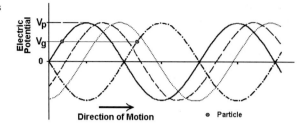

soon. Then the potential will be less than V_g, and the particle will gain less than the optimal energy. Therefore, it will travel to the next gap a little more slowly. This will let it experience a larger V_g, and hence it will gain an energy greater than intended. Thus, a continuous compensation between loss and gain occurs. This is called "phase stability."

10.3.3
Wave Guides

In electron accelerators, because the electron has a low rest energy (0.511 MeV), velocities comparable to the velocity of light c in vacuum are reached even at relatively low energies. The velocity of a 90-keV electron is 50% of c. At 2 MeV, it is 98% of c. (Heavy particles such as protons require several thousand MeV to reach similar velocities.) One can think of designing a single tubular metallic wave guide in which the RF travels, with the electron its cotraveler on the tube axis and both traveling at the velocity of light. However, this is not possible because the phase velocity of a wave in a tubular wave guide is greater than c and hence greater than the velocity of the electrons. To compensate for this, one can lower the phase velocity of the wave by the needed amount by designing wave guides (or cavities) that are "loaded" with distributed "reactive elements." These reactive elements may be one of the following: inserted metallic ribs, diaphragms, iris-loaded disks, tubes, stubs, corrugations, or layers of dielectric materials (as in the examples shown in Figure 10.6).

Fig. 10.6. Different designs of linear accelerator wave guides

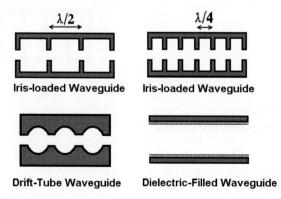

10.3.4
Standing Wave and Traveling Wave

Both standing-wave and traveling-wave linear accelerators have been used in medicine. In a traveling wave, the position of crests and troughs moves with time. In a standing wave, the positions remain steady. In a loaded wave guide, a wave can be propagated with the largest amplitude if the spacing between disks is $\lambda/2$ (Figure 10.7a). This is called π mode (i. e., phase angle $\pi^c = 180°$). If the wave guide terminates after a finite number of disks and the waves are reflected from the end, a standing wave results. The wave is a sum of the forward and reflected sinusoidal components, which are out of phase with each other by 180°. The guide acts like a resonance cavity at this frequency, with the diaphragms located at the nodes of the standing-wave pattern.

A different way of using a loaded wave guide is to employ diaphragms that are $\lambda/4$ apart, which leads to a nonreflecting termination by absorption of the RF at the forward end (Figure 10.7b). This produces a traveling wave. It is as though a sine wave and a cosine wave were present with a phase difference of $\pi/2$ (i. e., 90°). Hence this is called $\pi/2$ mode.

The standing-wave and traveling-wave systems have their respective advantages and disadvantages. In general, the standing-wave type has advantages at low energies. A standing wave is inefficient because it tries to combine two components that are out of phase. On the other hand, the traveling-wave guide employs more disks at closer intervals of 90° phase, and hence it incurs more resistive losses in the guide. The standing-wave guide employs only half as many diaphragms. Other comparisons may involve the dimensions of the diaphragms, methods of power input to the wave guide, and the power efficiency of the microwave cavity circuit.

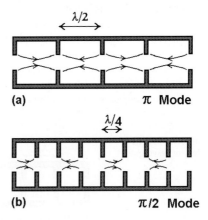

Fig. 10.7. Linear accelerator wave guides of π mode and $\pi/2$ mode

10.3.5
Clinical Linear Accelerator

A block diagram of the various sections of a clinical linear accelerator is shown in Figure 10.8. A power supply provides the necessary DC power to a pulse-forming network of capacitance and inductance. The pulses trigger both an electron gun (which

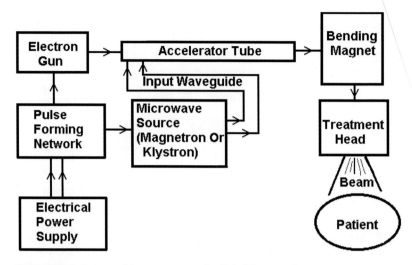

Fig. 10.8. Block diagram of the components of a clinical linear accelerator

is the source of electrons) and a microwave oscillator. The electrons released are accelerated through the wave guide. After the electrons gain their full energy, they are bent by a magnetic field. They are then made to pass through a treatment head, that is, a system for delivering a clinically useful beam.

Figure 10.9 shows the beam delivery system in the treatment head. The electrons can be made to strike a target to produce X-rays. The X-rays produced at megavoltage energies have a forward-peaked distribution of intensity (see Section 6.3.3) and thus do not cover a clinically useful area uniformly. Hence they are made to go through a suitably designed beam-flattening filter which is thick at its center and thin toward the edge. The system includes a primary collimator. The beam passes through one or more ionization chambers that monitor the beam intensity. The beam size is then restricted by a variable collimator before it strikes the patient.

Individual designs of accelerators and treatment heads vary widely. Some designs use no bending magnets, and others use 90° bending; and there are some others, as illustrated in Figure 10.9, that employ 270° bending. In modern accelerators designed for radiation therapy, the beam emerges from a treatment head that is mounted on a gantry which can be rotated around a patient. Such a system is referred to as isocentrically mounted.

Instead of striking a target to produce X-rays, the accelerated electron beam of small cross section can be spread out by a scattering foil to produce an electron beam that can cover a clinically useful area on the patient. An alternative method for spreading the electrons is to use a magnetic field to produce a scanning electron pencil beam (see Section 16.2).

The X-ray target, the flattening filter, the electron-scattering foils (with different foils for different electron energies), the monitor ion chambers, and the mirror of the light beam localizer can all be moved in and out of the path of the beam as needed. Appropriately designed interlocks are usually incorporated to ensure that no patient

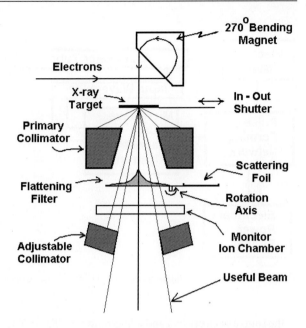

Fig. 10.9. Beam delivery system of a clinical electron accelerator

irradiation can be carried out with an improper combination of devices in the beam path.

The beam from an accelerator is emitted in pulses. It differs from a radioisotope therapy machine that gives a steady output and hence allows the use of timing of the irradiation to control the dose delivered. For accelerators, the signals from the monitoring ion chambers are needed for control of the patient dose and for terminating the irradiation at a preselected intensity level. The electron spectrum for a traveling-wave accelerator is shown in Figure 10.10.

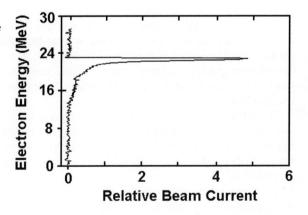

Fig. 10.10. Electron spectrum obtained from a traveling-wave linear accelerator. (Figure is based on Reference 6 cited for additional reading.)

10.4
Betatron

The betatron is an electron accelerator of the resonance type. It is a magnetic induction-type accelerator and uses a circular path of electrons. The path in the betatron is a circle of fixed radius, referred to as the equilibrium orbit. A ceramic high-vacuum chamber called a "donut" is placed between the truncated poles of a magnet that is powered by an alternating current of 50 to 200 Hz (Figure 10.11). The principle that a changing magnetic flux within a closed loop can create an electric field along the loop is used for acceleration of electrons in a betatron. First, the magnetic lines of force (shown by dashed lines in Figure 10.11a) exert a force on the electron normal to its path and keep it in its circular equilibrium orbit within the donut. A change in the magnetic flux through the orbit produces electric field lines that are in the shape of concentric circles. The electric field at the equilibrium orbit of the donut accelerates the electrons. (The betatron is analogous to a transformer in which the current through the primary coil excites the magnet. The secondary current is the electron beam current in the vacuum chamber. However, there is no conductor that carries the secondary current.) As the electron gains energy, it tends to move out of the equilibrium orbit. For the

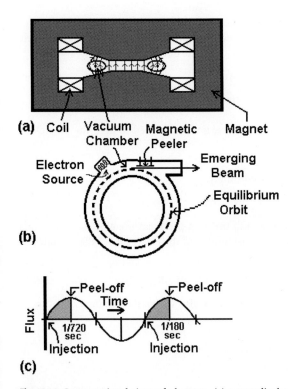

Fig. 10.11. Cross-sectional views of a betatron (a) perpendicular to the plane of particle motion, (b) in the plane of particle motion, and (c) magnetic flux vs. time with injection and ejection of the electron beam from a betatron

electron to be held in its orbit, the magnetic field must be increased. This increase in the magnetic field strength will produce an electric field, so that the electron will gain still more energy. Then a still stronger magnetic field will be needed to hold the electron in the equilibrium orbit. This further increase in the magnetic flux will make the electron experience a continuing electric field, and, thus, the electron gains more energy. The cycle continues until the alternating current exciting the magnet reaches its peak and starts to decrease. Before this instant, an iron "peeler" can be inserted which, by creating a magnetic-field-free region, lets the electrons emerge tangentially from the donut (Figure 10.11b).

The rate of increase of magnetic flux should be appropriate so that the path of the electron is the equilibrium orbit during the entire acceleration cycle. The electrons are injected in phase with the alternating current (AC) when the magnetic field at the orbit is near zero, and are allowed to circulate until the peak of the field is reached after a quarter period of the AC cycle. At this point, when the magnetic field is nearly maximum, the orbit is expanded by pulsing of a single coil, and the electrons are ejected. The betatron is idle for the next three quarters of the AC cycle, and then another bundle of electrons is injected and accelerated with the first quarter of the next cycle of the alternating current. Thus, the machine operates in a pulsed mode at the same frequency as the AC exciting the magnetic flux, as shown diagrammatically in Figure 10.11c.

The condition for the electron to remain in the equilibrium orbit can be derived mathematically. Let R be the radius of the equilibrium orbit and B the magnetic field at the orbit. The Lorentz force F_L acting on a particle of charge q is

$$\vec{F}_L = q\vec{v} \times \vec{B} \tag{10-6}$$

where v is the velocity of the orbiting electron. The magnitude of $\vec{F}_L$ is (qvB) when $\vec{v}$ is at right angles to $\vec{B}$.

The force F_L provides the centrifugal force, mv^2/R, needed to hold the particle in its orbit. Hence,

$$qvB = mv^2/R \tag{10-7}$$

The momentum p of the particle is, accordingly,

$$p = mv = qBR \tag{10-8}$$

The change of the magnetic flux Φ within the loop produces the electric field E that accelerates the electron. The rate of change of Φ and the electric field E are related to each other by the equation

$$2\pi RE = -d\Phi/dt = \pi R^2\, dB/dt \tag{10-9}$$

The force acting on the particle is qE, which is also the rate of change of momentum p.

Thus,

$$dp/dt = qE = (1/2\pi)(q/R)(d\Phi/dt) \tag{10-10}$$

From Equation (10-8), we also obtain

$$dp/dt = q(dB/dt)R \tag{10-11}$$

Equating (10-10) and (10-11), we obtain

$$d\Phi/dt = -2\pi R^2(dB/dt) \qquad (10\text{-}12)$$

This is the betatron resonance condition. The energy spectrum of the extracted electron beam is quite monoenergetic, i. e., at 20 MeV the spread is less than $\pm10\,kV$.

10.5
Cyclotron

In a cyclotron, a fixed magnetic field causes the particle under acceleration to travel in a spiraling orbit. The radius of the orbit changes with increasing energy of the particle. The energy is delivered by an alternating electric field of a fixed frequency. A schematic diagram is shown in Figure 10.12.

The ion source, which is the source of protons or other heavy particles, is located in the geometric center of the cyclotron. The two D-shaped electrodes (called "dees") are connected to an AC source. This creates an electric field E at the gap between the straight portions of the two dees. A constant magnetic induction is supplied by two magnetic poles lying above and below the vacuum chamber. After the positive ions leave the source, they are accelerated to position 1 in Figure 10.12. Here, they enter the dee. Due to the magnetic induction, the ions travel in a circle to reach position 2. The time, t, for an ion to go from position 1 to 2 is given by

$$t = \pi R/v \qquad (10\text{-}13)$$

where πR is the periphery of the semicircular orbit of radius R and v is the velocity of the particle. The value R is related to the magnetic induction B [see Equation (10-7)] by the balance of forces:

$$Bqv = mv^2/R$$

Fig. 10.12. Cross-sectional views of a cyclotron (a) perpendicular to the plane of particle motion and (b) in the plane of particle motion

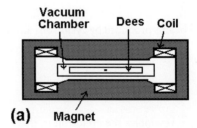

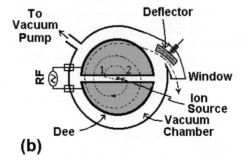

or

$$R = (mv)/(Bq) \qquad (10\text{-}14)$$

From (10-13) and (10-14), we obtain

$$t = (\pi m)/(Bq) \qquad (10\text{-}15)$$

This means that the orbital transit time from one gap to another in the dees is independent of the particle's velocity. For constant values of B, m, and q, if the value of t matches the half-period of the alternating current, the particle can pass from one dee to the other with the electric field in the proper direction to give it an acceleration. After acceleration to the required energy, a deflector is used which causes the particle to exit through a window.

The cyclotron's resonance condition fails at relativistic energies where the particle's velocity becomes comparable to the velocity of light, c. Then m, and hence t, becomes a function of v. Because of this, a cyclotron is suitable for accelerating heavy particles and not electrons. It can accelerate protons (ionized hydrogen), deuterons (ionized deuterium), or alpha particles (ionized helium). The cyclotron has been used for production of radioactive isotopes of many stable elements. For example, ^{32}P is a widely used beta source produced by the following reaction:

$$^{2}_{1}H + ^{31}_{15}P \rightarrow ^{32}_{15}P + ^{1}_{1}H$$

$^{32}_{15}P$ decays as follows:

$$^{32}_{15}P \rightarrow ^{32}_{16}S + e^{-}$$

Cyclotrons can be used for producing neutrons for therapy by bombardment of a low-atomic-number material with high-energy deuterons. A typical reaction used is

$$^{2}_{1}H + ^{9}_{4}Be \rightarrow ^{10}_{5}B + ^{1}_{0}n + 4.36\,MeV$$

The energy of 4.36 MeV is shared between the neutron and the recoiling boron nuclide. The neutron beams produced by cyclotrons are not monoenergetic.

10.6
Microtron

The microtron resembles the cyclotron in that charged particles are accelerated in a fixed-frequency resonant cavity. Also, as in a cyclotron, the particles move in a constant magnetic field B, describing circular trajectories of increasing radius. A schematic diagram of a microtron is shown in Figure 10.13.

As the particle passes through the resonant cavity, it gains energy. The radius R of the orbit and the transit time t for each turn change continuously. If R_n is the radius of the nth turn and T_n the transit time from exiting to reentering of the resonant cavity,

$$T_n = (2\pi E_n)/(c^2 qB) \qquad (10\text{-}16)$$

where q is the charge and E_n the particle energy at the nth cycle. If the particle encounters the field of the cavity in the same constant phase (ϕ), so that it is accelerated, the time T_n for all n must be integral multiples of the period (T_e) of the electric field. If E_o

Fig. 10.13. View of the microtron in the plane containing the particle track

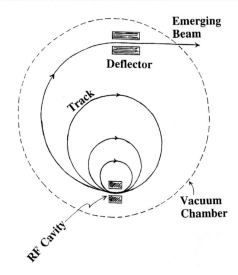

is the rest energy of the particle,

$$E_n = E_o + nqU \sin\phi \quad \text{for } n = 1, 2, \ldots \tag{10-17}$$

where U is the peak accelerating potential. The difference $[T_n - T_{n-1}]$ should be an integral multiple (say, j) of T_e for resonance to occur; i. e.,

$$T_n - T_{n-1} = jT_e \tag{10-18}$$

From (10-16) and (10-17),

$$T_n - T_{n-1} = 2\pi \left[E_n - E_{n-1}\right] / (c^2 qB) \tag{10-19}$$

$$= 2\pi U \sin\phi / (c^2 B) \tag{10-20}$$

From (10-18) and (10-20),

$$2\pi U \sin\phi / (c^2 B) = jT_e \tag{10-21}$$

This is the synchronization condition. If T_1 is an integral multiple of T_e, e. g., (kT_e), then, from (10-16) and (10-17),

$$T_1 = 2\pi \left[E_o + qU \sin\phi\right] / (c^2 qB) = kT_e \tag{10-22}$$

From (10-21) and (10-22), we can derive

$$U \sin\phi = (E_o/q) \left[j/(k-j)\right] \tag{10-23}$$

The frequency of the electric field f_e is

$$f_e = 1/T_e = (c^2 Bq)(k-j)/(2\pi E_o) \tag{10-24}$$

The value of k must be greater than j to result in a positive f_e. $k = 2$ and $j = 1$ are the smallest values possible. For example, for $B = 0.1$ Weber m^{-2} and $f_e = 2800$ MHz with 10.7 cm wavelength,

$$T_2 - T_1 = 1; \ j = 1; \ k = 2; \quad \text{and} \quad (k-j) = 1$$

we obtain, from (10-24),

$$E_o/q = \frac{c^2 B(k-j)}{2\pi f_e)} = \frac{[3.0 \times 10^8 \text{ m sec}^{-1}]^2 \times 0.1 \text{ Weber m}^{-2}}{2\pi \times 2800 \times 10^6 \text{ sec}^{-1}} = 511\,\text{kV}$$

From (10-23), for $|\sin \phi|$ to be ≤ 1, we need to satisfy the condition

$$U \geq E_o/q = 511\,\text{kV}$$

Such high voltages are possible with modern microwave technology. Smaller values of U can be chosen if a longer time for one orbit is used. If so, higher frequencies should be employed. Usually, a higher U needs a smaller number of turns and better separation between orbits.

The microtron enjoys the benefit of built-in phase stability (see Section 10.3.2). In some microtrons, the electrons to be accelerated are obtained directly by field emission from the walls of the cavity. In some others, the electrons are emitted from a small cathode located just outside the cavity.

Additional Reading

1. Karzmark, C.J., Nunan, C.S., Tanabe, E., Medical Electron Accelerators, McGraw-Hill, New York, 1993.
2. Ford, J.C., Advances in accelerator design, In Radiation Oncology Physics, 1986, Medical Physics Monograph No. 15 (Ed. Kereiakes, J. et al.), American Association of Physicists in Medicine, American Institute of Physics, New York, 1987.
3. Karzmark, C.J., Advances in linear accelerator design for radiotherapy, Med. Phys., Vol 11, p105–128, 1984.
4. Silverman, R., DiStasio, J. (Eds.) Radiation Therapy with Heavy Particles and Fast Electrons, Noyes Data Corporation, Park Ridge, New Jersey, 1980.
5. Karzmark, C.J., Electron linear accelerators for radiotherapy, history, principles and contemporary developments, Phys. Med. Biol., Vol 18, p321–354, 1973.
6. Lanzl, L.H., Magnetic and threshold techniques for energy calibration of high-energy radiations, Ann. N.Y. Acad. Sci., Vol 161, p101–108, July 3, 1969.
7. Green, D., an Willimas, P.C., Linear Accelerators for Radiation Therapy, Institute of Physics Publishing, Bristol, UK. 1997.

PART IV

Radiation Quantities, Units, and Detectors

Quantification of Radiation Field:
Radiation Units and Measurements

11.1
Radiation Field

In practical applications of radiation, the intensity of the radiation is a spatial variable, i. e., there is a radiation field. The radiation field comprises both the primary radiation coming directly from a source and any secondary emissions (Compton electrons, scattered photons, characteristic X-rays, etc.) arising due to the interactions of the primary radiation with matter. The radiation-induced processes of ionization and excitation of atoms and molecules in the irradiated medium cause the radiation effects that are observed. Charged particles such as electrons, protons, and alpha particles can ionize the medium directly; they are referred to as directly ionizing radiations. Photons and neutrons ionize indirectly by setting in motion, in various interactions, charged particles that do ionize directly. Hence, they are referred to as indirectly ionizing radiations. The purpose in radiation dosimetry is to correlate any radiation effect with the amount of radiation delivered. As a corollary, we would like to deliver a controlled amount of radiation so as to produce an intended effect.

The radiation field can be characterized by various well-defined physical quantities. "Radiation dosimetry" is a broad term which covers all of the evaluation and quantification processes that can be applied to irradiations. In this chapter, we deal with the definitions of the various dosimetric quantities and their units. The International Commission on Radiation Units and Measurements (ICRU) has been responsible for the development of the quantities and units over the years. The reader should use ICRU Reports 33, and 60 for additional study of the subject [1, 2].

11.2
Some Theoretical Concepts

11.2.1
Fluence

Figure 11.1 shows an irradiated medium that contains a point P. The beam causes N particles* to be incident on an area A, which is perpendicular to the direction of the beam. If a small area ΔA, chosen at point P, receives ΔN particles, then the fluence ψ_N at P (the number of particles per unit area) is given by

$$\psi_N = \frac{\Delta N}{\Delta A} \qquad (11\text{-}1)$$

---

* In Sections 11.2.1 to 11.2.4, the term "particle" is used to include photons.

Fig. 11.1. Example of fluence. N particles are incident on an area A. A mass Δm of material having a cross section ΔA is located at P

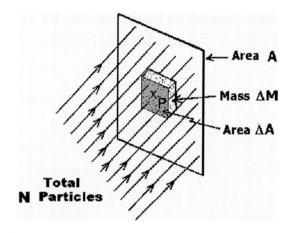

ψ_N can be expressed in units of m^{-2}. The ratio N/A is the average fluence over the entire area A. At a point, the fluence is dN/dA.

11.2.2
Energy Fluence

In the above geometry, if the energy incident on area ΔA is ΔE, then the energy fluence at P is given by

$$\psi_E = \frac{\Delta E}{\Delta A} \qquad (11\text{-}2)$$

For monochromatic radiation consisting of particles of a given energy E_v, the (number) fluence and energy fluence are related by

$$\psi_E = \psi_N E_v \qquad (11\text{-}3)$$

ψ_E can be evaluated in units of $J\,m^{-2}$. The average energy fluence over the entire area A is $(NE_v)/A$.

11.2.3
Fluence Rate

If ΔN particles arrive on area ΔA in a time interval Δt, the fluence rate is given by*

$$\dot{\psi}_N = \frac{\Delta N}{\Delta A}\frac{1}{\Delta t} \qquad (11\text{-}4)$$

$\dot{\psi}_N$ can be expressed in units of $m^{-2}\,s^{-1}$. The fluence rate at a point is expressed as

$$\dot{\psi}_N = \frac{d}{dt}\frac{dN}{dA}$$

---

* Placement of a dot over a variable (such as ψ_E or ψ_N) refers to the rate of change of that variable with time.

11.2.4
Energy Fluence Rate

If the photons have energy E_v, the energy fluence rate, $\dot{\psi}_E$, is given by

$$\dot{\psi}_E = \frac{\Delta N E_v}{\Delta A} \frac{1}{\Delta t} = \dot{\psi}_N E_v \qquad (11\text{-}5)$$

$\dot{\psi}_E$ can be expressed in units of $J\,m^{-2}\,s^{-1}$.

The above physical quantities are theoretical characteristics of a radiation field. Experimental radiation dosimetry in an actual field needs to rely on measurement of the effects caused by interactions of radiation with matter.

11.2.5
Energy Transferred and Kerma (k_{med})

We define the radiation quantity "kerma" to a medium as the initial kinetic energy transferred to the secondary charged particles in the medium per unit mass of the medium. From this definition, it is clear that kerma is defined for indirectly ionizing radiations. Let us say that a mass Δm of a medium of density ρ lies below the area ΔA at point P and that it is irradiated by a photon beam with a certain fluence. By interactions of the photons within the mass Δm, an amount of kinetic energy ΔT will be transferred to the charged particles. Then the kerma, k_{med}, in the medium at P is given by*

$$k_{med} = \frac{\Delta T}{\Delta m} \qquad (11\text{-}6)$$

The magnitude of ΔT can be evaluated as follows:

$\Delta T =$ (Photon energy falling on area ΔA) $\times$ (mass-energy transfer coefficient)
$\qquad \times$ (thickness in mass/unit area)

$\qquad = [\psi_E \Delta A][\mu_{tr}/\rho]\dfrac{\Delta m}{\Delta A}$

$\qquad = \psi_E[\mu_{tr}/\rho]\Delta m$

Thus,

$$k_{med} = \frac{\Delta T}{\Delta m} = \psi_E[\mu_{tr}/\rho] \qquad (11\text{-}7)$$

The kerma, which has the dimension energy/mass, can be measured in units of $J\,kg^{-1}$. The unit $J\,kg^{-1}$ is called by the special name "gray" (abbreviated Gy) in the Standard International (SI) System of units.

---

* In our convention, we add subscripts air, water, bone, etc. (such as k_{air}) to any physical variable (such as k) to refer to the material for which the variable (e. g., k) applies. Addition of a superscript and a subscript to a physical variable, such as $[\mu]_{air}^{water}$, refers to the ratio μ_{water}/μ_{air}. A bar over a variable indicates that it is a mean value.

11.2.6
Energy Absorbed and Dose (D_{med})

The radiation dose to a medium, D_{med}, is defined as the energy absorbed per unit mass of the medium. If ΔE is the energy absorbed within the mass Δm, D_{med} is the ratio

$$D_{med} = \frac{\Delta E}{\Delta m} \tag{11-8}$$

At a point, $D_{med} = dE/dm$.

The dose, like kerma, can be expressed in units of $J\,kg^{-1}$ or Gy. Although dose and kerma have the same physical dimensions, the difference between them should be understood. In expression (11-8) for dose, ΔE accounts for the energy dissipated within Δm, not only by the charged particles produced by photon interactions within Δm, but also by those originating outside Δm and passing through Δm. On the other hand, in expression (11-7) for kerma, ΔT accounts for the initial kinetic energy of the charged particles that originated due to interactions within Δm. (It may be that only a part of ΔT is dissipated within the mass Δm.) In a simple analogy, kerma is like the amount of rain striking a roof, whereas the dose is like the amount of water that actually accumulates on the roof, after some of the rain water that fell has run off and after more water has flowed in from elsewhere. Kerma and dose can be related numerically to each other under the special circumstance of a charged-particle equilibrium (CPE) around the mass Δm. CPE actually refers to the secondary-electron equilibrium for photons, because the charged particles released in photon interactions are electrons.

11.2.7
Charged-Particle Equilibrium

The energy transferred to the charged particles in a given mass is lost in collision and radiation events along their path. We will discuss CPE by considering photons as the primary radiation. The range of the electrons produced by the interaction of high-energy photons with tissue or water can be as high as several centimeters. For the present, let us assume that all of the energy transferred to the electrons is lost in collisions, with no bremsstrahlung losses. In general, any secondary electron produced in a mass Δm in an irradiated medium (as shown in Figure 11.2) may lose some part of its energy within the boundaries of Δm, and the rest outside. The track of an electron starting from point P in Figure 11.2 is an example. If we wish to account only for the part of the energy absorbed within the mass Δm (as distinct from the total energy transferred within Δm), we should disregard the energy expended by the electron outside Δm. But another electron that is released at point P_1 outside Δm can pass through Δm and dissipate a part of its energy within Δm. Thus, whatever energy the electron from **P** lost outside Δm has been compensated for. It is as if the entire energy of the electron from P had been absorbed within Δm. The same assumption of the total absorption of all the energy within Δm can become true for many other electron tracks originating from Δm. The part of the path of an electron originating at **Q** within Δm is compensated for in part by an electron from Q_1 and in part by one from Q_2. Then, if the photon fluence is the same at Q, Q_1, and Q_2 (Figure 11.2), we can be certain that, for every electron that originates at **Q**, there are corresponding compensating

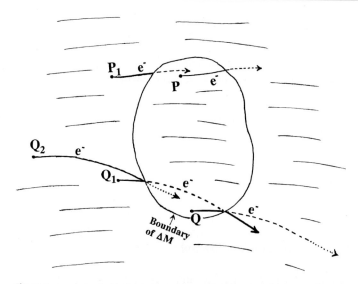

Fig. 11.2. A volume (with the indicated boundary) is crossed by secondary electron tracks. A part of the track from point **P** extends outside the boundary, but is compensated for by another track coming from point **P₁** outside the boundary. Likewise, the track from point **Q** that extends outside the volume is compensated for by tracks from **Q₁** and **Q₂**

electrons of similar energy and path from Q_1 and Q_2. If the photon fluence is uniform at least over one secondary electron range all around the mass Δm, CPE can exist. If so, the energy ΔE absorbed within Δm becomes equal to the energy transferred, ΔT, and the dose then becomes equal to the kerma.

CPE is possible if, and only if, the photon fluence does not change over at least one electron range in all directions. CPE exists only in an ideal situation. This is nearly achieved at low energies, but, as the energy increases, it becomes more and more of an approximation and becomes impossible at very high energies (see Section 11.3). The electron range becomes large at very high energies, and the attenuation of photon intensity can be significant over an electron range. This can cause spatial variation of the photon fluence over an electron range and defeat the uniformity of fluence needed for CPE.

11.2.8
Relationship between Kerma and Dose

Under conditions of CPE, the energy ΔE absorbed in Δm can be related to the energy fluence ψ_E and the energy absorption coefficient μ_{en} as follows:

$$\Delta E = [\text{total photon energy fluence over } \Delta A]$$
$$\times [\text{mass-energy absorption coefficient}]$$
$$\times [\text{thickness in mass/area}]$$

i. e.,

$$\Delta E = [\psi_E \Delta A][\mu_{en}/\rho][\Delta m/\Delta A]$$
$$= \psi_E[\mu_{en}/\rho]\Delta m = \psi_N E_v[\mu_{en}/\rho]\Delta m \qquad (11\text{-}9)$$

A fraction, g, of the energy of the electrons may be lost in producing bremsstrahlung x-rays. If we allow for g in dose evaluation, the dose D is given by

$$D = [\Delta E/\Delta m]$$
$$= \psi_E[\mu_{en}/\rho]$$
$$= \psi_E[\mu_{tr}/\rho][1 - g]$$
$$= \psi_N E_v[\mu_{tr}/\rho][1 - g] \qquad (11\text{-}10)$$

When the energy lost by bremsstrahlung is negligible (i. e., $g \approx 0$) and if CPE exists for Δm, the dose will be equal to the kerma.

11.3
Dose and Kerma Profiles – An Interface Example

Let us look at a situation in which a high-energy photon beam passes a vacuum-water interface, as shown in Figure 11.3. Here we assume that the beam is a monoenergetic photon beam with no charged-particle contamination. When the beam crosses the water surface, secondary electrons are released from successive layers of water. For simplicity, here the tracks are shown to be straight and proceeding in the forward direction, which is a reasonable assumption for high-energy photons. The energy is dissipated over the successive layers of water until each particle has traveled its full range. The range depends on the initial energy, which, in turn, is related to the incident photon energy. In the example of Figure 11.3, we have assumed (quite arbitrarily for illustration) that each layer of water generates seven secondary electron tracks, and

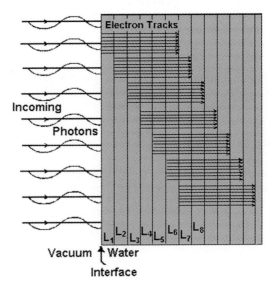

Fig. 11.3. Diagram illustrating the build-up of secondary electron tracks for a beam incident on a vacuum-water interface. Each of the layers L_1, L_2, etc. is assumed to release seven secondary electron tracks, resulting in a build-up of up to 42 tracks in layer L_6. Tracks originating beyond layer L_7 are not shown

that the electron tracks have a range of six layers. As we examine successive layers of water beyond the surface, the number of secondary electron tracks that cross them builds up from 7 in layer L_1 to 42 in layer L_7. Because the range of the electrons has been assumed to be six layers, it is not surprising that the maximum build-up to 42 tracks is reached in layer L_6. The build-up would be seen to be maintained in layers below L_6 (i. e., L_7, L_8, etc.).

In practice, the secondary electrons travel at various angles, and the depth of full build-up as measured from the interface would be less than the maximum electron range. In a simplistic way, we can picture that the dose delivered in any layer is directly proportional to the number of electron tracks passing through that layer. Thus, the build-up of secondary electron tracks also implies a dose build-up in successive layers. Likewise, because kerma is the energy transferred in any layer, the number of tracks originating in that layer is a measure of kerma. In our illustration, this is a constant number of seven tracks. In this example, the indication is that, whereas the dose can build up with depth to a maximum value, the kerma will remain constant. However, in reality, the photon fluence will be attenuated in water, resulting in a gradual decrease in the number of newly originating electron tracks with depth. Thus, the kerma will be maximum at the surface and decrease with depth, as shown by curve 1 in Figure 11.4. The dose build-up for a clean photon beam (which contains no electrons before reaching the water) can be expected to be like curve 2, with a very low surface dose. However, in practice a photon beam is never ideally clean, but contains electrons coming from the beam-collimating devices and from the air above the water. This contribution will increase the surface dose and make the dose build-up curve look like curve 3. Both curves 2 and 3 start with a low dose at the surface and increase to a maximum value with the build-up of secondary electrons.

We have seen that the dose at any depth is related to the number of electrons traveling from the material above. The photon flux is high in the layer where the beam enters the water and falls off in subsequent layers. For any layer, there are more electrons flowing down to it from layers above than there are electrons released in it to flow below. We know that the former governs the dose and the latter the kerma. Because of this, the dose is greater than the kerma after the depth of full build-up. In Figure 11.4, the dose at depth d_B is the same as the kerma at depth d_A, with the distance $(d_B - d_A)$ related to the

Fig. 11.4. Fall-off of kerma and build-up of dose with depth for a high-energy photon beam. Curves 1 and 2 give the kerma and dose, respectively, for a clean (i. e., electron-free) photon beam. Curve 3 is the dose build-up pattern for a typical therapy beam with a significant surface dose caused by electron contamination. The dose at depth d_B is the same as the kerma at depth d_A

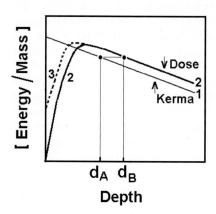

secondary electron range. The ratio of kerma to dose at depths beyond the maximum dose is related to the attenuation of the photon fluence over one secondary electron range. This situation leads to a constant ratio of dose to kerma beyond the depth of the dose maximum. This difference in the numerical values of dose and kerma indicates the absence of CPE caused by the decreasing photon fluence.

11.4
Air Kerma (k_{air}) and Water Kerma (k_{water})

The ions generated in an air volume by interaction of the radiation can be collected by application of an electric potential. This has been a useful approach to the measurement of radiation levels. On the other hand, water behaves almost like soft tissue in its interactions with radiation, and assessment of the dose to water is clinically useful. Hence, assessment of kerma in air and water is of special interest to radiation physicists.

Air (or water) kerma at any point in a medium is the energy transferred by photons to the charged particles per unit mass of air (or water) undergoing irradiation at that point. Air (or water) kerma can be conceptualized at any point, even if the medium irradiated is not air (or water). We first need to imagine that, at the point of interest, the medium is replaced by a tiny packet of air (or water). Then the energy transferred to the charged particles per unit mass of the air (or water) packet can be assessed. If ΔE is the photon fluence, the air kerma, k_{air}, and water kerma, k_{water}, are

$$k_{air} = \frac{\Delta T}{(\Delta m)_{air}} = \Psi_E(\mu_{tr}/\rho)_{air} = \Psi_N E_v(\mu_{tr}/\rho)_{air} \qquad (11\text{-}11)$$

$$k_{water} = \frac{\Delta T}{(\Delta m)_{water}} = \Psi_E(\mu_{tr}/\rho)_{water} = \Psi_N E_v(\mu_{tr}/\rho)_{water} \qquad (11\text{-}12)$$

11.5
Exposure

11.5.1
Concept of Exposure

Exposure is a radiation quantity of historical interest. Here, the word "exposure" is used in a special technical sense and not in the generic sense of "irradiation." Exposure was used originally for quantifying the radiation field in terms of the electrical charge in air produced by the secondary electrons generated by interaction of photons per unit mass of air. Let us visualize a uniform medium irradiated by photons (Figure 11.5a). To understand exposure, we consider that a packet of air of mass Δm is implanted in the medium (Figure 11.5b). The photons interacting with the atoms in this mass of air can release secondary electrons. Visualize (hypothetically) as if these electrons can continue to travel in air (and not in the medium), as in Figure 11.5c, and generate ions in air. If all the charges of one sign (created in air) are collected and gives a total accumulated charge ΔQ, then the exposure (X) at the site of the air packet of mass $(\Delta m)_{air}$ is given by

$$X = \frac{\Delta Q}{(\Delta m)_{air}} \qquad (11\text{-}13)$$

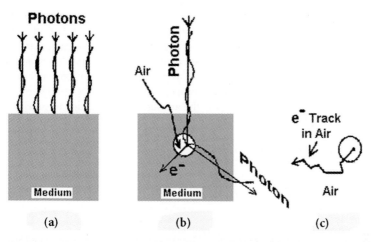

Fig. 11.5. Diagrams illustrating the concept of exposure at a point in an irradiated medium. (a) A photon beam is incident on a medium. (b) The photons interact with air in an air cavity visualized at the point where the exposure is to be determined and produce secondary electrons. (c) The secondary electrons produced are visualized to continue their travel in air, generating ions in air

The exposure has the dimension of charge/mass and can be evaluated in units of $C\,kg^{-1}$ (C is the charge unit coulomb in the SI system) [3].

The roentgen, R, is a special unit of exposure based on the CGS system of units and is equivalent to $2.58 \times 10^{-4}\,C\,kg^{-1}$. The special-odd number, 2.58×10^{-4}, that determines the roentgen's magnitude is derived from the following original definition of the roentgen unit. If photons interact with $1\,cm^3$ of air at normal temperature and pressure (NTP), i.e., 273 K and 760 mmHg, and if they generate secondary electrons which, as they continue to travel in air, produce a charge of 1 electrostatic unit (esu) of either sign, the exposure is 1 R. The density of air at NTP is known to be $1.293 \times 10^{-6}\,kg\,cm^{-3}$, and one esu is 3.333×10^{-10} C. Thus,

$$1\,R = \frac{3.333 \times 10^{-10}\,C}{1.293 \times 10^{-6}\,kg} = 2.58 \times 10^{-4}\,C\,kg^{-1} \tag{11-14}$$

(The odd magnitude of R of $2.58 \times 10^{-4}\,C\,kg^{-1}$ results, because in its definition neither the mass of air nor the charge is stated in terms of the SI units of kilogram and Coulomb.) The unit $C\,kg^{-1}$ is the preferred unit of exposure.

11.5.2
Relationship Among Exposure, Air Kerma, and Dose to Air

Because of its definition based on photon interactions in air, exposure is closely related to air kerma. We can derive a relationship between the exposure, X, and the air kerma, k_{air}. First, however, some distinctions between these two quantities should be understood. Whereas the air kerma is energy/mass, exposure is charge/mass. The air kerma is the amount of energy given to the secondary particles by interactions within a mass of air $(\Delta m)_{air}$. It does not concern itself with the details as to where the secondary particles travel or how they dissipate their energy. The exposure, X, on the other hand, is the amount of charge that will be generated by these particles if they continue to travel in air and lose all of their energy. A part, g, of the energy of the charged particles may be lost in bremsstrahlung and hence may not result in the generation of charges. We define a value $\bar{W}$ as the average energy needed to produce an ionization event that results in an ion pair. Because the production of each ion pair results in a charge e equal to that of an electron, the ratio $(\bar{W}/e)$ is the average energy needed to produce one unit of charge [4]. The exposure X is related to k_{air} by the ratio $(\bar{W}/e)_{air}$ applicable for air, as follows:

$$X = \frac{[k_{air}(1 - g)]}{(\bar{W}/e)_{air}} = [k_{air}(1 - g)](e/\bar{W})_{air}$$

$$= [\psi_N E_v (\mu_{tr}/\rho)_{air}(1 - g)](e/\bar{W})_{air} \qquad (11.15a)$$

which is the same as

$$X = [\psi_N E_v (\mu_{en}/\rho)_{air}](e/\bar{W})_{air} \qquad (11.15b)$$

Under CPE, the term in square brackets above is the dose to air, D_{air}. Thus, given CPE,

$$X = D_{air}(e/\bar{W})_{air} \qquad (11\text{-}16)$$

11.5.3
Relationship of Dose in Medium to Air Kerma and Exposure

The exposure X and k_{air} can be evaluated for a photon energy fluence ψ_E interacting with air. If the mass of air is replaced by a mass of medium, the same fluence will deliver a kerma k_{med} to the medium. The air-kerma to medium-kerma conversion factor, f_{akmk}, is defined by

$$(f_{akmk})_{med} = \frac{k_{med}}{k_{air}} = \frac{[\mu_{tr}/\rho]_{med}}{[\mu_{tr}/\rho]_{air}} \qquad (11\text{-}17)$$

When CPE exists, we can assess the air-kerma to medium-dose conversion factor, f_{akmd}, from the relationship

$$(f_{akmd})_{med} = \frac{D_{med}}{k_{air}} = \frac{[\mu_{en}/\rho]_{med}}{[\mu_{tr}/\rho]_{air}} \qquad (11\text{-}18)$$

From Equations (11-10) and (11.15b), the exposure-to-dose conversion factor, f_{xd}, for the medium is given by

$$(f_{xd})_{med} = \frac{D_{med}}{X} = (\bar{W}/e)_{air} \frac{[\mu_{en}/\rho]_{med}}{[\mu_{en}/\rho]_{air}} \qquad (11\text{-}19)$$

i. e.,

$$D_{med} = X \cdot (f_{xd})_{med} \qquad (11\text{-}20)$$

EXAMPLE 11.1

The average energy W required to produce an ion pair in air is 33.85 eV. Find the exposure-to-dose conversion factor for air, $(f_{xd})_{air}$.

When the medium is air, expression (11-19) becomes

$$(f_{xd})_{air} = (\bar{W}/e)_{air}$$

Given $W = 33.85\,eV = 33.85 \times 1.6 \times 10^{-19}\,J$ and the electron's charge $e = 1.6 \times 10^{-19}\,C$,

$$(f_{xd})_{air} = (\bar{W}/e)_{air} = 33.85\,J\,C^{-1}$$

EXAMPLE 11.2

Given that the special unit of dose, the "rad," equals 0.01 Gy, and the roentgen (R) is a special unit of exposure equal to $2.58 \times 10^{-4}\,C\,kg^{-1}$, calculate the rad/R conversion factor for air.

We use the information from Example 11.1, that an energy of 33.85 J is needed for generation of 1 C of charge in air. Because $1\,R = 2.58 \times 10^{-4}\,C\,kg^{-1}$, the corresponding energy absorbed per kg becomes

$$(f_{xd})_{air} = 2.58 \times 10^{-4}\,C\,kg^{-1}\,R^{-1} \times 33.85\,J\,C^{-1}$$
$$= 0.00873\,J\,kg^{-1}\,R^{-1} = 0.00873\,Gy\,R^{-1}$$

Because 1 rad = 0.01 Gy,

$$(f_{xd})_{air} = 0.873\,rad\,R^{-1} \qquad (11\text{-}21)$$

The quantity in (11-20) suggests that, if the exposure, X, due to an irradiating photon fluence is known from a charge measurement, the dose, D_{med}, at the same point at the same fluence under CPE can be derived by use of the conversion factor $(f_{xd})_{med}$. We point out in Section 11.7.7 why this is only an approximation, and that additional corrections to $(f_{xd})_{med}$ will be needed for an exact derivation of the dose in a medium.

EXAMPLE 11.3

The (μ_{tr}/ρ) values for air, water, and bone are given in Table 11.1 below for two photon energies. Calculate f_{akmk} for water and bone at these energies. If soft tissue behaves like water, what is the implication of the calculated f_{akmk} values for a clinical situation where bone and soft tissue are adjacent to each other and are irradiated by the same photon fluence at these energies?

At 60 keV:

$$[f_{akmk}]_{Water} = [\mu_{tr}/\rho]_{air}^{water} = 0.0320/0.0305 = 1.049$$

Table 11.1. Comparison of μ_{tr}/ρ (cm^2/g) for Air, Water, and Bone at Two Photon Energies

E_V (keV)	μ_{tr}/ρ (cm^2/g)		
	Air	Water	Compact Bone
60	0.0305	0.0320	0.0998
1250	0.0268	0.0298	0.0285

and

$$[f_{akmk}]_{Bone} = [\mu_{tr}/\rho]_{air}^{bone} = 0.0998/0.0305 = 3.272$$

The above values indicate that, if the same photon fluence is incident on bone and water, at 60 keV photon energy, the energy transferred to bone is $(3.27/1.049 =)$ 3.12 times that transferred to water. That is, the dose to bone is significantly higher than to water.

At 1250 keV:

$$[f_{akmk}]_{Water} = [\mu_{tr}/\rho]_{air}^{water} = 0.0298/0.0268 = 1.112$$

and

$$[f_{akmk}]_{Bone} = [\mu_{tr}/\rho]_{air}^{bone} = 0.0285/0.0268 = 1.063$$

The above values imply that, for the same incident photon fluence, at 1250 keV, the energy transferred to bone is $(1.063/1.112 =)$ 0.956 times that transferred to water. That is, the dose to bone is almost same, but marginally less, than to water.

11.6
Measurement of Exposure

11.6.1
Free-Air Ionization Chamber

The free-air ionization chamber [5] (Figure 11.6) is an instrument designed to measure exposure by collection of the electric charges created by radiation in a well-defined amount of air. An electric field is applied between two parallel plates, B and C. The field strength should be sufficiently large to provide a drift velocity so that the ions are collected without any recombination loss. At the same time, the field should not be so large that it adds energy to the ions by accelerating them. Plate C functions as the ion collector. The electric field lines of force between plates B and C define the air volume of ion collection. So that the volume is clearly defined, guard plates G are used, which are maintained at the same voltage as C. With the presence of guard plates, the electric lines of force run parallel to one another and perpendicular to plate C. The electric plates are enclosed in a lead-lined box, which has an aperture D formed by a diaphragm. A radiation beam from source S enters through the diaphragm. The separation between the plates and the chamber enclosure is large enough to provide enough air in all directions so that there is electronic equilibrium.

Let us say that the chamber operates at NTP and a charge ΔQ is collected in the chamber for an irradiation lasting a time t. The charge ΔQ is collected from a mass of air $(A_M L \rho)$, where A_M is the cross section of the beam at the mid-point M above the collecting electrode, L is the length of the collector plate, and ρ is the density of air at ambient temperature and pressure. The exposure X_M at point M is, accordingly, given by

$$X_M = \frac{\text{charge collected}}{\text{mass of air}} = \frac{\Delta Q}{A_M L \rho} \tag{11-22}$$

Let ΔQ, A_M, L, and ρ be in units of C, m^2, m, and $kg\,m^{-3}$, respectively. Because

Fig. 11.6. Schematic diagram of a free-air ionization chamber. S, Source of radiation; D, mid-point of diaphragm; A_D, area of diaphragm aperture; G, guard ring; L, length of sensitive volume; M, mid-point of sensitive volume; A_M, area of radiation beam at M

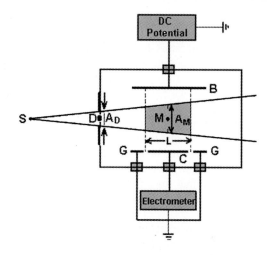

$1\,R = 2.58 \times 10^{-4}\,C\,kg^{-1}$, X_M stated in units of R will be

$$X_M = \frac{\Delta Q}{A_M L \rho} \frac{1}{2.58 \times 10^{-4}}\,R$$

The fluence falls off from D to M as per the inverse of the square of their distances SD and SM. (see Section 17.7) Hence, the exposure X_D at the diaphragm D is

$$X_D = X_M (SM/SD)^2$$

The areas A_D and A_M are related by

$$A_M = A_D (SM/SD)^2$$

Hence,

$$X_D = \frac{\Delta Q}{A_D L \rho} \qquad (11\text{-}23)$$

The above expression suggests as if, ions in a cylindrical volume of air of cross section A_D and length L located at the diaphragm, are collected to measure the exposure at the position of the diaphragm. Because the density ρ is affected by the ambient temperature and pressure of air, the free-air chamber measurements need to be corrected for temperature and pressure. Additional corrections are also needed for humidity, ion recombination losses, air attenuation of photons, and photon scatter.

11.6.2
Cavity Chambers

Free-air chambers are cumbersome for routine field applications. They are kept at standardization laboratories for calibration of the field instruments of institutional users, which are usually small cavity ionization chambers. The necessary dimensions of a free-air chamber increase rapidly as the X-ray energy increases. At high energies, the secondary electron range becomes as large as several meters and building free-air chambers becomes impractical. At such energies, cavity chamber principles need to be used even by standardization laboratories [6]. When the government of a country declares a laboratory to be the custodian of its standards, the free-air and cavity chambers of the laboratory are called the primary national standards for that country [7].

The principles of a cavity ionization chamber are discussed in greater detail in later sections of this chapter. For the present, we merely ask the question, is it possible to reduce the dimensions of a free-air chamber by using a high-density, air-equivalent plastic? In other words, can we design a chamber that consists of a small volume of air for collecting the ions, surrounded by a wall made of an "air-equivalent" material of high density, say, $\rho = 1\,\mathrm{g\,cm^{-3}}$? Ideally, the μ_{en}/ρ value for the wall material should be the same as that for air, and the wall thickness should be just large enough to provide CPE. Any plastic material that has the same Z_{eff} value as air can be used for the wall.

There are many kinds of cavity chambers. Among them, cylindrical (or thimble) chambers and parallel-plate chambers are common. A thimble chamber is shown in Figure 11.7a. The chamber has a central electrode and a wall of air-equivalent material. The inner wall is coated with a layer of conducting material and serves as the second electrode. An air volume is enclosed between the two electrodes and a collecting potential is applied between the electrodes. At any photon energy, the thickness of the wall should be sufficiently large to give CPE. Thus, different wall thicknesses will need to be used to provide CPE at different photon energies. In practice, it is possible to have a thin-walled chamber for use at low energies and to add a cap of appropriate

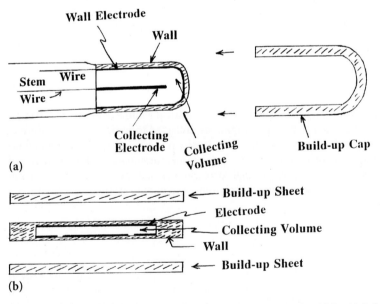

Fig. 11.7. Cross sections of cavity ionization chambers. (a) A cylindrical "thimble" chamber with a build-up cap for high-energy measurements. (b) A parallel-plate "pancake" chamber which can be used with build-up sheets

thickness, as shown in the right half of Figure 11.7a for use at higher energies. Such caps are referred to as "build-up caps," because they help to build up the secondary-electron fluence reaching the gas (usually air) cavity. Build-up caps of various thicknesses are kept to be appropriately chosen for use at different photon energies.

Figure 11.7b shows a cross section of a parallel-plate or "pancake" chamber. Such chambers can be sandwiched between build-up sheets of appropriate thickness to obtain CPE at different energies.

The cavity chamber is connected to an electrometer which measures the charge collected in an irradiation. In a particular irradiation, the electrometer may give a reading M. This can be related to the charge ΔQ collected by the relation

$$\Delta Q = M \cdot q_M \tag{11-24}$$

where q_M is the charge per meter reading. If the collecting volume of the chamber is ΔV and the density of air is ρ, the exposure X is given by

$$X = \frac{\Delta Q}{\rho \Delta V} = \frac{\Delta Q}{(\Delta m)_{air}} \tag{11-25}$$

where $(\Delta m)_{air}$ is the mass of air in the chamber.

11.6.3
Exposure Calibration Factor

Although the above equation is simple, in practice it is not easy to determine the value of ΔV or $(\Delta m)_{air}$ exactly. Furthermore, the so-called air-equivalent wall may not be exactly air-equivalent at all energies. Also, the photon interactions in the material of the central electrode can interfere with the air equivalency. This happens especially at low energies, where the photoelectric effect is important. At low keV, the strong influence of the atomic number Z of the different materials that make up the chamber can affect its response and render its air equivalence uncertain. For overcoming all of these uncertainties, it is an accepted practice to send any cavity chamber-electrometer system to an accredited dosimetry calibration laboratory (ADCL) [7–9]. At the ADCL, a comparison is made between a standard measurement chamber maintained there and the user's instrument, resulting in a calibration factor $N_{X,v}$ (in R/C) for the user's chamber. The subscripts X and v in $N_{X,v}$ refer to an exposure calibration factor obtained by the ADCL for a photon energy hv. In the USA, the ADCLs report the value of $N_{X,v}$ for the conditions of the chamber operating at the standard temperature and pressure (STP) of 295 K (i. e., 22°C) and 760 mmHg, respectively. Because the commonly used chambers are not hermetically sealed, one should allow for the fact that the mass of air contained in the chamber depends on the ambient temperature T (°C) and pressure P (mmHg). A meter reading of M', and charge $\Delta Q'$, measured at any ambient temperature and pressure, can be converted to corresponding meter readings of M and charge ΔQ that would be obtained at STP, as follows:

$$M = M' P_{tpf}; \quad \Delta Q' = M' \cdot q_M$$
$$\Delta Q = \Delta Q' \cdot P_{tpf} = M' \cdot q_M \cdot P_{tpf} \tag{11-26}$$

where P_{tpf} is a temperature-pressure correction factor, given by

$$P_{tpf} = \left[\frac{273 + T}{295} \right] \left[\frac{760}{P} \right] \tag{11-27}$$

When the chamber is irradiated by photons of the same energy under field conditions by the user, the exposure X can be derived from the charge $\Delta Q'$ collected as follows:

$$X = \left[\Delta Q' P_{tpf} \right] N_{X,v} = \left[M' q_M P_{tpf} \right] N_{X,v} \tag{11-28}$$

The value of X so derived is valid for the point occupied by the center of the ion chamber in the absence of the chamber. For use of the chamber at a low-kilovoltage X-ray energy, at which the photoelectric effect cannot be ignored, it is recommended that the calibration factor $N_{X,v}$ be obtained as close as possible to that energy [10]. For measurement at megavoltage X-ray energies, a calibration factor, $N_{X,Co}$, applicable to the energy of cobalt-60 photons, can be used, with methods outlined in Section 11.7.2 of this chapter. The value of $N_{X,Co}$ is valid when the chamber is used with a cobalt-60 build-up cap to ensure CPE.

The use of chambers with calibration factors obtained from an ADCL contributes to the traceability of the radiation standard unit to all clinics. The ADCLs, in their turn, maintain traceability to national standards laboratories in individual countries, and these national laboratories ensure traceability to the internationally accepted standard maintained by the Bureau International des Poids et des Mesures (BIPM), Sevres, France. Thus, the doses derived in clinics around the world can all be traced to the same radiation unit. Chambers calibrated in a radiation field which has been determined by the use of a primary national standard are called transfer, secondary, or field-standard chambers.

11.7
Use of Calibrated Ion Chamber in Therapy Beams

11.7.1
Need for Calibration of Beams

No radiation therapy beam can be used for patient treatment unless proper steps for ascertaining the dose received by the patient are established. It may be necessary to assess the dose delivered not only to the tumor, but also to a few other points of clinical interest in the patient. The absolute dose rate measured with a calibrated cavity ionization chamber at a chosen reference point in the therapy beam becomes the basis for derivation of the dose at any other point of interest. The factors and ratios useful for deriving the doses at points other than the reference point are covered in Chapter 13. Here, we concern ourselves with the process of absolute dose measurement at a chosen reference point. This is also referred to as calibration of the beam.

The reference point and the beam conditions to be adopted for the absolute calibration of radiation therapy beams from low kilovoltage x-rays to high-energy photon and electron beams have been discussed in various protocols [11–22]. Many of these protocols (which bear mutual alikeness) provide work sheets and a step-by-step approach for the derivation of the dose in beams of either X-rays or electrons of energies higher than that of cobalt-60 by using a chamber-electrometer system that has a known exposure calibration factor $N_{X,Co}$ at the cobalt-60 energy. It is not possible to deal with this subject in complete detail here; we will merely outline the overall principles. In the following sections, we first provide a simple discussion of the calibration of a cobalt-60 beam by using the cobalt calibration factor $N_{X,Co}$. Next, we discuss the general principles of the cavity ionization theory leading to a cavity gas calibration factor, N_{gas}. Next, we discuss the use of N_{gas} together with several correction factors for the calibration of photon beams according to modern protocols for high-energy beam calibration. Then we show how the value of N_{gas} can be derived from $N_{X,Co}$ for any particular cavity chamber. We follow this with an extension of the discussion to the calibration of electron beams. Finally, in Section 11.8, we cover the approach of the most recent protocols which use ion chambers that have an absorbed-dose-to water calibration factor $N_{D,Co}$ provided by a standard laboratory based on a water calorimeter as the primary standard instrument [19–21].

11.7.2
"Dose to Tissue in Air" for a Cobalt-60 Beam

Figure 11.8a illustrates an ionization chamber with its cobalt-60 build-up cap placed at a point P in air on the central axis of a cobalt-60 beam. The exposure X at P (in the absence of the chamber, as shown in Figure 11.8b) can be derived from expression (11-28) from the charge measured by the chamber. We would like to know the dose to a mass of tissue (or water) placed at P, as shown in Figure 11.8c. If CPE exists at the center of this mass, we can convert the measured exposure X into dose (to tissue or water) by applying the factor f_{xd}. To ensure CPE, the radius of the mass of tissue (or water) should be made sufficiently large so that it matches the range of the secondary electrons. We will refer to this mass as the equilibrium mass of tissue (or water). At

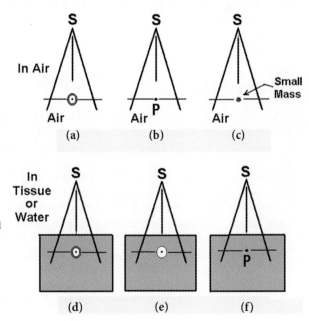

Fig. 11.8. Diagrams illustrating the concepts used for assessment of the dose delivered by a ^{60}Co beam with a calibrated ion chamber. (a) A cylindrical chamber with its build-up cap is placed in air for measurement of exposure. (b) The chamber is removed, and the position of the chamber center is marked as point **P**. (c) A small mass of tissue sufficient to produce CPE at its own center is placed at point **P**. (d) A cylindrical chamber is positioned in water for measurement of exposure. (e) The chamber is removed, and a hypothetical hole is left behind in the water. (f) The hole is filled with water; **P** marks the point where the dose is to be assessed

the cobalt-60 energy, the equilibrium mass has a diameter of about 10 mm. Because a mass of tissue (or water) has replaced air, the photon fluence at the center of this mass cannot correspond to the fluence for which X applies. If the attenuation and scatter of the photon fluence within the equilibrium mass can be accounted for by a correction factor A_{eq}, the dose D_{eq} at the center of the equilibrium mass is given by

$$D_{eq} = X_{fd} A_{eq} = \left[\Delta Q' P_{tpf} \right] N_{X,Co} f_{xd} A_{eq} \qquad (11\text{-}29)$$

At the cobalt-60 energy, A_{eq} is 0.99 [8]. At low photon energies (up to 500 keV), the equilibrium mass of tissue is very small, and the correction factor A_{eq} can be ignored (i. e., $A_{eq} = 1.0$).

11.7.3
Dose in Water for a Cobalt-60 Beam

Figure 11.8d illustrates a cobalt-60 beam incident on water. An ion chamber with its build-up cap for the cobalt-60 energy is positioned at point P at a depth on the central axis of the beam. The charge collected by the chamber can be converted to an exposure X, which, in turn, can be converted to dose by use of the factor f_{xd}. However, X applies to the location of the center of the chamber in the absence of the chamber. That is, X actually applies to the center of the hole in water, as shown in Figure 11.8e. Filling the hole can change the photon fluence and alter the dose. The dose, D_{water}, at point P in the medium when the hole is filled with water (as shown in Figure 11.8f) can be calculated by the expression

$$D_{water} = X f_{xd} A_c = \left[\Delta Q' P_{tpf} N_{X,Co} f_x A_c \right] \qquad (11\text{-}30)$$

with the factor A_c correcting for the change in fluence when the chamber and cap are replaced by water. The value of A_c for a chamber having a 6 mm inner diameter is about 0.993 [22].

11.7.4
Ideal Bragg-Gray Cavity

Cavity chamber theory has been discussed in detail by Burlin [23]. To determine the dose at any point in an irradiated medium, we introduce a gas cavity at the point of interest. The charged particles passing through the cavity will contribute to the ionization of the gas. We define an ideally small cavity as one in which (a) the direct interaction of the photons with the gas in the cavity is negligible and all the ions produced in the cavity can be attributed to the secondary particles that originate in the medium and cross the cavity, and (b) the range of the secondary particles is much larger than the dimensions of the cavity. Such an ideally small cavity is called a Bragg-Gray cavity and is illustrated in Figure 11.9a. Let us say that, at STP, the mass of gas in the cavity is $(\Delta m)_{gas}$ and the charge collected during an irradiation is ΔQ. Then the dose, D_{gas}, to the gas in the cavity is given by

$$D_{gas} = \frac{\Delta Q}{(\Delta m)_{gas}} (\bar{W}/e)_{gas} = \Delta Q \, N_{gas} \qquad (11\text{-}31)$$

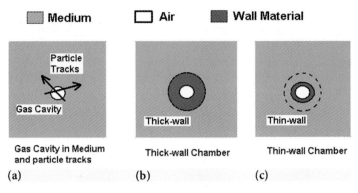

Fig. 11.9. Use of cavity theory for dosimetry in a medium. (a) A gas cavity traversed by ionizing particle tracks. (b) A cavity created by placement of a chamber with a wall thickness that is as large as the range of the secondary electrons (shown by dashed circle) around the gas cavity. (c) A cavity chamber with a wall thinner than that in (b)

where

$$N_{gas} = \frac{(\bar{W}/e)_{gas}}{(\Delta m)_{gas}} \qquad (11\text{-}32)$$

The above value, N_{gas}, is a characteristic of the cavity ion chamber called the cavity gas calibration factor.

All of the ions produced are due to the collision energy loss suffered by the charged particles in the gas, which is proportional to the mean mass collision stopping power of the gas. Hence, we can write the proportionality relation

$$D_{gas} \propto \left(\bar{S}_c/\rho\right)_{gas} \qquad (11\text{-}33)$$

The bar over S_c implies that the value has been averaged over the entire secondary-particle energy spectrum.

If the gas cavity is filled by the medium, the dose, D_{med}, to the medium replacing the gas will be proportional to the mean collision stopping power $(S_c/\rho)_{med}$ of the medium. Thus,

$$D_{med} \propto \left(\bar{S}_c/\rho\right)_{med} \qquad (11\text{-}34)$$

and

$$\frac{D_{med}}{D_{gas}} = \left[\bar{S}_c/\rho\right]_{gas}^{med} \qquad (11\text{-}35)$$

From (11-26), (11-31), and (11-35), we obtain

$$D_{med} = \left[\Delta Q' P_{tpf}\right] N_{gas} \left[\bar{S}_c/\rho\right]_{gas}^{med} \qquad (11\text{-}36)$$

The above expression applies irrespective of whether the medium is irradiated by a photon beam or an electron beam, or whether or not CPE exists.

Expression (11-36) suggests that, by introducing an ideal cavity at a point in an irradiated medium and collecting the ions produced, we can infer the dose delivered at this point if N_{gas} is known. According to (11-32), the value of N_{gas} is related to the mass of the collecting volume of gas, $(\Delta m)_{gas}$, at STP. Because it is difficult to know

$(\Delta m)_{gas}$ directly, in Section 11.7.7 we derive the value of N_{gas} from $N_{X,Co}$ indirectly. Furthermore, expression (11-36) is valid only for an ideally small cavity. Several other corrections are needed for less than ideal cavities used in practice so that the clinically required accuracy (of $\pm 2\%$) in dosimetry can be achieved. Readers who are not interested in understanding all of the details of cavity-ionization dosimetry are advised to skip to Section 11.8.

11.7.5
Less than Ideal (Larger) Cavity

In practice, the cavity needs to be sufficiently large so that it is sensitive and provides enough ions for collection. However, a large cavity can alter the photon fluence. This should be corrected for by a perturbation or replacement correction factor, P_{repl}. Furthermore, only secondary particles having a minimum energy Δ may be able to cross the cavity. However, the collision stopping power (S_c/ρ) includes secondary particles of all energies. Spencer and Attix [24] suggested that it is more appropriate to substitute S_c/ρ by a mean restricted mass stopping power $(L_c/\rho)_\Delta$ (see Section 6.3.5) in (11-36). Thus, in a practical situation,

$$D_{med} = \left[\Delta Q' P_{tpf}\right] N_{gas} \left[\left(\bar{L}_c/\rho\right)_\Delta\right]_{gas}^{med} P_{repl} \tag{11-37}$$

11.7.6
Walled Chamber in a Medium

In practice, cavity ionization is measured by placement of an ionization chamber in a medium. The ion chamber can have a wall, and the atomic composition of the wall material can be different from that of the medium. We will first address how the dose D_{med} can be related to the charge $\Delta Q'$ collected when the chamber is irradiated by a photon beam. The principles governing the use of a walled chamber in a medium as discussed here are fashioned after the American Association of Physicists in Medicine (AAPM) Task Group 21 protocol [11–13].

First, we identify a region around the cavity that extends to the range of the secondary charged particles, as shown by the dashed circle in Figure 11.9c. Only charged particles that originate within this region are considered to contribute to the ionization measured. The wall of the chamber forms a part of this region. We can divide the electron fluence crossing the cavity into two parts, namely, the part α that comes from the wall and the rest, $(1 - \alpha)$, that comes from the medium. If the wall contributes none of the secondary electrons, $\alpha = 0$ and expression (11-37) can be used. On the other hand, let us consider a thick-walled chamber (Figure 11.9b), for which the entire electron fluence comes from the wall and $\alpha = 1$. In this case, based on the same concepts as used for expression (11-37), the dose D_{wall} to the wall material of the chamber if the wall material fills the cavity is given by

$$D_{wall} = \left[\Delta Q' P_{tpf}\right] N_{gas} \left[\left(\bar{L}_c/\rho\right)_\Delta\right]_{gas}^{wall} P_{repl} \tag{11-38}$$

The secondary electron fluence from the wall is proportional to the energy absorption coefficient, $[\mu_{en/\rho}]_{wall}$, of the wall material. Our goal is to determine the dose delivered to the medium when the medium fills the cavity. If the chamber is removed and the cavity is filled by the medium, the secondary electron fluence will change to be proportional to the energy absorption coefficient $[\mu_{en}/\rho]_{med}$ of the medium. Thus, if the perturbation correction P_{repl} is assumed to be the same for both situations, we obtain the ratio

$$\frac{D_{med}}{D_{wall}} = \left[\bar{\mu}_{en}/\rho\right]_{wall}^{med} \tag{11-39}$$

From (11-38) and (11-39), we obtain, for $\alpha = 1$,

$$D_{med} = \left[\Delta Q' P_{tpf}\right] N_{gas} \left[(\bar{L}_c/\rho)_\Delta\right]_{gas}^{wall} \left[\bar{\mu}_{en}/\rho\right]_{wall}^{med} P_{repl} \tag{11-40}$$

In practical situations, a significant fraction of the ionization is attributable to the charged particles originating from the chamber wall. Then α is neither 0 nor 1. The expressions (11-40) for $\alpha = 1$ and (11-37) for $\alpha = 0$ should then be combined in the proportions of α and $(1 - \alpha)$ for derivation of D_{med}. In addition, we will need to incorporate a correction factor P_{ion} for a possible reduction in the charge collected due to ion recombination. With all of these refinements, D_{med} for a walled cavity chamber is given by

$$D_{med} = \left[\Delta Q' P_{ion} P_{tpf}\right] N_{gas} \left[(\bar{L}_c/\rho)_\Delta\right]_{gas}^{med} P_{wall} P_{repl} \tag{11-41}$$

where

$$P_{wall} = \frac{\alpha\left[(\bar{L}_c/\rho)_\Delta\right]_{gas}^{wall} \left[\bar{\mu}_{en}/\rho\right]_{wall}^{med} + (1 - \alpha) \left[(\bar{L}_c/\rho)_\Delta\right]_{gas}^{med}}{\left[(\bar{L}_c/\rho)_\Delta\right]_{gas}^{med}} \tag{11-42}$$

The wall correction factor P_{wall} becomes unity if the chamber has no wall or if its wall material is identical to the medium.

For a directed beam, the perturbation factor P_{repl} can be divided into a gradient correction, P_{gr}, and a fluence correction, P_{fl}; thus,

$$P_{repl} = P_{gr} P_{fl} \tag{11-43}$$

The gradient correction, P_{gr}, arises because the chamber does not provide a point measurement, but averages the dose over a region. If a radiation field is uniform and the measurement is made in a gradient-free condition, $P_{gr} = 1$. For example, this could be the case in the peak build-up region of a depth dose curve in a directed beam. The fluence correction, P_{fl}, allows for the change in the secondary-particle fluence caused by insertion of the cavity.

11.7.7
Determining N_{gas} from $N_{X,Co}$

Let us assume that the chamber and its electrometer are calibrated by an ADCL and a cobalt-60 exposure calibration factor $N_{X,Co}$ is obtained. The calibration factor is applicable to irradiation of the chamber in air with its cobalt-60 build-up cap in place to give CPE. We will first assume that the wall of the chamber and the build-up cap are made of the same material.

In a manner similar to expression (11-40), we can derive from the charge $\Delta Q'$ the dose, D_{air}, to the center of a mass of air replacing the chamber. When all secondary electrons originate in the wall of the chamber,

$$D_{air} = \left[\Delta Q' P_{ion} P_{tpf}\right] N_{gas} \left[\left(\bar{L}_c/\rho\right)_\Delta\right]_{gas}^{wall} \left[\bar{\mu}_{en}/\rho\right]_{wall}^{air} K_{fl} \qquad (11\text{-}44)$$

where K_{fl} is a correction factor that allows for a possible difference in photon fluence caused by the placement of the chamber in air. In practice, the wall material and the build-up cap material can be different. As already mentioned, a fraction α of the electron fluence may come from the wall material and the rest, $(1 - \alpha)$, from the cap material. In such a situation, D_{air} can be evaluated by addition of a correction factor K_{comp} in (11-44) to yield

$$D_{air} = \left[\Delta Q' P_{ion} P_{tpf}\right] N_{gas} \left[\left(\bar{L}_c/\rho\right)_\Delta\right]_{gas}^{wall} \left[\bar{\mu}_{en}/\rho\right]_{wall}^{air} K_{fl} K_{comp} \qquad (11\text{-}45)$$

with

$$K_{comp} = \frac{\left[\left(\bar{L}_c/\rho\right)_\Delta\right]_{gas}^{wall} \left[\bar{\mu}_{en}/\rho\right]_{wall}^{air} + (1 - \alpha) \left[\left(\bar{L}_c/\rho\right)_\Delta\right]_{gas}^{cap} \left[\bar{\mu}_{en}/\rho\right]_{cap}^{air}}{\left[\left(\bar{L}_c/\rho\right)_\Delta\right]_{gas}^{wall} \left[\bar{\mu}_{en}/\rho\right]_{wall}^{air}} \qquad (11\text{-}46)$$

Independently, we can also obtain D_{air} from $N_{X,Co}$ from the relation

$$D_{air} = \left[\Delta Q' P_{ion} P_{tpf}\right] N_{X,Co} \left(\bar{W}/e\right)_{air} \qquad (11\text{-}47)$$

From (11-45) and (11-47), after including K_{comp}, we obtain the following expression relating N_{gas} and $N_{X,Co}$:

$$N_{gas} = \frac{N_{X,Co} \left(\bar{W}/e\right)_{air}}{\left[\left(\bar{L}_c/\rho\right)_\Delta\right]_{gas}^{wall} \left[\mu_{en}/\rho\right]_{wall}^{air} K_{comp} K_{fl}} \qquad (11\text{-}48)$$

In (11-48) the (μ/ρ) and (L/ρ) ratios are for ^{60}Co energy. The factor K_{fl} can be considered as being made up of many correction factors, as follows:

$$K_{fl} = K_{wall} \times K_{st} \times K_{inv} \times K_{el} \times \ldots$$

where K_{wall}, K_{st}, K_{inv}, and K_{el} correct for any fluence changes caused by wall attenuation, stem scatter, beam divergence, the central metallic electrode, etc.

11.7.8
Dose Delivered by Electron Beams

For electron beams irradiating a medium, the dose D_{med} is related to the measured charge $\Delta Q'$ by

$$D_{med} = \left[\Delta Q' P_{ion} P_{tpf}\right] N_{gas} \left[\left(\bar{L}_c/\rho\right)_\Delta\right]_{gas}^{med} P_{repl} \qquad (11\text{-}49)$$

We know that P_{repl} can be divided into P_{gr} and P_{fl}. The values of P_{fl} for cylindrical cavities of different sizes have been reported. P_{fl} can be assumed to be unity for thin parallel-plate chambers which are recommended for electron beam measurements [13, 25, 26]. The correction P_{gr} can also be assumed to be unity if the dose gradient at the point of measurement is negligible, for example, at the peak dose of a depth dose curve. In the region of steep dose fall-off, the need for P_{gr} has been circumvented by some users by the assumption that the effective point of measurement is at one half-radius upstream from the geometric center of cylindrical cavities [11, 12, 27–29].

11.7.9
Converting Dose to Plastic to Dose to Water

For therapy dosimetry, water is recommended as the medium of dose assessment. However, solid plastic materials that behave almost like water are convenient for practical measurements. These may differ marginally (but not negligibly) from water in terms of their densities, and the actual photon fluence obtained at the point of dose measurement can be different from that which would be obtained in water.

For photon beams, the dose to water, D_{water}, is related to the D_{med} assessed in the plastic water-substitute medium by

$$\frac{D_{water}}{D_{med}} = D_{med} \left[\bar{\mu}_{en}/\rho\right]_{med}^{water} [SC]_{med}^{water} \qquad (11\text{-}50)$$

where SC is a correction factor that allows for a possible change in the scatter photon fluence due to the difference between the densities of the medium and of water.

The dose, D_{water}, for an electron beam can be related to the dose D_{med} as follows:

$$D_{water} = D_{med} \left[\bar{S}_c/\rho\right]_{med}^{water} \phi_{med}^{water} \qquad (11\text{-}51)$$

where ϕ_{med}^{water} is a correction factor for a possible fluence change between water and the medium of measurement. For accurate and consistent dose evaluations, the numerical values of various correction factors, ratios of stopping powers, and absorption coefficients should all conform to what has been recommended in any particular published protocol, such as those in References 11 to 21.

The discussion in this Section 11.7 has relied heavily on the use of N_{gas}, which was derived from the ^{60}Co exposure calibration factor $N_{X,Co}$, by using $(\bar{W}/e)_{air}$ (see Eq. 11-47). The discussion remained rather broad and general in order to explain all the intricacies involved. We will discuss next the more recent protocols that adopt restricted conditions in which the above process becomes simplified.

11.8
Calorimetry and Protocols Based on Absorbed Dose to Water

The radiation absorbed energy is degraded into thermal energy or heat with almost 100% efficiency. The temperature rise observed in an irradiated sample of known thermal capacity under adiabatic conditions is related to the radiation dose. Calorimetry relies on the measurement of the temperature rise and assessment of the heat energy delivered to an irradiated sample as a direct method of measurement of the absorbed energy. It does not rely on conversion factors such as $(\bar{W}/e)_{air}$, and its interpretation does not require attention to the physical details of the absorption or interaction processes. Its drawback is that it is a method of very low sensitivity. Even doses of several hundred Gy produce a temperature increase of only a fraction of a degree centigrade, as shown in the following example.

EXAMPLE 11.4

What is the expected rise in temperature of a sample of water that receives a radiation dose of 100 Gy under adiabatic (that is, thermally isolated) conditions? Given: specific heat of water $= 1$ calorie $g^{-1}\,^{\circ}C^{-1}$ and 1 calorie $= 4.18$ Joules.

First, we need to convert Gy to calories per gram.

$$100 \, \text{Gy} = 100 \, \text{J kg}^{-1} = [100/4.18] \, \text{calories kg}^{-1} = 23.92 \, \text{calories}/1000 \, \text{g}$$

$$= 0.024 \, \text{calories g}^{-1}.$$

The stated specific heat for water is 1 calorie $\text{g}^{-1} \, {}^\circ\text{C}^{-1}$, which means that 1 calorie received by 1 g of water will increase its temperature by 1°C. Hence, a dose of 100 Gy will increase the temperature by 0.024°C.

It is interesting to note that during radiotherapy doses in the range of 30–80 Gy is delivered in several fractions. The increase in temperature is so small during these treatments (as seen in the above example) that the patients do not feel the heat.

Hence, the techniques of calorimetry for dosimetry have been complex and have posed severe challenges to the standardization laboratories for developing them. Calorimetric determination needs an irradiation of a thermally isolated material element and observation of its rise in temperature, ΔT. Graphite has been used as a material. No significant heat loss or transfer should happen during the irradiation. The dose D_{med} is given by

$$D_{med} = (C_m \Delta T)/(1 - k_{HD}), \tag{11-52}$$

where C_m is the specific heat of the calorimetric material and k_{HD} is a correction for what is known as "heat defect" [30].

In recent times, it has been possible for some national standard laboratories to use water calorimeters that directly measure the heat generated, and thereby, the radiation energy absorbed in water [30–36].

In such a case, if D_{water} is the dose measured by a water calorimeter for a ${}^{60}\text{Co}$ beam, and $\Delta Q'$ is the charge measured by the ion chamber with its buildup cap for the same identical beam conditions, the following relation holds true:

$$D_{water} = \left[\Delta Q' P_{tpf}\right] N_{D,water,Co}, \tag{11-53}$$

where $N_{D,water,Co}$ is the absorbed-dose-to-water calibration factor at ${}^{60}\text{Co}$ energy. Such a possibility of a standard laboratory providing the value of $N_{D,water,Co}$ (rather than $N_{X,Co}$) is the basis of more recent protocols for high-energy beam calibration [19–21]. These protocols also advocate the use of water itself as the medium for dose measurement, and hence eliminate all additional corrections that may be warranted if any plastic material were used as a phantom. The dose to water when the ion chamber is used at any beam quality other than that of ${}^{60}\text{Co}$, is calculated by use of an ion chamber and beam-quality dependent multiplying factor k_Q, as shown below:

$$D_{water} = [\Delta Q' P_{tpf}] N_{D,water,Co} \, k_Q \tag{11-54}$$

The values of k_Q to be used are calculated and given by the protocols for various commercially available ion chambers and for different photon beam qualities. The value of k_Q changes from 1.000 for ${}^{60}\text{Co}$ to 0.945 ± 0.01 for 25 MV x-rays for typical cylindrical ion chambers.

For electron beams Ref. 19 regards the factor k_Q as made of three components as follows:

$$k_Q = P_{gr} \, k_{ecal} \, k_{R50} \tag{11-55}$$

in which P_{gr} is a gradient correction, k_{ecal} is a nominal first-level ion-chamber-specific factor to modify $N_{D,water,Co}$ to apply to high-energy electrons, and k_{R50} is an additional refining correction factor which is specific to an electron beam that has 50% of the maximum dose at a depth of R_{50} in water. All of these factors are chamber-specific. The value of k_{ecal} may be in the range of 0.897 to 0.916 for typical commercially available cylindrical chambers. The value of k_{R50} is 1.000 for an electron beam having R_{50} of 7.5 cm (and, hence, approximately 18 MeV). k_{R50} gradually reduces from 1.04 to 0.99 as R_{50} changes from 2 cm to 10 cm, that is, from about 4 MeV to 25 MeV. For both photon and electron beams, the protocols advocate the measurement of the depth-ionization fall off in water for a clearly defined beam geometry to identify the beam quality. To avoid the gradient correction, the protocols recommend the use of plane parallel chambers for electron beams, with the value of the product $[N_{D,water,Co}k_{ecal}]$ obtained through a cross-calibration with a cylindrical chamber having a known $N_{D,water,Co}$ [25, 26].

The value of $N_{D,water,Co}$ is related to $N_{X,Co}$ (used in the previous protocols) through $(\bar{W}/e)_{air}$ and other correction factors discussed in Section 11.7. The values of k_Q, k_{ecal}, and k_{R50} given by the later protocols are also calculated by means of the concepts discussed there.

The calibration protocols keep changing and improving. In the future it may become possible for the standard laboratories to use several different high-energy reference beams. They may be able to provide the dose-to-water calibration factor for any beam quality and any chamber [35–36]. Then, there can be even less reliance on calculated conversion factors. It is not within the scope of this book to detail a complete protocol and explain the significance of every step and correction factor used. Although the protocols have a lot of resemblance to each other, variation among them does exist [37–41]. Hence, we emphasize that any physicist called upon to calibrate a therapy beam for clinical application should study an entire protocol thoroughly. A chosen protocol should be followed in all of its details so that the beams are calibrated to an expected consistency and accuracy within a $\pm 2\%$ margin.

11.9
Air-Kerma Rate Constant for Radionuclide Sources

Some of the concepts developed for beams of photons and electrons are useful in the dose or kerma determinations for radioactive sources.

The air-kerma rate constant is a physical constant which has been defined in such a way as to be useful for dosimetry of discrete radioactive sources. It is related to the number and energy of the photons emitted per disintegration of the source nuclide.

First, we take a simple case of an isotropic point radioisotope source S located in air and emitting a discrete monoenergetic photon of energy E_v per disintegration. The activity of the source is A. We wish to calculate the air-kerma rate at point P at a distance r from the source (Figure 11.10). The attenuation of a photon in air between the source and point P can be regarded as negligible. The energy fluence rate at point P, $(\dot{\psi}_E)_{at\ P}$, is given by

$$(\dot{\psi}_E)_{at\ P} = \frac{\text{Photon energy emission rate of source}}{\text{Area of sphere of radius r}}$$

$$= \frac{AE_v}{4\pi r^2} \tag{11-56}$$

Fig. 11.10. A point-isotropic photon source S is located in air. Point P is on the surface of a sphere that has its center at the source and is of radius r

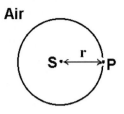

Air

The air-kerma rate at P, $(\dot{k}_{air})_{at\ P}$, is

$$(\dot{k}_{air})_{at\ P} = (\dot{\psi}_E)_{at\ P} \times [\bar{\mu}_{tr}/\rho]_{air}$$
$$= \frac{AE_v}{4\pi r^2}(\bar{\mu}_{tr}/\rho)_{air} \qquad (11\text{-}57)$$

EXAMPLE 11.5

Each disintegration of a radionuclide results in the emission of a photon of energy 660 keV. Calculate the hourly air-kerma rate at 1 cm from a source with an activity of 1 MBq (given that $(\mu_{tr}/\rho)_{air} = 0.0294\ cm^2\ g^{-1}$ at 660 keV and bremsstrahlung loss g is zero).

$$E_v = 660\ keV = 660 \times 1.6 \times 10^{-16}\ J$$
$$A = 1\ MBq = 1 \times 10^6\ disintegrations\ sec^{-1}$$

Because 1 h = 3600 sec,

$$A = 3.6 \times 10^9\ disintegrations\ h^{-1}$$

At the distance r = 1 cm,

$$\dot{\psi}_E = \frac{(3.6 \times 10^9) \times (660 \times 1.6 \times 10^{-16})}{4\pi(1)^2}$$
$$= \frac{3.802 \times 10^{-4}}{4\pi} = 3.026 \times 10^{-5}\ J\ cm^{-2}\ h^{-1}$$

$$\dot{k}_{air} = \dot{\psi}_E \times (\mu_{tr}/\rho)_{air}$$
$$= 3.026 \times 10^{-5}\ J\ cm^{-2}\ h^{-1} \times 0.0294\ cm^{-2}\ g^{-1} \times 10^3\ g/kg$$
$$= 8.896 \times 10^{-4}\ J\ kg^{-1}\ h^{-1}$$
$$= 889.6\ \mu Gy\ h^{-1}\ at\ 1\ cm$$

The above value of k_{air} is a characteristic of the particular source. It gives the air-kerma rate for a source having unit activity (1 MBq) at unit distance (1 cm) from the source. We denote this quantity by the symbol Γ_{ak} and call it the air-kerma rate constant. For the above radionuclide,

$$\Gamma_{ak} = 889.6\ \mu Gy\ MBq^{-1}\ h^{-1}\ cm^2$$

If Γ_{ak} is known, the value of k_{air} at any distance r from a source of activity A MBq, having the same photon spectrum of emission, can be calculated as follows:

$$\dot{k}_{air} = \frac{\Gamma_{ak} A}{r^2} \qquad (11\text{-}58)$$

EXAMPLE 11.6

For the radionuclide source of the previous example, calculate the exposure rate at 1.0 cm when the source has an activity of 1 mCi.

Because $g = 0$, $\mu_{en}/\rho = \mu_{tr}/\rho$, and the transferred energy rate in $\dot{k}_{air}$ can be assumed to be dissipated by ionization in air. We are given the following:

$\Gamma_{ak} = 889.6\,\mu\text{Gy MBq}^{-1}\,\text{h}^{-1}\,\text{cm}^2$;
$A = 1\,\text{mCi} = 3.7 \times 10^7$ disintegrations $\sec^{-1} = 37\,\text{MBq}$;
and $r = 1\,\text{cm}$

Substituting the values for Γ_{ak}, A, and r in expression (11-58), we obtain $\dot{k}_{air}$ at 1.0 cm for a 1 mCi source:

$$\dot{k}_{air} = \frac{889.6\,\mu\text{Gy MBq}^{-1}\,\text{h}^{-1}\,\text{cm}^2 \times 37\,\text{MBq}}{(1\,\text{cm})^2}$$

Because $1\,\mu\text{Gy} = 1 \times 10^{-6}\,\text{J kg}^{-1}$,

$$\dot{k}_{air} = 3.2915 \times 10^{-2}\,\text{J kg}^{-1}\,\text{h}^{-1}$$

The exposure rate is $\dot{X}_{air} = \dot{k}_{air}/(\overline{W}/e)_{air}$. Using $(\overline{W}/e)_{air} = 33.85\,\text{J C}^{-1}$,

$$\dot{X}_{air} = \frac{3.2915 \times 10^{-2}\,\text{J kg}^{-1}\,\text{h}^{-1}}{33.85\,\text{J C}^{-1}} = 9.72 \times 10^{-4}\,\text{C kg}^{-1}\,\text{h}^{-1}$$

Furthermore, $1\,\text{R} = 2.58 \times 10^{-4}\,\text{C kg}^{-1}$. Thus,

$$\dot{X}_{air} = \frac{9.72 \times 10^{-4}\,\text{C kg}^{-1}\,\text{h}^{-1}}{2.58 \times 10^{-4}\,\text{C kg}^{-1}\,\text{R}^{-1}} = 3.76\,\text{R h}^{-1}$$

The exposure rate calculated in the above example is specific to a source of activity 1 mCi, at a distance of 1 cm from the source. It is a constant that is characteristic for the radionuclide and is called the exposure rate constant. We will designate the exposure rate constant by Γ_x, i. e., $\Gamma_x = 3.76\,\text{R mCi}^{-1}\,\text{h}^{-1}\,\text{cm}^2$.

The value of Γ_{ak} is proportional to the product $[E_v(\mu_{tr}/\rho)_{air}]$. We know that $(\mu_{tr}/\rho)_{air}$ itself is a function of E_v. Initially, $(\mu_{tr}/\rho)_{air}$ decreases with an increase in E_v, but reaches a nearly constant value (of about $0.027 \pm 0.003\,\text{cm}^2\,\text{g}^{-1}$) between 80 keV and 2 MeV. Overall, the value of Γ_{ak} first decreases with the energy E_v of emission goes through a minimum at about 60 keV, and from there on increases monotonically with energy.

Thus far, we have discussed only the simplified case of a source emitting one discrete photon per disintegration. However, a radionuclide may emit several photons of different energies. The number of photons of different energies emitted per disintegration may vary. The overall value of Γ_{ak} (or Γ_x) for any actual source can be obtained by summing up, in the proper proportions, of the Γ_{ak} values for the individual photon energies emitted. We will illustrate this by two simple examples.

EXAMPLE 11.7

^{137}Cs emits a 662-keV photon in 86% of disintegrations, a 32-keV photon in 8% of disintegrations, and no photons in the remaining 6%. The Γ_{ak} values at 662 keV and 32 keV are $892\,\mu\text{Gy}\,\text{h}^{-1}\,\text{MBq}^{-1}\,\text{cm}^2$ and $193\,\mu\text{Gy}\,\text{h}^{-1}\,\text{MBq}^{-1}\,\text{cm}^2$, respectively. Evaluate the overall Γ_{ak} (in $\mu\text{Gy}\,\text{MBq}^{-1}\,\text{h}^{-1}\,\text{cm}^2$) and Γ_x (in $\text{R}\,\text{mCi}^{-1}\,\text{h}^{-1}\,\text{cm}^2$) for ^{137}Cs.

We will add the Γ_{ak} for 662 keV and 32 keV in the proportion of their yields.

$$\Gamma_{ak} = 892 \times 0.86 + 193 \times 0.08 = 783\,\mu\text{Gy}\,\text{MBq}^{-1}\,\text{h}^{-1}\,\text{cm}^2$$

The ratio Γ_{ak}/Γ_x as known from example 11.5, is $(3.76/889.6)\,\mu\text{Gy}^{-1}\,\text{MBq}\,\text{R}\,\text{mCi}^{-1}$. Hence,

$$\Gamma_x = 3.31\,\text{R}\,\text{mCi}^{-1}\,\text{h}^{-1}\,\text{cm}^2$$

EXAMPLE 11.8

^{60}Co emits one photon of energy 1170 keV and another of 1330 keV in each disintegration. Derive the value of Γ_{ak}. Assume that $(\mu_{tr}/\rho)_{air} = 0.0268\,\text{cm}^2\,\text{g}^{-1}$ for both photon energies. Use the result of Example 11.4.

In Example 11.4, using $(\mu_{tr}/\rho)_{air} = 0.0294\,\text{cm}^2\,\text{g}^{-1}$, we derived a value of 889.6 µGy $\text{MBq}^{-1}\,\text{h}^{-1}\,\text{cm}^2$ for Γ_{ak}, for a source that emitted one photon of 660 keV per disintegration. We know that Γ_{ak} increases with the weighted sum of the product $E_v\,(\mu_{tr}/\rho)_{air}$ for all photon energies emitted. At 660 keV, for one photon emitted per disintegration,

$$E_v(\mu_{tr}/\rho)_{air} = 660\,\text{keV} \times 0.0294\,\text{cm}^2\,\text{g}^{-1} = 19.4\,\text{keV}\,\text{cm}^2\,\text{g}^{-1}$$

This sum for ^{60}Co (which emits one photon of 1170 keV and another of 1330 keV for every disintegration), is

$$= 1170\,\text{keV} \times 0.0268\,\text{cm}^2\,\text{g}^{-1} + 1330\,\text{keV} \times 0.0268\,\text{cm}^2\,\text{g}^{-1}$$
$$= 67\,\text{keV}\,\text{cm}^2\,\text{g}^{-1}$$

Thus, the value of Γ_{ak} for ^{60}Co is

$$889.6 \times (67/19.4) = 3072\,\mu\text{Gy}\,\text{MBq}^{-1}\,\text{h}^{-1}\,\text{cm}^2$$

The corresponding value of Γ_x (this can be derived as in the preceding examples) is $12.98\,\text{R}\,\text{mCi}^{-1}\,\text{h}^{-1}\,\text{cm}^2$. It is to be noted that the Γ_x for ^{60}Co is about four times that for ^{137}Cs. This is related to the fact that ^{60}Co releases nearly four times more photon energy fluence ($\approx 1170 + 1330\,\text{keV}$) than ^{37}Cs (that emits on average only about 574 keV) per disintegration.

11.10
Reference Air-Kerma Rate for Specifying Brachytherapy Source Strength

11.10.1
Reference Air-kerma Rate (S_{ak})

In general, a point source may have an activity A, and emit photons of N different energies $E_1, \ldots, E_N$. Photons of a particular energy E_i may be emitted at the rate of n_i per disintegration. Then the air-kerma rate, $S_{ak}(r)$ at a distance r from the source is given by modifying Eq. (11-57) to be a summation as below:

$$S_{ak}(r) = \sum_{i=1} \left[A/(4\pi r^2)\right] [n_i E_i] \left[\mu_{tr}(E_i)/\rho\right]_{air} \qquad (11\text{-}59)$$

The air-kerma rate, $S_{ak}(r)$, can be measured at a distance r from a radioactive source. The value when multiplied by r^2 gives a normalized product $[r^2 S_{ak}(r)]$ that can be stated in units of $\mu Gy\, m^2\, h^{-1}$ (or $cGy\, cm^2\, h^{-1}$ which are equivalent). Some literature refers to $1\,\mu Gy\, m^2\, h^{-1}$ as 1 U. It has been recommended that the strengths of sources used for brachytherapy are specified in terms of the normalized air-kerma rate [42]. The relative merits of different quantities that have been used for the specification of source strength are discussed in more detail in Chapter 17. The National Institute of Standards and Technology (NIST) of the USA has recently commissioned a special wide-angle-free-air chamber (WAFC) for the assay of the air-kerma rate of brachytherapy sources (such as ^{125}I and ^{103}Pd) that emit low-energy photons [43]. It is a circular free-air chamber with a variable volume.

EXAMPLE 11.9

A ^{60}Co source having a reference air-kerma rate of $170\,\mu Gy\, m^2\, h^{-1}$ (or $cGy\, cm^2\, h^{-1}$ which is also approximately 15 mCi or 555 MBq). Calculate (a) the air-kerma rate at 2 cm from the source, and (b) the dose rate there in water taking into account the primary attenuation and scatter build-up (discussed in Section 7.10.2).

Given, for ^{60}Co photons in water: Attenuation coefficient $\mu = 0.064\, cm^{-1}$ (from Appendix B); air-kerma to dose conversion factor $(f_{amkd})_{water} = 1.112$ (from Example 11.3); and buildup factor at 2 cm, i. e., B (2 cm) = 1.12 (based on reference 44).

(a) $S_{ak} = 170\,\mu Gy\, m^2\, h^{-1}$; Distance from source r = 2 cm = 0.02 m.
Air-kerma rate at 2 cm in air $= S_{ak}/r^2 = 170\,\mu Gy\, m^2\, h^{-1}/(0.02\, m)^2 = 42.5\, cGy\, h^{-1}$.
(b) We need to evaluate the dose rate by expression:
Dose rate

$$D(r) = [\text{Air-kerma Strength } S_{ak}] \times [\text{Inverse Square factor } 1/r^2]$$
$$\times [\text{Primary attenuation factor } e^{-\mu r}] \times [\text{Buildup factor B}]$$
$$\times [\text{Air-kerma to dose conversion factor } (f_{amkd})_{water}]$$

That is,
$$D(r) = [S_{ak}/r^2] \times [e^{-\mu r} \times B] \times (f_{amkd})_{water} \qquad (11\text{-}60)$$

We have, $S_{ak} = 170\,\mu Gy\, m^2\, h^{-1}$; r = 2.0 cm = 0.02 m
Attenuation $e^{-\mu r} = \exp(-0.064\, cm^{-1} \times 2.0\, cm) = 0.880$;
Buildup factor B (2 cm) = 1.12; and $(f_{amkd})_{water} = 1.112$.
Substituting these values in (11-60), we obtain the dose rate at 2 cm as

$$D(\text{at } r = 2\, cm) = [170\,\mu Gy\, m^2\, h^{-1}/(0.02\, m)^2][(0.880)(1.12)](1.112)$$
$$= 4.66 \times 10^5\,\mu Gy\, h^{-1} = 0.466\, Gy\, h^{-1} = 46.6\, cGy\, h^{-1}.$$

11.10.2
Dose-Rate Constant (Λ)

In many therapeutic use of photon-emitting radioactive sources, the sources are embedded in tissue. Hence, the photon attenuation and buildup in tissue should be accounted for (as was done in Example 11.9 and also discussed in Section 7.10.2.) For our context here, we define an energy absorption buildup factor $B_{en}\{\mu(E_i)r\}$ as given by the ratio:

$$B_{en}\{\mu(E_i)r\} = \frac{\text{Total dose from both scatter and primary (at Energy } E_i)}{\text{Dose from primary only}} \qquad (11\text{-}61)$$

Buildup factors have been evaluated and published in the literature [44, 45]. Thus the dose rate, $D(r)$, at r can be evaluated as

$$D(r) = \sum_{i=1} \left[A/(4\pi r^2)\right] [n_i E_i] \left[\mu_{tr}(E_i)/\rho\right]_{water}$$

$$\cdot \exp\{-\mu(E_i)r\} \cdot B_{en}\{\mu(E_i)r\} \qquad (11\text{-}62)$$

Clinical dose evaluations are generally done for a water-equivalent medium. The ratio $[D(r)/S_{ak}(r)]$ in water at a distance of 1 cm from the source has been given the name "Dose rate constant" and designated by the symbol Λ. It is easy to prove that for a point-isotropic source emitting monoenergetic photons of energy E_v, the dose rate constant $\Lambda(E_v)$ is

$$\Lambda(E_v) = \left[\{\mu_{tr}(E_v)/\rho\}_{water}/\{\mu_{tr}(E_v)/\rho\}_{air}\right]$$

$$\cdot \exp\{-\mu(E_v)r\} \cdot B_{en}\{\mu(E_v)r\}/r^2 \qquad \text{at } r = 1 \text{ cm} \qquad (11\text{-}63)$$

Using the abbreviation U for source strength as referred to above, Λ can be stated in terms of cGy h^{-1} U^{-1} at 1 cm. The calculated values of Λ for bare, unfiltered, monoenergetic point sources are given in Table 11.2 [46]. The value of Λ is of use in brachytherapy dosimetry (covered in Chapter 17). Practical sources may have a finite length and usually have an encapsulation that may preferentially filter low-energy radiation emitted by the source. Hence, practical sources of same radioisotope, say, ^{125}I, but of different models or construction, may have different values of Λ.

EXAMPLE 11.10

For the source of ^{60}Co of Example 11.9, use the data from Table 11.2 and inverse square fall off, to derive the dose rate at 2 cm from the source. Assume the mean energy of ^{60}Co to be 1250 keV.

From Table 11.2, (by extrapolation) dose-rate constant Λ at 1250 keV is 1.090 cGy h^{-1} U^{-1} at 1 cm.

This value is valid for a distance of 1 cm from the source.
At 2 cm the inverse square correction factor is $= (1 \text{ cm}/2 \text{ cm})^2 = 0.25$.
The reference air kerma rate for the source is 170 μGy m^2 h^{-1} = 170 U.
The dose rate at 2 cm $= \Lambda \times S_{ak}/r^2 = 1.09$ cGy h^{-1} U$^{-1} \times 170$ U $\times 0.25$
$$= 46.3 \text{ cGy h}^{-1}.$$

The above answer is marginally different from the value obtained in Example 11.9. This is because of the difference in their ways of allowing for attenuation and scatter in water.

Table 11.2. Dose-rate constant Λ (cGy h^{-1} U^{-1}) for monoenergetic point sources in water*

Photon Energy E_V (keV)	Λ at 1cm.	Photon Energy E_V (keV)	Λ at 1cm.
20	0.649	100	1.259
30	1.086	120	1.229
40	1.250	150	1.193
50	1.300	180	1.169
55	1.310	200	1.159
60	1.312	300	1.133
65	1.312	400	1.122
70	1.308	500	1.114
75	1.301	600	1.107
80	1.294	800	1.097
90	1.277	1000	1.094

* $1\,U = 1\,\mu Gy\,m^2\,h^{-1} = 1\,cGy\,cm^2\,h^{-1}$. Values are reproduced with permission from Reference 46.

References

1. ICRU, Radiation Quantities and Units, ICRU Report 33, International Commission on Radiation Units and Measurements, Washington, D.C., 1980.
2. ICRU, Fundamental Quantities and Units for Ionizing Radiation, ICRU Report 60, International Commission on Radiation Units and Measurements, Bethesda, Maryland, USA, 1998.
3. NCRP, SI Units in Radiation Protection and Measurements, NCRP Report 82, National Council on Radiation Protection and Measurements, Bethesda, Maryland, 1985.
4. ICRU, Average Energy Required to Produce an Ion Pair, ICRU Report 31, International Commission on Radiation Units and Measurements, Washington, D.C., 1979.
5. Wyckoff, H.O., and Attix, F.H., Design of Free-Air Ionization Chambers, National Bureau of Standards, Handbook 64, U.S. Government Printing Office, Washington, D.C., 1957.
6. Loevinger, R., Realization of the unit of exposure: Cavity chambers, in Ionization Radiation Metrology, Casnati, E. (Ed.), Editrice Compositari, Bologna, Italy, 1977, p103.
7. Lanzl, L.H., World radiation therapy dosimetry network, Int. J. Radiat. Oncol. Biol. Phys., Vol 8, pp1607–1615, 1982.
8. Shalek, R.J., Humphries, L.J., and Hanson, W.F., The American Association of Physicists in Medicine Regional Calibration Laboratory System, in Proceedings of a meeting on Traceability for Ionizing Radiation Measurements, NBS Special Publication 609, National Bureau of Standards, Washington, D.C., 1981.
9. Lanzl, L.H., and Rozenfeld, M., Evaluation of the need for radiation calibrations in the United States of America, National and International Standardization of Radiation Dosimetry, Proceedings of a Symposium, Atlanta, Dec 5–9, 1977, Vol 1, p193–197, International Atomic Energy Agency, Vienna, Austria, 1978.
10. AAPM Task Group, Protocol for 40–300 kV X-ray beam dosimetry in radiotherapy and radiobiology, Med. Phys., Vol. 28, pp1868–893, 2001.
11. AAPM Task Group 21, A protocol for the determination of absorbed dose from high energy photon and electron beams, Med. Phys., Vol 10, p741–767, 1983, and Erratum for Figure 6, Med. Phys., Vol. 11, pp213, 1984.
12. Shultz, R.J., Almond, P.R., Kutcher, G., Loevinger, R., Nath, R., Rogers, D.W.O., Suntharalingham, N., Wright, K.A., and Khan, F.M., Clarification of the AAPM Task Group 21 Protocol, Med. Phys., Vol 13, pp756–759, 1986.
13. AAPM Task Group 25, Clinical Electron Beam Dosimetry, Med. Phys., Vol. 18, pp73–109, 1991.
14. IAEA, Absorbed Dose Determination in Photon and Electron Beams: An International Code of Practice, IAEA Technical Report Series 277, International Atomic Energy Agency, Vienna, Austria, 1987.
15. NACP, Procedures in external radiation therapy dosimetry with electron and photon beams with maximum energies between 1 and 50 MeV, Acta Radiol. Oncol., Vol 19, pp55–79, 1980.

16. NACP, Supplement to the recommendations of the Nordic Association of Clinical Physics: Electron beams with mean energies at the phantom surface below 15 MeV, Acta Radiol. Oncol., Vol 20, pp401–415, 1981.

17. SEFM, Procedimientos recommendatos para la dosimetria de fotones y electrones de energias comprendid entre 1 MeV y 50 MeV en radiotherapia de haces externos, Publication No. 1, Sociedad Espanola de Fisica Medica, Madrid, 1984.

18. SEFM, Supplemento al documento SEFM No. 1, 1984, Procedimientos recommendatos para la dosimetria de fotones y electrones de energias comprendid entre 1 MeV y 50 MeV en radiotherapia de haces externos, Publication No. 2, Sociedad Espanola de Fisica Medica, Madrid, 1987.

19. AAPM Task Group 51, Protocol for clinical reference dosimetry of high-energy photon and electron beams, Med. Phys., Vol. 26, pp1847–1870, 1999.

20. International Atomic Energy Agency (IAEA), Absorbed Dose Determination in External Beam Radiotherapy Based on Standards of Absorbed-Dose-to-Water, An International Code of Practice for dosimetry, Technical Report Series No. 398, IAEA, Vienna, 2001.

21. ICRU, Report 64, Dosimetry of High-Energy Photon Beams Based on Standards of Absorbed Dose to Water, International Commission on Radiological Units and Measurements, Journal of the ICRU, Vol. 1, 2001.

22. Holt, J.G., Fleischman, R.C., Perry, D.J., and Buffa, A., Examination of the factors A_c and A_{eq} for cylindrical ion chambers used in Co 60 beams, Med. Phys., Vol 6, pp280–284, 1979.

23. Burlin, T.E., Cavity chamber theory, Chapter 8, Radiation Dosimetry, Vol 1, Attix, F.H., and Roesch, W.C. (Eds.), Academic Press, New York, 1968.

24. Spencer, L.V., and Attix, F.H., A theory of cavity ionization, Radiat. Res., Vol 3, pp239-254, 1955.

25. AAPM Task Group 39, The calibration of and use of parallel-plate ionization chambers for dosimetry of electron beams, Med. Phys., Vol 21, pp1251–1260, 1994.

26. International Atomic Energy Agency (IAEA), The use of plane parallel ionization chambers in high energy electron and photon beams: An international code of practice for dosimetry, Technical Report Series No. 381, IAEA, Vienna, 1997.

27. Dutreix, J., and Dutreix, A., Etude comparee d'une serie de chambres d'ionisation dans des faisceaux d'electrons de 20 et 10 MeV, Biophysik, Vol 3, pp249–258, 1966.

28. Hettinger, G., Petterson, C., and Svensson, H., Calibration of thimble chambers exposed to a photon or electron beam from a betatron, Acta Radiol. (Therapy), Vol 6, pp61–64, 1967.

29. Weatherburn, H., and Stedeford, B., Effective measuring position for cylindrical ionization chambers when used for electron beam dosimetry, Br. J. Radiol., Vol 50, pp921–922, 1977.

30. Domen, S.R., A sealed water calorimeter for measuring absorbed dose, J. Res. Natl. Inst. Stand. Technol., Vol. 99, pp121–141, 1994.

31. C K Ross and N V Klassen , Water calorimetry for radiation dosimetry (Review Article), Phys. Med. Biol., Vol 41, 91–29, 1996. (Determination of absolute dose to water within a relative uncertainty of 0.5 to 1.0% is possible.

32. DuSautoy, A.R., The UK primary standard calorimeter for photon beam absorbed dose measurement, Phys. Med. Biol. Vol. 41, pp137–151, 1996.

33. McEwen, M.R., DuSautoy, A.R., and Williams, A.J., The calibration of therapy level electron beam ionization chambers in terms of absorbed dose to water, Phys. Med. Biol., Vol 43, pp2503-2519, Year 1998.

34. Seuntjens, J.P., and Palmans, H, Correction factors and performance of 4° sealed water calorimeter, Phys. Med. Biol., Vol 44, pp627–646, 1999.

35. Palmans, H., Mondelaers, W, and Thierens, H., Absorbed dose beam quality correction factors k_Q for the NE2571 chamber in a 5 MV and 10 MV photon beam, Phys. Med. Biol., Vol 44, pp647–663, 1999.

36. McEwen M.R., et al., Determination of absorbed dose calibration factors for therapy level electron beam ionization chambers, Phys. Med. Biol., Vol. 46, pp741–755, 2001.

37. Huq, S. M., and Andreo, P, Reference dosimetry in clinical high-energy photon beams: Comparison of the AAPM TG-51 and AAPM TG-21 dosimetry protocols, Med. Phys., Vol. 28. pp46–54, 2001

38. Dohm, O.S., Christ, G., Nusslin, F., Schule, E., Bruggmoser, G., Electron dosimetry based on the absorbed dose to water concept: A comparison of the AAPM TG-51 and DIN 6800-2 protocols, Med. Phys., Vol. 28, pp2258–2264, 2001.

39. Stewart, K.J. and Seuntjens, J.P., Comparing calibration methods of electron beams using plane-parallel chambers with absorbed-dose to water based protocols, Med. Phys., Vol. 29, pp284–289, 2002.

40. Araki, F and Kubo, H.D., Comparison of high-energy photon and electron dosimetry for various dosimetry protocols, Med. Phys., Vol.29, pp857–868, 2002.

41. Tailor, R.C., and Hanson, W.F., Calculated absorbed-dose ratios, TG51/TG21, for most widely used cylindrical and parallel-plate ion chambers over a range of photon and electron energies, Med. Phys., Vol. 29, pp1464–1472, 2002.

42. AAPM Task Group No. 43, Dosimetry of interstitial brachytherapy sources: Recommendations of the AAPM Radiation Therapy Committee Task Group No. 43, Med. Phys., Vol. 22, pp209–234, 1995.

43. Lamperti, P, Mitch, M., Soares, C., and Seltzer, S., Update on NIST Brachytherapy standards and calibrations, BIPM document CCRI (I)/01-15 (Bureau International des Poids ed Mesures, SËvres, France), 2001.

44. Berger, M.J., Energy deposition in water by photons from point isotropic sources, J. Nucl. Med., Suppl. 1, pp17–25, 1968.

45. Angelopulos, A, Perris, A., Sakellarious, K., Sakelliou, L., Sarigiannis, K., and Zarris, G., Accurate Monte Carlo calculations of the combined attenuation and buildup factors, for energies (20–1500 keV) at distances (0–10 cm) relevant in brachytherapy, Phys. Med. Biol., Vol. 36, pp763–778, 1991.

46. Chen, Z., and Nath, R., Dose rate constant and energy spectrum of interstitial brachytherapy sources, Med. Phys., Vol. 28, pp96–86, 2001.

Additional Reading

1. Attix, F H: Introduction to Radiological Physics and Radiation Dosimetry, John Wiley & Sons, New York, USA, 1986.

2. Kase, K. R. and Nelson, W.R., (Eds.) Dosimetry of Ionizing Radiation, Academic Press, New York, 1990.

3. Kase, K. R., Attix, F.H and Bjarngard, B. E., (Eds.), Dosimetry of Ionizing Radiation, Vol. I, Academic Press, New York, USA, 1985.

4. Kase, K. R., Attix, F.H and Bjarngard, B. E., (Eds.), Dosimetry of Ionizing Radiation, Vol. II, Academic Press, Orlando, Florida, USA, 1987.

5. ICRU, Radiation Quantities and Units, ICRU Report 33, International Commission on Radiation Units and Measurements, Washington, D.C., 1980.

6. ICRU, Fundamental Quantities and Units for Ionizing Radiation, ICRU Report 60, International Commission on Radiation Units and Measurements, Bethesda, Maryland, USA, 1998.

7. Domen, S R: Advances in Calorimetry for Radiation Dosimetry. In Kase, K.R., Bjärngard, B.E., and Attix, F.H., The Dosimetry of Ionising Radiation. Vol. II, Academic Press, Orlando, 1987.

CHAPTER 12

Instruments for Radiation Detection

12.1
Introduction

Radiation is detected by measurement of the effect of its interactions with target materials. The radiation-induced effect on a detector produces a signal that can be interpreted to give the radiation quantity of interest. We already discussed the use of ionization chambers and calorimeters for this purpose in Chapter 11. In this chapter, we will provide more details on ionization chambers and also discuss other devices used for radiation detection.

12.2
Ionization Detectors

12.2.1
Role of Applied Potential

Figure 12.1a shows a cylindrical ion chamber detector connected to a commercial electrometer of high sensitivity for measurement of nano-coulomb quantities of charge. The electrometer has a built-in power supply that provides the necessary polarizing voltage to the ion chamber detector. A simplified resistance-capacitance circuit is also shown. For routine use, the chamber and the electrometer are commercially available as an integrated system, with the polarizing voltage, V, preset for optimum operation. Let us assume that V can be varied. Figure 12.1b shows the effect of the applied voltage on the electrometer reading for alpha and beta radiations, representing densely and sparsely ionizing radiations, respectively. The figure suggests that an alpha particle crossing the chamber can be expected to cause more ion pairs than are produced by a relatively more penetrating beta particle.

When a low voltage is applied to the radiation detector, the ions are not collected quickly, and some may recombine prior to collection. The detector's response to a given amount of radiation (i. e., to a radiation pulse) will increase with increases in the applied voltage until a saturation level is reached. This is shown as plateau I in Figure 12.1b. At this plateau, all the ions are collected, without any recombination loss. An ionization chamber should operate at a voltage that corresponds to this plateau. Ion chambers used in practice operate at 150 to 300 V of applied potential. At such potentials, the ions are merely collected while they are drifting with no acceleration. If the voltage applied across the detector is increased further, the ions receive an acceleration and thus gain energy. Such ions of increased energy can produce even more secondary ions in the process of dissipating their energy. Such an increase in

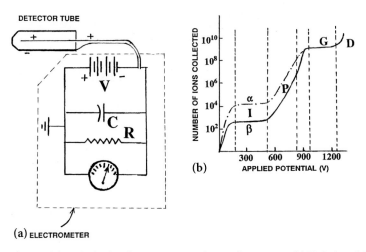

Fig. 12.1. (a) An ionization detector connected to an electrometer. (b) Variation of the number of ions collected with the potential applied

ionization is called "gas multiplication." This effect results in regions P and G in the curves of Figure 12.1b, which are called proportional counter and Geiger-Mueller (GM) counter regions, respectively.

Proportional counters and GM counters operate in pulsed mode; that is, a single photon or beta particle produces an avalanche or pulse of ions. Any single interaction in the detector creates an initial group of ions. At moderately high voltages (corresponding to region P), the size of the final pulse remains proportional to the size of the initial pulse. It is for this reason that the detector is called a proportional counter. A proportional counter can discriminate between a high-pulsed (i. e., a large number of ions) and a low-pulsed initializing event. Still higher potentials cause the detector to operate in the GM counter region G, where even a small initial ionizing event is amplified to such a degree as to ionize the entire gas volume. Here an avalanche of electrons is released which results in a large pulse, with no discrimination between alpha and beta particles and no dependence on the amount of energy that they lost in the initializing event. The region G is called the GM plateau. Still higher potentials, corresponding to region D of Figure 12.1b, will contribute to a direct discharge between the electrodes (caused by the potential itself). The direct-discharge principle is used in a device called a spark counter, which is used in high-energy particle physics.

12.2.2
Condenser Chamber

In Figure 12.1a, the chamber is connected to the electrometer by a cable. A different category of chambers, called condenser chambers, is designed to operate while detached from the electro-meter. Figure 12.2 illustrates a set of chambers of different sizes, designs, and sensitivities for use with a single electrometer. A detailed diagram of a condenser chamber is shown in Figure 12.3a. The two electrodes of the chamber are the central electrode and the conductive coating that is connected to the metallic

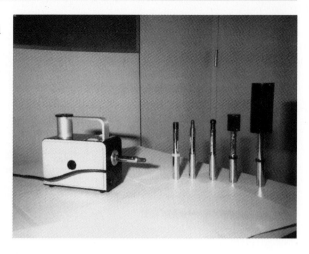

shield. The condenser, which has a high capacitance, is located in the stem. (For chambers that operate through a cable connection to an electrometer, the high-capacitance can be inside the electrometer.) The total capacitance C_t of the assembly is made up of the capacitance C_i of the ion chamber and the capacitance C_s built into the stem; i. e.,

$$C_t = C_i + C_s$$

The stem can be inserted into an electrometer and the capacitance C_t charged, resulting in a voltage V for a charge Q:

$$Q = (C_i + C_s)V$$

When the chamber and the stem are disconnected from the electrometer and irradiated in a beam, a voltage drop ΔV results, indicating an associated charge loss ΔQ, where

$$\Delta Q = (C_i + C_s)\Delta V$$

By measurement of ΔV, one can obtain the value of ΔQ. The value of C_s is sufficiently large to keep the voltage drop ΔV moderately low. Thus, with no resulting increase in ion recombination, the collection efficiency of the detector is maintained.

It may be desirable that the ion-collecting volume of a condenser chamber (such as that shown in Figure 12.3a) is strictly the same as the air volume of the chamber. This can be approximately, but not entirely, true. This is because the construction of the stem may not be perfect, and any tiny air paths in the insulator of the stem can also act as collecting volumes and thus enhance the signal. This increase in the signal, referred to as "stem effect," can depend on the length of the stem irradiated. One can measure the stem effect by irradiating the chamber at the center of a narrow rectangular field in two different ways, first orienting the long axis of the field perpendicular to the stem (Figure 12.3b) and then rotating the field by 90° (Figure 12.3c) to make its length parallel to the stem. The difference in the signal from the two geometries is the stem effect. In practice, the stem effect may either be negligible or amount to a few percent.

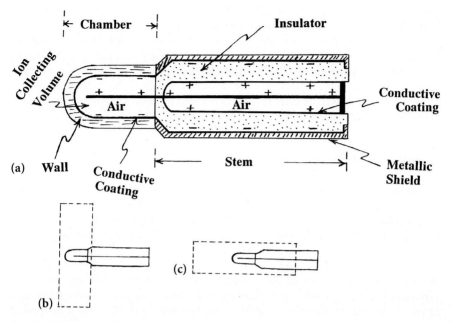

Fig. 12.3. (a) Schematic diagram of a condenser ionization chamber. (b) and (c) Chamber placed in a rectangular field in two different orientations

12.2.3
Cylindrical (Thimble) Chamber

Cylindrical chambers (see Section 11.6.1) have been widely used in radiotherapy. They have nearly cylindrical sensitive volumes and are available in different sizes. We already discussed, in Chapter 11, the perturbation corrections that will be needed for the interference of the air volume and the wall material when the chamber displaces a medium during measurement. In the selection of a chamber, a compromise always must be made in the selection of a chamber between the needed sensitivity and spatial resolution. Chambers of large volume have a high sensitivity for measurement of even small signals, but cannot give a point measurement. For ideal point measurements, small-volume chambers are preferable.

12.2.4
Parallel-Plate (Pancake) Chamber

Another ion chamber geometry uses a collecting volume between two parallel plastic sheets that form the walls of the chamber. The positive and negative electrodes are formed with a coating of a circular conducting layer on the two walls. These parallel-plate chambers (see Section 11.6.2) can be constructed with or without guard electrodes. A layer of gas of 1 to 2 mm thickness is formed between the plates to serve as the collecting volume. The air cavity can be so thin that its perturbation is minimal and much less than that of a cylindrical thimble chamber. The sensitive volume is normal to the radiation beam, and hence a measurement provides an average intensity over a larger cross section than is the case with a thimble chamber. This causes no problem if the chamber is used for measurements at locations in clinical radiotherapy beams where the intensity is expected to be uniform (for example, at the central axis of a typical radiotherapy beam of large cross section). However, it can become a problem if the measurement is to be done in a radiation field (such as a beam modified by the insertion of a wedge filter) that has a dose gradient.

12.2.5
Extrapolation Chamber

Extrapolation chambers use the principles of parallel-plate chambers, but provide for a change of separation between the plates. These chambers are designed for fields that have a uniform intensity across the area of the parallel plates, but vary sharply in the perpendicular direction. This is so, for example, for a planar strontium-90 (^{90}Sr), β-emitting eye applicator. Ideally, one would like to measure the ionization in the thinnest possible cavity, causing a minimum perturbation. However, a very thin cavity with a minimal volume of air cannot offer enough ions to give the required sensitivity. The extrapolation chamber helps to circumvent this difficulty by allowing the estimation of the charge collectible in a negligibly thin collecting layer of air by a method of extrapolation.

In Figure 12.4, a ^{90}Sr source is shown placed above a typical extrapolation chamber. A back-scattering layer of material is located behind the chamber, and a spacer of thickness S is located between the ^{90}Sr applicator and the chamber. Any suitable tissue substitute material can be used for the spacer and the backscatterer. Let us say that the separation (t_i) between the plates is finite and not negligible. It can be varied in a controlled way by the micrometer screw. Measurements of the charge collected per unit time per unit volume for gradually reduced values of t_i can be obtained. Graphic extrapolation of these values can yield an interpreted value for $t_i = 0$. The measurements can be repeated for as many values of S as desired. These chambers can precisely increase the collecting volume by ΔV and ascertain the resultant incremental ionization, ΔQ. The mass of air, Δm, corresponding to volume ΔV can be derived, and the ratio [$\Delta Q/\Delta m$] can be converted to dose (see Section 11.7.4). Hence, well-constructed extrapolation chambers have been used for measuring the dose without depending on

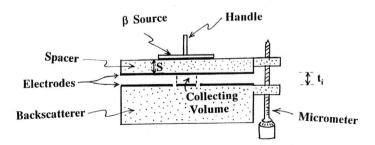

Fig. 12.4. Schematic diagram of an extrapolation chamber

a calibration factor provided by a standard laboratory. Since early years extrapolation chambers have found many useful applications in radiotherapy contexts [1–9].

12.3
Photographic Film Detector

12.3.1
Photographic Process

A photographic emulsion is made of a polyester base coated with photosensitive silver halide (predominantly silver bromide) grains. The radiation or light energy absorbed in the grains forms a latent image. The grains can be developed to become pure silver by treatment of the emulsion in a chemical developer. The developing solution makes use of the latent absorbed energy in the grains for a chemical reaction that reduces the silver halide to silver. Next, the film is treated with a chemical solution that fixes some of the silver to the film base and washes away the silver halide. At places on the film that received a high absorbed energy from the radiation, the silver concentration will be high, and the film consequently will be dark. At sites on the film that received negligible radiation, the film will appear clear and transparent. Hence, the film will give an overall image of the radiation energy absorption pattern [11].

12.3.2
Optical Density

The darkness (or response) of the film is evaluated in terms of optical density, which can be determined quantitatively with a densitometer. The densitometer (Figure 12.5) has a collimated light source below a light-sensing detector. Let us consider that the light intensity measured initially (i. e., with no film in place) is I_0. When a film is placed between the light source and the detector, the intensity may decrease to a value I. Then the optical density D is defined by

$$D = \log_{10}[I/I_0]$$

A density value of 1.0 means that the transmitted light intensity is $(1/10)I_0$. A density of zero means 100% transmission of light by the film. However, this does not happen in practice. The film base can filter some amount of light even without any darkening

Fig. 12.5. Schematic diagram of an optical densitometer

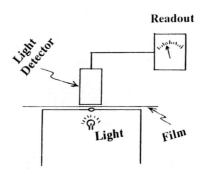

contributed by radiation. This darkness inherent in the film base is referred to as "fog" density. The measured density minus the fog density is called the net density and is relevant for dosimetry.

12.3.3
Calibration of a Film

Film is not an absolute dosimeter. The grain size, the developing time, developer concentration, temperature, and humidity all influence the outcome. Film should be considered to be merely a radiation sensor. For use of the film as a dosimeter, it is necessary to calibrate the response (i. e., the darkening) produced at different doses. For such a calibration, the film should be irradiated by a therapy beam of known dose rate. The conditions of irradiating the film should closely match the conditions under which the calibration of the therapy beam holds. Photon beams are calibrated for conditions of full secondary-electron build-up. While the film is irradiated for calibration by photon beams, the film must be covered above and below with tissue- or air-equivalent materials of a thickness sufficient to give the needed secondary-electron build-up. Different irradiation times will match different dose or exposure levels for calibration purposes.

12.3.4
Film Response Curves

Figures 12.6a and b present the typical variation of the film density with exposure and with the logarithm of exposure, respectively. It can be seen from Figure 12.6a that the density is proportional to exposure for low exposures and low densities. At higher exposures, the film density becomes less than proportional to exposure and finally saturates to a maximum value, when all grains have been developed. The shape of this curve should be known for any particular film for that film to be used as a dosimeter.

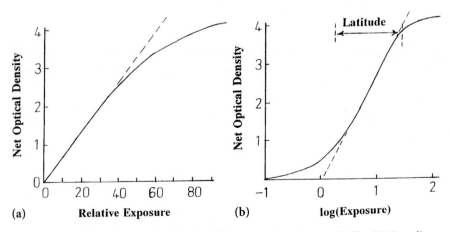

Fig. 12.6. Typical variation of net optical density with exposure for a photographic film. (a) Linear-linear graph; (b) log-linear graph

Ideally, the exposure range used should lie in the region of linear response. Some films have a low sensitivity and wide range, and others may saturate quickly.

The curve of Figure 12.6b is useful for the diagnostic application of films. This curve (which was first published in 1890 by F. Hurter and V.C. Driffield, in England) is referred to as "H & D curve" or "characteristic curve." It can be drawn for any film with or without intensifying screens (see Section 12.3.5). Diagnostic films are viewed with the help of a lighted box. Because the eye responds to light on a logarithmic scale, the level of exposure of the diagnostic film should be in the linear region of the curve in Figure 12.6b. The extent of the straight-line region is the "latitude" of the film. The slope of the curve is called "gamma" and is a measure of the film sensitivity. "Speed" is another term used in reference to sensitivity. "High speed" and "low speed" mean high and low sensitivities. At extremely high exposures (not shown in the figure), the density is known to decrease. (This phenomenon can be exploited for copying an exposed film onto another film by keeping them in contact and shining intense light through them.)

12.3.5
Intensifying Screens and Grids

Figure 12.7 illustrates schematically the geometry of exposure of a patient to a diagnostic X-ray beam imaged by a film. Diagnostic films are often used with intensifying screens. The intensifying screens are held in a light-tight cassette together with the film during the exposure. These screens absorb the X-rays and emit visible and ultraviolet light which, in turn, irradiates the film. The intensification results in increased

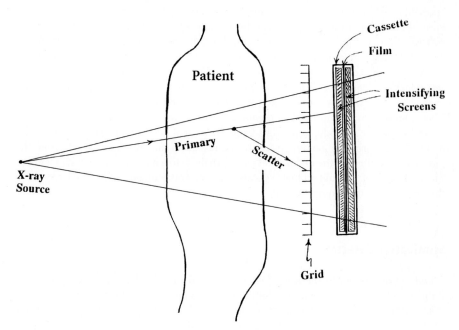

Fig. 12.7. Relative positions of X-ray source, patient, grid, cassette with its intensifying screens, and film during radiography

darkening of the film for the same incident quantity of X-rays and helps to reduce the patient dose.

Intensifying screens are of different designs for different applications and offer different levels of intensification. They can be placed either in front of the film only or in the back as well. Sometimes, it is advantageous to interpose a "grid" between the patient and the film to cut off the scattered radiation (as shown in the figure) and hence reduce the blurring of the image. The grid is made up of radio-opaque ribs. Because the scattered photons travel at angles with respect to the incident direction, they strike the ribs and are prevented from reaching the film. The efficiency of the grid in improving the image will depend on the grid position, spacing, and construction. Some cassettes contain a built-in grid.

12.3.6
High-Energy Port Films

Radiotherapy beams used for treatment of patients are initially localized and simulated with the use of a diagnostic X-ray beam of a radiotherapy simulator that mimics the motions, adjustments, and features of the therapy machine with which the patient will be treated. After the simulation, the actual treatment can be carried out under the therapy machine.

It is necessary to verify the anatomic coverage provided by the therapy beam at the beginning of treatment and also at weekly intervals thereafter. This verification is done with the use of a film that images the treatment port on the patient. Such "port filming" or imaging with a high-energy therapy beam has inherent problems. First, therapy beams are megavoltage beams and produce less contrast between air, soft tissue, and bone than do diagnostic X-ray beams in the 80- to 120-kV range. Second, image blur caused by scatter cannot be reduced by the use of a grid, because no grid can be designed to cut off photons of high energy and penetration. Third, the secondary electrons emanating from the back surface of the patient may have enough energy to penetrate the cassette and join the scattered radiation to blur the image. The situation can be improved by the use of lead or other metal sheets above the film, which cut off the secondary electrons from the patient before they reach the film. The metal also absorbs the low-energy scattered radiation preferentially. In addition, the photoelectric effect in the metal sheet can contribute to a modest image enhancement. Thus, cassettes with built-in metal sheets can give better images of high-energy ports than do those not so equipped [11].

12.4
Scintillation Detector

"Scintillation" refers to the light flashes observed in special crystals activated with impurities (or activators) when radiation energy is absorbed in them. Without the activating impurities, the inorganic crystals do not exhibit any appreciable luminescence. Rutherford used a thin zinc sulfide layer activated by silver to observe scintillations caused by alpha particles. Anthracene crystals have been used for detection of beta particles. Thallium-activated sodium iodide (NaI(Tl)) is a rather commonly used and

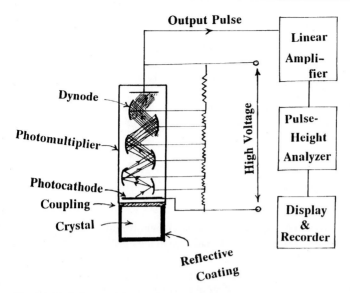

Output Pulse

Dynode

Photomultiplier

Photocathode

Coupling

Crystal

Reflective Coating

High Voltage

Linear Amplifier

Pulse-Height Analyzer

Display & Recorder

Fig. 12.8. Block diagram of a scintillation detector circuit

proven gamma detector. Tissue-equivalent plastic scintillators have been used for quality assurance in radiotherapy [12–14].

Figure 12.8 is a schematic diagram of a scintillation spectrometer. The fluorescent emission from a scintillator can be detected by a photomultiplier tube coupled to the crystal. The photomultiplier has a cathode that releases photoelectrons on being exposed to light. The photoelectron current is amplified within the photomultiplier by a succession of coated metal surfaces shaped for focusing, called "dynodes," which are subjected to a gradually increasing electric potential. A potential of several hundred volts may be used across a photomultiplier tube. The photocurrent amplification results in a detectable pulse, which can be amplified further by an electronic linear amplifier. The potential of the final pulse is dependent on the radiation energy absorbed within the scintillation crystal. The pulses can be fed into a pulse-height discriminator or a multichannel pulse-height analyzer. The observed pulse-height spectrum can be interpreted to yield the energy spectrum of the radiation incident on the crystal. This is the basis of a scintillation spectrometer.

12.5
Solid-State Electrical Conductivity Detectors

Radiation-induced changes in electrical conductivity in semiconductors and crystals can be used for radiation detection [15]. A semiconductor is a substance that has electrical conduction between that of a good conductor and that of an insulator. Silicon and germanium are well-known semiconductors that have found wide applications. Normally, a semiconducting substance will have an equal number of electrons and "holes" ("holes" refer to the presence of a local net positive charge

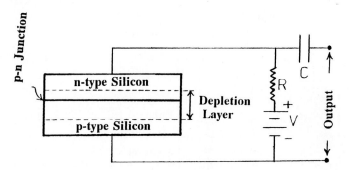

Fig. 12.9. Diagram of a p-n junction semiconductor detector

caused by the absence of an electron in a crystal site). Semiconductor materials can be modified or doped with impurities which make them have either excess electrons or excess "holes." A material with excess electrons is referred to as "n-type" and that with excess holes as "p-type." A semiconductor diode is a junction of p-type and n-type materials. If an electric field is applied across the p-n junction to have a forward bias with the positive terminal connected to the p-type, a current can flow across the junction. If a reverse bias is applied, as shown in Figure 12.9, no current is observed. The excess electrons and holes are swept away from the junction, forming a thin charge "depletion layer" at the interface. When charged particles cross the depletion layer, electron-hole pairs are produced. These cause a current across the junction and produce a signal. Thus, the p-n junction functions like an ion chamber with a sensitive volume corresponding to the depletion layer. Commercially available metal-oxide semiconductor field-effect transistors (MOSFET) [16–19] and diamond crystals have been studied for dosimetry in radiotherapy situations [20–23].

12.6
Thermoluminescent Dosimeters (TLDS)

12.6.1
Thermoluminescence

Thermoluminescence is the phenomenon of light emission from solid crystals that are subjected to heating. The heat acts as an agent to shake off the excited electrons trapped in any metastable energy states in the solid. The electronic transition during the release of the trapped electrons results in emission of light. The traps are metastable states created in the crystal lattice by the addition of impurities. An example is the addition of manganese or magnesium as an impurity to an otherwise regular crystal lattice of LiF, with alternating lithium and fluorine atoms. The impurity sites have electron traps. Irradiation of the crystal lifts some of the electrons from normal energy levels to traps. These electrons contribute to the thermoluminescence observed on subsequent heating of the irradiated sample.

12.6.2
TLD Instrumentation

In practice, the thermoluminescent signal is rather weak and has to be measured with an instrument called a TLD reader (shown in Figure 12.10a), which consists of a dark enclosure with a heating pad, a photomultiplier light sensor coupled to an amplifier, a meter for reading the integrated signal, and a circuit for heating the sample. The intensity of light emission with raised temperature of the sample is called a glow curve (Figure 12.10b). The glow curve may have one or more peaks. The area under that glow curve represents the integrated light output due to the radiation-induced thermoluminescence. This signal can be correlated to dose. However, it should be recognized that the light output is an arbitrary measure, which is influenced by several arbitrarily chosen parameters, including the reflectivity of the heating pad, the heating cycle, the position of the photomultiplier sensor, and the amplification of the photomultiplier output. Furthermore, different thermoluminescent materials have different sensitivities. The amount of impurities added can affect the thermoluminescence yield. In fact, the same crystal may show different yields with differences in thermal treatment (or annealing) prior to use.

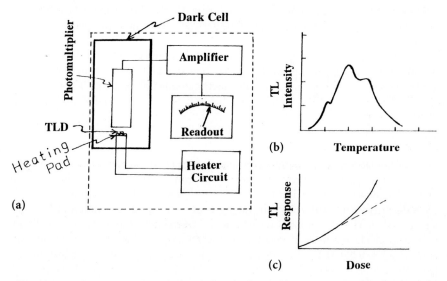

Fig. 12.10. (a) Block diagram of a thermoluminescent dosimeter (TLD) reader. (b) A thermoluminescent glow curve. (c) A typical thermoluminescence (TL) vs. dose-response curve

12.6.3
Measuring an Unknown Dose by TLD

Before being used to measure an unknown dose, the TLD material should be irradiated to known doses and a correlation established between its signal and the dose. The dose vs. response correlation should be established by use of the same quality of the radiation as that in which the unknown dose is to be measured. Generally, the known doses used are applicable to irradiation conditions with charged-particle equilibrium. Thus, for calibration purposes, the TLD sample also should be irradiated under charged-particle equilibrium. This is usually achieved by covering of the TLD on all sides with a plastic material of adequate thickness. Ideally, the TLD material chosen should have the same mass stopping power, attenuation, and absorption characteristics as the medium in which the unknown dose is to be measured. This is somewhat difficult at low energies, where the photoelectric effect plays an important role. The effective Z of the material should be kept in mind for the selection of any one TLD material over another for a given application. It is also possible to vary the effective Z by changing the amount of the added impurities in the TLD material.

TLD materials respond linearly to dose up to a certain dose level, as illustrated in Figure 12.10c. Above that dose level, the response becomes supralinear; that is, it gives a signal that rises more rapidly than proportionally to the dose. The signal from TLD materials fades rapidly in the first 24 h even when these are stored at room temperature. The fading is attributed to the release of electrons in low-lying traps. These electrons contribute to the light emission observed in the low-temperature portion of the glow curve. One way of overcoming the uncertainty caused by the fading is to wait for 24 to 48 h after irradiation and then to read the TLDs. Alternatively, the reading cycle in the TLD reader can be set to ignore the signal during the initial stage of the heating cycle, up to 80–100°C. Then the glow yield will be derived only from the deeper traps, which are not influenced by decay.

Teflon rods or disks impregnated with a thermoluminescent material such as LiF are convenient for use in patients for dosimetry in vivo. LiF phosphor in plastic capsules has been used for intercomparison of dosimetry among different clinics [24–26].

12.7
Chemical Dosimeters

The fact that absorbed radiation energy can induce chemical reactions is the basis of chemical dosimetry [27–28]. We will discuss mainly the ferrous sulfate dosimeter or Fricke dosimeter, introduced in 1927 by H. Fricke, because it continues to be a highly accurate instrument. The Fricke dosimeter is an aerated dilute solution of 0.001 M* ferrous sulfate ($FeSO_4$) in 0.8 N sulfuric acid. (This concentration was originally intended to produce a mass absorption coefficient close to that of air for low-energy X-rays.) Also, 0.001 M NaCl is added, which desensitizes the system against any organic impurities to give improved reproducibility. The solution is placed in a cell and, when irradiated, yields ferric sulfate (Fe_3SO_4) by radiation-induced oxidation of $FeSO_4$. Chemical titration may be used for evaluation of the ferric-ion yield.

A more common method of chemical dosimetry is to measure the absorbance (i. e., optical density) of ultraviolet radiation of 304 nm wavelength in the cell by placing the cell in a spectrophotometer. If the measured absorbance is A, it is related to the concentration C (in moles per liter) of the absorbing species by the expression

$$A = \varepsilon \ell C \qquad (12\text{-}1)$$

---

* M is moles per liter.

where ℓ is the path length through the cell and ε is a constant of proportionality referred to as the molar extinction coefficient. Let us assume that the mass density of the solution is ρ and the concentration of the chemical species monitored per unit volume increases by ΔC due to dose D. Then the chemical yield per unit mass is $(\Delta C/\rho)$. We define the radiation chemical yield (G) as the number of molecules of the chemical product resulting per unit of absorbed energy. Then the dose D is

$$D = \Delta C/(\rho G) \qquad (12\text{-}2)$$

If the absorbance of the cell prior to irradiation is A, it will be $(A + \Delta A)$ subsequent to receiving the dose D. From (12-1)

$$\Delta A = \varepsilon \ell \Delta C \qquad (12\text{-}3)$$

Thus,

$$D = \Delta A/(\varepsilon \ell \rho G) \qquad (12\text{-}4)$$

The value of G varies slowly with the energy of the radiation and is approximately 1.61×10^{-6} mol/J for cobalt-60 gamma rays for 0.4 N sulfuric acid.

The G value of a chemical dosimeter is akin to the W value for the ion chambers discussed in Section 11.5.2. With a known G value, the chemical dosimeter can function as a direct dosimeter. (This is unlike film or TLDs, which need a calibration of their signal with an already known dose.) Chemical dosimeters, in general, are not very sensitive and require high doses (several gray). Chemical species are formed by radiation only indirectly, through several intermediate reactions. Another chemical dosimeter system uses the reduction of ceric sulfate, with a useful range up to 10^8 rad. Other chemical dosimetry systems have used oxalic acid or benzene.

12.8
Optically Stimulated Luminescence (OSL) Dosimetry

The phenomenon of optically stimulated luminescence is similar to thermoluminescence. OSL dosimetry differs from TLD in that the trapped charges from the irradiated sample are released, not by thermal heat, but by an optical laser beam of an appropriate wavelength [29–34]. Like TL, OSL also relates to the dose received by the sample under controlled conditions.

Light emission that is proportional to the radiation dose may occur during the laser stimulation (luminescence) and also continue after the stimulation (phosphorescence). An OSL dosimeter unlike a TLD, can be read several times. Every readout of an OSL sample may release only a small fraction of the trapped energy. At storage temperatures of less than 22°C, the OSL dosimter can maintain the latent signal for more than one year.

A typical OSL reader is somewhat like a TLD reader. However, because the exciting laser beam is a bright light beam, and the luminescent emission is a weak light signal, a pulsed read-out method has been preferred [30–32]. A calibration of the OSL output to a known radiation dose is needed for deriving the dose from a measured luminescence output (as in section 12.6.3).

A very successful OSL dosimetry system uses a layer of anion-deficient aluminum oxide doped with carbon (Al_2O_3: C) [31, 32]. This OSL system offers a wide range from as low a dose as $10\,\mu Gy$ up to $10\,Gy$. Recently, it has been adopted by R.S. Laundauer Inc., Glenwood, Illinois, USA, with the proprietary name Luxel, to provide commercial personnel monitoring for radiation safety [33].

OSL can have other applications in clinical situations in future. Plastic sheets with embedded OSL material can act like radiographic films and can be scanned with a laser beam to produce image patterns. Similar layers can be used for mapping the depth-dose distributions in radiation beams. Fiber-optic probes with OSL phosphors can be used for *in vivo* dosimetry.

12.9
Nuclear Magnetic Resonance (NMR) Dosimetry

Magnetic resonance imaging (MRI) devices have become common in hospitals and clinics around the world. In a previous section, we already discussed chemical dosimetry with ferrous sulfate. NMR dosimetry also depends on the radiation-induced oxidation of ferrous ion to ferric ion as stabilized in a near-tissue-equivalent ferrous sulfate gel. Such a transition also changes the nuclear magnetic resonance spin-lattice (T_1) and spin-spin (T_2) relaxation times. Relaxation times govern the change of MR signal with time. One obtains diagnostic MR images by placing the subject in a strong external magnetic field, applying an "imaging sequence", and measuring the relaxation times. Quantitative evaluation of such relaxation times is also the basis of MRI dosimetry [35–39]. An entire gel phantom is irradiated and imaged to act as a dosimeter [40–42]. The gel structure should be such that there is no transport or migration of the resultant chemical product between irradiation and imaging. MRI produces a three-dimensional (3D) image of the chemical change for visualization. Thus, a "3D" dose image can be recorded even for a complex irradiation with many radiation beams [43–44]. The magnetic relaxation times (both T_1 and T_2) at a point in the gel are inversely proportional to the dose and can be quantitatively evaluated by an MRI scanner. The gel needs to be calibrated with a known radiation dose for a well-defined imaging sequence [45–47]. The sensitivity of this method of dosimetry is such that a dose in the range of 3 to 10 Gy may be needed to double the value of $(1/T_1)$ or $(1/T_2)$. A commercial brand is the 'BANG' gel made by MGS Research Inc., Guilford, Connecticut, USA.

12.10
Radiochromic Film Dosimetry

Radiochromic film is a plastic film impregnated with radiosensitive chemicals or radiochromic dyes [18, 48–57]. A commercial brand produced by GAF Chemical Corporation, Wayne, New Jersey, USA, has the name GafChromic film. On irradiation, the film changes color from a light blue to a denser blue roughly proportional to the absorbed dose. The density (or darkening) of the irradiated region happens with a time delay post irradiation [48, 52, 57]. No chemical processing in a darkroom or development is needed. A delay of about 24 hours is suggested between irradiation and readout for the density to stabilize. The optical density is measured with a special densitometer using a laser blue light of wavelength around 634 nm. Irradiation of a film sample with a known radiation dose is necessary to establish a calibration (as in Section 12.6.3). The test samples should be measured and evaluated under the same conditions as the calibration film. Radiochromic film has been reported to display a response nonuniformity as high as $\pm15\%$ [52, 55]. The dose needed to achieve a net optical density of 1 can vary from 15 Gy to 150 Gy, depending on the exact wavelength of light used and method of densitometry [58].

Radiochromic film, unlike conventional silver halide film, enjoys the merit of near tissue equivalence, making it an energy-independent dosimeter suitable for radiotherapy situations. However, as it is not as sensitive as silver halide emulsions, it requires larger radiation doses for measurements. Radiochromic films have been used to monitor heavy radiation doses associated with industrial irradiations. Multiple layers of films can be used, if need be, to increase the sensitivity in radiotherapy applications. As a planar film, it can be used for mapping a two-dimensional dose distribution with high resolution [55]. Flat-bed scanners coupled to a personal computer have also been used for mapping the dose distribution [54]. Dose evaluation of very small fields is possible due to the high resolution [56].

12.11
Concluding Remarks

For clinical dosimetry, it is important to bear in mind the role of energy absorption coefficients and stopping powers. The amount of radiation energy absorbed or transferred to a dosimeter may or may not represent the dose to tissue, muscle, or bone in a patient that may be sought to be ascertained. This difference is influenced by the energy of the radiation, the stopping power ratios, the effective atomic number, and the electron density of the detector material. The detector's surroundings and embedding may play a role also, as has been discussed in the case of cavity ionization in Section 11.7. In fact, any detector can be thought of as a 'cavity detector' perturbing the medium. Always, attention should be paid to the presence (or lack) of charged-particle equilibrium condition as it can affect the signal, and the interpreted dose. A reliable calibration of the measured signal to a known dose may often be necessary (as outlined in Sections 12.3.3 and 12.6.3 for film and TLD, respectively.) The linearity of the response to dose should be ascertained along with the dose rate independence of the response. Neither of these can be taken for granted. There can be nonlinearity, energy dependence, directional dependence, and background variations. Every dose-measuring device has its own merits and shortcomings for various contexts of application. In this chapter, we have merely abstracted some of the known methods of radiation detection with minimum detail. The reader is advised to study the references cited and the suggested additional readings for a deeper understanding.

References

1. Failla, G., Measurement of tissue dose in terms of the same unit for all ionizing radiations, Radiology, Vol. 29, pp202–215, 1937.
2. Loevinger, R., Extrapolation chamber for the measurement of beta sources, J. Sci. Instrum., Vol. 24, pp907–914, 1953.
3. Rase, S., and Pohlit, W., Eine Extrapolationskammer als Standardmessegerat for energiereiche Photonen und Electronen Strahlung, Strahlentherapie, Vol. 119, pp266–275, 1962.
4. Bohm, J., and Schneider, U., Review of extrapolation chamber measurements of beta rays and low energy x-rays, Rad. Prot. Dosim., Vol. 14, pp 193–198, 1986.
5. Soares, C.G., Calibration of ophthalmic applicators at NIST: A revised approach, Med. Phys., Vol. 18, pp787–793, 1991.

6. Manson, J., Verkley, D., Purdy, J.A., and Oliver, G.D., Measurement of surface dose using buildup curves obtained with an extrapolation chamber, Radiology, Vol. 115, pp473–474, 1975.
7. Klavenhagen, S.C., Determination of absorbed dose in high-energy electron and photon radiation by means of an uncalibrated ionization chamber, Phys. Med. Biol., Vol. 36, pp239–253, 1991.
8. Zankowski, C.E., and Podgorsak, E.B., Calibration of photon and electron beams with an extrapolation chamber, Med. Phys., Vol. 24, pp497–503, 1997.
9. DeBlois, F., Abdel-Rahman, W., Seuntjens, J.P., and Podgorsak, E.B., Measurement of absorbed dose with a bone equivalent extrapolation chamber, Med. Phys., Vol. 29, pp433–439, 2002.
10. Becker, K, Photographic Film Dosimetry, The Focal Press, London and New York, 1966.
11. AAPM Task Group 28, Radiotherapy Port Film Quality, AAPM Report 24, American Association of Physicists in Medicine, American Institute of Physics, New York, 1988.
12. Beddar, A.S., Mackie, T.R., and Attix, F. H., Water equivalent plastic scintillation detectors for high-energy beam dosimetry, I. Physical characteristics and Theoretical Considerations, Phys. Med. Biol., Vol. 37, pp1883–1992.
13. Beddar, A.S., Mackie, T.R., and Attix, F. H., Water equivalent plastic scintillation detectors for high-energy beam dosimetry, II Properties and Measurements, Phys. Med. Biol., Vol. 37, pp1901–1913, 1992.
14. Beddar, A.S., A new scintillator detector system for the quality assurance of ^{60}Co and high-energy therapy machines, Phys. Med. Biol., Vol. 39, pp253–263, 1994.
15. Fowler, J.F., Solid state electrical conductivity dosimeters, In Radiation Dosimetry, Vol. II, (Ed.: Attix, F.H. and Roesch, W.), Academic Press, New York, 1966.
16. Soubra, M., Cygler, J., and MacKay, G.F., Evaluation of a dual bias metal-oxide-silicon field effect transistor detector as a radiation dosimeter, Med. Phys., Vol. 21, pp567–572, 1994.
17. Ramani, R., Russell, S.,and O'Brien, P., Clinical dosimetry using MOSFETs, Int. J. Radiat. Oncol. Biol. Phys., Vol. 37, pp956–964, 1997.
18. Francescon, P., Cora, S., Cavendon, C., Scalchi, P., Reccanello, S., and Colombo, F., Use of a new type of radiochromic film, a new parallel-plate micro-chamber, MOSFETs, and TLD 800 microcubes in the dosimetry of small beams, Med. Phys., Vol. 25, pp503–511, 1998.
19. Scalchi, P, and Fransescon, P., Calibration of a MOSFET detection system for 6-MV in-vivo dosimetry, Int. J Radiat. Oncol. Biol. Phys., Vol. 40, pp987–993, 1998.
20. Planskoy, B., Evaluation of diamond radiation dosemeters, Phys. Med. Biol., Vol. 25, pp519-532, 1980.
21. Hoban, P.W., Heydarian, M., Beckham, W.A., and Beddoe, A.H., Dose rate dependence of a PTW diamond detector in the dosimetry of a 6 MV photon beam, Phys. Med. Biol., Vol. 39, pp1219–1229, 1994.
22. Vatnitsky, S., and Jarvinesan, H., Application of a natural diamond detector for the measurement of relative dose distributions in radiotherapy, Phys. Med. Biol., Vol. 38, pp173–184, 1993.
23. Rustgi, S. N., Application of a diamond detector to brachytherapy dosimetry, Phys. Med. Biol., Vol. 43, pp2085–2094, 1998.
24. Izewska, J and Andreo, P., The IAEA/WHO TLD postal programme for radiotherapy hospitals, Radiother. Oncol., Vol. 54, pp65–72, 2000.
25. Eisenlohr, H.H. and Jayaraman, S., IAEA-WHO cobalt-60 teletherapy dosimetry programme using mailed LiF dosimeters, A survey of results obtained during 1970–1975, Phys. Med. Biol., Vol. 22, pp18–28, 1977.
26. Pfalzner, P.M., and Jayaraman, S., TLD intercomparison of absorbed dose in cobalt-60 teletherapy, Acta Radiologica (Ther., Phys., Biol.), Vol. 9, pp501–512, 1970.
27. Fricke, H., and Hart, E., Chemical Dosimetry, pp167–239, In Radiation Dosimetry, Vol. II, Ed. Attix, F.H. and Roesch, W., Academic Press, New York, 1966.
28. Ellis, S C: The dissemination of absorbed dose standards by chemical dosimetry. Mechanism and use of the Fricke dosimeter, in Ionization Radiation Metrology, in Dosimetry of Ionizing Radiation, Vol. II, Ed., Kase, K., Attix, F.H., Bjarngard, B. E., Academic Press, Orlando, 1987.
29. McKeever, S.W.S., Optically stimulated luminescence dosimetry, SPIE, Vol. 3534, pp531–541, 1999.
30. Akselrod, M.S. and McKeever, S.W.S., A radiation dosimetry system using pulsed optically stimulated luminescence, Rad. Prot. Dosim., Vol. 81, pp167–176, 1999.
31. Akselrod, M.S. and McKeever, S.W.S., Radiation dosimetry using pulsed optically stimulated luminescence of aluminium oxide, Rad. Prot. Dosim., Vol. 84, pp317–320, 1999.
32. McKeever, S.W.S., Akselrod, M.S., Colyott, L.E., Agersnap Larsen, N., Polf, J.C., and Whitley, V.H., Characterization of Al_2O_3 for use in thermally stimulated and optically stimulated luminescence dosimetry, Radiat. Prot. Dosim., Vol. 84, pp163–168, 1998.
33. Technology Monitor, Optically stimulated luminescence dosimeters, Health Phys., Vol. 80, pp108–109, 2001.
34. Bötter-Jensen, L., Bullur, E., Duller, G.A.T., and Murray, A.S., Advances in luminescence instrument systems, Radiation Measurements, Vol. 32, pp523–528, 2000.

35. Olsson, L.E., Petersson, S., Ahlgren, L. and Mattsson, S, 1989, Ferrous suplphate gels for determination of absorbed dose dostribution using MRI technique: basic studies, Phys. Med. Biol., Vol 34, pp43–52, 1989.
36. Day, M.J., Radiation dosimetry using nuclear magnetic resonance: An introductory review, Phys. Med. Biol., Vol 35., pp1605–1609, 1990.
37. Olsson, L.E., Fransson, A., Ericson, A, and Mattsson, S, MR imaging of absorbed dose distributions for radiotherapy using ferrous sulphate gels, Phys. Med. Biol., Vol.35, pp1623–1631, 1990.
38. Maryanski, M.J., Shultz, R.J., Ibbott, G.S., Gatenby, J.C., Xie. J., Horton, D., Gore, J.C., Magnetic resonance imaging of radiation dose distributions using a polymer-gel dosimeter, Phys. Med. Biol., Vol. 39, pp14337–1455, 1994.
39. Chu, W.C., (Invited review paper) Radiation dosimetry using Fricke-infused gels and magnetic resonance imaging, Proc. Natl. Sci. Counc. ROC(B), Vol. 25, pp1–11, 2001.
40. Maryanski, M.J., Gore, J.C., Kennan, R.P., and Shultz, R.J., NMR relaxation enhancement in gels ploymerized and cross-linked by ionizing radiation: A new approach to 3D dosimetry by MRI, Magn. Reson. Imaging, Vol 11, pp253–258, 1993.
41. Kron, T., and Pope, J.M., Dose distribution measurements in superficial x-ray beams using NMR dosimetry, Phys. Med. Biol., Vol. 39, pp1337–1349, 1994.
42. Maryanski, M.J., Ibbott, G.S., Eastman, P., Shultz, R.J., and Gore, J.C., Radiation therapy dosimetry using magnetic-resonance imaging of polymer gels, Med. Phys., Vol 23, pp699–705, 1996.
43. Oldham, M., Baustert, I., Lord, C., Smith, T.A.D., McJury, M., Warrington, A.P., Leach, M.O., and Webb, S., An investigation into the dosimetry of nine-field tomotherapy irradiation using BANG-gel dosimetry, Phys. Med. Biol., Vol. 43, pp1113–1132, 1998.
44. Ibbott, G.S., Maryanski, M.J., Eastman, P., Holcomb, S.D., Zhang, Y.S., Avison, R.G., Sanders, M., and Gore, J.C., 3D visualization and measurement of conformal dose-distributions using MRI of BANG-gel dosimeters, Int. J. Radiat. Ocol. Biol. Phys., Vol 38, pp1097–1103, 1997.
45. Schultz, R.J., deGuzman, A.F., Nguyen, D.B., and Gore, J.C., Dose-response curves for Fricke-infused agarose gels as obtained by nuclear magnetic resonance, Phys. Med. Biol., Vol. 35, pp1611–1622, 1990.
46. Hazle, J.D., Hefner, L., Nyerick, C.E., Wilson, L., Boyer, A., Dose-response characteristics of a ferrous-sulphate-doped gelatin system for determining radiation absorbed dose distributions by magnetic resonance imaging (Fe MRI), Phys. Med. Biol., Vol. 36, pp1117–1125, 1991.
47. Oldham, M., McJury, M., Baustert, I.B., Webb, S., Leach, M.O., Improving calibration accuracy in gel dosimetry, Phys. Med. Biol., Vol. 43, pp2709–2720, 1998.
48. Chu, R.D.H., Van Dyk, G, Lewis, D.F., O'Hara, K.P., Buckland, B.W., and Dinelle, F., GafChromic dosimetry media: A new high dose, thin film, routine dosimeter and dose mapping tool, Radiat. Phys. Chem., Vol 35, pp767–773, 1990.
49. Muench, P.J., Meigooni, A.S., Nath, R., McLaughlin, W.L., Photon energy dependence of the sensitivity of radiochromic film and comparison with silver halide film and LiF TLD's used for brachyterapy dosimetry, Med. Phys., Vol. 18, pp769–775, 1991.
50. McLaughlin, W.L., Chen Yun-Dong, Soares, C.G., Miller, A., Van Dyk, G., Lewis, D.F., Sensitometry of the response of a new radiochromic film dosimeter to gamma radiation and electron beams, Nucl. Instr. and Meth., Vol. A302, pp165–176, 1991
51. AAPM Task Group 55, Radiochromic Dosimetry: Recomendations of AAPM Radiation Therapy Committee Task Group 55, Med. Phys., Vol. 25, pp2093–2115, 1998.
52. Meigooni, A.S., Sanders, M.F. and Ibbott, G.S. Dosimetric characteristics of an improved radiochromic film, Med. Phys., Vol. 23; 11, pp1883–1888, 1996.
53. Klassen, N.V., van der Zwan, L., and Cygler, J., GafChromic MD-55: Investigated as a precision dosimeter, Med. Phys. Vol. 24, pp1924–1934, 1997.
54. Stevens, M.A., Turner, J.R., Hugtenburg, R.P., and Butler, P.H., High-resolution dosimetry using radiochromic film and a document scanner, Phys. Med. Biol., Vol 41, pp2357–2365, 1996.
55. Zhu, Y., Kirov, A.S., Mishra, V., Meigooni, A.S., Williamson, J.F., Quantitative evaluation of radiochromic film response for two-dimensional dosimetry, Med. Phys. Vol. 24; pp223–231, 1997.
56. Caporali, C., Guerra, A.S., Laitano, R.F., Pimpinella, M., Possenti, L., Study of the characteristics of a radiochromic film for dosimetry of small radiation beams, Physica Medica, Vol. XIII; pp87-89, 1997.
57. Reinstein, L.E., Gluckman, G.R., and Meek, A.G., A rapid colour stabilization technique for radiochromic film dosimetry, Phys. Med. Biol., Vol. 43, pp2703–2708, 1998.
58. Reinstein, L.E., and Gluckman, G.R., Comparison of dose response of radiochromic film measured with He-Ne laser, broadband, and filtered light densitometers, Med. Phys., Vol. 24, pp1531–1533, 1997.

Additional Reading

1. Knoll, G.F., Radiation Detection and Measurement, 3rd edition, John Wiley & Sons, New York, 2000.
2. Shani, Gad, Radiation Dosimetry Instrumentation and Methods, CRC Press, Boca Raton, Florida, USA, 1991.
3. Attix, F H: Introduction to Radiological Physics and Radiation Dosimetry. John Wiley & sons, New York, 1986.
4. Kase, K. R., Attix, F.H and Bjarngard, B. E., (Eds.), Dosimetry of Ionizing Radiation, Vol. II, Academic Press, Orlando, Florida, USA, 1987.
5. Kase, K. R., Attix, F.H, and Bjarngard, B. E., (Eds.), Dosimetry of Ionizing Radiation, Vol. III, Academic Press, New York, Hartcourt College Publishers, 1990.
6. Furetta, C., and Pao-Shan Weng, Operational Thermoluminescence Dosimetry, Imperial College Press, London, 1998.
7. Marshall, T.O., and Dennis, J.A., (Ed.) Proceedings of 8th International. Conference on Solid State Dosimetry, Oxford, 1986, Radiat. Prot. Dosim., Vol. 17, 1986.
8. Kron, T., Thermoluminescence Dosimetry and its application in Medicine – Physics, materials, and equipment, Sciences in Med., Vol. 17, pp 175–199, 1994.

PART V

Dosimetry of Radiation Beams

Basic Ratios and Factors for the Dosimetry of External Beam

13.1
Introduction

Radiotherapy machines are of different kinds and are capable of producing beams of various qualities. Conventional X-ray machines, radioisotope teletherapy machines, and accelerators were discussed in the earlier chapters. Any radiotherapy clinic may equip itself with one or more of these machines, suitably selected to meet its requirements. The quality (meaning the type, energy, and penetration) of the beam produced by any particular radiotherapy machine should be understood so that the machine will be used properly on patients. The penetration characteristics of any beam should be evaluated by experimental measurements.

Several physical quantities have been defined for characterizing radiation beams to aid in their practical use. The experimentally measured values of these quantities are useful for carrying out patient-specific day-to-day calculations of the doses delivered during treatment. They are also of help in the comparison of beams of different qualities so that the most suitable beam is selected for a particular clinical situation. In this chapter, we define and discuss these physical quantities, and use them to study the behavior of radiation beams of different qualities. We also discuss how some of these quantities are interrelated and are useful for calculation of the patient dose. In the current chapter, most of our discussion is concerned with photon beams.

In this discussion, unless otherwise stated, we regard the patient's body as consisting of water-equivalent, unit-density material. We use the word "phantom" for a configuration of materials, including water, that can serve as patient substitutes for experimental measurements. Because the measured quantities are for use in patient dosimetry, we may use the words patient, phantom, water, and tissue interchangeably.

13.2
Defining the Beam Geometry

The controlled delivery of a radiation dose to a patient requires that the patient is properly positioned with respect to the radiation source. Figure 13.1 shows a beam emerging from a source S and collimated by a diaphragm D. Point P is at the center of the tumor being treated. The various parameters that specify the treatment geometry are

(1) The location of the dashed line at the geometric center of the beam, referred to as the central axis of the beam

(2) The distance at which the source is located, as specified by the source-to-skin distance (SSD)

Fig. 13.1. Diagram showing the geometric parameters of a beam irradiating a patient who has a tumor centered at point P

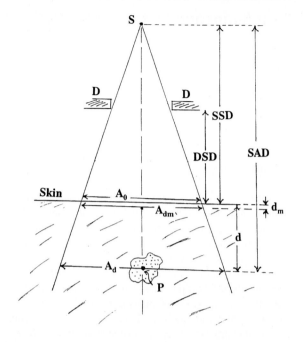

(3) The treatment depth d

(4) The cross section of the beam, commonly referred to as the field size, which can be specified, for example, by its dimension A_d at depth d from the patient's surface.

Adding the SSD and the depth d gives the distance of the source from point P, which we will call the source-to-axis distance (SAD). The term "axis" is used because, in treatment with machines that provide an isocentric rotation, the axis of rotation will commonly be at point P, the center of the tumor. Because SAD = SSD + d, any two of the three variables SSD, d, and SAD can define the third uniquely. One of the two distances, SSD or SAD, is selected in advance for setting up the patient. The other is determined by the treatment depth d for the particular situation. Setups for isocentric machines are conveniently done at a preselected SAD. For nonisocentric machines, a preselected SSD may be used. The above two methods are referred to as "fixed-SAD" and "fixed-SSD" techniques, respectively.

In practice, the beam cross section can be circular, square, or rectangular. For simplicity, we use the symbol A for the field size without reference to any particular shape. Most modern therapy machines produce fields of rectangular cross section that can be specified as having a field size W × L, where W is the width and L is the length. When W and L are given, it is important to recognize not only the distance from the source at which their values are specified, but also the fact that radiation beams do not have a sharp edge (see also Section 15.3.2), but have a penumbra (see Figure 13.2). In radiologic terms, W and L are defined to be the distance between the 50% beam intensity levels, with the 100% level defined to be that at the center of the field. This corresponds to the geometric width (and length) in most practical instances.

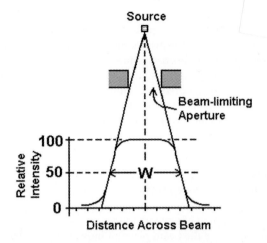

Fig. 13.2. Profile of intensity vs. distance normal to central axis of beam

The symbol A which we use for the field dimension is a collective reference to both L and W.

In general, the beam dimension, **A**, can be specified at any depth or at any distance from the source. A can be specified by A_d at depth d, or by A_0 at the surface. It can also be specified by A_{dm} at the depth d_m at which full secondary electron build-up and the peak dose result. In practice, it is convenient to use the value A_d at depth d at SAD for fixed-SAD setups, and the value A_0 at the surface at SSD for fixed-SSD setups. A_d and A_{dm} are related to A_0 by

$$A_d = A_0 \frac{(SSD + d)}{SSD} = A_0 \frac{SAD}{SSD}$$

$$A_{dm} = A_0 \frac{(SSD + d_m)}{SSD} \tag{13-1}$$

13.3
Quality of Beams

In radiologic physics, we use the term "quality of a radiation beam" to refer to the type of radiation of which the beam consists. Different types of radiations, such as photons, electrons, protons, heavy ions, π mesons, neutrons, etc., may be used for therapy. For our present purpose, quality refers not only to the type of radiation, but also to the penetration and absorption properties of the beam. In this sense, photon beams of different energies have different qualities, and so do electron beams of different energies.

Many parameters are useful for specifying and understanding beam quality. For monoenergetic beams, the energy of the radiation can be stated for specifying the quality. For non-monoenergetic beams, such as X-ray beams modified by filters (see Section 8.6), a measured half-value thickness (HVT) can be used for specifying the quality. At megavoltage energies, the beam quality can be stated in terms of the nominal acceleration voltage corresponding to the peak energy (such as 6-MV X-rays or 10-MeV electrons). For X-rays, because a spectrum of photon energies up to a maximum energy constitutes the beam, specification by the peak MV (such as 25-MV X-rays) is appropriate. For electron beams, specification by MeV (such as 22-MeV electrons) can be used, as these beams are more monoenergetic. These are nominal specifications. However, two different machines producing beams of the same stated nominal quality may have marginally different penetrations. The practical clinical significance of this should not be ignored. Any clinic should carry out actual measurements to ascertain the quality of the beams which they have available, rather than depending on any nominal specifications. In the ensuing discussion, we use Q to refer to beam quality in a broad sense.

13.4
Central-Axis Dose Profile

In the planning of any radiation treatment, the nature of the dose variation along the central axis of the beam plays an important role. Three broad categories of radiation beams are in common use, as indicated by the distinct features of their central-axis dose profiles. These are (i) low-energy kilovoltage (also called orthovoltage) X-rays, (ii) high-energy megavoltage X-rays, and (iii) high-energy electrons. The typical shapes of the central-axis dose profiles of these beams are compared in Figure 13.3 for 3.0-mm Cu HVT X-rays, 10-MV X-rays, and 10-MeV electrons as typical examples of each category.

The 3-mm Cu HVT X-ray beam has a high skin dose and a monotonic and rapid decrease of dose with depth. The 10-MV X-rays have an initial region of rapid dose build-up near the surface up to depth d_m, which is followed by a gradual fall-off. The 10-MeV electron beam shows a gradual and modest dose build-up to a maximum dose, which is followed by a rather steep fall-off that ends in a flat tail. The reasons for the features observed for any high-energy electron beam will be discussed in Chapter 16. The physical basis for the dose build-up observed with high-energy photon beams was discussed in Section 11.3. The depth, d_m, of the peak dose is related to the secondary

Fig. 13.3. Comparison of central-axis depth vs. dose of 3 mm Cu HVT X-rays, 10-MV X-rays, and 10-MeV electrons. SSD is 50 cm for HVT 3 mm Cu, and 100 cm for the others

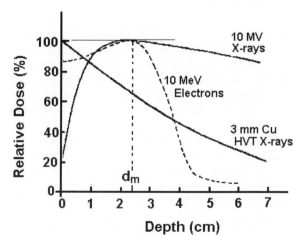

Table 13.1. Depth of the Peak Dose from Water Surface for Different Photon Beam Qualities	Nominal Beam Quality (Q-MV)	Depth of Peak Do d_m (cm)
	Cobalt-60	0.5
	4	1.2
	6	1.5
	8	2.0
	10	2.5
	16	3.0
	18–21	3.5–4.0
	25	4.0–4.5

electron range. The nominal values of d_m for photon beams of different qualities are given in Table 13.1.

The superficial layers of the skin are known to be very radiation-sensitive. With orthovoltage X-rays, the skin dose is higher than the dose delivered in the depth. In the early days of radiotherapy with low-energy X-rays, the skin tolerance limited the dose that could be delivered to a deep-lying tumor. The surface build-up of dose that occurs with high-energy beams eliminates this problem, besides providing improved penetration. The actual surface dose is a complex function of the distance of the collimator from the skin, the field size, the energy of the radiation, and the presence of any material interposed in or located near the beam.

In practical instances, the skin dose from high-energy (megavoltage) X-ray beams can be about 20 to 50% of the peak dose. A significant skin dose is contributed by the secondary electrons produced by photon interactions in materials that are located between the source and the skin. This means that some electron contamination exists in any photon beam. The level of electron contamination should be kept low in order for the skin dose to be low.

The electron contamination dose to the skin increases with decreasing distance of the collimator from the skin. It also increases with increase in field size. The field size cannot be compromised in practice because of the need to cover the volume to be treated; however, it is recommended that a distance of at least 20 cm be maintained between the collimator (or any other device in the beam) and the skin.

13.5
Calculation of Dose in the Depth: General Approach

In clinical practice, the treatment duration should be such that a preselected dose is delivered to a point P at the center of the tumor volume. The most direct way of obtaining the dose rate at P is to place a radiation detector there and measure its response rate, R. If the detector has a response-to-dose conversion factor, C_{sp} (with the subscript sp added to imply that it is specific for this condition of use of the detector), the dose rate $\dot{D}_P$ at P will be

$$\dot{D}_P = R \cdot C_{sp} \tag{13-2}$$

However, making a special measurement for every treatment situation is not practical. Furthermore, it may not be sufficient to know the dose at one site only. Hence, concepts for creating generalized data tables that can be used for varying treatment contexts have been developed. The numerical values in these data sets are ratios (or conversion factors) that relate the dose rate possible under one condition of irradiation to another. The ratios to be used can be ascertained with any convenient, sensitive, small-volume ionization chamber. However, an absolute assessment of a reference dose rate for at least one well-defined "calibration" condition should be made by adhering to a recommended protocol, as has been discussed in Chapter 11. Then one can use the tabulated ratios to derive the dose estimates for any treatment condition.

13.6
Dose to Tissue in Air

Let us consider a collimated radiation beam that diverges and is propagated in air (Figure 13.4). Let us think of a volume of tissue large enough to provide a full secondary-electron build-up at its center (see Section 11.7.2), placed on the central axis of the beam at a distance f_1 from the source. We will refer to the dose at the center of such an equilibrium mass of tissue as "dose to tissue in air." The photons that travel directly from the source to the tissue mass are primary photons. Some photons from the source may interact with objects above the tissue, such as the collimating diaphragm or air. The resulting scattered photons or secondary electrons (as shown by two different Compton interactions in the diaphragm in Figure 13.4) may travel toward the irradiated tissue. Thus, the irradiated tissue sees the following three radiation components:

(1) The primary photons coming directly from the source
(2) The photons scattered from the diaphragm
(3) The secondary electrons resulting from interactions in the diaphragm and in air.

In practice, most of the photon fluence is due to the primary photon component. The secondary electrons do not penetrate the equilibrium mass of tissue and thus do not contribute to the dose at its center. As to photon scatter, in addition to component (2), the scattered photons due to scatter events occurring within the small mass of tissue will add marginally to the dose. The dose contributed at the center of the volume

Fig. 13.4. A collimated photon beam diverging in air, illustrating scattered photon and secondary electron tracks from the diaphragm

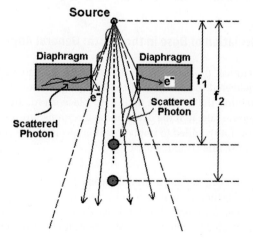

of tissue by such scatter can be considered to be directly proportional to the prim fluence.

13.7
Inverse-Square Fall-Off

The photons from a near-point source travel through air, diverge, and spread over surfaces of increasing area. Attenuation and scatter in air can be discounted because of the low density of air ($0.00129 \, g \, cm^{-3}$). About 80 cm of air will be equivalent to a 1-mm layer of water. If the scatter from the diaphragm is also negligible, the fall-off of the dose to tissue in air with distance from the source will be governed directly by the fall-off of the primary photon fluence. The diverging primary photons from the source will cover areas proportional to f_1^2 and f_2^2 at distances f_1 and f_2 from the source, respectively. Accordingly, the primary fluence should be inversely proportional to f_1^2 and f_2^2 at distances f_1 and f_2. Thus,

$$\text{Dose to tissue in air at distance } f_1 \propto (1/f_1)^2$$
$$\text{Dose to tissue in air at distance } f_2 \propto (1/f_2)^2$$

$$\frac{\text{Dose to tissue in air at distance } f_1}{\text{Dose to tissue in air at distance } f_2} = \left(\frac{f_2}{f_1}\right)^2$$

The above expression is the inverse of the ratio of the square of the distances f_1 and f_2. This ratio (which is a geometrical beam divergence correction) is referred to as the inverse-square distance correction or inverse-square factor (ISqF). The ISqF relates fluence in air (and hence the dose to tissue in air) at two different distances from any given point source under scatter-free conditions. The geometric divergence from the source point that is applicable to primary photons is not true for the scattered photons. Because there are also scattered photons from the diaphragm that irradiate the patient, in reality the photon fluence does not diverge from an ideal point source. In spite of this, the dose fall-off in air can be considered to be proportional to the inverse-square distance from the source without much loss of accuracy. This is shown by the following example.

EXAMPLE 13.1

A ^{60}Co beam has a dose rate to tissue in air of 100 cGy min^{-1} at 80 cm distance from the source. It is known that the collimator scatter contributes 6% of the total dose. The source-to-diaphragm distance is 50 cm. Calculate the dose rate to tissue in air at 100 cm distance from the source, assuming (i) that the entire dose resulted only from the primary photons from the source and (ii) that the contribution of scattered photons came from an effective source located 25 cm below the primary source.

(i) The inverse-square correction for the primary beam is

$$[80/100]^2 = 0.64$$

Applying this correction, we obtain the following dose rate at a distance of 100 cm from the source:

$$100 \, \text{cGy min}^{-1} \times 0.64 = 64.0 \, \text{cGy min}^{-1}$$

(ii) The above factor of 0.64 can be used only for the primary component, which amounts to $(100 - 6 =)$ 94% of the dose. The "effective source" for the scattered photons is 25 cm closer. The inverse-square correction for the scatter part alone is

$$[(80 - 25)/(100 - 25)]^2 = [55/75]^2 = 0.538$$

The primary and scatter contributions at 100 cm are as follows:

$$\text{From primary} = 0.94 \times 100 \, \text{cGy min}^{-1} \times 0.64 = 60.16 \, \text{cGy min}^{-1}$$
$$\text{From scatter} = 0.06 \times 100 \, \text{cGy min}^{-1} \times 0.538 = 3.23 \, \text{cGy min}^{-1}$$

Hence,

$$\text{Total} = 60.16 + 3.23 = 63.4 \, \text{cGy min}^{-1}$$

(Note that the difference is only 1% between the results in (i) and in (ii). This example has been constructed to represent a particularly adverse situation for the approximation to hold.)

13.8
Irradiation Parameters

The dose rate at any point, such as P in Figure 13.1, is related to the fluence of secondary electrons and the energy losses suffered by them at that point. We can assume that, at depths greater than the depth of the peak dose, secondary-electron equilibrium exists and the secondary-electron fluence is directly proportional to the photon fluence. The photon fluence at point P is affected by three main parameters:

(1) The distance SP of point P from the source, which governs the loss of fluence due to the beam divergence (i. e., inverse-square fall-off)
(2) The depth d of point P, which governs the loss of fluence due to the attenuation of radiation in the medium
(3) The field size A_x (with x chosen according to one of the conventions discussed in Section 13.2), which governs the volume irradiated and hence the gain in fluence of the scattered photons.

For the discussion that follows, we will use Figure 13.5, in which the middle diagram shows a water phantom representing a patient. The water phantom is set up with point P at depth d. Our purpose is to devise ways of calculating the dose delivered at point P. On the left and right sides of Figure 13.5, two other beams are shown for comparison. These beams have a size and divergence identical to those of the beam in the middle diagram, but represent two different attenuation and scatter conditions. The beam on the left is a beam in air. The beam on the right has the surface of the water phantom set up so as to have point P at depth d_m at the peak dose. Points 1, 2, 3, and 4 have been identified to help us in defining various transfer factors (or ratios) in setting up procedures for the derivation of the dose rate at point P. We adopt the general notation

$$D(\text{medium, SP, d, } A_x)$$

to refer to the dose (and $\dot{D}$ for dose rate) to a central-axis point such as P in any medium. The parameters listed in parentheses specify, in sequence, the medium (either air or water) in which point P lies, the distance SP of the point from the source, the depth d of

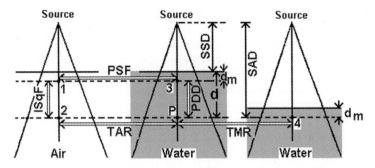

Fig. 13.5. Three different attenuation and scatter geometries for photon beams are shown side by side

the point from the water surface, and the field size A_x. If the medium is air, the depth d is specified from the level in air corresponding to the level of the water surface in the middle diagram. In fixed-SSD geometries, SP = SSD + d. In isocentric geometries, SP = SAD. Thus, following this notation,

$$\text{Dose at P} = D(\text{water}, \text{SAD}, d, A_d)$$
$$\text{Dose at point 1} = D(\text{air}, \text{SSD} + d_m, d_m, A_{dm})$$
$$\text{Dose at point 2} = D(\text{air}, \text{SAD}, d, A_d)$$
$$\text{Dose at point 3} = D(\text{water}, \text{SSD} + d_m, d_m, A_{dm})$$
$$\text{Dose at point 4} = D(\text{water}, \text{SAD}, d_m, A_d) \tag{13-4}$$

Depending upon whether SSD or SAD is fixed, the field size lends itself to a convenient specification by either A_0 at the surface or A_d at the depth. The approximation $A_{dm} = A_0$ can usually be made for all practical purposes. The doses to tissue in air at points 1 and 2 in air are related by an ISqF given by

$$\text{ISqF} = \frac{\text{Dose to tissue in air at point 2}}{\text{Dose to tissue in air at point 1}} = \left(\frac{\text{SSD} + d_m}{\text{SSD} + d} \right)^2 \tag{13-5}$$

13.9
Tissue-Air Ratio (TAR)

The tissue-air ratio (TAR) is a concept that is especially useful in isocentric or fixed-SAD treatment situations. We use A_d for specification of the field size. The TAR at any point is the ratio of the dose in water at that point to the dose to tissue in air, at the same geometric point, with the water phantom replaced by air. In terms of Figure 13.5,

$$\text{TAR at point P} = \frac{\text{Dose in water at P}}{\text{Dose to tissue in air at point 2}}$$

i.e.,

$$\text{TAR} = \frac{D(\text{water}, \text{SAD}, d, A_d)}{D(\text{air}, \text{SAD}, d, A_d)} \tag{13-6}$$

ıse points P and 2 are at the same distance from the source, the fluence as
by beam divergence (i. e., the inverse-square fall-off) is identical for them.
ııowever, the fluence reaching point 1 is also affected by the attenuation and scatter in
water. Thus, TAR links the dose at point 2 to the dose at P, allowing for the differences
caused by attenuation and scatter. The attenuation of the primary photons from the
source is a function of depth d. The accumulation of scattered photon fluence, which
depends on the volume irradiated, is a function of the field size.

We know that attenuation and scatter vary with the beam quality Q. For any particular beam quality, it has been observed that the scatter contribution is more or less
uniquely defined by the field size A_d measured at depth d, irrespective of the SSD used.
In summary, the TAR depends on Q, d, and A_d. The functional dependence of the TAR
can then be stated as

$$TAR = TAR(Q, d, A_d) \tag{13-7}$$

For any given beam quality, the TAR values can be presented in tabular form for
different depths and field sizes. TAR values for cobalt-60 are given in Table 13.2. TAR
tables use the field size A_d specified at depth d. For all practical purposes, the TAR is
independent of the source-to-skin distance (SSD). The TAR increases with the beam
energy and decreases with depth. It increases with field size. The increase of the TAR
with field size is considerable for small fields, but becomes insignificant for large fields.
This is because, with large fields, the field edges are far away from the central axis of the
beam. Any increase in field size adds a scattering volume at a distance too far from the
central axis, and hence it adds negligibly to the scattered photon fluence at the central
axis.

13.10
Peak Scatter Factor (PSF)

The tissue-air ratio specific for the depth of the peak dose, d_m, has been given the
special name "peak scatter factor" (PSF). In terms of the diagram in Figure 13.5,

$$PSF = \frac{\text{Dose in water at point 3}}{\text{Dose to tissue in air at point 1}}$$

i. e.,

$$PSF = TAR(Q, d_m, A_{dm}) = \frac{D(\text{water}, SSD + d_m, d_m, A_{dm})}{D(\text{air}, SSD + d_m, d_m, A_{dm})} \tag{13-8}$$

It is the scattering from the large volume of water surrounding point 3 that causes the
difference in doses between points 1 and 3. Because point 3 is almost at the surface,
the scattered photons come mostly from the medium behind that point, i. e., they are
contributed mainly by backscattered photons. Because of this, the PSF is sometimes
also referred to as the back-scatter factor (BSF). PSF values are always greater than 1.
PSF values are dependent upon beam quality and field size:

$$PSF = PSF(Q, A_{dm}) \tag{13-9}$$

At very low X-ray energies, the photoelectric effect is more significant than Compton
scatter. With increasing energy, the proportion of scattering events increases, but the
absolute number of interactions decreases due to the more penetrating nature of the

Table 13.2. Tissue-Air-Ratios for Cobalt-60 Beams

Depth (cm)	Field Size (cm × cm)														
	0 × 0	4 × 4	5 × 5	6 × 6	7 × 7	8 × 8	9 × 9	10 × 10	12 × 12	15 × 15	20 × 20	25 × 25	30 × 30	35 × 35	40 × 40
0.5	1.000	1.014	1.018	1.022	1.025	1.029	1.033	1.035	1.041	1.049	1.059	1.066	1.070	1.074	1.077
1.0	0.968	0.998	1.004	1.011	1.016	1.021	1.025	1.029	1.035	1.044	1.054	1.062	1.067	1.071	1.076
2.0	0.906	0.961	0.972	0.981	0.988	0.994	0.999	1.005	1.013	1.024	1.036	1.045	1.051	1.056	1.060
3.0	0.849	0.919	0.932	0.944	0.953	0.961	0.968	0.974	0.984	0.996	1.013	1.022	1.029	1.034	1.038
4.0	0.795	0.877	0.892	0.905	0.915	0.925	0.933	0.940	0.953	0.967	0.985	0.996	1.004	1.010	1.017
5.0	0.744	0.832	0.849	0.864	0.876	0.888	0.897	0.905	0.919	0.936	0.957	0.969	0.978	0.984	0.990
6.0	0.697	0.787	0.805	0.820	0.835	0.847	0.858	0.868	0.884	0.904	0.925	0.940	0.950	0.958	0.964
7.0	0.652	0.743	0.763	0.780	0.795	0.808	0.820	0.830	0.848	0.870	0.893	0.908	0.920	0.928	0.935
8.0	0.611	0.702	0.721	0.738	0.754	0.768	0.780	0.791	0.810	0.834	0.861	0.879	0.892	0.900	0.907
9.0	0.572	0.660	0.680	0.699	0.715	0.729	0.742	0.755	0.775	0.799	0.828	0.847	0.861	0.871	0.879
10.0	0.536	0.620	0.642	0.659	0.676	0.692	0.706	0.718	0.738	0.765	0.795	0.816	0.830	0.841	0.850
11.0	0.502	0.585	0.604	0.623	0.639	0.654	0.663	0.680	0.702	0.729	0.762	0.784	0.800	0.811	0.821
12.0	0.470	0.550	0.570	0.587	0.603	0.618	0.632	0.646	0.668	0.696	0.730	0.753	0.770	0.782	0.792
13.0	0.440	0.517	0.536	0.553	0.569	0.584	0.598	0.612	0.635	0.663	0.699	0.723	0.741	0.755	0.765
14.0	0.412	0.487	0.505	0.521	0.539	0.553	0.566	0.579	0.602	0.630	0.668	0.693	0.711	0.726	0.737
15.0	0.386	0.457	0.474	0.491	0.507	0.520	0.533	0.547	0.571	0.600	0.638	0.664	0.683	0.698	0.710
16.0	0.361	0.431	0.448	0.463	0.477	0.491	0.505	0.518	0.542	0.571	0.609	0.636	0.655	0.671	0.684
17.0	0.338	0.403	0.420	0.436	0.450	0.463	0.477	0.490	0.512	0.542	0.580	0.607	0.627	0.644	0.657
18.0	0.317	0.380	0.395	0.410	0.425	0.439	0.451	0.463	0.485	0.514	0.553	0.580	0.600	0.618	0.630
19.0	0.297	0.356	0.370	0.385	0.399	0.412	0.425	0.438	0.459	0.488	0.526	0.553	0.575	0.592	0.606
20.0	0.278	0.335	0.348	0.362	0.375	0.387	0.399	0.411	0.433	0.462	0.500	0.527	0.548	0.566	0.580
22.0	0.244	0.297	0.308	0.321	0.333	0.344	0.356	0.367	0.388	0.416	0.453	0.481	0.503	0.522	0.535
24.0	0.214	0.260	0.272	0.284	0.295	0.305	0.316	0.326	0.346	0.373	0.409	0.437	0.458	0.477	0.492
26.0	0.187	0.230	0.239	0.250	0.261	0.270	0.281	0.291	0.309	0.335	0.370	0.396	0.417	0.436	0.451
28.0	0.164	0.203	0.212	0.222	0.231	0.240	0.250	0.260	0.276	0.299	0.334	0.360	0.382	0.400	0.414
30.0	0.144	0.178	0.187	0.196	0.205	0.213	0.221	0.229	0.245	0.268	0.300	0.326	0.347	0.365	0.378

Reprinted with permission from Br. J. of Radiol., Supplement 17, Central Axis Depth Dose Data for Use in Radiotherapy, British Institute of Radiology, London, 1983.

Table 13.3. Peak Scatter Factors (PSFs)* for Different Beam Qualities and Field Sizes

Beam Quality Q	Field Size (cm × cm)								
	4 × 4	6 × 6	8 × 8	10 × 10	12 × 12	14 × 14	16 × 16	18 × 18	20 × 20
1.0 mm Al HVT	1.13	1.17	1.19	1.20	1.21	1.22	1.23	1.24	1.24
1.0 mm Cu HVT	1.18	1.25	1.31	1.36	1.39	1.42	1.45	1.47	1.49
2.0 mm Cu HVT	1.16	1.22	1.27	1.31	1.35	1.38	1.40	1.42	1.44
^{60}Co	1.014	1.022	1.029	1.035	1.041	1.046	1.051	1.055	1.059

* Based on data from Reference 2.

radiation. The former indicates that the PSF can increase with energy, but the latter indicates that the PSF should decrease with energy. The overall effect of energy on PSF is shown in Table 13.3, which gives the PSF values for different photon energies. The PSF initially increases with the energy of the beam, reaches a maximum at a medium quality of HVT 0.8 mm to 1.0 mm Cu, and then decreases. It is only a few percent more than 1.0 at megavoltage energies. For any given beam quality, the PSF (like the TAR) increases with field size and reaches a saturation value for very large fields.

13.11
Normalized PSF (NPSF)

The peak scatter factor for any field size, A_{dm}, expressed as the ratio of the peak scatter factor for a chosen "standard" field size A_{St} (i. e., with $A_{dm} = A_{St}$) is referred to as the normalized peak scatter factor (NPSF):

$$NPSF = NPSF(Q, A_{dm}) = \frac{PSF(Q, A_{dm})}{PSF(Q, A_{St})} \qquad (13\text{-}10)$$

A_{St} is often selected in practice to be a square field with 10 cm sides.

13.12
Percent Depth Dose (PDD)

This parameter is defined for use with fixed-SSD setups. Hence we can use A_0 for the specification of field size. The PDD at any point in water is the dose at that point expressed as percentage of the peak dose on the central axis of the beam. From Figure 13.5, the PDD for point P is given by

$$PDD = \frac{\text{Dose in water at point P}}{\text{Dose in water at point 3}} \times 100$$

i. e.,

$$PDD = \frac{D(\text{water}, SSD + d, d, A_0)}{D(\text{water}, SSD + d_m, d_m, A_0)} \times 100 \qquad (13\text{-}11)$$

The PDD links the doses at points 3 and P. Tables 13.4, 13.5, and 13.6 provide the PDD data for cobalt-60 beams used at different SSDs. The data in Table 13.7 are for a

Table 13.4. Percent Depth Doses for Cobalt-60 Beams with SSD = 60 cm

Depth (cm)	Field Size (cm × cm)												
	0 × 0	4 × 4	5 × 5	6 × 6	7 × 7	8 × 8	9 × 9	10 × 10	12 × 12	15 × 15	20 × 20	25 × 25	30 × 30
PSF	1.000	1.014	1.018	1.022	1.025	1.029	1.033	1.035	1.041	1.049	1.059	1.066	1.070
0.5	100.0	100.0	100.0	100.0	100.0	100.0	100.0	100.0	100.0	100.0	100.0	100.0	100.0
1.0	95.2	96.8	97.0	97.3	97.5	97.6	97.7	97.8	97.8	97.9	97.9	98.0	98.1
2.0	86.3	90.3	91.0	91.5	91.9	92.2	92.4	92.6	92.8	93.0	93.2	93.4	93.6
3.0	78.3	83.8	84.7	85.4	86.0	86.3	86.6	87.0	87.3	87.7	88.2	88.5	88.8
4.0	71.0	77.6	78.6	79.4	80.1	80.6	81.0	81.5	82.1	82.6	83.3	83.7	84.0
5.0	64.4	71.5	72.7	73.7	74.6	75.2	75.7	76.2	76.9	77.7	78.6	79.0	79.4
6.0	58.6	65.8	67.0	68.1	69.1	69.8	70.5	71.1	71.9	72.9	73.8	74.5	74.9
7.0	53.2	60.4	61.8	63.0	64.0	64.8	65.5	66.2	67.2	68.2	69.3	69.9	70.5
8.0	48.4	55.5	56.9	58.1	59.2	60.0	60.7	61.4	62.5	63.7	65.0	65.9	66.4
9.0	44.0	50.9	52.4	53.6	54.7	55.6	56.4	57.1	58.2	59.5	60.9	61.8	62.5
10.0	40.0	46.7	48.1	49.3	50.5	51.5	52.2	53.0	54.2	55.5	57.0	58.0	58.7
11.0	36.5	42.8	44.3	45.4	46.4	47.3	48.2	49.0	50.3	51.6	53.3	54.3	55.1
12.0	33.2	39.4	40.7	41.8	42.9	43.9	44.7	45.5	46.8	48.2	49.8	50.9	51.7
13.0	30.2	36.1	37.3	38.5	39.6	40.5	41.4	42.2	43.4	44.9	46.6	47.8	48.6
14.0	27.5	33.2	34.3	35.6	36.5	37.4	38.2	39.0	40.3	41.8	43.6	44.7	45.6
15.0	25.1	30.4	31.6	32.6	33.6	34.5	35.3	36.1	37.4	38.9	40.7	41.9	42.8
16.0	22.9	28.0	29.1	30.0	31.0	31.9	32.7	33.5	34.8	36.3	38.1	39.2	40.2
17.0	20.9	25.7	26.7	27.7	28.7	29.5	30.3	31.0	32.3	33.7	35.5	36.7	37.6
18.0	19.1	23.6	24.6	25.6	26.5	27.3	28.0	28.7	29.9	31.4	33.1	34.3	35.2
19.0	17.4	21.6	22.6	23.5	24.4	25.2	25.9	26.6	27.8	29.2	30.9	32.1	33.1
20.0	15.9	19.9	20.8	21.6	22.4	23.2	23.9	24.6	25.7	27.2	28.8	30.0	31.0
22.0	13.3	16.8	17.7	18.4	19.2	19.9	20.5	21.2	22.2	23.6	25.2	26.4	27.3
24.0	11.1	14.3	15.0	15.7	16.4	17.0	17.6	18.2	19.2	20.5	22.0	23.2	24.0
26.0	9.3	12.0	12.7	13.4	14.0	14.6	15.1	15.7	16.6	17.8	19.2	20.3	21.1
28.0	7.8	10.3	10.8	11.4	12.1	12.5	13.0	13.5	14.4	15.5	16.9	17.9	18.6
30.0	6.5	8.7	9.3	9.7	10.2	10.7	11.2	11.7	12.4	13.4	14.8	15.7	16.3

Reprinted with permission from Br. J. of Radiol., Supplement 17, Central Axis Depth Dose Data for Use in Radiotherapy, British Institute of Radiology, London, 1983.

Table 13.5. Percent Depth Doses for Cobalt-60 Beams with SSD = 80 cm

Depth (cm)	Field Size (cm × cm)															
	0 × 0	4 × 4	5 × 5	6 × 6	7 × 7	8 × 8	9 × 9	10 × 10	12 × 12	15 × 15	20 × 20	25 × 25	30 × 30	35 × 35	40 × 40	45 × 45
PSF	1.000	1.014	1.018	1.022	1.025	1.029	1.033	1.035	1.041	1.049	1.059	1.066	1.070	1.074	1.077	1.079
0.5	100.0	100.0	100.0	100.0	100.0	100.0	100.0	100.0	100.0	100.0	100.0	100.0	100.0	100.0	100.0	100.0
1.0	95.6	97.2	97.5	97.7	97.8	97.9	98.0	98.1	98.2	98.3	98.3	98.4	98.5	98.5	98.6	98.7
2.0	87.3	91.4	92.1	92.6	93.2	93.2	93.4	93.7	93.9	94.1	94.3	94.5	94.7	94.8	94.9	95.0
3.0	79.9	85.4	86.3	87.0	87.6	88.0	88.4	88.7	89.1	89.5	90.1	90.3	90.5	90.6	90.7	90.8
4.0	73.0	79.7	80.7	81.6	82.3	82.8	83.2	83.7	84.3	84.9	85.6	86.0	86.3	86.5	86.7	86.9
5.0	66.7	73.9	75.2	76.2	77.1	77.8	78.3	78.8	79.5	80.3	81.3	81.7	82.1	82.4	82.7	82.9
6.0	61.1	68.4	69.7	70.8	71.9	72.6	73.3	73.9	74.9	75.9	76.9	77.5	78.1	78.4	78.7	78.9
7.0	55.8	63.3	64.7	66.0	67.0	67.9	68.6	69.3	70.3	71.5	72.6	73.3	73.9	74.3	74.7	74.9
8.0	51.1	58.5	59.9	61.2	62.3	63.2	64.0	64.7	65.8	67.1	68.6	69.5	70.1	70.5	70.9	71.2
9.0	46.0	53.9	55.5	56.8	57.9	58.8	59.7	60.5	61.7	63.0	64.6	65.6	66.3	66.8	67.2	67.5
10.0	42.9	49.7	51.2	52.5	53.8	54.8	55.7	56.4	57.7	59.2	60.8	61.9	62.6	63.2	63.7	64.1
11.0	39.3	45.9	47.4	48.7	49.8	50.7	51.6	52.5	53.8	55.3	57.2	58.3	59.1	59.8	60.3	60.7
12.0	36.0	42.4	43.8	45.0	46.2	47.2	48.1	48.9	50.3	51.9	53.7	55.0	55.8	56.5	57.0	57.4
13.0	33.0	39.1	40.4	41.6	42.8	43.8	44.7	45.6	47.0	48.6	50.5	51.8	52.8	53.4	54.0	54.5
14.0	30.2	36.1	37.3	38.7	39.7	40.7	41.6	42.4	43.7	45.4	47.4	48.7	49.8	50.5	51.1	51.6
15.0	27.7	33.2	34.5	35.7	36.7	37.6	38.5	39.4	40.8	42.5	44.5	45.9	46.9	47.6	48.2	48.7
16.0	25.4	30.8	31.9	33.0	34.0	35.0	35.9	36.8	38.1	39.7	41.8	43.2	44.2	45.0	45.7	46.3
17.0	23.3	28.3	29.5	30.5	31.5	32.5	33.3	34.1	35.5	37.1	39.2	40.5	41.6	42.4	43.1	43.7
18.0	21.4	26.2	27.3	28.3	29.3	30.2	30.9	31.7	33.1	34.7	36.7	38.1	39.2	39.9	40.6	41.2
19.0	19.6	24.1	25.1	26.1	27.1	28.0	28.8	29.5	30.8	32.4	34.4	35.8	36.9	37.7	38.4	39.0
20.0	18.0	22.2	23.2	24.1	25.0	25.8	26.6	27.4	28.7	30.2	32.2	33.5	34.7	35.5	36.2	36.8
22.0	15.2	19.0	19.9	20.7	21.5	22.3	23.0	23.7	25.0	26.5	28.4	29.8	30.8	31.5	32.1	32.7
24.0	12.8	16.2	17.0	17.7	18.5	19.2	19.9	20.5	21.7	23.1	24.9	26.2	27.3	28.1	28.7	29.3
26.0	10.8	13.8	14.5	15.2	15.9	16.6	17.2	17.8	18.9	20.2	21.9	23.2	24.2	24.9	25.4	25.9
28.0	9.1	11.8	12.5	13.1	13.8	14.4	14.9	15.4	16.4	17.7	19.3	20.6	21.5	22.1	22.6	23.0
30.0	7.7	10.1	10.7	11.2	11.8	12.3	12.8	13.3	14.2	15.4	17.0	18.2	19.0	19.6	19.9	20.2

Reprinted with permission from Br. J. of Radiol., Supplement 17, Central Axis Depth Dose Data for Use in Radiotherapy, British Institute of Radiology, London, 1983.

Table 13.6. Percent Depth Doses for Cobalt-60 Beam with SSD = 100 cm

Depth (cm)	Field Size (cm × cm)															
	0 × 0	4 × 4	5 × 5	6 × 6	7 × 7	8 × 8	9 × 9	10 × 10	12 × 12	15 × 15	20 × 20	25 × 25	30 × 30	35 × 35	40 × 40	50 × 50
PSF	1.000	1.014	1.018	1.022	1.025	1.029	1.033	1.035	1.041	1.049	1.059	1.066	1.070	1.074	1.077	1.080
0.5	100.0	100.0	100.0	100.0	100.0	100.0	100.0	100.0	100.0	100.0	100.0	100.0	100.0	100.0	100.0	100.0
1.0	95.8	97.5	97.7	98.0	98.2	98.3	98.4	98.5	98.5	98.6	98.6	98.7	98.7	98.8	98.9	99.3
2.0	88.0	92.1	92.8	93.2	93.6	93.8	94.0	94.3	94.5	94.8	95.0	95.2	95.4	95.5	95.6	96.0
3.0	80.8	86.4	87.3	88.1	88.6	89.0	89.3	89.7	90.1	90.5	91.1	91.4	91.6	91.7	91.8	92.4
4.0	74.2	81.0	82.0	82.9	83.6	84.1	84.5	85.0	85.7	86.3	87.0	87.4	87.7	88.0	88.3	88.8
5.0	68.2	75.4	76.7	77.7	78.6	79.3	79.8	80.4	81.1	82.0	83.0	83.4	83.9	84.1	84.4	85.2
6.0	62.7	70.1	71.4	72.6	73.6	74.4	75.1	75.8	76.7	77.8	78.8	79.5	80.0	80.4	80.7	81.4
7.0	57.5	65.1	66.6	67.8	68.9	69.8	70.5	71.2	72.3	73.5	74.7	75.5	76.1	76.5	76.9	77.7
8.0	52.9	60.4	61.9	63.1	64.3	65.2	66.0	66.8	68.0	69.3	70.8	71.8	72.5	72.9	73.3	74.3
9.0	48.6	55.9	57.5	58.8	60.0	61.0	61.9	62.7	64.0	65.3	67.0	68.0	68.8	69.3	69.8	70.7
10.0	44.7	51.7	53.3	54.6	55.9	57.0	57.9	58.7	60.0	61.6	63.3	64.4	65.2	65.8	66.3	67.3
11.0	41.1	47.9	49.4	50.8	52.0	52.9	53.9	54.8	56.2	57.8	59.7	60.9	61.8	62.5	63.0	64.0
12.0	37.8	44.4	45.9	47.1	48.3	49.4	50.4	51.2	52.7	54.3	56.3	57.6	58.6	59.2	59.8	60.9
13.0	34.8	41.1	42.5	43.7	44.9	46.0	47.0	47.9	49.3	51.0	53.1	54.5	55.6	56.2	56.8	57.9
14.0	32.0	38.1	39.4	40.7	41.9	42.8	43.7	44.6	46.1	47.8	50.0	51.4	52.5	53.3	53.9	54.9
15.0	29.5	35.2	36.5	37.7	38.8	39.7	40.7	41.6	43.1	44.9	47.1	48.6	49.7	50.5	51.1	52.1
16.0	27.1	32.7	33.9	35.0	36.0	37.1	38.0	38.9	40.4	42.1	44.3	45.8	47.0	47.9	48.5	49.5
17.0	24.9	30.1	31.4	32.5	33.5	34.5	35.4	36.2	37.7	39.4	41.6	43.2	44.4	45.3	46.0	46.9
18.0	23.0	27.9	29.1	30.2	31.3	32.1	33.0	33.8	35.2	37.0	39.2	40.7	41.9	42.7	43.4	44.3
19.0	21.1	25.8	26.9	27.9	28.9	29.9	30.7	31.5	32.9	34.6	36.8	38.4	39.6	40.4	41.2	42.1
20.0	19.5	23.9	24.9	25.9	26.8	27.6	28.5	29.3	30.7	32.4	34.5	36.0	37.3	38.1	38.9	39.7
22.0	16.6	20.5	21.5	22.3	23.2	24.0	24.7	25.5	26.9	28.4	30.6	32.1	33.3	34.1	34.8	35.7
24.0	14.1	17.6	18.4	19.2	20.0	20.7	21.4	22.2	23.4	24.9	27.0	28.4	29.7	30.5	31.2	32.0
26.0	11.9	15.0	15.8	16.5	17.3	18.0	18.6	19.3	20.5	21.9	23.8	25.2	26.4	27.2	27.9	28.5
28.0	10.1	12.9	13.6	14.3	15.0	15.7	16.2	16.8	17.8	19.3	21.1	22.5	23.6	24.3	24.9	25.5
30.0	8.6	11.1	11.8	12.3	12.9	13.5	14.0	14.6	15.6	16.9	18.6	19.9	20.9	21.6	22.1	22.6

Reprinted with permission from Br. J. of Radiol., Supplement 17, Central Axis Depth Dose Data for Use in Radiotherapy, British Institute of Radiology, London, 1983

3.7. Percent Depth Doses for 4-MV X-Ray Beam (Lead Flatness Filter) with SSD = 80 cm

(cm)	Field Size (cm × cm)										
	3 × 3	4 × 4	5 × 5	6 × 6	8 × 8	10 × 10	12 × 12	15 × 15	20 × 20	25 × 25	30 × 30
1.2	100.0	100.0	100.0	100.0	100.0	100.0	100.0	100.0	100.0	100.0	100.0
2.0	95.8	96.3	96.6	96.7	96.7	96.8	96.8	96.8	96.8	96.9	97.0
3.0	89.4	90.3	90.9	91.2	91.6	92.2	92.4	92.6	93.0	93.2	93.5
4.0	83.1	84.3	85.3	86.0	86.5	87.4	87.8	88.1	88.6	88.9	89.3
5.0	77.2	78.8	79.9	80.6	81.6	82.4	83.0	83.7	84.3	84.8	85.3
6.0	71.5	73.3	74.5	75.5	76.8	77.9	78.8	79.5	80.3	80.9	81.6
7.0	66.4	68.2	69.7	70.7	72.1	73.8	74.5	75.2	76.2	77.0	77.8
8.0	61.7	63.2	64.7	65.8	67.6	68.8	70.0	71.2	72.2	73.0	73.9
9.0	57.1	58.7	60.1	61.3	63.0	64.6	66.0	67.2	68.4	69.2	70.1
10.0	53.0	54.6	56.0	57.2	59.1	60.8	62.2	63.6	64.8	65.7	66.8
11.0	49.3	50.8	52.2	53.3	55.1	57.0	58.6	59.9	61.2	62.4	63.3
12.0	45.7	47.0	48.3	49.8	51.7	53.4	55.0	56.2	58.0	59.0	60.1
13.0	42.4	43.7	45.0	46.3	48.2	50.0	51.8	52.9	54.8	56.0	57.2
14.0	39.3	40.5	41.7	43.1	45.1	46.7	48.5	49.9	52.0	53.0	54.2
15.0	36.5	37.8	38.9	40.1	42.1	43.9	45.5	47.0	48.9	50.2	51.2
16.0	33.9	35.1	36.2	37.4	39.3	41.0	42.7	44.2	46.0	47.3	48.5
17.0	31.4	32.6	33.7	34.9	36.7	38.3	40.0	41.6	43.3	44.5	45.7
18.0	29.3	30.4	31.4	32.5	34.3	35.7	37.5	39.0	40.9	42.1	43.3
19.0	27.2	28.2	29.2	30.3	32.0	33.5	35.0	36.8	38.4	39.7	41.0
20.0	25.2	26.2	27.2	28.3	30.0	31.4	32.7	34.4	36.3	37.8	38.8
21.0	23.4	24.3	25.3	26.3	28.0	29.3	30.8	32.4	34.1	35.4	36.4
22.0	21.7	22.6	23.5	24.5	26.3	27.4	28.7	30.3	32.1	33.3	34.4
23.0	20.2	21.1	22.0	22.9	24.5	25.7	26.9	28.5	30.2	31.2	32.4
24.0	18.8	19.6	20.4	21.4	22.9	24.1	25.4	26.7	28.5	29.5	30.5
25.0	17.4	18.2	19.1	19.8	21.4	22.6	23.8	25.0	26.8	27.8	28.8
26.0	16.2	16.9	17.8	18.6	20.0	21.1	22.2	23.5	25.3	26.2	27.1
27.0	14.9	15.7	16.5	17.3	18.6	19.7	20.9	22.0	23.8	24.7	25.6
28.0	13.8	14.6	15.4	16.2	17.4	18.6	19.6	20.7	22.4	23.2	24.1
29.0	12.9	13.5	14.4	15.0	16.3	17.3	18.3	19.4	21.2	21.9	22.8
30.0	11.9	12.6	13.4	14.0	15.2	16.2	17.2	18.2	19.9	20.6	21.4

Reprinted with permission from Peterson, M. and Golden, R., Dosimetry of Varian Clinac-4 Linear Accelerator, Radiology, Vol. 103, p675–680, 1972.

4-MV beam. The PDD is a ratio of doses at two points that are at two different distances from the source. Points 3 and P are at distances $(SSD + d_m)$ and $(SSD + d)$ from the source, respectively. Accordingly, the ratio PDD inherently includes an inverse-square factor $[(SSD + d_m)/(SSD + d)]^2$. The PDD also corrects for the attenuation of the primary photons passing through depth d and the scatter accumulation from the irradiated volume of water, which, in turn, depend on both the depth and the field size. Because the attenuation and scatter vary with the beam quality, the overall functional dependence of the PDD can be stated as

$$PDD = PDD[Q, SSD, d, A_0] \qquad (13\text{-}12)$$

PDD increases with energy. Because the inverse-square divergence correction is lower for larger SSDs, for any given beam quality the PDD increases with SSD. The PDD decreases with depth due to the increase in beam attenuation, and it increases with field size due to the increase in scatter.

It is possible to measure the PDD values for a particular SSD and multiply the values by the term $[(SSD+d)/(SSD+d_m)]^2$, thereby removing the inverse-square component.

Table 13.8. Percent Depth Doses for 25-MV X-Ray Beam with an Infinite SSD

Depth (cm)	Field Size (cm × cm)											
	5 × 5	6 × 6	7 × 7	8 × 8	9 × 9	10 × 10	12 × 12	15 × 15	20 × 20	25 × 25	30 × 30	35 × 35
1.0	65.0	65.9	66.9	68.3	69.5	70.7	73.1	76.5	79.2	82.5	84.2	84.3
2.0	89.8	90.1	90.4	90.9	91.4	91.9	92.7	93.7	94.7	95.5	95.7	95.8
3.0	100.0	100.0	100.0	100.0	100.0	100.0	100.0	100.0	100.0	100.0	100.0	100.0
4.0	102.1	102.1	102.0	102.0	102.0	102.0	101.0	100.2	98.9	98.9	98.9	98.9
5.0	103.4	103.0	102.8	102.2	101.8	101.4	100.7	98.8	97.8	97.6	97.6	97.7
6.0	102.3	102.2	101.9	101.6	101.1	100.6	99.6	98.3	96.3	95.9	95.8	95.8
7.0	100.1	100.1	100.1	99.7	99.3	98.8	97.7	96.1	94.1	93.7	93.7	93.7
8.0	98.0	98.2	98.2	97.9	97.4	96.8	95.7	94.3	92.5	92.0	92.0	92.2
9.0	96.2	96.3	96.2	95.8	95.5	95.1	94.1	92.7	90.9	90.3	90.3	90.6
10.0	93.5	93.6	93.7	93.6	93.2	92.7	91.7	90.5	88.8	88.2	88.0	88.1
11.0	91.2	91.4	91.5	91.4	91.2	90.8	89.9	88.7	87.1	86.6	86.5	86.5
12.0	88.8	89.1	89.2	89.1	88.9	88.6	87.8	86.7	85.4	84.9	84.9	84.9
13.0	86.6	86.9	87.1	87.1	86.9	86.6	86.0	85.0	83.9	83.5	83.6	83.9
14.0	84.3	84.7	85.0	85.0	84.7	84.5	83.8	83.0	82.0	81.8	81.9	82.2
15.0	82.1	82.6	83.0	83.0	82.6	82.6	82.0	81.3	80.5	80.3	80.5	80.8
16.0	80.1	80.6	80.9	80.9	80.7	80.4	80.1	79.5	78.9	78.7	78.8	79.0
17.0	77.9	78.3	78.7	78.7	78.7	78.6	78.3	77.7	77.0	76.8	77.0	77.4
18.0	75.8	76.2	76.6	76.6	76.5	76.4	76.2	75.6	75.0	75.0	75.3	75.6
19.0	73.9	74.5	75.0	75.0	74.9	74.8	74.5	74.2	73.7	73.7	74.0	74.4
20.0	72.1	72.6	73.0	73.0	73.0	72.9	72.4	71.8	71.6	72.0	72.4	72.9
22.0	68.4	68.8	69.1	69.4	69.5	69.5	69.3	69.1	68.9	69.1	69.5	69.8
24.0	64.9	65.4	65.8	66.0	66.2	66.2	66.1	65.9	65.8	66.1	66.7	67.1
26.0	61.4	61.9	62.4	62.7	62.9	63.0	63.2	63.0	63.0	63.5	63.9	64.4
28.0	58.4	58.8	59.1	59.4	59.7	59.9	60.1	60.1	60.2	60.7	60.9	61.6
30.0	55.3	55.8	56.3	56.7	57.0	57.2	57.3	57.5	57.7	58.1	58.7	59.3

Reprinted with permission from Br. J. of Radiol., Supplement 17, Central Axis Depth Dose Data for Use in Radiotherapy, British Institute of Radiology, London, 1983.

Then the resulting PDD data will apply for an infinite-SSD condition of a non-diverging parallel beam. Table 13.8 gives the PDD data for a 25-MV X-ray beam for an infinite SSD.

13.13
Tissue Maximum Ratio (TMR)

The TAR was defined for low X-ray energies at a time when high-energy beams were rare. The TMR is a variation of the TAR that makes it suitable for use at high energies. TAR and TMR are alike, but not identical, concepts.

The TAR uses the dose to tissue in air under conditions of minimum tissue absorption and scatter as the reference denominator. Because, for high-energy photons, the secondary-electron ranges become large, the tissue mass in air satisfying the condition of electronic equilibrium at its center also becomes large, measuring several centimeters in diameter. Such a large mass can also contribute a considerable amount of scattered photon fluence. With such a mass of tissue placed in air, it is a misnomer to refer to the reference denominator in (13-6) as a dose in air and the ratio as tissue-air ratio. This prompted the definition of a tissue maximum ratio (TMR). TMR adopts, for the reference denominator, the peak dose received at that same point for the same field size and distance from the source, with a thickness d_m of overlying water under

tions of full backscatter. In terms of Figure 13.5, TMR is given by

$$\text{TMR} = \frac{\text{Dose in water at point P}}{\text{Dose in water at point 4}}$$

i. e.,

$$\text{TMR} = \frac{D(\text{water, SAD, d, } A_d)}{D(\text{water, SAD, } d_m, A_{dm} = A_d)} \tag{13-13}$$

TMR is the link between the doses at points 4 and P. TMR, like TAR, is insensitive to the SSD and depends on the depth d and the field size A_d at depth d;

$$\text{TMR} = \text{TMR}(Q, d, A_d)$$

It will be noticed that TAR and TMR use the doses at points 2 and 4 as reference denominators, respectively. The dose at point 4 differs from that at point 2 only in the scatter fluence added by water. This is like the difference between points 1 and 3, which was accounted for by the PSF. Thus, the relationship between TMR and TAR is

$$\text{TMR} = \text{TAR/PSF} \tag{13-14}$$

Because PSF values are greater than 1.0, TARs are larger than TMRs for the same depth and field size. Tables 13.9, 13.10, and 13.11 give the TMR data for 4-MV, 6-MV, and 18-MV X-ray beams.

Under infinite-SSD conditions (with no beam divergence and no inverse-square fall-off), the dose at point 4 can be the same as the dose at point 3. Hence, TMR can also be derived by TMR = (PDD for infinite SSD)/100.

13.14
Tissue-Phantom Ratio

If the reference denominator in (13-13) is changed to be the dose at an arbitrarily chosen reference depth d_r, a different ratio (allied to TMR), called the tissue-phantom ratio (TPR), is obtained. The TPR is given by

$$\text{TPR} = \text{TPR}(Q, d, A_d) = \frac{D(\text{water, SAD, d, } A_d)}{D(\text{water, SAD, } d_r, A_{dr} = A_d)} \tag{13-15}$$

13.15
Dose Output Factors

13.15.1
Calibrated Dose Output

In the sense that the machine provides a dose output, the terms "dose" and "output" have been used interchangeably in the literature. ISqF, TAR, TMR, TPR, PSF, and PDD are factors that relate the dose obtained under one condition of distance, depth, absorption, and scatter to that obtained for another set of conditions. We refer to them collectively as depth-dose data. These are merely ratios or percentages and do not provide clues to the absolute dose rates. Machines in different clinics that produce

Table 13.9. Tissue Maximum Ratios for 4-MV X-Ray Beams (through Lead Flattening Filter)

Depth (cm)	Field Size (cm × cm)															
	0 × 0	4 × 4	5 × 5	6 × 6	7 × 7	8 × 8	9 × 9	10 × 10	11 × 11	12 × 12	14 × 14	16 × 16	18 × 18	20 × 20	25 × 25	30 × 30
1.2	1.000	1.000	1.000	1.000	1.000	1.000	1.000	1.000	1.000	1.000	1.000	1.000	1.000	1.000	1.000	1.000
2.0	0.935	0.978	0.980	0.981	0.983	0.984	0.985	0.985	0.986	0.986	0.987	0.988	0.989	0.989	0.990	0.990
3.0	0.900	0.940	0.945	0.950	0.953	0.956	0.959	0.962	0.963	0.964	0.965	0.966	0.968	0.969	0.971	0.972
4.0	0.840	0.897	0.907	0.913	0.918	0.923	0.927	0.930	0.933	0.936	0.940	0.942	0.944	0.946	0.950	0.955
5.0	0.792	0.854	0.867	0.878	0.884	0.890	0.895	0.900	0.904	0.908	0.915	0.918	0.921	0.923	0.929	0.935
6.0	0.751	0.812	0.827	0.838	0.846	0.855	0.862	0.868	0.873	0.878	0.885	0.890	0.894	0.896	0.904	0.912
7.0	0.715	0.771	0.787	0.801	0.810	0.820	0.828	0.835	0.841	0.846	0.855	0.862	0.866	0.871	0.879	0.888
8.0	0.670	0.735	0.750	0.765	0.775	0.785	0.794	0.802	0.809	0.815	0.825	0.833	0.839	0.844	0.855	0.865
9.0	0.634	0.696	0.713	0.728	0.740	0.752	0.761	0.770	0.777	0.783	0.795	0.805	0.813	0.819	0.830	0.841
10.0	0.600	0.661	0.678	0.693	0.705	0.718	0.728	0.738	0.745	0.752	0.764	0.775	0.783	0.791	0.805	0.816
11.0	0.565	0.625	0.643	0.659	0.672	0.685	0.695	0.705	0.713	0.720	0.733	0.745	0.755	0.763	0.779	0.791
12.0	0.535	0.592	0.609	0.627	0.640	0.653	0.663	0.673	0.681	0.689	0.703	0.717	0.729	0.737	0.754	0.761
13.0	0.505	0.562	0.579	0.595	0.607	0.620	0.631	0.642	0.651	0.660	0.674	0.688	0.701	0.710	0.728	0.741
14.0	0.477	0.534	0.550	0.565	0.578	0.591	0.602	0.613	0.623	0.633	0.647	0.661	0.674	0.683	0.702	0.715
15.0	0.450	0.505	0.520	0.535	0.548	0.561	0.572	0.583	0.593	0.603	0.618	0.634	0.648	0.658	0.677	0.692
16.0	0.425	0.480	0.493	0.508	0.520	0.533	0.544	0.555	0.565	0.575	0.592	0.608	0.621	0.631	0.652	0.668
17.0	0.404	0.454	0.468	0.482	0.494	0.506	0.518	0.529	0.535	0.550	0.565	0.581	0.596	0.605	0.627	0.648
18.0	0.380	0.430	0.443	0.457	0.468	0.480	0.491	0.502	0.511	0.520	0.538	0.554	0.569	0.580	0.603	0.623
19.0	0.359	0.408	0.421	0.434	0.446	0.457	0.471	0.478	0.484	0.500	0.516	0.533	0.547	0.556	0.579	0.600
20.0	0.338	0.386	0.399	0.412	0.424	0.435	0.441	0.456	0.466	0.475	0.492	0.508	0.523	0.533	0.557	0.577
21.0	0.319	0.366	0.378	0.390	0.401	0.412	0.423	0.434	0.444	0.453	0.469	0.485	0.500	0.511	0.535	0.554
22.0	0.302	0.346	0.358	0.370	0.381	0.392	0.403	0.413	0.422	0.431	0.448	0.464	0.478	0.489	0.513	0.533
23.0	0.284	0.328	0.340	0.351	0.363	0.372	0.383	0.393	0.414	0.411	0.427	0.443	0.457	0.468	0.490	0.513
24.0	0.269	0.310	0.322	0.333	0.344	0.354	0.364	0.373	0.382	0.391	0.407	0.423	0.436	0.447	0.471	0.492
25.0	0.254	0.294	0.305	0.316	0.326	0.336	0.346	0.355	0.364	0.372	0.389	0.405	0.416	0.427	0.450	0.470
30.0	0.191	0.224	0.233	0.242	0.251	0.260	0.271	0.276	0.284	0.291	0.308	0.323	0.332	0.342	0.364	0.383
35.0	0.143	0.171	0.178	0.186	0.193	0.200	0.213	0.218	0.222	0.228	0.243	0.257	0.265	0.274	0.294	0.312
40.0	0.107	0.130	0.136	0.143	0.148	0.155	0.167	0.168	0.173	0.179	0.192	0.205	0.212	0.220	0.237	0.254

Based on data from Peterson, M. and Golden, R., Dosimetry of Varian Clinac-4 linear accelerators, Radiology, Vol 103, p675-680, 1972.

Table 13.10. Tissue Maximum Ratios for 6-MV X-Ray Beams

Depth (cm)	Field Size (cm × cm)															
	0 × 0	4 × 4	5 × 5	6 × 6	7 × 7	8 × 8	9 × 9	10 × 10	11 × 11	12 × 12	14 × 14	16 × 16	18 × 18	20 × 20	25 × 25	30 × 30
0.0	0.160	0.208	0.220	0.232	0.244	0.256	0.268	0.280	0.289	0.297	0.314	0.332	0.349	0.367	0.411	0.455
0.4	0.661	0.667	0.668	0.673	0.679	0.684	0.690	0.695	0.697	0.705	0.715	0.726	0.737	0.747	0.768	0.795
0.8	0.832	0.847	0.851	0.854	0.858	0.862	0.866	0.870	0.873	0.876	0.882	0.888	0.895	0.901	0.915	0.929
1.2	0.957	0.961	0.962	0.963	0.964	0.965	0.966	0.967	0.968	0.968	0.968	0.971	0.975	0.979	0.983	0.985
1.5	1.000	1.000	1.000	1.000	1.000	1.000	1.000	1.000	1.000	1.000	1.000	1.000	1.000	1.000	1.000	1.000
2.0	0.977	0.983	0.984	0.985	0.986	0.987	0.988	0.988	0.989	0.990	0.992	0.992	0.993	0.994	0.994	0.995
3.0	0.932	0.956	0.960	0.963	0.965	0.967	0.969	0.970	0.971	0.971	0.972	0.973	0.974	0.976	0.976	0.977
4.0	0.889	0.923	0.929	0.934	0.937	0.940	0.943	0.945	0.947	0.948	0.951	0.952	0.954	0.955	0.956	0.957
5.0	0.848	0.889	0.895	0.902	0.906	0.910	0.914	0.917	0.919	0.922	0.925	0.927	0.929	0.931	0.934	0.936
6.0	0.809	0.856	0.864	0.870	0.876	0.882	0.887	0.891	0.894	0.897	0.901	0.904	0.907	0.910	0.915	0.918
7.0	0.772	0.823	0.832	0.847	0.850	0.853	0.857	0.862	0.866	0.870	0.875	0.879	0.882	0.885	0.893	0.900
8.0	0.737	0.787	0.796	0.805	0.813	0.820	0.826	0.832	0.837	0.842	0.849	0.854	0.859	0.864	0.871	0.877
9.0	0.703	0.756	0.765	0.774	0.781	0.788	0.794	0.800	0.806	0.811	0.819	0.826	0.833	0.839	0.849	0.854
10.0	0.671	0.721	0.731	0.740	0.748	0.756	0.763	0.770	0.776	0.782	0.791	0.800	0.807	0.814	0.827	0.832
11.0	0.640	0.691	0.701	0.712	0.721	0.729	0.739	0.745	0.751	0.756	0.766	0.775	0.783	0.790	0.803	0.809
12.0	0.610	0.666	0.676	0.686	0.695	0.704	0.717	0.719	0.726	0.732	0.742	0.751	0.759	0.767	0.778	0.788
13.0	0.582	0.637	0.648	0.658	0.667	0.675	0.684	0.690	0.696	0.702	0.713	0.723	0.732	0.741	0.757	0.765
14.0	0.556	0.607	0.614	0.628	0.638	0.647	0.655	0.663	0.670	0.676	0.688	0.698	0.707	0.716	0.730	0.743
15.0	0.530	0.582	0.593	0.604	0.614	0.623	0.631	0.639	0.646	0.653	0.665	0.674	0.683	0.691	0.706	0.719
16.0	0.506	0.556	0.566	0.576	0.585	0.594	0.603	0.612	0.619	0.626	0.637	0.647	0.658	0.669	0.686	0.699
17.0	0.483	0.531	0.542	0.552	0.561	0.571	0.579	0.587	0.595	0.603	0.617	0.627	0.637	0.647	0.666	0.680
18.0	0.460	0.508	0.519	0.529	0.539	0.549	0.557	0.564	0.572	0.589	0.598	0.607	0.616	0.626	0.644	0.657
19.0	0.439	0.484	0.499	0.509	0.518	0.527	0.536	0.544	0.552	0.560	0.573	0.584	0.591	0.598	0.621	0.635
20.0	0.419	0.466	0.476	0.487	0.496	0.506	0.514	0.522	0.530	0.537	0.550	0.562	0.572	0.582	0.600	0.615
21.0	0.400	0.447	0.458	0.467	0.477	0.486	0.494	0.502	0.510	0.518	0.531	0.542	0.551	0.561	0.580	0.596
22.0	0.381	0.426	0.436	0.446	0.455	0.464	0.472	0.480	0.487	0.494	0.508	0.520	0.531	0.542	0.560	0.575
23.0	0.364	0.408	0.418	0.428	0.437	0.446	0.454	0.463	0.470	0.477	0.490	0.502	0.512	0.522	0.542	0.557
24.0	0.347	0.391	0.400	0.410	0.418	0.426	0.435	0.444	0.451	0.458	0.472	0.484	0.494	0.504	0.524	0.538
25.0	0.331	0.373	0.382	0.391	0.400	0.409	0.417	0.425	0.432	0.440	0.453	0.464	0.475	0.485	0.505	0.517
30.0	0.261	0.299	0.307	0.314	0.323	0.331	0.338	0.346	0.352	0.361	0.371	0.383	0.394	0.404	0.425	0.435
35.0	0.207	0.239	0.246	0.252	0.260	0.267	0.274	0.282	0.287	0.295	0.304	0.316	0.328	0.337	0.358	0.365
40.0	0.163	0.191	0.197	0.202	0.210	0.216	0.223	0.229	0.233	0.242	0.249	0.261	0.272	0.281	0.301	0.307

Data from collection of author Subramania Jayaraman as found applicable to tailored 6-MV x-ray beams of Varian Clinac-1800 dual-energy accelerators. Values for depths less than 1.5 cm are strongly dependent on electron contamination from accessories. They are presented here merely to give an approximate trend of the dose build-up.

Table 13.11. Tissue Maximum Ratios for 18-MV X-Ray Beams

Depth (cm)	Field Size (cm × cm)															
	0 × 0	4 × 4	5 × 5	6 × 6	7 × 7	8 × 8	9 × 9	10 × 10	11 × 11	12 × 12	14 × 14	16 × 16	18 × 18	20 × 20	25 × 25	30 × 30
0.0	0.030	0.060	0.080	0.097	0.115	0.132	0.150	0.167	0.182	0.196	0.226	0.258	0.289	0.316	0.386	0.457
0.5	0.443	0.507	0.523	0.539	0.555	0.572	0.589	0.605	0.617	0.629	0.653	0.677	0.701	0.724	0.757	0.790
1.0	0.610	0.630	0.633	0.643	0.655	0.667	0.681	0.695	0.709	0.722	0.747	0.773	0.791	0.810	0.839	0.858
2.0	0.885	0.890	0.889	0.889	0.894	0.900	0.908	0.915	0.922	0.929	0.941	0.960	0.965	0.969	0.983	0.988
3.0	0.975	0.975	0.974	0.976	0.977	0.978	0.982	0.985	0.987	0.989	0.993	0.998	1.001	1.004	1.008	1.008
4.0	1.000	1.000	1.000	1.000	1.000	1.000	1.000	1.000	1.000	1.000	1.000	1.000	1.000	1.000	1.000	1.000
5.0	0.965	0.989	0.994	0.996	0.996	0.995	0.994	0.993	0.992	0.991	0.988	0.997	0.986	0.986	0.985	0.984
6.0	0.940	0.971	0.980	0.980	0.980	0.979	0.978	0.977	0.975	0.974	0.972	0.970	0.968	0.967	0.970	0.968
7.0	0.921	0.951	0.957	0.959	0.959	0.959	0.958	0.957	0.956	0.955	0.954	0.952	0.951	0.950	0.953	0.951
8.0	0.902	0.932	0.935	0.938	0.939	0.939	0.939	0.939	0.938	0.937	0.936	0.935	0.935	0.934	0.936	0.936
9.0	0.878	0.908	0.912	0.916	0.917	0.917	0.918	0.918	0.919	0.919	0.918	0.916	0.916	0.915	0.918	0.920
10.0	0.855	0.884	0.889	0.895	0.896	0.896	0.897	0.898	0.899	0.899	0.898	0.898	0.898	0.898	0.901	0.904
11.0	0.824	0.856	0.865	0.870	0.873	0.875	0.876	0.877	0.878	0.878	0.879	0.879	0.880	0.880	0.884	0.887
12.0	0.794	0.830	0.842	0.847	0.851	0.854	0.855	0.856	0.857	0.858	0.859	0.861	0.862	0.862	0.867	0.870
13.0	0.770	0.809	0.821	0.826	0.830	0.834	0.835	0.836	0.838	0.839	0.841	0.844	0.845	0.846	0.851	0.854
14.0	0.746	0.788	0.800	0.805	0.810	0.814	0.815	0.816	0.819	0.821	0.824	0.826	0.828	0.830	0.835	0.839
15.0	0.723	0.768	0.780	0.785	0.790	0.794	0.795	0.797	0.800	0.803	0.807	0.809	0.811	0.813	0.820	0.824
16.0	0.698	0.747	0.760	0.765	0.770	0.774	0.777	0.779	0.782	0.785	0.789	0.792	0.794	0.796	0.803	0.808
17.0	0.673	0.727	0.740	0.745	0.750	0.755	0.757	0.760	0.764	0.767	0.771	0.774	0.776	0.779	0.787	0.792
18.0	0.650	0.707	0.720	0.726	0.731	0.736	0.740	0.743	0.746	0.749	0.753	0.757	0.759	0.762	0.771	0.777
19.0	0.630	0.689	0.701	0.708	0.713	0.718	0.721	0.724	0.727	0.730	0.735	0.739	0.741	0.746	0.755	0.760
20.0	0.615	0.670	0.682	0.690	0.695	0.700	0.703	0.706	0.709	0.712	0.718	0.722	0.724	0.730	0.739	0.744
21.0	0.597	0.651	0.664	0.672	0.677	0.681	0.685	0.689	0.692	0.695	0.700	0.705	0.709	0.714	0.723	0.729
22.0	0.579	0.633	0.646	0.655	0.659	0.664	0.668	0.671	0.675	0.679	0.684	0.688	0.693	0.698	0.708	0.715
23.0	0.562	0.615	0.629	0.638	0.643	0.647	0.652	0.655	0.659	0.663	0.669	0.673	0.678	0.683	0.693	0.701
24.0	0.546	0.602	0.618	0.622	0.627	0.632	0.636	0.640	0.643	0.647	0.653	0.659	0.664	0.669	0.678	0.687
25.0	0.530	0.588	0.598	0.606	0.611	0.617	0.621	0.625	0.629	0.633	0.639	0.644	0.649	0.654	0.664	0.673
30.0	0.457	0.516	0.524	0.532	0.537	0.544	0.549	0.553	0.558	0.563	0.569	0.574	0.582	0.586	0.597	0.609
35.0	0.394	0.453	0.460	0.467	0.472	0.479	0.485	0.490	0.495	0.500	0.506	0.512	0.522	0.525	0.536	0.551
40.0	0.339	0.397	0.403	0.411	0.415	0.423	0.428	0.434	0.439	0.445	0.450	0.457	0.467	0.470	0.482	0.498

Data from collection of author Subramania Jayaraman as found applicable to tailored 18-MV x-ray beams of Varian Clinac-1800 dual-energy machines. Values for depths less than 4 cm are strongly dependent on electron contamination from accessories. They are presented here merely to give an approximate trend of the dose build-up.

beams of identical quality and use the same conditions for treatment can all use the same depth-dose data set. For example, for several cobalt-60 machines of identical design that are used for treatment of patients at an SSD of 80 cm, one may be able to use the same set of depth-dose data. However, the absolute dose rate outputs for the different machines can be different, as they depend on the strength of the source used, the radiation emission rate from the source, and collimator scatter. Thus, for absolute dose calculations, we need to carry out an absolute dose rate measurement on the particular treatment machine for at least one standard condition with a clearly defined distance from the source, depth, field size, and scattering geometry. Then the doses received under conditions differing from the standard condition can be derived by application of the appropriate ratios and factors. The dose rate measured for the standard condition is the calibrated output rate. The calibration of dose output should be an absolute dose determination made with a dosimeter having traceability to a primary national and international dosimetry standard according to a recommended protocol. (See Sections 11.7 and 11.8 of Chapter 11.)

For the calibration of dose output, we use a standard field size, A_{St}, as measured at the distance SAD for isocentric machines and at SSD for fixed-SSD machines. Commonly, A_{St} is taken to be 10 cm × 10 cm. The distance at which the output measurement is made can be standardized conveniently to be the SAD for the isocentric case and $(SSD + d_m)$ for the fixed-SSD case.

13.15.2
In-Air Output and Peak Output

The output can be chosen to be either the dose to tissue in air or the peak dose at depth d_m in a phantom. We will refer to the former as the "in-air output" and to the latter as the "peak output." Accordingly, we will speak of the "calibrated air output rate" (CAOR) and the "calibrated peak output rate" (CPOR). CPOR and CAOR are related by the PSF for the field A_{St}; that is,

$$CPOR = CAOR \cdot PSF(A_{St}) \tag{13-16}$$

The calibrated output rate can apply only to the standard field size A_{St}. For radioisotope machines and conventional X-ray machines, the duration of treatment is controlled by time, and the output rate can be expressed in cGy min^{-1}. For accelerators, the duration of treatment is controlled by the monitor unit (Mu) counts from a monitor ionization chamber (see Section 10.3.5), and the output rate is expressed in cGy Mu^{-1}. Usually an adjustment of the sensitivity of the monitor chamber is done to obtain a calibration output rate (CAOR or CPOR) of 1.0 cGy Mu^{-1}.

In general, the output rate changes when the field is changed from one size, A_{St}, to another, A_X. To calculate the ouput rate for any field size A_X, we define a normalized output factor (NOF) as

$$NOF(A_X) = \frac{\text{Output rate for field size } A_X}{\text{Output rate for field size } A_{St}} \tag{13-17}$$

For any machine, one set of NOFs covering the entire range of possible field sizes should be measured and made available.

For the discussion that follows, we will find it convenient to make a distinction between NOF values for which air output is used and those for which peak output is used.* We will call these the normalized air output factor (NAOF) and the normalized peak output factor (NPOF), respectively. NPOF and NAOF are related to each other through the PSF by

$$\begin{aligned} NPOF(A_X) &= \frac{\text{Peak output for field } A_X}{\text{Peak out for field } A_{St}} \\ &= \frac{\text{Air output for field } A_X \cdot PSF(A_X)}{\text{Air output for field } A_{St} \cdot PSF(A_{St})} \\ &= NAOF(A_X) \cdot \frac{PSF(A_X)}{PSF(A_{St})} \end{aligned}$$

i. e.,

$$NPOF(A_X) = NAOF(A_X) \cdot NPSF(A_X) \qquad (13\text{-}18)$$

Tables 13.12 and 13.13 provide output calibration data for a ^{60}Co machine and a 4-MV X-ray machine, respectively.

Table 13.12. Output Factors (Typical) for a Cobalt-60 Machine

Quantity	Field Size (cm × cm)								
	4 × 4	6 × 6	8 × 8	10 × 10	12 × 12	14 × 14	16 × 16	18 × 18	20 × 20
NAOF	0.964	0.977	0.989	1.00	1.010	1.019	1.027	1.035	1.040
PSF[a]	1.014	1.022	1.029	1.035	1.041	1.046	1.051	1.055	1.059
NPSF[a]	0.972	0.987	0.994	1.000	1.006	1.011	1.015	1.020	1.025
NPOF	0.944	0.965	0.983	1.000	1.016	1.030	1.043	1.055	1.064

[a] Based on data from Reference 2.

CAOR = 93.0 cGy min^{-1} to tissue in air at 80 cm distance from source for 10 × 10 cm field.
CPOR = CAOR × PSF(10 × 10) = 96.3 cGy min^{-1} at depth d_m at SAD = 80 cm for 10 × 10 cm field.

Table 13.13. Output Factors (Typical) for a 4-MV X-Ray Machine

Quantity	Field Size (cm × cm)								
	4 × 4	6 × 6	8 × 8	10 × 10	12 × 12	14 × 14	16 × 16	18 × 18	20 × 20
NAOF	0.938	0.958	0.981	1.000	1.004	1.014	1.021	1.025	1.027
PSF[a]	1.007	1.023	1.031	1.037	1.043	1.048	1.053	1.058	1.063
NPSF[a]	0.972	0.987	0.994	1.000	1.006	1.011	1.015	1.020	1.025
NPOF	0.911	0.945	0.975	1.00	1.010	1.025	1.036	1.046	1.053

[a] Based on data from Reference 2.

CAOR = 1.0 cGy Mu^{-1} to tissue in air at 100 cm distance from source for 10 × 10 cm field.
CPOR = CAOR × PSF(10 × 10) = 1.037 cGy Mu^{-1} at depth d_m at SAD = 100 cm for 10 × 10 cm field.

---

* Using a different nomenclature, some published literature uses an equation equivalent to (13-18) of the form $S_t(A_X) = S_c(A_X) \cdot S_p(A_X)$. They refer to S_t, S_c, and S_p, as total output factor, collimator output factor, and phantom-scatter factor, respectively. It is useful to note that S_t, S_c, and S_p, respectively, correspond to the acronyms, NPOF, NAOF, and NPSF, used in this book.

13.16
Methods of Deriving the Dose Rate $\dot{D}_P$ at Point P

We have stated that our purpose in defining the various ratios is to use them to derive the dose rate, $\dot{D}_P$, at any point, such as P at any depth d in water for any field size A_X. We will now show how a procedure for routine patient dose calculations can be set up by one of six different methods. The relationships provided by the factors ISqF, PSF, TAR, TMR, and PDD as shown in Figure 13.5 are to be referred to by the reader for understanding the ensuing discussion.

We recall that A_0, A_{dm}, and A_d denote the field sizes at distances of SSD, SSD + d_m, and SAD (= SSD + d), respectively. Only PDD uses the field size A_0. In many practical contexts, the sizes A_{dm} and A_0 are almost the same. For simplicity, therefore, we will consider only two field sizes, A_{dm} at (SSD + d_m) and A_d at SAD.

Method 1: This method is tailored to a fixed-SSD technique. The calibrated air output rate is the dose to tissue in air at point 1 at a distance of (SSD + d_m) for a field size $A_{dm} = A_{St} = 10\,cm \times 10\,cm$. That is, we are given

$$CAOR = \dot{D}(air, SSD + d_m, d_m, 10\,cm \times 10\,cm)$$

Step 1: Multiply CAOR by NAOF(A_{dm}) to obtain the dose rate at point 1 for the actual field size A_{dm} in use.
Step 2: Multiply by PSF to obtain the dose rate at point 3.
Step 3: Multiply by PDD/100 to obtain the dose rate at point P.
Combining all of the above steps, we obtain

$$\dot{D}_P = CAOR \cdot NAOF(A_{dm}) \cdot PSF(A_{dm}) \cdot [PDD(SSD, A_d, d)/100] \qquad (13\text{-}19)$$

Method 2: This method is also intended for a fixed-SSD technique, but the calibrated output rate is the peak dose in water at point 3 at a distance of (SSD + d_m) for a field size $A_{dm} = A_{St} = 10\,cm \times 10\,cm$. That is, we are given

$$CPOR = \dot{D}(water, SSD + d_m, d_m, 10\,cm \times 10\,cm)$$

Step 1: Multiply CPOR by NPOF(A_{dm}) to obtain the dose rate at point 3 for the actual field size A_{dm} used.
Step 2: Multiply by PDD/100 to obtain the dose rate at point P. Combining the above steps, we obtain

$$\dot{D}_P = CPOR \cdot NPOF(A_{dm}) \cdot [PDD(SSD, A_m, d)/100] \qquad (13\text{-}20)$$

Method 3: Here we consider the isocentric or fixed-SAD technique. The calibrated output rate is the dose rate to tissue in air at point 2 at a distance of SAD (= SSD + d) for a field size $A_d = A_{St} = 10\,cm \times 10\,cm$. That is, we are given

$$CAOR = \dot{D}(air, SAD, d, 10\,cm \times 10\,cm)$$

Step 1: Multiply CAOR by NAOF to obtain the dose rate at point 2 for the actual field size A_d in use.

Step 2: Multiply by TAR to obtain the dose rate at point P. Then

$$\dot{D}_P = CAOR \cdot NAOF(A_d) \cdot TAR(A_d, d)$$

Method 4: This method is also intended for an isocentric or fixed-SAD technique. The calibrated output rate is the peak dose in water at point 4 at a distance of SAD ($=$ SSD $+$ d) for a field size $A_d = A_{St} = 10\,cm \times 10\,cm$. That is, we are given

$$\dot{D}_P(water, SAD, d_m, 10\,cm \times 10\,cm)$$

Step 1: Multiply CPOR by NPOF(A_d) to obtain the dose rate at point 4 for the field size A_d.

Step 2: Multiply by TMR to obtain the dose rate at P. Combining the above steps yields

$$\dot{D}_P = CPOR \cdot NPOF(A_d) \cdot TMR(A_d, d) \tag{13-22}$$

Method 5: Here, the known calibrated output rate is (as in Method 1) the dose in air at point 1 at a distance of (SSD $+ d_m$) for a field size $A_{dm} = A_{St} = 10\,cm \times 10\,cm$. That is, we are given

$$CAOR = \dot{D}(air, SSD + d_m, d_m, 10\,cm \times 10\,cm)$$

Step 1: Multiply CAOR by NAOF(A_{dm}) to obtain the output rate at point 1 for the actual field size A_{dm} used.

Step 2: Multiply by ISqF $= [(SSD + d_m)/(SSD + d)]^2$ to obtain the dose rate at point 2 in air.

Step 3: Multiply by TAR to obtain the dose rate at point P. Combining all the above steps, we obtain

$$\dot{D}_P = CAOR \cdot NAOF(A_{dm}) \left[(SSD + d_m)/(SSD + d)\right]^2 \cdot TAR(d, A_d) \tag{13-23}$$

Method 6: Here, the known calibrated output rate is (as in case 2) the peak dose in water at point 3 at a distance of SSD $+ d_m$ for a field size $A_{dm} = A_{St} = 10\,cm \times 10\,cm$. That is, we are given

$$CPOR = \dot{D}(water, SSD + d_m, d_m, 10\,cm \times 10\,cm)$$

Step 1: Multiply by NPOF(A_{dm}) to obtain the dose rate at point 3 for the actual field size A_{dm} used.

Step 2: Divide by PSF to obtain the dose rate at point 1.

Step 3: Apply the inverse-square factor ISqF to obtain the dose rate at point 2.

Step 4: Multiply by TAR to obtain the dose rate at point P. Combining all of these steps, we obtain

$$\dot{D}_P = CPOR \cdot NPOF(A_{dm}) \frac{1}{PSF(A_{dm})} \left[(SSD + d_m)/(SSD + d)\right]^2 \cdot TAR(d, A_d) \tag{13-24}$$

Because TMR$(d, A_d) = [TAR(d, A_d)/PSF(A_d)]$, we can also write the above equation as follows:

$$\dot{D}_P = CPOR \cdot NPOF(A_{dm}) \frac{PSF(A_d)}{PSF(A_{dm})} \left[(SSD + d_m)/(SSD + d)\right]^2 \cdot TMR(d, A_d)$$

$$(13.24a)$$

Furthermore, by (13-18) $NPOF(A_{dm}) = NAOF(A_{dm}) \times NPSF(A_{dm})$. Hence (13.24a) can be changed and written as

$$\dot{D}_P = CPOR \cdot NAOF(A_{dm}) \cdot NPSF(A_d) \cdot \left[(SSD + d_m)/(SSD + d)\right]^2 \cdot TMR(d, A_d)$$

$$(13.24b)$$

Methods 5 and 6 show how inverse-square corrections can be incorporated where necessary.

In practice, it is desirable to set up the procedure for dose calculation so as to conform to one of the first four approaches. In all of these, the distance of calibration matches either a fixed SSD or a fixed SAD of choice. The approaches in Methods 5 and 6 are more general. The inverse-square term used in these two methods makes it possible to derive the dose rate for any arbitrary distance of point P, unrestricted by the SSD or SAD chosen for the calibration.

13.17
Calculation of Treatment Duration

We devised methods for the derivation of the dose rate at P as a step for calculating the duration of treatment for delivery of any intended dose to point P. The treatment duration, T, for delivery of a prescribed dose, D_{Pr}, to point P is given by

$$T = \frac{D_{Pr}}{\text{dose rate at P}} \qquad (13\text{-}25)$$

T can be expressed in minutes or monitor units (Mu). Any one of the different expressions from (13-19) to (13.24a) can be used for calculating the dose rate at P. When this is done, the expression for T will have the form

$$T = \frac{D_{Pr}}{\text{calibrated output rate} \times tf_1 \times tf_2 \times tf_3 \times K} \qquad (13\text{-}26)$$

where tf_1, tf_2, etc. are various transfer factors such as NAOF, NPOF, TMR, TAR, PSF, ISqF, etc. Sometimes, in addition to the factors that we described in Section 13.16, a factor may be needed that corrects for any material such as a plastic sheet or a wedge inserted in the beam in special treatment situations. Different notations and formalisms have been evolved using factors and ratios that are mutually consistent and coherent for use in a form resembling equation (13-26) [1–7]. It is advised that, for day-to-day work, any clinic adopt one of the available formalisms and follow it consistently.

13.18
Equivalent Squares and Circles

The standard depth dose tables are typically set up for a set of square-field cross sections ranging from $4\,cm \times 4\,cm$ to $40\,cm \times 40\,cm$. These tables cannot be used

Fig. 13.6. (Top) A rectangular field of size $W \times L$ with its equivalent square field of side E_{Sq}. The scatter from areas A and B is compensated for by that from areas A_1 and B_1 of the equivalent square field. (Bottom) The square field is compared with its equivalent circular field which produces the same amount of scatter

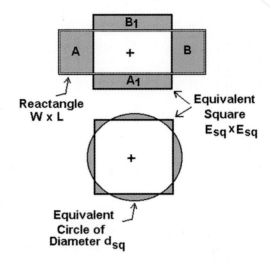

directly for rectangular fields. Square fields and rectangular fields of the same area do not contribute the same amount of scatter. This is illustrated in Figure 13.6. The square field irradiates a volume spread evenly around the central axis. On the other hand, a rectangular field of total area identical to that of the square field will have more irradiated volume that is far removed from the central axis. The remote areas contribute less scatter to the center. Overall, the rectangular field is a poorer scatterer than is a square field having the same area. Table 13.14 gives the equivalent square fields for rectangular fields in a more general way. The data applicable to an equivalent square field of side E_{sq} as read from this table can be used for a rectangular field of dimensions $W \times L$.

An approximate formula for E_{sq} can be derived based on the empirical premise that the ratio of area A to perimeter p correlates better with the scatter than does area alone. For a given field area A, large elongated fields have a large p. A rectangular field of size $W \times L$ can be approximated by an equivalent square field of side E_{sq} that has the same ratio A/p, as follows:

$$A/p = (WL)/[2(W + L)] = [E_{Sq} \times E_{Sq}]/[4E_{Sq}] = E_{Sq}/4$$

Hence,

$$E_{Sq} = 4(A/p) = 2[(WL)/(W + L)] \tag{13-27}$$

The above formula is reasonably accurate except for very elongated fields. A circular field of equivalent diameter E_{dia} can also be derived by the approximate relation

$$E_{dia} = 1.1E_{Sq} \tag{13-28}$$

The equivalent-square and equivalent-circle concepts address photon scatter geometry and should be used only for photon beams. They may not hold for electron beams (see Chapter 16, Sect. 16.9.2).

Table 13.14. Side of Equivalent Square for Beams of Rectangular Cross Section

Second Side of Rectangle (cm)	First Side of Rectangle (cm)																											
	1.0	2.0	3.0	4.0	5.0	6.0	7.0	8.0	9.0	10.0	11.0	12.0	13.0	14.0	15.0	16.0	17.0	18.0	19.0	20.0	22.0	24.0	26.0	28.0	30.0	34.0	36.0
1.0	1.0																										
2.0	1.4	2.0																									
3.0	1.6	2.4	3.0																								
4.0	1.7	2.7	3.4	4.0																							
5.0	1.8	2.9	3.8	4.5	5.0																						
6.0	1.9	3.1	4.1	4.8	5.5	6.0																					
7.0	2.0	3.3	4.3	5.1	5.8	6.5	7.0																				
8.0	2.1	3.4	4.5	5.4	6.2	6.9	7.5	8.0																			
9.0	2.1	3.5	4.6	5.6	6.5	7.2	7.9	8.5	9.0																		
10.0	2.2	3.6	4.8	5.8	6.7	7.5	8.2	8.9	9.5	10.0																	
11.0	2.2	3.7	4.9	6.0	6.9	7.8	8.5	9.3	9.9	10.5	11.0																
12.0	2.2	3.7	5.0	6.1	7.1	8.0	8.8	9.6	10.3	10.9	11.5	12.0															
13.0	2.2	3.8	5.1	6.2	7.2	8.2	9.1	9.9	10.6	11.3	11.9	12.5	13.0														
14.0	2.3	3.8	5.1	6.3	7.4	8.4	9.3	10.1	10.9	11.6	12.3	12.9	13.5	14.0													
15.0	2.3	3.9	5.2	6.4	7.5	8.5	9.5	10.3	11.2	11.9	12.6	13.3	13.9	14.5	15.0												
16.0	2.3	3.9	5.3	6.5	7.6	8.6	9.6	10.5	11.4	12.2	12.9	13.7	14.3	14.9	15.5	16.0											
17.0	2.3	3.9	5.3	6.5	7.7	8.8	9.8	10.7	11.6	12.4	13.2	14.0	14.7	15.3	15.9	16.5	17.0										
18.0	2.3	3.9	5.3	6.6	7.8	8.9	9.9	10.9	11.8	12.6	13.5	14.3	15.0	15.7	16.3	16.9	17.5	18.0									
19.0	2.3	4.0	5.4	6.6	7.8	8.9	10.0	11.0	11.9	12.8	13.7	14.5	15.3	16.0	16.7	17.3	17.9	18.5	19.0								
20.0	2.3	4.0	5.4	6.7	7.9	9.0	10.1	11.1	12.1	13.0	13.9	14.7	15.5	16.3	17.0	17.7	18.3	18.9	19.5	20.0							
22.0	2.4	4.0	5.5	6.8	8.0	9.1	10.2	11.3	12.3	13.3	14.2	15.1	16.0	16.8	17.6	18.3	19.0	19.7	20.3	20.9	22.0						
24.0	2.4	4.0	5.5	6.8	8.1	9.2	10.4	11.4	12.5	13.5	14.5	15.4	16.3	17.2	18.0	18.8	19.6	20.3	21.0	21.7	22.9	24.0					
26.0	2.4	4.1	5.5	6.9	8.1	9.3	10.5	11.6	12.6	13.7	14.7	15.7	16.6	17.5	18.4	19.3	20.1	20.9	21.6	22.4	23.7	24.9	26.0				
28.0	2.4	4.1	5.5	6.9	8.2	9.4	10.5	11.7	12.7	13.8	14.8	15.8	16.8	17.8	18.7	19.6	20.5	21.3	22.1	22.9	24.4	25.7	26.9	28.0			
30.0	2.4	4.1	5.6	6.9	8.2	9.4	10.6	11.7	12.8	13.9	15.0	16.0	17.0	18.0	18.9	19.9	20.8	21.6	22.5	23.3	24.9	26.4	27.7	28.9	30.0		
32.0	2.4	4.1	5.6	6.9	8.2	9.4	10.6	11.8	12.9	14.0	15.0	16.1	17.1	18.1	19.1	20.1	21.0	21.9	22.8	23.7	25.4	26.9	28.4	29.7	30.9	32.0	
34.0	2.4	4.1	5.6	6.9	8.2	9.5	10.7	11.8	13.0	14.1	15.1	16.2	17.2	18.2	19.2	20.2	21.2	22.1	23.1	24.0	25.7	27.4	29.0	30.4	31.7	32.9	34.0
36.0	2.4	4.1	5.6	7.0	8.2	9.5	10.7	11.8	13.0	14.1	15.2	16.2	17.3	18.3	19.3	20.3	21.3	22.3	23.3	24.2	26.0	27.8	29.4	31.0	32.4	33.7	36.0
38.0	2.4	4.1	5.6	7.0	8.3	9.5	10.7	11.9	13.0	14.1	15.2	16.3	17.4	18.4	19.4	20.4	21.3	22.4	23.4	24.4	26.3	28.1	29.8	31.4	33.0	34.4	36.9
40.0	2.4	4.1	5.6	7.0	8.3	9.5	10.7	11.9	13.0	14.1	15.2	16.3	17.4	18.5	19.5	20.5	21.5	22.6	23.5	24.5	26.4	28.3	30.1	31.8	33.5	35.0	37.7
50.0	2.4	4.1	5.6	7.0	8.3	9.5	10.7	11.9	13.1	14.2	15.3	16.4	17.5	18.6	19.7	20.7	21.8	22.8	23.8	24.9	26.9	28.9	30.9	32.8	34.7	36.6	40.2
60.0	2.4	4.1	5.6	7.0	8.3	9.5	10.7	11.9	13.1	14.2	15.4	16.5	17.6	18.6	19.7	20.8	21.8	22.9	23.9	25.0	27.0	29.1	31.0	33.1	35.1	37.1	41.0
Inf.	2.4	4.1	5.6	7.0	8.3	9.5	10.8	11.9	13.1	14.2	15.4	16.5	17.6	18.6	19.7	20.8	21.9	22.9	24.0	25.0	27.1	29.2	31.2	33.3	35.3	37.3	41.4

Reprinted with permission from Br. J Radiol., Supplement 17, Central Axis Depth Dose Data for Use in Radiotherapy, British Institute of Radiology, London, 1983.

13.19
Relationship of TAR and TMR to PDD

If we compare the following expressions for the dose rate at P in methods 1 and 5,

$$\dot{D}_P = \text{CAOR} \cdot \text{NAOF}(A_{dm}) \cdot \text{PSF}(A_{dm}) \cdot [\text{PDD}(\text{SSD}, A_d, d)/100] \qquad (13\text{-}19)$$

$$\dot{D}_P = \text{CAOR} \cdot \text{NAOF}(A_{dm}) \left[(\text{SSD} + d_m)/(\text{SSD} + d)\right]^2 \cdot \text{TAR}(d, A_d) \qquad (13\text{-}23)$$

we obtain the relation

$$\text{TAR}(d, A_d) = [\text{PSF}(A_{dm})] \cdot [\text{PDD}(\text{SSD}, A_{dm}, d)/100]$$
$$\cdot [(\text{SSD} + d)/(\text{SSD} + d_m)]^2 \qquad (13\text{-}29)$$

Because $\text{TMR}(d, A_d) = \text{TAR}(d, A_d)/\text{PSF}(A_d)$,

$$\text{TMR}(d, A_d) = [\text{PSF}(A_{dm})/\text{PSF}(A_d)] \cdot [\text{PDD}(\text{SSD}, A_{dm}, d)/100]$$
$$\cdot [(\text{SSD} + d)/(\text{SSD} + d_m)]^2 . \qquad (13\text{-}30)$$

If a set of PDD values for a chosen SSD covering a range of depths and field sizes is available, these, together with a set of PSF values, can be utilized in (13-29) or (13-30) for derivation of the TAR (or TMR) values. It is to be noted that a PDD value for a field size A_{dm} (that is specified at depth d_m) gives a TAR (or TMR) for a different field size A_d (that is specified at depth d) by the above conversion.

13.20
Converting PDD for One SSD to that for Another

Let us assume that we already know the PDD values for a particular SSD and that we need to create a new table of percent depth dose values, PDD$'$, for SSD $=$ SSD$'$. For this we write the relation of TAR to PDD$'$ in a way similar to (13-29):

$$\text{TAR}(d, A_d) = [\text{PSF}(A'_{dm})] \cdot [\text{PDD}'(\text{SSD}', A'_{dm}, d)/100]$$
$$\cdot [(\text{SSD}' + d)/(\text{SSD}' + d_m)]^2 \qquad (13\text{-}31)$$

where A'_{dm} is the field size at (SSD$'$ + d_m) if the field size is A_d at (SSD$'$ + d). Equating (13-29) and (13-31) for TAR and transposing the terms gives the relation

$$\text{PDD}'(\text{SSD}', A'_{dm}, d) = \text{PDD}(\text{SSD}, A_{dm}, d) \cdot [\text{PSF}(A_{dm}/\text{PSF}(A'_{dm})]$$
$$\cdot \left\{ [(\text{SSD} + d)/(\text{SSD} + d_m)]^2 [(\text{SSD}' + d_m)/(\text{SSD}' + d)]^2 \right\}$$
$$(13\text{-}32)$$

The PSF changes slowly with field size. Therefore, the PSF ratio in the first square bracket above can be assigned a value of 1.0 without much error. The term in the curly brackets has been given the name Mayneord F factor. The F factor is

$$F = [(\text{SSD} + d)/(\text{SSD} + d_m)]^2 \cdot [(\text{SSD}' + d_m)/(\text{SSD}' + d)]^2 \qquad (13\text{-}33)$$

This factor essentially removes the inverse-square fall-off between (SSD + d_m) and (SSD + d) applicable to the old SSD and incorporates the inverse-square fall-off from (SSD$'$ + d_m) to (SSD$'$ + d) applicable to the changed SSD.

It should be noted that PDD for field size A_{dm} converts by (13-32) to give the PDD′ applicable to a different field size, A'_{dm}. If this change in field size is not recognized, the approximation $A_{dm} = A'_{dm}$, can result in errors of 0.5 to 3% in the derived PDD′ values in some practical situations.

EXAMPLE 13.2

The PDDs at 10 cm depth for ^{60}Co beams of field sizes 8 cm × 8 cm and 9 cm × 9 cm used at SSD = 80 cm are 54.8 and 55.7, respectively. Derive the corresponding TAR values and the field sizes at the depth for which they apply. Use the PSF data from Table 13.3.

Field widths of 8 cm and 9 cm at SSD result in the following field widths at a depth of 10 cm at SAD = 90 cm:

$$8 \times \frac{90}{80} = 9.0 \, \text{cm}; \; 9 \times \frac{90}{80} = 10.1 \, \text{cm}$$

Relation (13-29) can be used for deriving the TARs for the above two field sizes at a depth of 10 cm. The inverse-square term in (13-29) is

$$\left(\frac{\text{SSD} + d}{\text{SSD} + d_m} \right)^2 = \left(\frac{80 + 10}{80 + 0.5} \right)^2 = 1.25$$

The PSF values (from Table 13.3) for the above two field sizes are 1.029 and 1.033, respectively. Substituting in (13-29), we obtain the following TARs:

$$\text{TAR}(^{60}\text{Co}, d = 10 \, \text{cm}, A_d = 9.0 \, \text{cm} \times 9.0 \, \text{cm})$$
$$= (54.8/100) \times 1.029 \times 1.25 = 0.705$$
$$\text{TAR}(^{60}\text{Co}, d = 10 \, \text{cm}, A_d = 10.1 \, \text{cm} \times 10.1 \, \text{cm})$$
$$= (55.7/100) \times 1.033 \times 1.25 = 0.719$$

EXAMPLE 13.3

The PDD for 10 cm depth for a ^{60}Co beam of 10 cm × 10 cm used at SSD = 60 cm is 53.0. Convert this PDD value to apply to SSD = 100 cm and calculate the field size at the surface for which the converted PDD is valid.

We will use relation (13-32), a part of which is the F factor given by (13-33). Substituting SSD = 60 cm, SSD′ = 100 cm, $d_m = 0.5$ cm, and d = 10 cm in (13-33), we obtain

$$F = \left(\frac{60 + 10}{60 + 0.5} \right)^2 \times \left(\frac{100 + 0.5}{100 + 10} \right)^2$$
$$= (1.157)^2 \times (0.914)^2 = 1.118$$

SSD = 60 cm and A_0 is a 10 cm square.

We know that the scatter component depends on the field size A_d at depth d. For 10 cm depth,

$$A_d = A_0 \times (\text{SSD} + d)/\text{SSD} = 10.0 \times (60 + 10)/60 = 11.7 \, \text{cm}$$

Another part of (13-32) is a ratio of PSFs. The PSFs are to be selected based on field sizes at depth d_m.

The field size A'_{dm} at depth d_m, when the field size is 11.7 cm at depth d and SSD is 100 cm, is

$$A'_{dm} = A_d \times (100 + d_m)/(100 + d) = 11.7 \times (100.5/110) = 10.7\,\text{cm}$$

The corresponding field size at the surface is

$$A_0 = A_d \times SSD/(SSD + d) = 11.7 \times (100/110) = 10.6\,\text{cm}$$

The field size A_{dm} at depth d_m when SSD = 60 cm is

$$A_{dm} = A_0 \times (SSD + d_m)/SSD = 10.0 \times (60.5/60) = 10.1\,\text{cm}$$

From the PSF data in Table 13.3, the ratio $PSF(A_{dm})/PSF(A'_{dm})$ to be used in (13-32) is:

$$\frac{PSF(^{60}Co, A_{dm})}{PSF(^{60}Co, A'_{dm})} = \frac{PSF(Co^{60}, 10.1\,\text{cm} \times 10.1\,\text{cm})}{PSF(Co^{60}, 10.7\,\text{cm} \times 10.7\,\text{cm})} = \frac{1.035}{1.037} = 0.998$$

By substitution in (13-32), the given PDD value of 53.0 at 10 cm depth for SSD = 60 cm gives the following:

$$PDD(^{60}Co, SSD = 100\,\text{cm}, d = 10\,\text{cm}, A_0 = 10.6 \times 10.6\,\text{cm})$$
$$= 53.0 \times 0.998 \times 1.118 = 59.1$$

It will be noticed that the term involving the ratio of PSFs is almost unity, implying a minimal correction and a negligible change in backscatter.

EXAMPLE 13.4

The internal mammary nodes of a patient are treated with a single ^{60}Co beam having a field size of 5 cm × 20 cm at SSD = 80 cm (see Figure 13.7). A dose of 200 cGy per treatment to the nodes at 3 cm depth is prescribed. Calculate (i) the treatment time and (ii) the dose delivered to the spinal cord at 15 cm depth. Use the data from Tables 13.5 and 13.12.

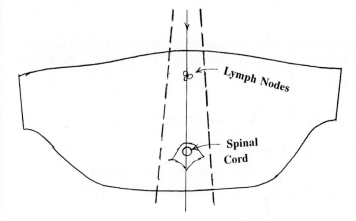

Fig. 13.7. Cross section of a patient treated with a single beam passing through the anterior nodes and the spinal cord

Treatment geometry: SSD $= 80$ cm, field size $A_0 = 5$ cm $\times 20$ cm at SSD. We will assume $A_{dm} = A_0$.

(i) Time to deliver 200 cGy to 3 cm depth
From (13-27), the side of the equivalent square is

$$E_{sq} [(5 \times 20)/(5 + 20)] \times 2 = 8.0 \text{ cm}$$

From the footnote to Table 13.12, the dose rate to tissue in air for $A_{St} = 10$ cm $\times$ 10 cm is

$$CAOR = 93.0 \text{ cGy min}^{-1}$$

The peak dose is to be determined at a distance of $(SSD + d_m)$, which in this case is

$$(80 + 0.5) \text{ cm} = 80.5 \text{ cm}$$

The inverse-square factor applicable to a change in distance from 80.0 cm to 80.5 cm is

$$ISqF = [80/80.5]^2 = 0.988$$

The normalized air output factor is

$$NAOF(8 \text{ cm} \times 8 \text{ cm}) = 0.989 \quad \text{(from Table 13.12)}$$

The peak scatter factor is

$$PSF(^{60}Co, A_{dm} \approx 8 \text{ cm} \times 8 \text{ cm}) = 1.029 \quad \text{(from Table 13.12)}$$

The peak dose rate (i. e., 100% dose rate) is

$$CAOR \cdot ISqF \cdot NAOF \cdot PSF = 93.0 \text{ cGy min}^{-1} \times 0.988 \times 0.989 \times 1.029$$
$$= 93.5 \text{ cGy min}^{-1}$$

The percent depth dose is

$$PDD(^{60}Co, SSD = 80 \text{ cm}, A_0 = 8 \text{ cm} \times 8 \text{ cm}, d = 3 \text{ cm}) = 88.0$$
$$\text{(from Table 13.5)}$$

The dose rate at 3 cm depth $= 93.5 \text{ cGy min}^{-1} \times (88.0/100) = 82.3 \text{ cGy min}^{-1}$
The time to deliver 200 cGy $= 200 \text{ cGy}/82.3 \text{ cGy min}^{-1} = 2.43 \text{ min} = 2 \text{ min } 26 \text{ sec}$

(ii) Dose to spinal cord:
From Table 13.5,

$$PDD(^{60}Co, SSD = 80 \text{ cm}, A_0 = 8 \text{ cm} \times 8 \text{ cm}, d = 15 \text{ cm}) = 37.6$$

Dose rate to spinal cord at 15 cm depth $=$ peak (100%) dose rate $\times (37.6/100)$
$$= 93.5 \text{ cGy min}^{-1} \times 0.376$$
$$= 35.2 \text{ cGy min}^{-1}$$

The dose to the spinal cord in each treatment is

$$2.43 \text{ min} \times 35.2 \text{ cGy min}^{-1} = 85.4 \text{ cGy}$$

Alternatively, we can use the ratio of PDDs to derive the dose to the spinal cord as follows:

$$200 \text{ cGy} \times [\text{PDD at 15 cm depth}]/[\text{PDD at 3 cm depth}]$$
$$= 200 \times 37.6/88.0 = 85.4 \text{ cGy}$$

EXAMPLE 13.5

Solve the previous example for a treatment situation in which a 4-MV X-ray beam and an isocentric setup having an SAD $= 100$ cm are used. Use the data from Tables 13.9 and 13.13.

(i) Monitor units to deliver 200 cGy at 3 cm depth:
The setup uses SAD $= 100$ cm, depth d $= 3$ cm
SSD $=$ SAD $-$ d $= 97$ cm
Field size $A_d = 5$ cm $\times$ 20 cm at SAD $= 100$ cm
From (13-27), the side of the equivalent square is

$$E_{Sq} = 2 \times (5 \times 20)/(5 + 20) = 8 \text{ cm}$$

$$\text{CPOR} = 1.037 \text{ cGy Mu}^{-1} \quad \text{(from footnote to Table 13.13)}$$

$$\text{NPOF}(A_{dm} = 8 \text{ cm} \times 8 \text{ cm}) = 0.975 \quad \text{(from Table 13.13)}$$

$$\text{TMR}(4 \text{ MV}, d = 3 \text{ cm}, A_d = 8 \text{ cm} \times 8 \text{ cm}) = 0.956 \quad \text{(from Table 13.9)}$$

From (13-22), the dose rate at 3 cm depth is

$$\text{CPOR} \times \text{NPOF} \times \text{TMR} = 1.037 \text{ cGy Mu}^{-1} \times 0.975 \times 0.956$$
$$= 0.967 \text{ cGy Mu}^{-1}$$

Mu to deliver 200 cGy $= 200 \text{ cGy}/0.967 \text{ cGy Mu}^{-1} = 207$ Mu

(ii) Dose delivered to spinal cord:

Peak dose rate for field size in use at 100 cm distance
$$= \text{CPOR} \times \text{NPOF} = 1.037 \text{ cGy Mu}^{-1} \times 0.975 = 1.011 \text{ cGy Mu}^{-1}$$

$$\text{PSF}(4 \text{ MV}, 8 \text{ cm} \times 8 \text{ cm}) = 1.031 \quad \text{(from Table 13.13)}$$

Dose per monitor unit to tissue in air at 100 cm from source for 8 cm $\times$ 8 cm field:

Peak dose rate/PSF $= 1.011 \text{ cGy Mu}^{-1}/1.031 = 0.981 \text{ cGy Mu}^{-1}$

Distance of spinal cord from source:

$$\text{SAD} - 3 \text{ cm} + 15 \text{ cm} = 100 \text{ cm} - 3 \text{ cm} + 15 \text{ cm} = 112 \text{ cm}$$

ISqF for the distance 112 cm $= (100/112)^2 = 0.797$.
Dose per monitor unit to tissue in air at 112 cm distance is

$$0.981 \text{ cGy Mu}^{-1} \times 0.797 = 0.782 \text{ cGy Mu}^{-1}$$

The field width (W) and length (L) at 112 cm distance from the source at the depth of the spinal cord are

$$W = 5 \times 112/100 = 5.6\,\text{cm}; \quad L = 20 \times 112/100 = 22.4\,\text{cm}$$

From (13-27), the side of the equivalent square is

$$E_{Sq} = 2 \times (5.6 \times 22.4)/(5.6 + 22.4) = 9.0\,\text{cm}$$

$$PSF(4\,\text{MV}, 9\,\text{cm} \times 9\,\text{cm}) = 1.034 \quad \text{(from Table 13.13)}$$

Peak dose rate at 112 cm distance from source for field size 5.6 × 22.4 cm:

$$\text{Dose rate in air} \times PSF = 0.782\,\text{cGy Mu}^{-1} \times 1.034$$
$$= 0.809\,\text{cGy Mu}^{-1}$$

TMR for spinal cord at 15 cm depth for $A_d = 5.6\,\text{cm} \times 22.4\,\text{cm}$ (i. e., 9 cm^2 equivalent square):

$$TMR(4\,\text{MV}, d = 15\,\text{cm}, A_d = 9\,\text{cm} \times 9\,\text{cm}) = 0.572 \quad \text{(from Table 13.9)}$$

Dose rate at the spinal cord = peak dose rate at 112 cm × TMR = $0.809\,\text{cGy Mu}^{-1} \times 0.572 = 0.463\,\text{cGy Mu}^{-1}$.
Dose delivered to spinal cord for 207 Mu irradiation:

$$207\,\text{Mu} \times 0.463\,\text{cGy Mu}^{-1} = 96\,\text{cGy}$$

EXAMPLE 13.6

A patient is treated on a 4-MV X-ray machine with an isocentric setup with parallel opposed beams, each having a field size 12 cm × 20 cm at SAD = 100 cm (see Figure 13.8). The patient thickness is 38 cm in the direction of the beams. (i) What should be the monitor units for delivering a daily treatment giving 100 cGy by each beam at point P_{mid}, at the patient's midline? (ii) If the treatment is continued to deliver 5000 cGy at P_{mid}, estimate the dose at point P_{Sk} located at depth d_m from the skin. Use the data for 4 MV in Tables 13.9 and 13.13.

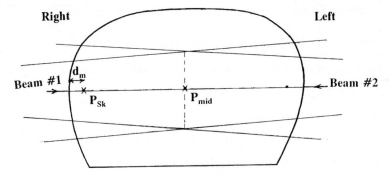

Fig. 13.8. Cross section of a patient treated with parallel opposed lateral beams. P_{mid} is a point at the patient's midline. P_{Sk} is at a depth of d_m from the right lateral skin

(i) Dose rate at P_{mid}:

Field $W_d = 12.0$ cm, field length $L_d = 20$ cm.

From (13-27), the side of the equivalent square is

$$E_{Sq} = \frac{W_d \times L_d}{(W_d + L_d)} \times 2 = \frac{12 \times 20}{(12 + 20)} \times 2 = 15 \text{ cm}$$

The depth of midline point P_{mid} is

$$d = 38.0/2.0 = 19.0 \text{ cm}$$

$$TMR(4\,MV, d = 19 \text{ cm}, A_d = 15 \text{ cm} \times 15 \text{ cm}) = 0.524 \quad \text{(from Table 13.9)}$$

$$CPOR = 1.037 \text{ cGy Mu}^{-1} \quad \text{(from footnote to Table 13.13)}$$

$$NPOF(15 \text{ cm} \times 15 \text{ cm}) = 1.031 \quad \text{(from Table 13.13)}$$

From Equation (13-22), the dose rate at P_{mid} is

$$CPOR \times NPOF \times TMR = 1.037 \text{ cGy Mu}^{-1} \times 1.031 \times 0.524$$
$$= 0.560 \text{ cGy Mu}^{-1}$$

Mu to deliver $100 \text{ cGy} = 100 \text{ cGy}/0.560 \text{ cGy Mu}^{-1} = 179$ Mu

Thus, each beam should be turned on for 179 monitor units.

(ii) Dose at point P_{Sk}:

For both beams, point P_{Sk} is at a distance different from the distance of 100 cm where the calibrated output is applicable. Because of this, we will use explicit inverse-square distance corrections. First, we derive the output rate to tissue in air at P_{mid} at $SAD = 100$ cm as given by

$$\frac{\text{peak output rate at } P_{mid}}{\text{peak scatter factor}} = \frac{CPOR \times NPOF(A_d)}{PSF(A_d)}$$
$$= \frac{1.037 \text{ cGy Mu}^{-1} \times 1.031}{1.050}$$
$$= 1.018 \text{ Gy Mu}^{-1} \quad \text{(to tissue in air)}$$

For Beam 1

Distance of point P_{Sk} from the source:

$$(SAD - 19 \text{ cm} + d_m) = (100 \text{ cm} - 19 \text{ cm} + 1.2 \text{ cm}) = 82.2 \text{ cm}$$

Corresponding ISqF:

$$ISqF = (100.0/82.2)^2 = 1.48$$

Output rate at the distance of P_{Sk} in air
$= 1.018 \text{ cGy Mu}^{-1} \times 1.48 = 1.507 \text{ cGy Mu}^{-1}$ in air.

We multiply this by the PSF to obtain the peak output rate at the distance of P_{Sk}. The field width and length for beam 1 at P_{Sk} are

$$W_{dm} = (12 \times 82.2/100) = 9.9 \text{ cm}$$
$$L_{dm} = (20 \times 82.2/100) = 16.4 \text{ cm}$$

From (13-27), the side of the equivalent square is

$$E_{Sq} = 2 \times 9.9 \times 16.4/(9.9 + 16.4) = 12.3 \text{ cm}$$

and

$$PSF(4 \text{ MV}, 12.3 \text{ cm} \times 12.3 \text{ cm}) = 1.044$$

The peak output rate at the distance of P_{Sk} is

$$1.507 \text{ cGy Mu}^{-1} \times 1.044 = 1.573 \text{ cGy Mu}^{-1}$$

This should be multiplied by the TMR applicable to point P_{Sk} to give the output rate at P_{Sk}.

$$TMR(4 \text{ MV}, d = 1.2 \text{ cm}, A_d = 12.3 \text{ cm} \times 12.3 \text{ cm}) = 1.0 \quad \text{(from Table 13.9)}$$

Thus, the output rate at P_{Sk} for beam 1 is

$$1.573 \text{ cGy Mu}^{-1} \times 1.000 = 1.573 \text{ cGy Mu}^{-1}$$

For Beam 2
We calculate the same factors as for beam 1.
Distance of P_{Sk} from the source:

$$(SAD + 39 \text{ cm} - d_m) = (100 \text{ cm} + 38 \text{ cm} - 1.2 \text{ cm}) = 117.8 \text{ cm}$$

Corresponding ISqF:

$$ISqF = (100/117.8)^2 = 0.721$$

The output rate at the distance of P_{Sk} in air
$= 1.018 \text{ CGy Mu}^{-1} \times 0.721 = 0.734 \text{ cGy Mu}^{-1}$
At P_{Sk}, the field width and length are:

$$W_d = 12 \times 117.8/100 = 14.1 \text{ cm}$$
$$L_d = 20 \times 117.8/100 = 23.6 \text{ cm}$$

The equivalent square from (13-27) is

$$E_{Sq} = 2 \times (14.1 \times 23.6)/(14.1 + 23.6) = 17.65 \text{ cm}$$

The PSF is

$$PSF(4 \text{ MV}, 17.6 \text{ cm} \times 17.6 \text{ cm}) = 1.057 \quad \text{(from Table 13.13)}$$

The peak output rate at the distance of P_{Sk}
$= 0.734 \text{ cGy Mu}^{-1} \times 1.057 = 0.776 \text{ cGy Mu}^{-1}$

Point P_{Sk} is at a depth of $39 \text{ cm} - d_m = 37.8 \text{ cm}$ for beam 2. The applicable TMR is

$TMR(4 \text{ MV}, d = 37.8 \text{ cm}, A_d = 17.6 \text{ cm} \times 17.6 \text{ cm}) = 0.237 \quad \text{(from Table 13.9)}$

Hence, the dose rate at P_{Sk} is

$$0.776 \text{ cGy Mu}^{-1} \times 0.237 = 0.184 \text{ cGy Mu}^{-1}$$

5000 cGy will be delivered to point P_{mid} in 25 treatments of 200 cGy each. The total Mu for beam 1 and beam 2 will be

$$179 \, \text{Mu/treatment/beam} \times 25 \, \text{treatments} = 4475 \, \text{Mu per beam}$$

Dose at P_{Sk}:

Dose from beam 1 + dose from beam 2
$$= 4475 \, \text{Mu} \times 1.573 \, \text{cGy Mu}^{-1} + 4475 \, \text{Mu} \times 0.184 \, \text{cGy Mu}^{-1}$$
$$= 7039 \, \text{cGy} + 823 \, \text{cGy} \approx 7862 \, \text{cGy}$$

A total of 7862 cGy will be received at P_{Sk} when 5000 cGy is delivered at P_{mid}.

An Alternate (Approximate) Approach for Solving Example 13.6

An approximate approach for calculating the dose received at point P_{Sk} is to derive it from the dose delivered to P_{mid} by allowing for the facts that P_{Sk} and P_{mid} (i) are at different distances from the source and (ii) are at different depths and hence are being subjected to differences in attenuation and scatter. The role of distance can be accounted for by an inverse-square factor. The role of attenuation and scatter can be taken into account by a ratio of TAR or, less exactly, by a ratio of TMR.

Point P_{mid} is at 100 cm from the source and at a depth of 19 cm for both beams. It has

$$\text{TMR}(4 \, \text{MV}, d = 19 \, \text{cm}, A_d = 15 \, \text{cm} \times 15 \, \text{cm}) = 0.524 \quad \text{(from Table 13.9)}$$

for both beams.

For Beam 1
Point P_{Sk} is at a depth of 1.2 cm and at a distance of 82.2 cm from the source. Hence, the TMR for P_{Sk} for beam 1 is

$$\text{TMR}(4 \, \text{MV}, d = 1.2 \, \text{cm}, A_d = 12.3 \, \text{cm} \times 12.3 \, \text{cm}) = 1.000$$

Ratio of TMRs for point P_{Sk} and P_{mid}:

$$1.000/0.524 = 1.908$$

The change resulting from distance is the ISqF

$$(100/82.2)^2 = 1.48$$

Combining the above two factors, the overall ratio for beam 1 is

$$(\text{dose at } P_{Sk}/\text{dose at } P_{mid}) = 1.908 \times 1.48 = 2.824$$

For Beam 2
Point P_{Sk} is at a depth of 37.8 cm and a distance of 117.8 cm from the source. The corresponding TMR for P_{Sk} is

$$\text{TMR}(4 \, \text{MV}, d = 37.8 \, \text{cm}, A_d = 17.4 \, \text{cm} \times 17.4 \, \text{cm}) = 0.237$$

Ratio of TMRs for points P_{Sk} and P_{mid}:

$$0.237/0.524 = 0.452$$

The change resulting from distance is the ISqF given by

$$(100/117.8)^2 = 0.721$$

Combining the above two factors, the overall ratio for beam 2 is

$$(\text{dose at } P_{Sk}/\text{dose at } P_{mid}) = 0.452 \times 0.721 = 0.326$$

Both Beams Together
A total of 5000 cGy is received at P_{mid}, with 2500 cGy contributed by each of beams 1 and 2.

$$\text{Dose at } P_{Sk} = 2500\,\text{cGy}(\text{ratio for beam } 1 + \text{ratio for beam } 2)$$
$$= 2500(2.824 + 0.326) \approx 7875\,\text{cGy}$$

EXAMPLE 13.7

A tumor is treated with a moving 4-MV X-ray beam spanning a 280° arc with a field size of 6 cm × 12 cm at SAD = 100 cm. The lengths of the different radii from the isocenter to the surface of the patient at 20° angular intervals are as shown in Figure 13.9. Use this information to evaluate (i) an effective TMR for the arc, (ii) the monitor units to deliver 200 cGy, and (iii) the monitor units per degree of arc needed. Use data from Tables 13.9 and 13.13.

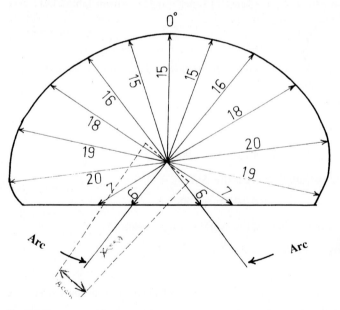

Fig. 13.9. Treatment with a moving beam covering a 280° arc. The depths to the isocenter along different radii of the arc (in cm) are indicated

(i)   TMR for arc:
      Field width $W_d = 6.0$ cm, field length $L_d = 12.0$ cm.

Table 13.15. Weighted Summation

Radius i	Angle[a] ϕ_i	Radius $r_{i\,(cm)}$	$TMR(r_i)$[b]	Weight w_i
1	$-140°$	6.0	0.855	0.5
2	$-120°$	7.0	0.820	1.0
3	$-100°$	20.0	0.435	1.0
4	$-80°$	19.0	0.457	1.0
5	$-60°$	18.0	0.480	1.0
6	$-40°$	16.0	0.533	1.0
7	$-20°$	15.0	0.561	1.0
8	$0°$	15.0	0.561	1.0
9	$+20°$	15.0	0.561	1.0
10	$+40°$	16.0	0.533	1.0
11	$+60°$	18.0	0.480	1.0
12	$+80°$	20.0	0.435	1.0
13	$+100°$	19.0	0.457	1.0
14	$+120°$	7.0	0.820	1.0
15	$+140°$	6.0	0.855	0.5

[a] $\phi = 0°$ corresponds to vertically downward direction.
[b] Values based on data in Table 13.9.

Side of equivalent square $E_{Sq} = 2(6 \times 12)/(6 + 12) = 8.0$ cm.
We can approximate the arc by individual beams at 20° angular intervals. We tabulate the angles, radii, and TMRs and find an average TMR for the arc.
During the arc motion, the beams entering along the first and last radii have only one half of the full field width. Along all of the other radii, the beams have full field width. Hence we have done a weighted summation in the above table by assigning a weight of 0.5 to the TMRs for the first and last radii and 1.0 for the others.

TMR for arc = weighted mean TMR for 15 listed radii in Table 13.15

$$= \frac{w_i \times TMR(r_i, 8 \times 8\,cm)}{15} = \frac{7.988}{15} = 0.532$$

(ii) Mu for 200 cGy:
From Table 13.13,
CPOR $= 1.037$ cGy Mu^{-1}; NPOF(8×8 cm) $= 0.975$;

$$\text{Arc output rate} = 1.037\,\text{cGy Mu}^{-1} \times 0.975 \times 0.532$$
$$= 0.538\,\text{cGy Mu}^{-1}$$

$$\text{Mu for 200 cGy} = \frac{200}{0.538\,\text{cGy Mu}^{-1}} = 372\,\text{Mu}$$

(iii) Monitor units per degree of arc:
Monitor units/arc angle $= 372\,\text{Mu}/280° = 1.33\,\text{Mu/degree}$.

13.21
Concluding Remarks

In this chapter we defined various ratios and factors useful for relating the treatment time (or monitor units) to the radiation dose to any point on the central axis of a radiation beam. The various calculated examples used the values of factors from the data tables provided for the purpose. Any radiation therapy clinic should have similar sets of data tables and methodology of its own for the beams produced by its machines for routine patient dosimetry. It is the duty of the clinical physicist to establish the data base and procedure. Such depth-dose data tables can be prepared by the physicist based on either direct measurements for a given machine, or by adoption of a set of readily available values of PDD, TAR, or TMR in the published literature. It may be possible to get the beam energy fine-tuned to obtain a close match to an available and reliable TMR data for a machine of the same model.

For direct detailed measurements, it is convenient to set up a rectangular water phantom with the water surface at a selected SSD, and to measure at different depths along the central axis with an ionization chamber. Commercially available automatic scanning equipment consisting of an ion chamber and a water phantom can be either leased or purchased for rapid collection of data. Alternatively, unit-density water-equivalent plastic can be used. In this manner, a direct assessment of peak outputs, NPOF, and PDD can be done. The intent is to derive the values of TAR (or TMR) from the PDD through concepts outlined in Section 13.19.

It is relatively more difficult to make measurements in air. Measurement of the "dose to tissue" in air will call for the use of a mini-phantom of appropriate size suspended in air. It is in general an experimental challenge to ascertain the values of in-air output factors. Thus, ascertaining the values of PSF, NAOF, and NPSF can pose a problem. Fortunately, it happens that the values of NPSF remain nearly the same for all energies of x-ray beams above that of ^{60}Co [2–3]. Hence, knowing the NPOF values by measurement and adopting the published values of NPSF(A), the NAOF values may be derived by the relation NAOF(A) = NPOF(A)/NPSF(A).

In all cases, the reliability of the finalized dataset should be ascertained experimentally. This can be done by first using the dataset to calculate the treatment times (or Mus) needed to deliver a specified dose (of say 200 cGy) for a few field sizes and depths. Then by placing an ion chamber in a water phantom it can be verified that the calculated times (or Mus) indeed deliver the expected dose for the respective field sizes and depths. The field sizes and depths chosen should encompass the entire range of the anticipated clinical use.

Glossary of Abbreviations

CAOR Calibrated air output rate
CPOR Calibrated peak output rate
ISqF   Inverse square factor
Mu   Monitor Unit
NAOF Normalized air output factor (Equivalent to Sc in some published literature)

NBSF Normalized backscatter factor
NOF   Normalized output factor
NPOF Normalized peak output factor
      (Equivalent to St in some published literature)
NPSF Normalized peak scatter factor
      (Equivalent to Sp in some published literature)

PDD Percent depth dose
PSF   Peak scatter factor
TAR Tissue-air ratio
TMR Tissue maximum ratio
TPR Tissue phantom ratio

References

1. Massey, J.B., A Manual of Dosimetry in Radiotherapy, Technical Report Series No. 110, International Atomic Energy Agency, Vienna, Austria, 1970.
2. Joint Working Party of the British Institute of Radiology and Hospital Physicists' Association, U.K., Central Axis Depth Dose Data for Use in Radiotherapy, British Journal of Radiology Supplement 17, British Institute of Radiology, London, U.K., 1983.
3. Joint Working Group of British Institute of Radiology and Institute of Physics and Engineering in Medicine, Central Axis Depth Dose Data for Use in Radiotherapy, British Journal of Radiology, Supplement 25, British Institute of Radiology, London, 1996.
4. Dutreix, A., Bjangard, B.E., Bridier, A., Mijnheer, B., Shaw, J.E., and Svensson, H., Monitor unit calculation for high energy photon beams, Physics for clinical radiotherapy, ESTRO Booklet no. 3, Leuven, Garant, 1997.
5. Netherlands Commission on Radiation Dosimetry, Determination and use of scatter correction factors of megavoltage photon beams, NCS Report 12, Delft, NCS, 1998.
6. Venselaar, J. L. M., van Gasteren, J. J.M., and Heukelom, S., A consistent formalism for the application of phantom and collimator scatter factors, Phys. Med. Biol. Vol. 44, p365–381, 1999.
7. Georg, D, Heukelom, S, and Venselaar, J., Formalisms for MU calculations, ESTRO Booklet 3, versus NCS report 12, Radiother. Oncol., Vol. 60, p319–328, 2001.

CHAPTER 14

Beam Dosimetry: Additional Corrections – Special Situations

14.1
Introduction

In the previous chapter, we covered the various factors and ratios that are useful for calculating the output rate and treatment time under standard conditions. The standard definition restricted the calculations to (i) beams of rectangular cross section, (ii) points on the central axis of the beam, (iii) a flat surface of incidence, (iv) a homogeneous water-equivalent, unit-density medium, and (v) uniform intensity across the beam. In this chapter, we address practical situations in which there can be deviations from the above conditions.

14.2
Scatter Considerations

14.2.1
Scatter in Blocked Fields

In practice in many patient situations, the normal rectangular fields possible with the built-in adjustable collimators of the treatment machine may not conform ideally to the shape of the cross section of the target volume to be treated. In such cases, it is usual to insert shielding blocks in the beam and modify the field outline to fit the target volume. In recent years, technical advancement has produced multi-leaf collimators (MLC) that provide irregularly shaped fields without the need for insertion of blocks [1–4]. MLC, as the name suggests, has several metal leaves that can be inserted into the beam to block the radiation. Successive leaves are connected by tongue-and-grove joints, but each leaf can move with some independence allowed by the design. Any contoured block can be substituted by the successive steps of the MLC leaves. The width of the leaves, which may be in the range of 3 mm to 10 mm depending on the model, governs the accuracy with which an MLC can substitute a custom-fabricated block. As a corollary, any field blocked by an MLC can be approximated by a contoured block. Hence, in this chapter no distinction is made between fields shaped by MLC and by custom-blocks.

Two cases of shaped fields are illustrated in Figures 14.1 and 14.2. In both cases, the outlines of the rectangular field defined by the collimators have been identified by A. Some areas within A have been protected by placement of shaped shielding blocks. The outlines marked B indicate the odd-shaped cross section of the actual scattering medium after the blocked areas and the air volume outside the patient's body are omitted from A. With such a change in the scattering volume, the standard depth-dose

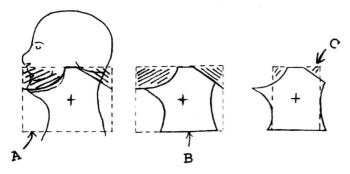

Fig. 14.1. A blocked field used for treatment of a tumor in the neck region. Outline *A* represents the rectangular collimator field. Outline *B* is the irregular shape of the cross section of the scattering volume when the blocked areas and air volumes within *A* are omitted. Outline *C* is the effective rectangular field giving the same scatter as *B* to the points of dose calculation indicated by +

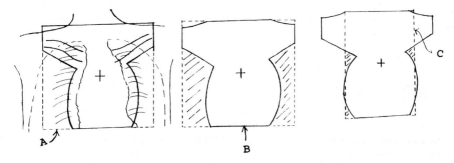

Fig. 14.2. A blocked field used for treatment of the chest. Outlines *A*, *B*, and *C* are defined as in Figure 14.1

data applicable for beams of rectangular and square cross sections cannot be used for patient dosimetry. We will discuss both simple and more accurate methods that are available to account for the change in scatter.

14.2.2
Effective Rectangular Field

Sometimes it is possible to configure an effective rectangular field with its center at the point of dose calculation. "Effective rectangle" here means that the dose at its center is very close to the dose at the point of interest in the actual field shape. The rectangular field outlines **C** in Figures 14.1 and 14.2 are effective rectangles. These leave out some areas covered by outlines **B**, but include some of the blocked areas to compensate for the loss. If an effective rectangle is drawn in such a way that the scatter missed from the areas left out is compensated for by the scatter from the additional areas included, the depth-dose data applicable to the effective rectangle can be used for patient dosimetry. Such compensation is possible only if the areas left out of **B** and the corresponding compensating areas included within **C** are at about the same geometric location in relation to the point of dose calculation (which is indicated by crosses in Figures 14.1

and 14.2). Thus, the effective rectangle **C** should be drawn judiciously so that

$$TAR(d, B) = TAR(d, C)$$
$$PSF(B) = PSF(C)$$
$$TMR(d, B) = TMR(d, C)$$

where d is the treatment depth and where TAR, PSF, and TMR are the tissue-air ratio, peak scatter factor, and tissue maximum ratio, respectively, as defined in Chapter 13. For fixed source-to-axis distance (SAD) conditions, with the output factors determined in air, the dose rate $\dot{D}_P$ (at point P in Figure 13.5) can be calculated from a relation that adopts the logic of Equation (13-21). As we recall, the normalized air output factor, NAOF(A), is affected by the photons scattered from the materials in the treatment head.* Such scatter, called head scatter, depends in a complicated manner on the design of the treatment head [5–7]. Because it is influenced mainly by the scatter from the collimating diaphragms, a practical approximation is to assume that the head scatter is unique for a given collimator opening. Hence, we will use the NAOF applicable for the unblocked collimator field **A** (and not the effective field **C**). However, the patient scatter depends on the effective scattering cross section as indicated by the rectangular outline **C**. Hence, it is proper to use the TAR value applicable to field **C**. Thus,

$$\dot{D}_P = CAOR \times NAOF(A) \times TAR(d, C) \tag{14-1}$$

where CAOR is the calibrated air output rate.

The situation is different if peak output rates are used in the calibration and if the dosimetry is based on the calibrated peak output rate (CPOR), normalized peak output factor (NPOF), and TMR data. The value NPOF(A) is affected by both head scatter and patient scatter. The patient scatter comes from effective field **C**. Hence, the NPOF for the blocked field can be derived as follows:

$$\text{Dose rate to tissue in air for field A} = CPOR \times NPOF(A)/PSF(A)$$

$$NPOF(\text{blocked field}) = (\text{dose rate to tissue in air for field A}) \times PSF(C)$$
$$= CPOR \cdot [NPOF(A)/PSF(A)] \cdot PSF(C) \tag{14-2}$$

Multiplying this by TMR(d, C) for field **C**, we obtain

$$\dot{D}_P = CPOR \cdot [NPOF(A)/PSF(A)] \cdot PSF(C) \cdot TMR(d, C)$$

that is,

$$\dot{D}_P = CPOR \cdot NPOF(A) \cdot TMR(d, C) \cdot [PSF(C)/PSF(A)] \tag{14-3}$$

Expression (14-3) contains more terms than does (14-1). The ratio of PSFs in (14-3) is an additional correction needed for the system of dosimetry that is based on the use of peak outputs measured with backscatter and TMRs. Expression (14-3) can be rewritten in a different way (see Chapter 13) by substitution of

$$NPOF(A) = NAOF(A) \cdot NPSF(A)$$
$$NPSF(A) = [PSF(A)/PSF(A_{St})]$$

---

* Some publications use notations S_t, S_c, and S_p, in lieu of acronyms NPOF, NAOF, and NPSF, respectively.

and

$$NPSF(C) = [PSF(C)/PSF(A_{St})].$$

Then we obtain,

$$\dot{D}_P = CPOR \cdot NAOF(A) \cdot TMR(d, C) \cdot NPSF(C) \qquad (14.3a)$$

EXAMPLE 14.1

A patient is treated by having the diaphragms set to give a square field of 15 cm × 15 cm size at the tumor at a depth of 10 cm and an SAD of 80 cm. However, the field is blocked to give an effective field area of 4 cm × 4 cm, as shown in Figure 14.3. Calculate the monitor units required to deliver a dose of 200 cGy by using (i) the TAR data of Table 13.2 and the calibration data of Table 13.12 for a ^{60}Co machine and (ii) the TMR data of Table 13.9 and the calibration data of Table 13.13 for a 4-MV X-ray machine.

Fig. 14.3. A collimator field 15 cm × 15 cm in size is blocked to give a treatment field 4 cm × 4 cm in size

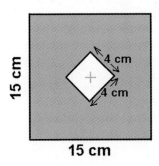

(i) We obtain
    CAOR = 93.0 cGy min^{-1} (from footnote to Table 13.12)
    NAOF(A_m = 15 cm × 15 cm) = 1.023 (from Table 13.12)
    TAR(d = 10 cm, A_d = 4 cm × 4 cm) = 0.620 (from Table 13.2)
    Substituting in Equation (14-1), we obtain

$$\dot{D}_P = 93.0 \times 1.023 \times 0.620 = 59.0\,cGy\,min^{-1}$$

Time to deliver 200 cGy = 200/59.0 = 3.39 min = 3 min 23 sec.
(ii) We obtain
    CPOR = 1.037 cGy Mu^{-1} (from footnote to Table 13.13)
    NPOF(A_m = 15 cm × 15 cm) = 1.031 (from Table 13.13)
    PSF(A_m = 15 cm × 15 cm) = 1.051 (from Table 13.13)
    PSF(A_m = 4 cm × 4 cm) = 1.007 (from Table 13.13)
    TMR(d = 10 cm, A_d = 4 cm × 4 cm) = 0.661 (from Table 13.9)
    Substituting in Equation (14-3), we obtain

$$\dot{D}_P = 1.037\,cGy\,Mu^{-1} \times 1.031 \times [1.007/1.051] \times 0.661$$
$$= 0.677\,cGy\,Mu^{-1}$$

Mu to deliver 200 cGy = 200/0.677 = 295 Mu.

Alternately we can use (14.3a) as follows:

CPOR $= 1.037$ cGy Mu^{-1} (from footnote to Table 13.13)
NAOF($A_m = 15$ cm $\times$ 15 cm) $= 1.018$ (for open field from Table 13.13)
TMR($d = 10$ cm, $A_d = 4$ cm $\times$ 4 cm) $= 0.661$ (for blocked field from Table 13.9)
NPSF($A_m = 4$ cm $\times$ 4 cm) $= 0.972$ (for blocked field from Table 13.13)

$$\dot{D}_P = 1.037 \text{ cGy Mu}^{-1} \times 1.018 \times 0.661 \times 0.972 = 0.678 \text{ cGy Mu}^{-1}$$

Mu to deliver 200 cGy $= 200/0.678 = 295$ Mu.

14.2.3
Scatter-Air Ratio, SAR(d, A$_d$)

As we discussed in Section 13.9, the tissue-air ratio corrects for (i) the attenuation of the primary photon fluence by the overlying thickness d of tissue and (ii) the augmentation of the scattered photon fluence from the volume covered by the field A_d. We call the former the primary component and the latter the scatter component of the TAR. For a given beam quality, the primary component is unique for a given depth d, but the scatter component will increase with the field size. As the limit of the field size approaches zero (i. e., as A_d reaches zero), the TAR can be construed to be made up entirely of the primary component, with negligible scatter. Such a limiting value of TAR is the "zero-field TAR," which can also be called the primary-air ratio (PAR). Thus,

$$\text{PAR} = \text{PAR}(d) = \text{TAR}(d, 0 \times 0) \tag{14-4}$$

We define the scatter-air ratio (SAR) as the scatter component of the tissue-air ratio [8]. Thus,

$$\begin{aligned} \text{SAR} = \text{SAR}(d, A_d) &= \text{TAR}(d, A_d) - \text{PAR}(d) \\ &= \text{TAR}(d, A_d) - \text{TAR}(d, 0 \times 0) \end{aligned} \tag{14-5}$$

SAR, like TAR, depends on the quality of the radiation, the depth, and the field size and is practically independent of the source-to-skin distance (SSD). The SAR rapidly increases with field size for small fields and gradually saturates for very large fields.

A listing of SARs for circular fields of different radii is called scatter radius data. The scatter radius data can be derived from the TAR data. Figure 14.4 shows the increase of the TAR with field radius for one selected depth of 9 cm for cobalt-60 radiation. The data points for five field sizes have been plotted. Because a "zero field size" is a theoretical concept, it is difficult to measure the PAR directly. However, PAR for any depth can be inferred indirectly by graphic extrapolation to a zero field size, for data measured at that depth for larger field sizes, or by a theoretical estimation [9–13]. An example of the derivation of PAR by graphic extrapolation is shown in Figure 14.4. If one knows the PAR for any particular depth, the SAR value for any field size can be obtained by subtraction of the PAR from the TAR. SAR values for ^{60}Co for a depth of 9 cm are listed in Table 14.1.

Fig. 14.4. Increase of TAR and SAR with field radius at 9 cm depth for a cobalt-60 beam. The level of TAR for zero field radius (derived by extrapolation) divides the primary and scatter components of the TAR

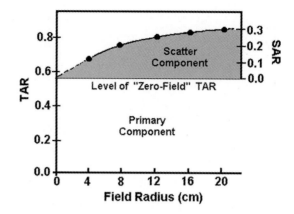

Table 14.1. Scatter-Air Ratios for Circular Fields of Cobalt-60 at 9 cm Depth

Radius (cm)	SAR
0.0	0.000
1.0	0.050
2.0	0.085
3.0	0.115
4.0	0.145
5.0	0.170
6.0	0.190
7.0	0.208

14.2.4
Scatter-Radius Integration

The scatter radius data are useful for inferring the scatter at any point in a field of any shape by a sector integration method, attributed to Clarkson [14]. Let SAR(d, r) designate the scatter-air ratio for a circular field of radius r and depth d. Figure 14.5a shows a field of irregular shape. The field has been divided into N sectors in Figure 14.5b. Let us assume that the sector radii are $r_1, r_2, \ldots, r_N$ and that they are drawn at angular intervals of $\Delta\theta$. A full circle subtends an angle 2π at its center. The scatter volume under a sector of a particular radius is $\Delta\theta/2\pi$ times that under a full circle of the same radius. The SAR contribution due to a volume under a full circle of radius r_i (Figure 14.5c) is SAR(d, r_i). The partial SAR contributed by a sector of angle $\Delta\theta$ will be

$$\text{SAR}(d, r_i) \times (\Delta\theta/2\pi)$$

The total SAR for the entire irregular field is the sum for all sectors 1 to N:

$$\text{SAR}(d, \text{irregular field}) = \sum_{i=1}^{N} \text{SAR}(d, r_i)(\Delta\theta/2\pi) \tag{14-6}$$

The TAR for the irregular field is the sum of SAR and PAR (given by zero-field TAR). That is,

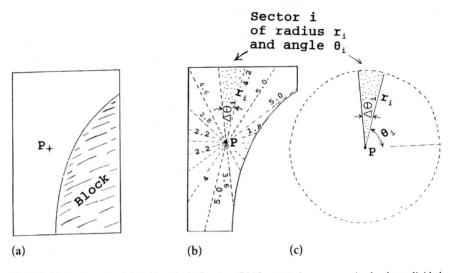

Fig. 14.5. (a) A rectangular field with a blocked region. (b) The scattering cross section has been divided into sectors, each of angle $\Delta\theta$, with sector i having radius r_i at angle θ_i. (c) Sector i is shown as a part of a full circle

$$
\begin{aligned}
\text{TAR}(d, \text{irregular field}) &= \text{PAR}(d) + \text{SAR}(d, \text{irregular field}) \\
&= \text{TAR}(d, 0) + \text{SAR}(d, \text{irregular field}) \\
&= \text{TAR}(d, 0) + \sum_{i=1}^{N} \text{SAR}(d, r_i)(\Delta\theta/2\pi) \qquad (14\text{-}7)
\end{aligned}
$$

An expression similar to (14-7) should apply for the PSF, which is a special case of the TAR for depth d_m. For a zero field size, PSF has its minimum possible value of 1.0. Hence,

$$
\begin{aligned}
\text{PSF}(d_m, \text{irregular field}) &= \text{PSF}(d_m, 0) + \text{SAR}(d_m, \text{irregular field}) \\
&= 1.0 + \sum_{i=1}^{N} \text{SAR}(d_m, r_i) \times \Delta\theta/2\pi
\end{aligned}
$$

TMR can be derived from TAR and PSF by the relation TMR = TAR/PSF.

EXAMPLE 14.2

The rectangular field in Figure 14.5 is of size 6 cm × 9 cm. After the block is added, 18 sector radii are drawn at 20° angular intervals. The consecutive radii are 4.2, 5.0, 5.0, 1.8, 1.5, 1.4, 1.5, 1.8, 3.6, 5.0, 4.0, 2.5, 2.2, 2.1, 2.2, 2.8, 4.6, and 4.2 cm. Estimate the TAR at point P at 9 cm depth located in the central region of the unblocked field by sector integration, using the scatter radius data of Table 14.1. Compare the result with the TAR applicable to the same point for the unblocked field.

We first tabulate the sector number, radius, and the corresponding SAR in sequence.

Substituting,

Sector i	Radius r_i (cm)	$SAR(d, r_i)$	Sector i	Radius r_i (cm)	$SAR(d, r_i)$
1	4.2	0.150	10	5.0	0.170
2	5.0	0.170	11	4.0	0.145
3	5.0	0.170	12	2.5	0.100
4	1.8	0.079	13	2.2	0.091
5	1.5	0.068	14	2.1	0.088
6	1.4	0.064	15	2.2	0.091
7	1.5	0.068	16	2.8	0.109
8	1.8	0.078	17	4.6	0.160
9	3.6	0.133	18	4.2	0.150

$$\text{Sum} = \sum_i SAR(d = 9\,\text{cm}, r_i) = 2.05$$

$$SAR(d = 9\,\text{cm, irregular field}) = \sum_i SAR(d, r_i) \times \Delta\theta/2\pi .$$

$$\Delta\theta/2\pi = 20°/360° \quad \text{and} \quad \sum_i SAR(d = 9\,\text{cm}, r_i) = 2.05$$

$$SAR(d = 9\,\text{cm, irregular field}) = 2.05 \times 20°/360° = 0.114$$

Primary component PAR is zero-field TAR.

$$PAR = TAR(d = 9\,\text{cm, zero field}) = 0.572 \quad \text{(from Table 13.2)}$$

$$TAR(d = 9\,\text{cm, irregular field}) = PAR + SAR(d, \text{irregular field})$$
$$= 0.572 + 0.114 = 0.686$$

TAR for unblocked field:
The side of an equivalent square for an unblocked rectangular field of size 6 cm × 9 cm is 7.2 cm (from Table 13.12). The TAR at 9 cm depth for a 7.2 cm × 7.2 cm field (as obtained from Table 13.2) is 0.718, which is 4.7% higher than the irregular-field TAR derived above.

14.2.5
Day's Method

The standard tables of depth-dose data apply only to points on the central axis of rectangular or square fields. They are not valid for off-central axis points. The sectors for deriving the SAR for an off-central axis point Q in a rectangular field are illustrated in the upper right diagram of Figure 14.6. The sector integration method is the most general method for determining the SAR. It can be used for any field shape and for any point.

A different method, called Day's method [15], is a simpler procedure that can be used for any off-central axis point when the field shape is a rectangle. The upper left diagram in Figure 14.6 illustrates the basis of the method. Four rectangular areas marked a, b,

Fig. 14.6. (Top left) The four
rectangular scattering areas a, b, c, and d around an
off-central axis point Q in a
rectangular field. (Top right)
Scattering sectors (see Figure 14.5) around Q. (Bottom)
Four full rectangles of which
a, b, c, and d are each one
quarter, as visualized in Day's
method

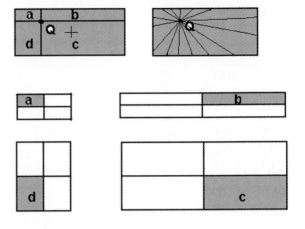

Fig. 14.6. (Top left) The four rectangular scattering areas a, b, c, and d around an off-central axis point Q in a rectangular field. (Top right) Scattering sectors (see Figure 14.5) around Q. (Bottom) Four full rectangles of which a, b, c, and d are each one quarter, as visualized in Day's method

c, and d are selected so that all four have a common corner Q. Each of these areas, in turn, is one quarter of the larger rectangles that are shown in the bottom part of Figure 14.6. Hence, each contributes one quarter of the total scatter that its respective full rectangle contributes. Thus, we can write

$$\text{SAR for point Q} = \frac{\text{Sum of SARs for the four larger rectangles}}{4}$$

and

$$\text{TAR for point Q} = \text{PAR} + \text{SAR}$$
$$= \text{PAR} + \frac{\text{Sum of SARs for the four larger rectangles}}{4}$$

14.3
General Approach for Off-Central Axis Points

14.3.1
Surface Curvature, Distance, and Depth

Figure 14.7 shows a beam incident on a curved surface of a patient. The point of interest for dose calculation is Q, which, for generality, can be anywhere within a field of any shape. The position of the patient may be set up such that a particular preselected SSD or SAD is obtained at the central ray of the beam. The SSDs at other points on the surface will depend on the curvature of the patient's surface. The SSDs of different surface locations can usually be read by an optical distance indicator (see Section 9.4.2). If the SSD read at the surface point directly above Q is SSD_Q and the depth of Q is d_Q, then, as a practical approximation, the distance of point Q from the source during the irradiation can be taken to be $[\text{SSD}_Q + d_Q]$. (Although this ignores the divergence of the ray from the source, it gives the accuracy needed in practice.) Let us assume here that (i) the patient has been set up with an $\text{SSD} = \text{SSD}_C$, at the central axis, and (ii) the system of dosimetry uses calibration and output factors that are obtained in air at a distance of $(\text{SSD}_N + d_m)$, where SSD_N is the normal SSD of choice. That is, the value of

Fig. 14.7. A beam diverging from source S is incident on a patient contour. Q_c is on the central axis, and Q is an off-central axis point

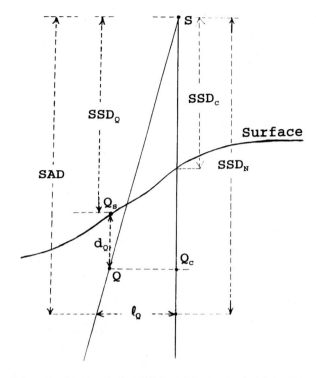

CAOR applies to the distance $(SSD_N + d_m)$, and all of the output factors are NAOF(A) values, with the field size A defined at the SSD_N. The dose rate, $(\dot{D}_Q)_{air}$, to tissue in air at Q is then given by

$$(\dot{D}_Q)_{air} = CAOR \cdot NAOF(A) \times \left[(SSD_N + d_m)/(SSD_Q + d_Q)\right]^2 \qquad (14\text{-}8)$$

The TAR_Q for point Q at depth d_Q for the field shape used can be obtained by sector integration or any other approximate method which has already been discussed. The above value of $(\dot{D}_Q)_{air}$ is not always sufficiently accurate to be multiplied by the TAR_Q to give the correct dose rate at Q. This is because, for broad, extended fields, we also need to account for a possible lack of beam flatness.

14.3.2
Off-Center Ratios in Air, OCR$_{air}$

The photon beams produced by high-energy accelerators pass through a beam-flattening filter (see Section 10.3.5). Although the flattening filter improves the uniformity of the intensity across the beam, the beam obtained may not be ideally flat. This lack of flatness can be measured with a detector and by scanning of the beam from the center outward on a plane at the standard distance of SSD_N. The ratio of the intensity at distance ℓ from the central axis to that obtained at the central axis is defined as the off-center ratio in air, OCR$_{air}(\ell)$. Apart from the effect of the flattening filter, the penumbra at the beam edge also can be included as part of the OCR. In general, OCR$_{air}$

can be regarded as a function of both the off-center distance and the geometric field size A; i. e.,

$$OCR_{air} = OCR_{air}(\ell_Q, A)$$

For points not close to the geometric edge of the field (and hence not in the penumbra), OCR_{air} can be regarded as a function of ℓ alone. If point Q is located on a ray at distance ℓ_Q from the central axis, the OCR value that will apply for deriving the dose rate at Q is $OCR_{air}(\ell_Q)$.

14.3.3
Dose Rate at Off-Center Point Q

Taking into account both TAR and OCR, the dose rate, $(\dot{D}_Q)_{water}$ at point Q in water is given by

$$(\dot{D}_Q)_{water} = (\dot{D}_Q)_{air} \cdot OCR_{air}(\ell_Q, A) \cdot TAR_Q$$

Substituting for $(\dot{D}_Q)_{air}$ from (14-8) gives

$$(\dot{D}_Q)_{water} = CAOR \cdot NAOF(A) \cdot \left[(SSD_N + d_m)/(SSD_Q + d_Q)\right]^2$$
$$\cdot OCR_{air}(\ell_Q, A) \cdot TAR_Q \tag{14-9}$$

The method discussed above is based on Reference 16. Other investigators [17–19] have reported a softening of the beam (resulting in poor penetration) at off-central locations and have suggested that different PAR values may apply for different off-central rays. Whereas the jaws of traditional collimators move symmetrically with respect to the central axis of the beam, newer collimator designs have independent jaws that allow asymmetric jaw arrangements. This offers the possibility of blocking one half of the beam and using only the other half for irradiation. This produces a non-diverging field edge at the central axis and offers a geometrical advantage in some clinical situations. Also, with independent jaws, it is possible to reduce the volume of coverage of the beam at progressive stages of treatment by only changing the diaphragms without changing the patient's position. With asymmetric collimation, the central axis of the useful beam is not the mechanical central axis of the source-head assembly. The significance of softening of the beam has been studied in the context of modern machines equipped with asymmetric collimators [20–23]. These studies suggest some finer improvements in dosimetry by suitably modifying one or more among the values of PARs, output factors, and off-axis ratios for asymmetric collimation.

14.4
Correction for Body Inhomogeneities

14.4.1
Inhomogeneities

Different body tissues differ in their atomic composition and density. At megavoltage energies, because of the dominance of the Compton effect, the density (more specifically, the electron density) of the structures is more important than the atomic compo-

Table 14.2. Effective Atomic Number and Density of Body Constituents

Constituent	Effective Atomic Number (Z_{eff})	Density ($g\,cm^{-3}$)
Blood	7.74	1.06
Muscle	7.63	1.0–1.04
Adipose tissue	6.43	0.92
Lung	7.72	0.26–1.05
Cortical bone	13.3	1.85
Inner bone	9.27	1.12
Bone marrow	6.94	1.03

Values are from White, D.R., and Constantinou, C., Anthropomorphic phantom materials, Chapter 3, in Progress in Medical Radiation Physics, Vol. 1, Orton, C.G. (Ed.), Plenum Press, New York, 1982.

sition. The densities and effective atomic numbers of different body constituents are listed in Table 14.2.

Historically, the dosimetry in radiotherapy was carried out with the simple assumption that the body is uniform and water-equivalent. Advances have been made in recent years in two different aspects that can impact positively on the future capacity to account properly for the presence of inhomogeneities. These are (i) the availability of computed tomographic scanners by which full anatomic and density details of the body cross sections can be determined, and (ii) the availability of more computer power and advanced algorithms for carrying out inhomogeneity corrections.24

14.4.2
Inhomogeneity Correction Factor (ICF)

Although the above developments are under way, it is necessary to keep in perspective the fact that the knowledge of the relationship between dose and clinical response comes from clinical experience of the past, and that the current dose prescriptions for treatments are based on this past experience. No inhomogeneity corrections were made in the past. Evaluating and recording the doses without the inhomogeneity corrections should be continued, because this serves as a link to the earlier clinical experience. Until we understand exactly how the prescriptions should be revised based on the inhomogeneity-corrected doses, this link should be maintained. Therefore, it is appropriate to consider the correction for the presence of inhomogeneities as a two-stage process in which the dose is first stated without the inhomogeneity correction and subsequently is modified by an inhomogeneity correction factor (ICF), defined as

$$\text{ICF} = \frac{\text{(dose estimated allowing for inhomogeneities)}}{\text{(dose estimated in water-equivalent medium)}}$$

14.4.3
Lung and Bone

A look at the figures in Table 14.2 suggests that the lung and cortical bone are structures in the body that have densities very different from that of water. The lung is a large organ, and radiotherapy beams may pass through 5 to 20 cm of lung. The corrections for the presence of the low-density lung volume in radiotherapy beams can be very significant. Although cortical bone has a high density, its interior structures, consisting of the inner bone and bone marrow, have densities closer to water. Furthermore, the lung, being a more voluminous organ, occupies larger volumes in a beam than does bone. The thickness of bones traversed by radiotherapy beams is less than that of the lungs. However, at low energies at which the photoelectric interaction is important, bone causes another type of perturbation due to its higher effective atomic number. In our discussion, we first pay detailed attention to the problem of correcting for the presence of the low-density lung. Later, we discuss the effect of the presence of bone.

14.4.4
Lung Phantom Geometry

Figure 14.8a shows a cross section of a patient that includes a low-density lung volume and is irradiated by an X-ray beam. Figure 14.8b shows a corresponding laboratory setup made with slabs of water-equivalent and lung-equivalent material, in which measurements can be made. Point P is at a geometric depth d in the central region of the lung. The ray from the source to point P passes through thicknesses d_W of water and d_L of lung. In the next sections, we discuss some of the existing, simple-to-use methods for deriving the ICF for the lung. Such simple methods do not account exactly for the alterations in the scatter photon fluence caused by the low-density lung. There are also other complex models, based on Monte Carlo calculations or differential scatter analysis, that can predict the scatter changes more reliably. However, these are too difficult and cumbersome to be performed routinely. These methods are beyond the scope of this text.

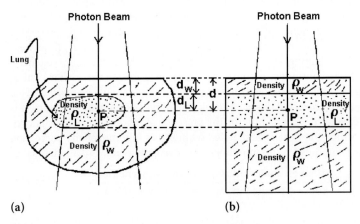

(a)   (b)

Fig. 14.8. (a) A patient-like phantom with a medium of density ρ_L in a water-equivalent medium of density ρ_W. (b) A similar situation represented by rectangular slabs

14.4.5
Effective Depth (d_{eff})

The variation in density results in a change of the mass-equivalent thickness of the medium overlying point P. Let us use ρ_L and ρ_W to denote the densities of lung and water, respectively. Then the effective water-equivalent depth, d_{eff}, for estimation of the TAR is given by

$$d_{eff} = \frac{\text{actual mass-equivalent depth}}{\rho_W} = \frac{[(d - d_L)\rho_W + d_L\rho_L]}{\rho_W} \tag{14-10}$$

14.4.6
ICF Based on Accounting for d_{eff}

An ICF value can be derived based on the simple assumption that the TAR applicable to the water-equivalent depth d_{eff} is more appropriate than that for the geometric depth d. The ICF then would be the ratio of TARs for the depths d_{eff} and d, for the same stated field size A_d. Thus,

$$ICF = \frac{TAR(d_{eff}, A_d)}{TAR(d, A_d)} \tag{14-11}$$

The above method of deriving the ICF is called the ratio-of-TAR method [24]. This method is rather simplistic, because it assumes that the geometric field size A_d is adequate to define the scatter, even when nonunit-density structures are present within the field.

14.4.7
Effective Field Size (A_{eff})

In a uniform water-equivalent medium, the field size A_d at the depth d gives an adequate measure of the mass of the scattering volume. However, if there are non-unit-density structures in the beam, the geometric field size A_d cannot uniquely define the mass of the scattering volume. It is better to determine an effective field size to reflect the effective mass of the scattering volume based on an effective density. Let us say that the geometric length and width of the field (at depth d) are L_d and W_d, respectively. Assuming that the medium behaves as if the effective density were ρ_{eff}, the effective (or water-equivalent) field length L_{eff} and width W_{eff} can be obtained by density scaling as follows:

$$W_{eff} = (W_d\rho_{eff})/\rho_W \tag{14.12a}$$
$$L_{eff} = (L_d\rho_{eff})/\rho_W \tag{14.12b}$$

Corresponding to W_{eff} and L_{eff}, there is an effective field size, A_{eff}, that can be used for finding the appropriate value of the TAR. The value of ρ_{eff} adopted can depend on the location of the point of interest in the medium.

14.4.8
ICF Based on Equivalent TAR, with d_{eff} and A_{eff}

The ICF based on a new TAR that takes into account both the effective depth and the field size is

$$\text{ICF} = \frac{\text{TAR}(d_{\text{eff}}, A_{\text{eff}})}{\text{TAR}(d, A_d)} \qquad (14\text{-}13)$$

The above method of deriving the ICF is called the "equivalent TAR method" [24].

14.4.9
ICF by Batho's Method

This empirical method, also called the power law of TAR method, was originally evolved by Batho [25]. Later, it was presented in a more generalized and modified form by Sontag and Cunningham [26, 27]. In this approach, the correction factor for a point such as R in Figure 14.9 is derived from a generalized formula,

$$\text{ICF} = \frac{[\text{TAR}(d_1, A_d)]^{(\rho_1 - \rho_2)}}{[\text{TAR}(d_2, A_d)]^{(1-\rho_2)}} \qquad (14\text{-}14)$$

where ρ_1 = density of the structure in which the point R lies; d_1 = depth of point R from the interface above; ρ_2 = density of the structure above; and d_2 = depth of R from the surface of the structure above. Likewise, for a point R' (see Figure 14.9), behind a medium of density ρ_1 and in a medium of density ρ_3, the ICF is given by

$$\text{ICF} = \frac{[\text{TAR}(d_1, A_{d'})]^{(\rho_3 - \rho_1)}}{[\text{TAR}(d_{2'}, A_{d'})]^{(1-\rho_1)}} \qquad (14\text{-}15)$$

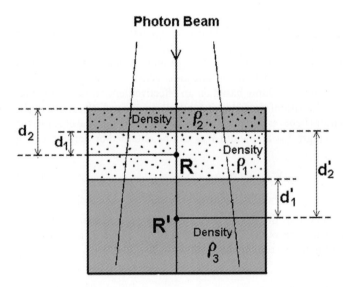

Fig. 14.9. A phantom made of three slabs of materials of three different densities to illustrate Batho's method of inhomogeneity correction

Near an interface, Batho's method suggests a transition and discontinuity in the value of the correction factor across the interface, as is evident from the fact that the formulas for R and R′ are different. Such a discontinuity cannot be real. Hence, Batho's method should not be used close to an interface. It applies more accurately to points well inside the region of inhomogeneity. In the application of Equation (14-14), the TARs used should belong to depths greater than the depth of the peak dose d_m. If the depths happen to be less than d_m, TAR values determined by extrapolation from depths higher than d_m should be used [27].

Point P in Figure 14.8 lies in a low-density lung-equivalent region. There is a layer of water above point P through which the radiation beam is incident. To calculate an ICF by Batho's method for point P, by substituting in Equation (14-14), $\rho_1 = \rho_L$; $\rho_2 = \rho_W = 1.0\,\mathrm{g\,cm^{-3}}$; $d_1 = d_L$; $d_2 = d$, we obtain

$$ICF = \frac{[TAR(d_L, A_d)]^{(\rho_L - \rho_W)}}{[TAR(d, A_d)]^{(1-\rho_W)}}$$

$$= [TAR(d_L, A_d)]^{(\rho_L - 1)} = \frac{1}{[TAR(d_L, A_d)]^{(1-\rho_L)}} \tag{14.16a}$$

Alternatively, in terms of TMR,

$$ICF = \frac{1}{[PSF(A_d) \times TMR(d_L, A_d)]^{(1-\rho_L)}} \tag{14.16b}$$

14.4.10
Comparison of ICF Obtained by Different Methods

For this discussion, we use a set of experimentally measured data published by Mauceri and Kase [28]. The top part of Figure 14.10 shows the inhomogeneous phantom that they employed. A beam is incident on a 5-cm layer of water backed by an extended medium of a low density of $0.32\,\mathrm{g\,cm^{-3}}$. ICF values for cobalt-60 measured at different depths in the low-density region for a field size of $10\,\mathrm{cm} \times 10\,\mathrm{cm}$ and an SAD of 80 cm are shown in the graph in the lower part of Figure 14.10. The graph also shows the estimates of ICF calculated by the various methods. Let us consider a specific point at 10 cm depth from the surface. For this point,

$$d = 10\,\mathrm{cm},\ d_L = 5\,\mathrm{cm},\ A_d = 10\,\mathrm{cm} \times 10\,\mathrm{cm}$$

$$d_{eff} = [(d - d_L)\rho_W + d_L\rho_L]/\rho_W$$
$$= [(10 - 5)1.0 + 5 \times 0.32]/1.0 = 6.6\,\mathrm{cm}$$

We can evaluate the ICF for the above point by the various methods.

Ratio of TAR: From Equation (14-11),

$$ICF = \frac{TAR(d_{eff}, A_d)}{TAR(d, A_d)} = \frac{TAR(6.6\,\mathrm{cm}, 10\,\mathrm{cm} \times 10\,\mathrm{cm})}{TAR(10\,\mathrm{cm}, 10 \times 10\,\mathrm{cm})} = \frac{0.845}{0.718} = 1.18$$

Equivalent TAR: For this method, one needs an effective field size A_{eff} in addition to the d_{eff}. To determine A_{eff}, we must obtain an effective density ρ_{eff} for use in expressions

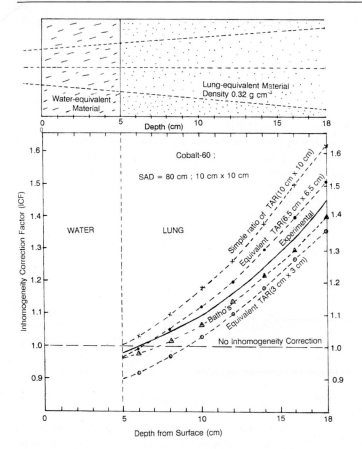

Fig. 14.10. (Top) A beam (dashed lines) is incident on a phantom that consists of a layer of water-equivalent medium on the left followed by a low-density medium simulating lung. (Bottom) The ICFs obtained by different methods at different depths in the lung for a cobalt-60 beam of 10 cm × 10 cm size at SAD 80 cm. (Experimental values are taken from Reference 28.)

(14.12a) and (14.12b). If we make the extreme assumption that the effective density is the low density of $0.32\,\mathrm{g\,cm^{-3}}$ applicable to the lung, the field of 10 cm × 10 cm will be reduced to an effective square field of sides

$$10\,\mathrm{cm} \times \rho_{\mathrm{eff}}/\rho = 10\,\mathrm{cm} \times 0.32\,\mathrm{cm^{-3}}/1.0\,\mathrm{cm^{-3}} = 3.2\,\mathrm{cm}$$

Using TAR data from Table 13.2, we obtain

$$\mathrm{ICF} = \frac{\mathrm{TAR}(d_{\mathrm{eff}}, A_{\mathrm{eff}})}{\mathrm{TAR}(d, A_d)} = \frac{\mathrm{TAR}(6.6\,\mathrm{cm}, 3.2 \times 3.2\,\mathrm{cm})}{\mathrm{TAR}(10\,\mathrm{cm}, 10 \times 10\,\mathrm{cm})} = \frac{0.743}{0.718} = 1.03$$

A more reasonable assumption for ρ_{eff} would be to take it to be the mean density of water and lung. Then, $\rho_{\mathrm{eff}} = (1.0 + 0.32)/2 = 0.66\,\mathrm{g\,cm^{-3}}$. This gives an effective square field of sides

$$10 \times 0.66/1.0 = 6.6\,\mathrm{cm} \approx 6.5\,\mathrm{cm}$$

Using the TAR data from Table 13.2, we obtain

$$\text{ICF} = \frac{\text{TAR}(d_{\text{eff}}, A_{\text{eff}})}{\text{TAR}(d, A_d)} = \frac{\text{TAR}(6.6\,\text{cm}, 6.6\,\text{cm} \times 6.6\,\text{cm})}{\text{TAR}(10\,\text{cm}, 10\,\text{cm} \times 10\,\text{cm})} = \frac{0.803}{0.718} = 1.12$$

Batho's Method: We substitute in (14.16a)

$$d_L = 5\,\text{cm}, \quad A_d = 10 \times 10, \quad \rho_L = 0.32\,\text{g cm}^{-3}$$

and use the TAR data from Table 13.2 to obtain

$$\text{ICF} = \frac{1}{\text{TAR}(d_L, A_d)^{(1-\rho_L)}} = \frac{1}{[\text{TAR}(5\,\text{cm}, 10\,\text{cm} \times 10\,\text{cm})]^{(1-0.32)}}$$

$$= \frac{1}{(0.905)^{0.68}} = 1.070$$

We have thus derived ICF values of 1.18, 1.03, 1.12, and 1.07 for the same situation by using different methods and assumptions. The experimentally measured ICF for the above situation is 1.10 (see Figure 14.10). The variations in the ICFs obtained by the different methods are attributable to the different assumptions they make with regard to the change in scatter caused by the presence of inhomogeneities. Figure 14.11 presents similar results (for the same experimental setup) for 10-MV X-rays. At 10 MV, the influence of scatter is less than that for ^{60}Co; therefore, the disagreement between different methods is reduced. Figures 14.10 and 14.11 do not cover regions beyond the lung-equivalent segment. Experimental results [29] show that, for points in a unit-density region behind a low-density region, the disagreements among the various methods are reduced.

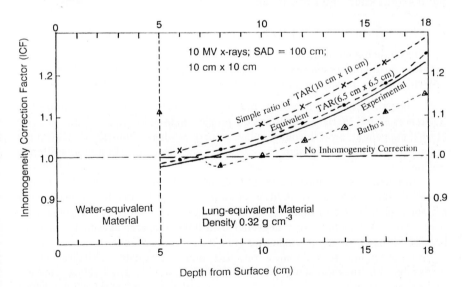

Fig. 14.11. The ICFs obtained by different methods (for the phantom at the top in Figure 14.10) at different depths in the lung for a 10-MV X-ray beam of 10 cm × 10 cm size at SAD 100 cm. (Experimental results are from Reference 28.)

We suggest that, before any of these methods are applied in practice, the suitability of the method be ascertained experimentally for scatter conditions with both large and small field sizes. An acceptable approach can be to consult the published values of experimentally measured correction factors for a variety of energies and phantom geometries [29–32].

14.4.11
Lung Density and Lateral Electronic Equilibrium

The above methods do not address in any explicit detail the secondary electron fluence. They endeavor mainly to correct the changes in photon fluence, assuming that charged-particle equilibrium is always present. The change in electron density at an interface can be expected to destroy charged particle equilibrium. Calculations that allow for secondary electron disequilibrium are more complex [33–36]. At high photon energies, secondary electron disequilibrium can occur inside low-density structures if the field sizes used are small. For a 15-MV photon beam of $5\,cm \times 5\,cm$ size, it has been observed [30, 33] that about a 15 to 20% reduction in dose can occur inside a medium of density $0.18\,g\,cm^{-3}$, because of the absence of lateral electronic equilibrium. At 15 MV, the secondary electron ranges are such that a thickness of nearly $3.0\,g\,cm^{-2}$ is needed all around a point to establish charged-particle equilibrium at that point. A square field of 5-cm sides in a medium of density $0.18\,g\,cm^{-3}$ provides for only $(5/2) \times 0.18\,g\,cm^{-2} = 0.45\,g\,cm^{-2}$ build-up thickness in the lateral directions from the central axis.

14.5
Bone Attenuation and Absorption

Bony regions in the body differ from soft-tissue regions in three respects:

(i)   They have higher mean densities, in the range of 1.1 to $1.5\,g\,cm^{-3}$
(ii) They have a higher effective atomic number than do soft tissue and water
(iii) The electron density for bone is less than that for soft tissue and water

To understand the problem of the presence of bone, the reader is advised to study References 37 and 38. Here, we discuss the problem in brief in two parts: first in terms of what happens at low (kilovoltage) photon energies where photoelectric absorption is important and then for high (megavoltage) energies where Compton scattering predominates.

The higher density of bone causes increased attenuation compared to water (or muscle) at all photon energies. In addition, at low kV, the higher effective atomic number of bone compared to soft tissue contributes to increased photoelectric absorption in bone. Therefore, a higher dose is delivered to the bone compared to water (or muscle), because the μ_{en}/ρ values are higher for bone than for water. Table 14.3 compares the μ_{en}/ρ for water, muscle, and bone at various photon beam qualities. The last column in the table gives the ratio of μ_{en}/ρ for bone to that for muscle. These ratios at low energies indicate that the total amount of energy absorbed per unit mass of bone (which governs the absorbed dose to bone) can be up to 4.5 times more, depending on the energy. The expected change in the depth dose profile of a 4-mm Cu HVT X-ray beam

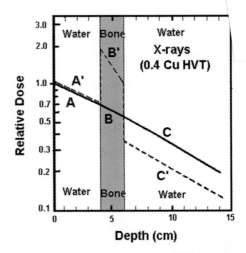

Fig. 14.12. A, B, and C are the depth-dose profile of a cobalt-60 beam in a homogeneous water-equivalent medium. A', B', C' is the profile when a 2 cm thick bone is introduced

in the presence of bone is shown in Figure 14.12. The continuous curve with sections A, B, and C is the pattern observed in the absence of bone. The dashed curve with sections A', B', and C' illustrates the expected change when a 2 cm thick bone is introduced. Parts A and A' are nearly identical. Inside the bone, curve B' is at a higher dose level, with nearly twice the dose of B, due to the increased photoelectric absorption in bone. (See also Example 11.3.) The fall-off of B' is steeper than that of B, because of the higher linear attenuation coefficient of bone. Sections C and C' are nearly parallel to each other, with a separation that is related to the excess attenuation which the beam suffered when it passed through the bony region.

At MeV photon energies, the situation is different than at keV X-ray energies. At such high energies, the photoelectric effect can be disregarded and the Z_{eff} of bone becomes unimportant. Compton scattering, which depends on the electron density of the absorbing material, predominates. In Figure 14.13, two depth-dose profiles are

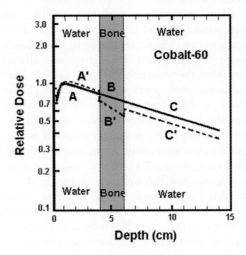

Fig. 14.13. A, B, and C are the depth-dose profile of a cobalt-60 beam in a homogeneous water-equivalent medium. A', B', C' is the profile when a 2 cm thick bone is introduced

Table 14.3. Mass-Energy Absorption Coefficients for Water, Soft Tissue, and Bone at Different Photon Energies*

Photon Energy E_v (MeV)	μ_{en}/ρ (cm^2 g^{-1})			$[\mu_{en}/\rho]^{Bone}_{Muscle}$
	Water	Muscle (*striated*)	Bone	
0.01	4.79	4.87	19.2	3.94
0.015	1.28	1.32	5.84	4.42
0.02	0.512	0.533	2.46	4.62
0.03	0.149	0.154	0.720	4.68
0.04	0.0677	0.0701	0.304	4.34
0.05	0.0418	0.0431	0.161	3.74
0.06	0.0320	0.0328	0.0998	3.04
0.08	0.0262	0.0264	0.0537	2.03
0.10	0.0256	0.0256	0.0387	1.51
0.15	0.0277	0.0275	0.0305	1.11
0.2	0.0297	0.0294	0.0301	1.02
0.3	0.0319	0.0317	0.0310	0.98
0.4	0.0328	0.0325	0.0315	0.97
0.5	0.0330	0.0328	0.0317	0.97
0.6	0.0329	0.0325	0.0314	0.97
0.8	0.0321	0.0318	0.0306	0.96
1.0	0.0309	0.0306	0.0295	0.96
1.5	0.0282	0.0280	0.0270	0.96
2.0	0.0260	0.0257	0.0249	0.97
3.0	0.0227	0.0225	0.0219	0.97
4.0	0.0206	0.0204	0.0200	0.98
5.0	0.0191	0.0189	0.0187	0.99
6.0	0.0180	0.0178	0.0178	1.00
8.0	0.0166	0.0164	0.0167	1.02
10.0	0.0157	0.0155	0.0159	1.03

* From Evans. R.D., X-ray and γ-ray interactions, Chapter 3, Table XXII, in Radiation Dosimetry, Vol. 1, Fundamentals, Attix, F.H., and Roesch, W.C. (Eds), Academic Press, New York, 1968.

shown for cobalt-60 gamma rays. The profile with sections **A**, **B**, and **C** applies to a uniform water-equivalent medium. The profile **A′**, **B′**, **C′** is obtained when bone is included. Parts **A** and **A′** are identical. Section **B′** in bone has a marginally (about 4%) lower dose than does **B**. (In Table 14.3, it will be noticed that the ratio of μ_{en}/ρ of bone to water is 0.96.) This is because the slightly lower electron density of bone reduces the mass absorption in bone, resulting in a lower dose to the bone. The increased slope of **B′** compared to **B** is due to the higher linear attenuation in bone caused by its higher density. After the beam exits through the bone, curves **C** and **C′** run a parallel course. The separation between them is due to the higher attenuation in bone.

The sharp discontinuities shown in the profiles **A′**, **B′**, **C′** of Figures 14.12 and 14.13 at the water-bone interfaces do not occur in reality. Because of the unavoidable cross-over and sharing of the secondary electrons between the two media, the dose profile will have a continuity at any boundary. Furthermore, any tissue surrounded by bone (such as the bone marrow), and subjected to the secondary-electron shower from the bone, will receive a dose similar to that for bone.

In Table 14.3, the ratio of μ_{en}/ρ of bone to water exceeds 1.0 by 2% and 3% at 8 and 10 MeV, respectively. This indicates a marginally higher energy absorption in bone compared to muscle. This is because at such high energies the role played by pair production is not to be ignored and pair production increases with Z.

14.6
Beams of Non-Uniform Intensity

We already discussed (in Section 14.2) beams with blocked regions. For scatter evaluation, it was assumed that the blocked regions received zero or negligible intensity, and
the unblocked regions received a maximum possible uniform intensity. We will now
address a more complex situation of a beam with a varying intensity, as can happen
when a wedge or compensating filter is interposed in the beam.

It is easy to discern that the contribution to SAR from the annular region between
circles of radii r and $(r + \Delta r)$ as shown in Fig. 14.14 (a) is $[SAR(d, r + \Delta r) - SAR(r)]$.
Dividing this by the area of the annulus $(2\pi r \Delta r)$ gives the differential scatter air ratio
(DSAR) given by,

$$DSAR(d, r) = [SAR(d, r + \Delta r) - SAR(r)]/(2\pi r \Delta r)$$

DSAR is actually the incremental contribution to SAR from a narrow pencil beam
of unit area located at a distance r away from a point of calculation at depth d for a
normal beam of uniform intensity incident on a water equivalent medium. In general,
any beam can be conceived as composed of N adjacent pencil beams. The point of
calculation, P, itself may fall within a pencil beam, k. A particular pencil beam, m, may
be at a distance r_m, and have a cross section of ΔA_m (Fig. 14.14 (b)). If a wedge filter
is interposed (Fig. 14.14 (c)) and it changes the intensity of the pencil beam m by an
attenuation factor w_m, the incremental scatter air ratio, $(\Delta SAR)_m$, contributed by the
pencil beam will be

$$(\Delta SAR)_m = DSAR(d, r_m) \Delta A_m w_m \qquad (14\text{-}17)$$

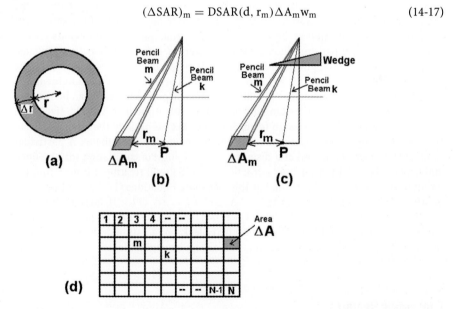

Fig. 14.14. (a) Shows the annular region between two circular fields of radii r and $(r + \Delta r)$, (b) shows a
pencil beam of area ΔA_m at distance r_m from pencil beam k which contains the calculatioin point P,
(c) shows a wedge inserted in the beam to modify the beam, (d) A beam is viewed as divided into N
modules! of area ΔA

We should address pencil beam k separately, as it will also contribute primary radiation. The total SAR due to all pencil beams, other than beam k, is obtained as the sum

$$SAR = \sum_{m=1, m\neq k}^{N} (\Delta SAR)_m \qquad (14.18a)$$

To this we will add the contribution to SAR by pencil beam k, which is

$$SAR(d, \Delta A_k)w_k \qquad (14.18b)$$

The factor w_k will also affect the zero-field TAR and, hence, the primary dose. The zero-field TAR changes to

$$TAR(d, 0)w_k \qquad (14.18c)$$

The sum of (14.18a) and (14.18b) gives the TAR for pencil beam k. Hence the total effective TAR for the point of calculation for the beam is

$$TAR(d, \text{non-uniform field}) = TAR(d, \Delta A_k)w_k + \sum_{m=1, \ m\neq k}^{N} (\Delta SAR)_m \qquad (14\text{-}19)$$

The values $w_1, w_2, \ldots, w_N$, act as weights for the different pencil beams. This approach of dividing a beam into weighted pencil beams can find many applications. Many computerized treatment-planning systems are known to use this approach.

In recent times, use of beams with a computer-optimized modular intensity pattern is being investigated. The method relies on superposing several sub-beams within the same directed beam. Each sub-beam may be planned to have its own (MLC produced) cross-section and duration of irradiation. The combination of all sub-beams creates a modular intensity pattern. Such a beam is referred to as an intensity-modulated radiation therapy (IMRT) beam. Although the irradiation times are provided by the computer algorithms used, it is advisable to verify its accuracy by a measurement and an independent hand calculation [39, 40]. For this purpose, the beam can be thought of as made up of an array of rectangular modules of identical area ΔA. The size of the module is governed by the design features of the MLC, especially the leaf width, and the size of the pencil beams assumed for the mathematical optimizing. A particular module at a position, m, and at a distance r_m from point of calculation may be open and deliver the radiation for only a fraction f_m of the total treatment time T min (or monitor units M Mu) of the beam. For this situation, Equations (14-17) to (14-19) can be used by assuming $\Delta A_m = \Delta A_k = \Delta A$, and $w_m = [f_m T]$ (or $[f_m M]$). It should be noted that for a time $\{(1 - f_k)T\}$ (or $\{(1 - f_k)M\}$) the beam is on, but the pencil beam k is blocked. Hence it will receive an amount of leakage radiation dose as transmitted through the leaves of the MLC. This may not always be negligible.

14.7
Concluding Remarks

We outlined in this chapter only the simple approaches for carrying out inhomogeneity corrections. There are more advanced theoretical models, which include Monte Carlo techniques [36, 41–44], volume integration, and convolution approaches [45–52]. Another advance has been the advent of CT scanners and the possibility of transferring CT data to treatment-planning computers. This has offered a great potential to incorporate inhomogeneity corrections in an accurate manner on a routine basis [53–55]. CT scans give the electron densities of various volume elements and their geometric location in the body through what are called CT numbers. It is not within the scope of this book to discuss these sophisticated approaches. They hold great promise for the future, but have not become routine in clinical practice not only for reasons of complexity, but also due to the clinical reasons already explained in Section 14.4.2.

Glossary of Acronyms

PAR   Primary air ratio
SAR   Scatter air ratio
OCR_{air} Off-center ratio in air
ICF   Inhomogeneity correction factor
MLC   Multi-leaf collimators
DSAR   Differential Scatter air ratio
IMRT   Intensity-modulated radiation therapy
See also the list at the end of Chapter 13.

References

1. Zhu, Y., Boyer, A.L., and Desobry, G.E., Dose distributions of x-ray fields as shaped with multi-leaf collimators, Phys. Med. Biol., Vol. 37, pp163–174, 1992.
2. Jordan, T., and Williams, P.C., The design and performance characteristics of a multileaf collimator, Phys. Med. Biol., Vol. 39, p231–251, 1994.
3. Klein EE, Tepper J, Sontag M, Franklin M, Ling C, and Kubo D, Technology assessment of multileaf collimation: a North American users survey, Int. J. Radiat. Oncol. Biol. Phys., Vol. 44, pp705–710, 1999.
4. AAPM Report No. 72, Basic applications of multileaf collimators, Report of Task Group 50, Radiation Therapy Commmittee, for American Association of Physicists in Medicine, College Park, MD, USA by Medical Physics Publishing, Madison, Wisconsin, USA, 2001.
5. Chaney, E.L., Cullip, T.J., and Gabriel, T.A., A Monte Carlo study of accelerator head scatter, Med. Phys., Vol 21, p1383–1390, 1994.
6. Kase, K.R., and Svenson, G.K., Head scatter data for several linear accelerators (4–18 MV), Med. Phys., Vol 13, p530–532, 1986.
7. Dunscombe, P.B., and Nieminen, J.M., On the field-size dependence of relative output from a linear accelerator, Med. Phys., Vol 19, p1441–1444, 1992.
8. Cunningham, J.R., Scatter-air ratios, Phys. Med. Biol., Vol 17, p42–51, 1972.
9. Nizin, P. S., and Kase, K.R., Determination of primary dose in ^{60}Co beam using a small attenuator, Med. Phys., Vol 17, p92–94, 1985.
10. Kijewski, P.K., Bjarngard, B.E., and Petti, P.L., Monte Carlo calculations of scatter dose for small field sizes in a ^{60}Co beam, Med. Phys., Vol 13, p74–77, 1986.
11. Bjarngard, B.E., and Petti, P.L., Description of the scatter component in photon beam data, Phys. Med. Biol., Vol 33, p21–32, 1988.
12. Nizin, P.S., Geometrical aspects of scatter-to-primary ratio and primary dose, Med. Phys., Vol 18, p153–160, 1991.
13. Nizin, P., Qian, G.-X., and Rashid, H., "Zero field" dose data for ^{60}Co and other high-energy photon beams in water, Med. Phys., Vol 20, p1353–1360, 1993.
14. Clarkson, J.R., A note on depth-doses in fields of irregular shape, Br. J. Radiol., Vol 14, p265–268, 1941.
15. Day., M.J., A note on the calculation of dose in X-ray fields, Br. J. Radiol., Vol 23, p368–369, 1950.
16. Cundiff, J.H. et al., A method for the calculation of dose in the radiation treatment of Hodgkin's disease, Am. J. Roentgenol., Vol 117, p30–44, 1973.

17. Hanson, W.F., and Berkley, L.W., Off-axis beam quality change in linear accelerator X-ray beams, Med. Phys., Vol 7, p145–146, 1980.
18. Horton, J.L., Dosimetry of Siemens Mevatron 67 linear accelerator, Int. J. Radiat. Oncol. Biol. Phys., Vol 9, p1217–1223, 1983.
19. Yu, M.K., Sloboda, R.S., and Murray, B., Linear accelerator photon quality at off-axis points, Med. Phys., Vol. 24, pp233–239, 1997.
20. Marinello, G., Dutreix, A., A general method to perform dose calculations along the axis of asymmetrical photon beams, Med. Phys., Vol. 19, pp275–281, 1992.
21. Gibbons, J.P., and Khan, F. M., Calculation of dose in asymmetric photon fields, Med. Phys., Vol.22, pp1451–1457, 1995.
22. Loshek, D.D., and Keller, K.A., Beam profile generator for asymmetric fields, Med. Phys., Vol. 15, pp604–610, 1988.
23. Palta, J.R., Ayyangar, K.M., and Suntharalingam, N., Dosimetric characteristics of a 6 MV photon beam from a linear accelerator with asymmetric collimator jaws, Int. J. Radiat. Oncol. Biol. Phys., Vol 14, pp383–387, 1988.
24. Cunningham, J.R., Tissue heterogeneity corrections in photon beam treatment planning, In Progress in Medical Physics, Vol 1, C.G. Orton (Ed.), Plenum Press, New York, 1982.
25. Batho, H.F., Lung corrections in ^{60}Co beam therapy, J. Can. Assoc. Radiol., Vol 15, p79–83, 1964.
26. Sontag, M.R., and Cunningham, J.R., Corrections to absorbed dose calculations for tissue inhomogeneities, Med. Phys., Vol 4, p431–436, 1977.
27. Thomas, S.J., A modified power law formula for inhomogeneity corrections in beams of high energy X-rays, Med. Phys., Vol 18, p719–723, 1991.
28. Mauceri, T., and Kase, K., Effects of ionization chamber construction on dose measurements in a heterogeneity, Med. Phys., Vol 14, p653–656, 1987.
29. Wingate, C.L., Gross, W., and Failla, G., Experimental determination of absorbed dose from X-rays near the interface of soft tissue and other materials, Radiology, Vol 79, p984–1000, 1962.
30. Rice, R.K., Mijnheer, B.J., and Chin, L.M., Benchmark measurements for lung dose corrections for X-ray beams, Int. J. Radiat. Oncol. Biol. Phys., Vol 15, p399–409, 1988.
31. Farahani, M., Eichmiller, F.C., and McLaughlin, W.C., Measurement of absorbed doses near metal and dental material interfaces irradiated by x- and gamma-ray therapy beams, Phys. Med. Biol., Vol 35, p369–385, 1990.
32. Klein, E.E., Chin, L.M., Rice, R.K., and Mijnheer, B.J., The influence of air-cavities on interface doses for photon beams, Int. J. Radiat. Oncol. Biol. Phys., Vol 27, p419–427, 1993.
33. Mackie, T.R., El Khatib, E., Battista, J.J., and Scrimger, J., Lung dose corrections for 6 and 15 MV X-rays, Med. Phys., Vol 12, p327–332, 1985.
34. van de Geijn, J., The extended net fractional depth-dose: Correction for inhomogeneities, including effects of electron transport in photon beam dose calculations, Med. Phys., Vol 14, p84–92, 1987.
35. Werner, B.L., Das, I.J., Khan, F.M., and Meigoni, A.S., Dose perturbation at interfaces in photon beams, Med. Phys., Vol 14, p585–595, 1987.
36. Petti, P.L., Rice, K.P., Mijnheer, B.J., Chin, L.M., and Bjarngard, B.E., A heterogeneity model for photon beams incorporating electron transport, Med. Phys., Vol 19, p349–354, 1987.
37. Spiers, F.W., Transition zone dosimetry, in Radiation Dosimetry, Vol III, Sources, Fields, Measurements, and Applications, Attix, F.H., and Tocilin, E. (Eds.), Academic Press, New York, 1969.
38. Dutreix, J., and Bernard, M., Dosimetry at interfaces for high energy x and gamma rays, Br. J. Radiol., Vol 39, p205–210, 1966.
39. Kung, J.H., Chen, G.T.Y., and Kuchnir, F.K., A monitor unit verification calculation in intensity modulated radiotherapy as a dosimetry quality assurance, Med. Phys., Vol. 27, pp2226–2230, 2000.
40. Xing, L., Chen, Y., Luxton, G., Li, J.G., and Boyer, A.R., Monitor unit calculation for an intensity modulated photon field by a simple scatter-summation algorithm, Phys. Med. Biol., Vol. 45, pp N1–N7, 2000.
41. Webb, S., and Fox, R.A., Verification of Monte Carlo methods of a power law of tissue-air ratio algorithm for inhomogeneity corrections in photon beam dose calculation, Phys. Med. Biol., Vol 25, p225–240, 1980.
42. Webb, S., and Parker, R.P., A Monte Carlo study of the interaction of external beam x-radiation with inhomogeneous media, Phys. Med. Biol., Vol 23, p1043–1059, 1978.
43. Morin, R.L., Monte Carlo Simulation in Radiological Sciences, CRC Press, Boca Raton, Florida, 1988.
44. Mackie, T.R., Bilelajew, A.F., Rogers, D.W.O., and Battista, J.J., Generation of photon energy deposition kernels using EGS Monte Carlo code, Phys. Med. Biol., Vol. 33, p1–20, 1988.
45. Zhu, Y., and Boyer, A.L., X-ray dose computations in heterogeneous medium using 3-dimensional FFT convolution, Phys. Med. Biol., Vol 35, p351–368, 1990.

46. Ahenesjo, A., Collapsed cone convolution of radiant energy for photon dose calculation in heterogeneous media, Med. Phys., Vol 16, p577–591, 1989.

47. Boyer, A.L., and Mok, E.C., Calculation of photon dose distributions in an inhomogeneous medium using convolutions, Med. Phys., Vol 13, p503–509, 1986.

48. Mackie, T.R., Scrimger, J.W., and Battista, J.J., A convolution method for calculating dose for 15 MV X-rays, Med. Phys., Vol 12, p188–196, 1985.

49. Bourland, J.D., and Chaney, E.L., A finite size pencil beam model for photon dose calculations in three dimensions, Med. Phys., Vol 19, p1401–1412, 1992.

50. Ahnesjo, A., Saxner, M., and Trepp, A., A pencil beam model for photon dose calculation, Med. Phys., Vol 19, p263–273, 1992.

51. Mohan, R., Chui, C.S., and Lidowski, L., Differential pencil beam dose computation models for photons, Med. Phys., Vol 13, p64–73, 1986.

52. O'Conner, J.E., and Malone, D.E., An equivalent shape approximation for photon doses in lung, Phys. Med. Biol., Vol 35, p223–234, 1990.

53. Wong, J.W., and Henkelman, R.M., A new approach to CT pixel-based photon dose calculation in heterogeneous media, Med. Phys., Vol 10, p199–208, 1983.

54. Siddon, R.L., Fast calculation of the exact radiological path for a three dimensional CT array, Med. Phys., Vol 12, p252–255, 1985.

55. Cassell, K.J., Hobday, P.A., and Parker, R.P., The implementation of a generalized Batho inhomogeneity correction for radiotherapy planning with direct use of CT numbers, Phys. Med. Biol., Vol 26, p825–833, 1981.

Radiation Treatment Planning

PART VI

Radiation Treatment Planning

Treatment Dose Distribution Planning: Photon Beams

15.1
Introduction

Before a patient is treated with radiation, the target volume for delivery of the radiation dose is delineated by the physician, who takes into account the stage and extent of the tumor and the clinical objective of palliation or cure. The methods and processes available for delivery of radiation, as well as the mechanisms of radiation interaction, are such that we cannot restrict the dose delivery strictly to the target volume alone, with no incidental irradiation elsewhere.

After a target volume is decided upon and designated to receive a prescribed dose, an acceptable or optimum treatment strategy needs to be worked out. The treatment should be planned in such a way that (i) the designated target volume, which includes the tumor, is given a uniform dose; (ii) incidental irradiation of the surrounding normal structures is minimal; and (iii) the dose to any vital body organ does not exceed its tolerance level. The entire dose distribution pattern made possible by a particular treatment plan should be evaluated carefully before the plan is accepted for implementation on a patient. Several different treatment strategies can be compared and the optimum one selected.

In this chapter, we restrict the subject of dose distribution planning to the use of photon beams. Planning for the use of electron beams and discrete sealed radioactive sources in the brachytherapy mode will be covered in the two chapters that follow.

15.2
Isodose Surfaces and Curves

When a beam passes through a patient, different points within the patient will receive different doses; that is, there will be a spatial dose distribution. Because it is convenient to think in terms of relative rather than absolute doses, it is usual to select a particular point in the irradiated field as a reference point and to designate the dose it receives as 100%. Let us say that a particular point in the field receives a dose of p% (relative to 100%). Then there may be several other points in the field that receive a dose of p%. The surface formed when all of these points are connected is referred to as an isodose surface for p%. Isodose surfaces are three-dimensional (3D) constant-value surfaces, just like isotherms and isobars in weather maps. The line or curve obtained at the intersection of a plane with an isodose surface is an isodose curve. Isodose curves are two-dimensional (2D) entities because they lie in a plane intersecting the 3D dose distribution. Because of the fact that the isodose surfaces or curves represent a specific dose value, the isodose surfaces or curves for two different dose levels cannot cross one another. Isodose curves have been used more commonly than isodose surfaces for analysis of dose distributions, because the fact that they are 2D allows them to be displayed on paper. Three-dimensional displays and surface representations are becoming feasible with the use of computed tomography (CT) and graphic work stations [1–9].

15.3
Single-Beam Isodose Curves

15.3.1
General Features

In Chapters 13 and 14, we discussed the dose calculation at points on and away from the central axis. Calculation of the dose received at many points in the beam can reveal the geometric dose distribution pattern for any radiotherapy beam. The dose distribution obtained for any beam will depend on its geometric divergence, energy and depth-dose characteristics, off-central-axis fall-off of intensity and penumbra, and the influence of any beam-modifying filters such as wedge filters or beam-flattening filters inserted in the beam.

Figure 15.1a is a 3D view of a radiation beam of rectangular cross section. Figures 15.1b and c represent two mutually perpendicular planes through this beam – a plane perpendicular to the central axis of the beam, and the plane that contains the central axis and a major axis of the rectangular cross section, respectively. The

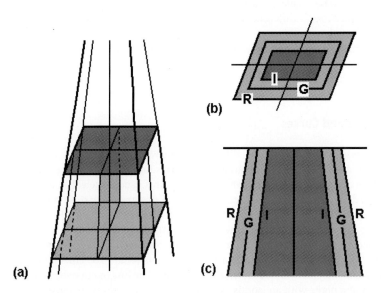

Fig. 15.1. (a) Three-dimensional view of a beam of rectangular cross section. (b) View of a plane perpendicular to the central axis of the beam. (c) View of a plane containing the central axis of the beam and a principal axis of the rectangle. G is the geometric edge. Lines I and R are drawn to define the inner region (within I) and the remote region (beyond R), respectively

lines marked G on both of these diagrams are the geometric edges of the beam (see Section 9.3.5).

For the purpose of understanding and analyzing the dose distribution, any single radiation beam can be visualized as consisting of three zones. These are (i) the useful inner region lying between lines I, covering up to 80 or 90% of the geometric width of the beam; (ii) a penumbra or fall-off region lying between lines I and R on either side of the geometric edge; and (iii) a distal or remote region that lies well beyond lines R, where most of the dose is contributed by radiation leaking through the diaphragms and by scattered radiation. The ideal would be to have a cross-beam radiation intensity profile that is highly uniform in the inner region, with a rapid and abrupt fall-off in the penumbra and a negligible magnitude in the remote regions. In practice, beams are not so perfect, as our further discussion will reveal. Single-beam isodose curves have been published in the form of atlases for academic study [10, 11].

15.3.2
Low-Energy Kilovoltage X-Ray Beam

Figure 15.2a is a schematic diagram of the source and diaphragm geometry for a low-energy X-ray beam. A small X-ray focal spot gives a near-point source of radiation emission. The beam size is limited by thin diaphragms made of lead, which need to be only a few millimeters thick because of the high efficiency of absorption in lead at low energies. Figure 15.2b presents the isodose curves for such a beam. The peak dose at the surface on the central axis has been designated as 100% for normalization.

The isodose curves are concave upward in the central region of the beam. This indicates a reduction in the dose from the central axis outward, because the amount of scattered radiation falls off from the central axis toward off-axis points. As we know, the scatter dose at any point depends on the location of the point in the irradiated

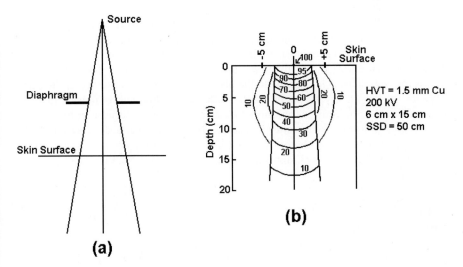

Fig. 15.2. (a) Schematic diagram of a low-energy X-ray beam emerging from a near-point source through a thin beam-limiting diaphragm. (b) Isodose curves for a 200-kV X-ray beam

field and on the geometry of the scattering volume. The central-axis point at a given depth receives more scatter than does an off-central-axis point. The scattered dose component for low-energy X-rays is considerably greater than that at megavoltage energies.

Looking at the penumbral region in Figure 15.2b, we notice that the isodose curves have a sharp cut-off at the geometric edge of the beam. In low-energy X-ray beams, the combination of a near-point source and thin collimating diaphragms produces such sharp beam edges, with almost no penumbra.

At low energies, outside the geometric beam edge, the primary radiation levels are reduced to negligible amounts by the beam-limiting diaphragms. However, in Figure 15.2b we observe 20% and 10% isodose curves in the regions outside the edges. This dose comes from the photons scattered sideways from the beam. At such low energies, Compton-scattered photons spread over a wide angle and make the lateral scatter prominent. These isodose curves are concave toward the central axis, giving an appearance of a beam that is being propagated laterally outward from the central axis and perpendicular to it.

15.3.3
^{60}Co Beam

Figure 15.3a is a schematic diagram of a beam produced by a ^{60}Co teletherapy machine. The source has a finite size, often in the range of 1.0 to 2.0 cm in diameter. Collimating a beam of high-energy photons (1.17 MeV and 1.33 MeV) requires thick diaphragms made of several centimeters of a heavy metal such as lead, tungsten, or uranium. The overall geometry is such that (i) a geometric penumbra is caused by the finite size of the source, and (ii) the partial transmission of some oblique rays from the source through the corners of the diaphragms adds a transmission penumbra (see also Section 9.3.6).

Figure 15.3b presents a typical isodose pattern for a ^{60}Co beam. The isodose curves are normalized to 100% at the peak dose on the central axis. In the inner regions, the curves are flat and perpendicular to the central axis. Near the beam edge, the curves are parallel to the edge and go all the way up to the surface. The dose fall-off is gradual across the edge. This is in contrast to the discontinuity that we observed at the beam edge for the low-energy X-rays in Figure 15.2b. The isodose curves outside the field edges are not as prominent as are those for low-energy X-rays because, at this energy, there is no significant lateral scatter. Outside the beam edges, some dose is contributed by direct transmission of photons through the collimator diaphragms. Such leakage through the collimator diaphragms usually amounts to about 0.5 to 3% of the peak dose on the central axis.

15.3.4
Megavoltage X-Rays

In Sections 6.3 and 10.3.5, we discussed the fact that the high-energy X-ray emission has a forward peak and that the X-ray intensity needs to be flattened by an interposed beam-flattening filter. Figure 15.4a is a schematic diagram of the geometric features of

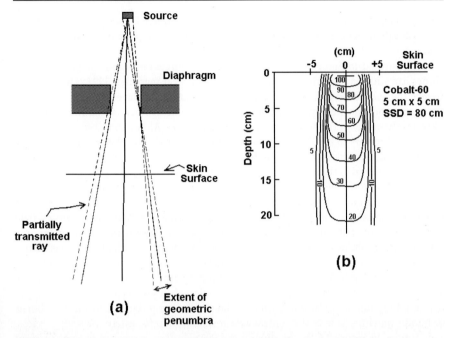

Fig. 15.3. (a) Schematic diagram of a cobalt-60 beam emerging from a source of finite size through a thick beam-limiting diaphragm. The geometric penumbra and a partially transmitted ray are shown on the right and left edges of the beam, respectively. (b) Isodose curves for a cobalt-60 beam

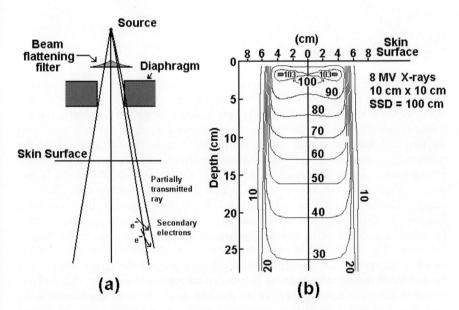

Fig. 15.4. (a) Schematic diagram of a megavoltage X-ray beam showing the source of emission, the beam flattening filter, the thick beam-limiting diagram, a partially transmitted ray through the diaphragm, and secondary electron spill over the beam edge. (b) Isodose curves for an 8-MV X-ray beam

gavoltage photon beam. The isodose curves for an 8-MV X-ray beam are shown
Figure 15.4b. The 100% dose has been taken to be the peak dose on the central
axis.

As illustrated in Figure 15.4a, the focal spots (sources) in megavoltage X-ray machines are smaller than the size of the sources in ^{60}Co machines [12]. This helps to
reduce the geometric penumbra. However, the diaphragms have to be thick, as with
^{60}Co, and hence, a transmission penumbra cannot be avoided. In addition, at high
energies the range of the secondary electrons increases. Although the secondary electrons travel mostly in the forward direction, they can spill over the geometric edge of
the beam and blur the edge. Most high-energy beams have less penumbra than does a
^{60}Co beam, but exceptions cannot be ruled out.

In the design of the beam-flattening filter, the presence of scatter fluence in an
irradiated medium is also taken into account. The flattening filter is usually optimized
to give a flatness of $\pm 3\%$ in the inner region covering about 80% of the geometric field
width at a depth of about 10 cm in water. This depth is chosen with the understanding
that the target volume is usually located at about that depth in patients. Because scatter
accumulates with depth, its contribution to the total dose is low at the surface and
increases with depth. The scatter aids in beam flattening because it tends to disperse
the fluence. A beam-flattening filter that is designed to give beam flatness at 10 cm
depth, taking into account the scatter at that depth, can produce a beam with horns
or humps on either side of the central axis at shallow depths, where the scatter is less.
This is why, in Figure 15.4b, the dips in the 90% isodose curve and the hot spots of
103% near the surface occur. The humps may be particularly prominent in beams of
large width.

15.4
Concept of Combining Beams

The tolerance of sensitive tissues through which a beam may pass from its entrance
to its exit in the patient can limit the total tumor dose that can be delivered by that
beam. When a beam is directed to irradiate a tumor located in the depth, the entrance region (just beyond the build-up) will receive a much higher dose than does
the tumor. A beam in transit will give a higher dose on the entrance side of the
target volume than on its exit side. (Some exceptions occur in rare contexts when
photon beams of very high energies, 40 MV and above, are used.) Often, the higher
dose received by the subcutaneous tissues near the entrance surface limits the total
tumor dose that can be delivered by a single beam. By using more than one beam
focused and directed toward the tumor, one can distribute the doses along multiple entrance and exit paths around the target volume and concentrate the dose at
the tumor. The positions and paths of the beams can be planned so as not to exceed the tolerance dose of normal tissues that lie around the target volume and
are irradiated incidentally. Multiple beams can be combined with the added objective of molding the dose distribution to conform to the shape of the volume to be
treated and to make the dose uniform within the target volume. The aim should
be to create an optimum or at least an acceptable dose distribution in the patient.

15.5
Derivation of Dose Distribution

15.5.1
General Approach

Single-beam isodose curves are the basis for inferring the dose distribution for a combination of beams. In the early days of the practice of external-beam therapy, physicists added the dose distributions of single beams manually to obtain the composite dose distribution for multiple-beam arrangements. In the modern practice of radiation oncology, dose distribution calculations and plotting of isodose curves are done by computerized treatment-planning systems, and the arduous and time-consuming manual calculations have mostly been dispensed with. Although computers speed up the process, manual methods form the basis of computer calculations. Hence, we cover these methods here next.

The dose distribution in a patient is a 3D entity. 3D dose calculations and 3D display of dose distributions are rather voluminous and complex. In many situations, for practical purposes, a simpler dose distribution plotted in a 2D mid-transverse section of the patient provides useful insight for dose distribution planning. Figure 15.5a shows a transverse contour of a patient. A total of M beams, $1, 2, 3, \ldots, M$, are set up to converge at a point T inside the patient. Let us assume that all are beams of rectangular cross section. It is common to refer to the field dimension in the direction of the long axis of the patient as "field length" and to that in the transverse plane of the contour as "field width." To find the dose distribution, we set up a rectangular grid of points $P_1, P_2, P_3, \ldots$ to cover the region of interest (Figure 15.5a). Our approach is to determine the doses received at the individual grid points for each individual beam and to add them to obtain the total dose for the beam combination. From knowing the doses at the grid points, it should be possible to designate a particular dose level as 100% and to plot the isodose curves for the combination of beams. Usually, the 100% level is selected to be the dose at the center of the target volume to be treated. Many times it may be the dose at point T, where the beam axes converge.

The field widths, $W_1, W_2, \ldots, W_M$, of the individual beams are generally planned to cover the width of the target volume as seen from the direction of the beam. After other aspects of the plan (the beam angles, widths, treatment times, etc.) have been accepted in a review of the 2D plan, the field lengths (which may have the same value, L, for all beams) can be selected to cover the length of the target volume. It is worth reiterating that the dose distribution in this central 2D transverse plane need not necessarily represent the dose distribution obtainable in other transverse sections along the length of the patient. However, this information, when used with caution, has proved to be useful in the practice of radiotherapy.

15.5.2
Dose at P_I for Fixed-SSD Technique

For the fixed source-to-skin distance (SSD) technique, we set up all of the beams to have a constant, preselected SSD. The set of isodose curves appropriate for the chosen SSD for a field width W_1 and length L is placed on the patient contour to provide the

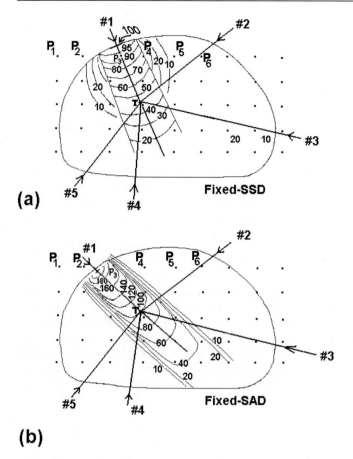

Fig. 15.5. A patient's transverse contour with the grid of points chosen for dose estimation and an isodose curve placed at the position of a beam. (a) Use of isodose charts with 100% at the peak dose, as applicable for a fixed-SSD-type setup. (b) Use of isodose charts that have 100% at the depth of the isocenter, as applicable to an isocentric setup

dose distribution from beam 1, as shown in Figure 15.5a. The percentage (depth) dose $PDD_{i,1}$ as shown by the isodose curve at point P_i is read with the 100% being the peak dose. If the treatment duration for beam 1 is such that the 100% dose (also called the 'given dose') is G_1, then the dose $D_{i,1}$ at P_i due to beam 1 is given by

$$D_{i,1} = PDD_{i,1}\frac{G_1}{100}$$

The procedure can be carried out first for beam 1 for all grid points and then for all M beams. The total dose D_i at point P_i is given by the sum

$$D_i = \sum_{j=1}^{j=M} PDD_{i,j} \cdot \frac{G_j}{100}$$

15.5.3
Dose at P_i for Isocentric Technique

For treatment with a machine that is capable of isocentric rotation, the central point T can be chosen to be at the isocenter for all of the M beams. During treatment, the patient needs to be positioned only once for the first beam to have T at the isocenter. Subsequently, a mere rotation of the gantry of the machine can give the other beam locations without any need for moving the patient. (This is not possible for the fixed-SSD technique, which requires a movement of the patient for each individual beam so that the chosen SSD is obtained.)

To infer the dose distribution for isocentric situations, we need to use special isodose curves that are normalized to have the 100% dose level at the depth of the isocenter (Figure 15.5b). This means that, for a given field width, we will need many different isodose patterns with 100% chosen to be at various depths of normalization. In theory, all depths of normalization are possible. Although this implies that innumerable isodose charts covering every possible depth of normalization should be available, this is not so in practice. Fortunately, percent depth doses read from isodose charts normalized at a particular depth are not too sensitive to the depth of the normalization (i. e., the position of the surface). This is because the different points in the beam remain at the identical distances from the source, irrespective of the depth of normalization. The isodose curves merely reflect the differences in dose caused by attenuation and scatter. Hence, it is possible to do the treatment planning with a limited number of isodose charts for a few discrete depths of normalization without losing much accuracy. The percent (depth) dose at point Pi can be read to be $PDD_{i,1}$ for beam 1. The absolute value of the 100% dose is a function of the time of irradiation with beam 1. If the 100% dose (or given dose) for beam 1 is G_1, the dose $D_{i,1}$ at point p_1 from beam 1 is

$$D_{i,1} = G_1 \cdot (PDD_{i,1}/100)$$

G_1 is given by the product of the dose to tissue in air, $(D_{air})_1$, and the tissue-air ratio TAR_1 for beam 1. Thus,

$$D_{i,1} = (D_{air})_1 \cdot TAR_1 \cdot (PDD_{i,1}/100)$$

The evaluation can be carried out first for beam 1 for all of the grid points and then for the rest of the M beams. The total dose D_i at point p_i then is given by the sum

$$D_i = \sum_{j=1}^{j=M} (D_{air})_j \cdot TAR_j \cdot (PDD_{i,j}/100)$$

The values of G_j for the different beams can be optimally selected so that a good dose distribution results.

15.5.4
Correction for Contour Shape

The isodose charts that we used in the previous examples are for beams incident on a flat surface. In practice, the patient's contour may be curved, or the beam may be incident obliquely on the surface, as shown in Figure 15.6. The data read from the

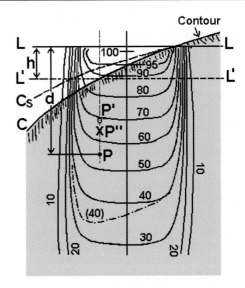

Fig. 15.6. A beam incident on a curved contour C. P is the point where the dose is estimated. Line L is at the level of the SSD. Line L′ is at the level of the surface point directly above P. The depth of P is d, and h is the thickness of the 'missing' tissue. C_s is the effective contour obtained by the 2/3 shift method. P′ and P″ are effective positions of point P in two different interpretations

standard isodose curves need to be modified for nonstandard situations. This is also referred to as the 'missing tissue' problem. A solution can be to flatten the surface by filling the 'missing tissue' with a tissue-equivalent material or bolus. However, this will have the negative effect of producing a build-up of secondary electrons on the patient's surface, and of enhancing the skin dose, with the resulting loss of skin sparing. Here we present different methods of correcting the standard isodose curves for incidence on a flat surface to allow for the presence of body curvature [13].

The diagram in Figure 15.6 shows a standard set of isodose curves positioned as if the body surface were flat and located at the level of line L. Let us say that we desire to know the percent depth dose (PDD) at point P, which is at depth d below line L. Line L′ is drawn through the actual point on the surface (on contour C) directly above P. The thickness of 'missing tissue' is h, and the actual depth of P is (d − h). (The 'missing tissue' problem discussed here is only a part of the overall problem of off-central-axis and inhomogeneity corrections discussed in Sections 14.3 and 14.4.)

Ratio-of-TAR Correction Method

If A_d is the field size at the level of point P in Figure 15.6, a correction factor CF for the value of PDD as read from the normal isodose chart can be worked out from the ratio of TARs as follows:

$$CF = \frac{\text{TAR for the effective depth (d − h)}}{\text{TAR for depth d implied in the isodose curve}}$$
$$= \frac{TAR(d - h, A_d)}{TAR(d, A_d)}$$

PDD actual = PDD read from isodose chart × CF

Isodose Shift and Effective SSD Correction Method

We could slide the isodose chart down so that its surface matches the line L′ and read a PDD value at P. Then the PDD value read will correspond to that for the point P′. Although this value is for the true depth $(d - h)$, the distance of the 100% reference value in the isodose curve has changed from $(SSD + d_m)$ to $(SSD + h + d_m)$. Because this change of distance is not really true for point P, we obtain the PDD at P by applying an inverse square distance correction to the PDD read at P′, as follows:

$$\frac{\text{PDD at P}}{\text{(Surface L′)}} = \frac{\text{PDD read at P′}}{\text{(Surface L)}} \times \left[\frac{(SSD + d_m)}{(SSD + h + d_m)}\right]^2$$

The above method, although it uses a different route, is the same in principle as the ratio-of-TAR method discussed previously.

Partial Isodose Shift Correction Method

In this method also, the isodose chart is shifted down, not through the entire distance h to the level of line L′, but through a fractional distance $k \times h$. Table 15.1 gives the values of k recommended for different energies in Report 24 of the International Commission on Radiation Units and Measurements (ICRU) [13]. These values of k are empirical and are designed to allow for the net effect of primary, scatter, and inverse-square fall-off, as observed in practical cases. For ^{60}Co, k can be taken as 2/3, and hence this method is also referred to as the '2/3 shift method.' A 2/3 shift will move point P to P′ in the dose distribution of Figure 15.6.

Table 15.1. Isodose Shift Factors, k, for Different Beam Qualities

X-Ray Quality	150 kV to 1 MV	1 MV to 5 MV	5 MV to 15 MV	15 MV to 30 MV	30 MV and Above
k	0.8	0.7	0.6	0.5	0.4

From ICRU-24 [13].

This method can be used easily for generating an entire isodose distribution for a change in contour shape. In Figure 15.6, the 40% isodose curve has been redrawn based on this method. The 2/3 shifts for the missing tissue result in an effective contour CS in Figure 15.6.

EXAMPLE 15.1

Derive the percent depth dose at point P in Figure 15.6 by the three methods of correction discussed above. The beam is from ^{60}Co. Point P is at 10 cm depth from line L, but is at an actual depth of 7 cm. The SSD = 90 cm and the field size is 9 cm × 9 cm at SSD.

Ratio of TAR:
In this example, $d = 10$ cm, the field size at depth d is $A_d = 10$ cm × 10 cm, $h = 3$ cm, and the beam is from ^{60}Co.

The PDD read from the isodose curves at P is 55%.

$$\text{TAR}(d, A_d) = \text{TAR}(d = 10\,\text{cm}, A_d = 10\,\text{cm} \times 10\,\text{cm}) = 0.718 \quad \text{(Table 13.2)}$$

$$\begin{aligned} \text{TAR}(d - h, A_d) &= \text{TAR}(d = 10 - 3\,\text{cm}, A_d = 10\,\text{cm} \times 10\,\text{cm}) \\ &= \text{TAR}(7, 10 \times 10) = 0.830 \quad \text{(Table 13.2)} \end{aligned}$$

$$\text{Correction factor, CF} = 0.830/0.718 = 1.156$$
$$\begin{aligned} \text{Corrected PDD} \quad &= \text{PDD read} \times \text{CF} \\ &= 55 \times 1.156 = 63.6\% \end{aligned}$$

Isodose Shift and Effective SSD:
After the isodose chart is shifted down by h = 3 cm, the position of P will move up to P′.

$$\text{PDD read at P}' = 68\%$$
$$\text{SSD} = 90\,\text{cm}, \ \text{SSD} + d_m = 90 + 0.5 = 90.5\,\text{cm}$$
$$\text{SSD} + d_m + h = 90 + 0.5 + 3.0 = 93.5\,\text{cm}$$
$$[(\text{SSD} + d_m)/(\text{SSD} + d_m + h)]^2 = [90.5/93.5]^2 = 0.937$$
$$\text{PDD actual} = \text{PDD read} \times 0.937 = 68.0 \times 0.937 = 63.7\%$$

Partial (2/3) Shift Method:
For h = 3 cm, 2/3 of h is 2 cm. The isodose chart shifted by 2 cm places the point P at P′ (Figure 15.6). A vertical interpolation between the 60 and 70% isodose curves gives a PDD at point P′ of 64%. In this example, the three methods give nearly the same result.

15.5.5
Influence of Obliquity on Dose Build-Up

The corrections for contour shape and obliquity of the surface that we discussed above are applicable at points that lie beyond the depth of the peak dose. At depths closer to the surface, where full secondary electron build-up has not been attained, the dose estimation becomes more complex. The secondary-electron build-up and the depth at which the peak dose occurs are influenced by the obliquity of the surface with respect to the direction of incidence of the beam [14–18]. In Figure 15.7, a beam is incident on an oblique surface S. The dashed line S′ indicates a flat surface perpendicular to the direction of the beam. We know from Chapter 7 that secondary electrons from Compton scatter can emerge up to a maximum angle of 90° with respect to the direction of an incident photon. Points P′ and P have been chosen on a vertical ray below each other on surfaces S′ and S, respectively. Points Q′ and Q have also been chosen on these surfaces, on a vertical ray displaced laterally, but within a secondary-electron range. If the surface is S, P can receive secondary electrons from several points between Q and Q′, but if it is S′, P′ can receive secondary electrons only from Q′. Thus, the secondary electron fluence at P on surface S can be greater than that at point P′ on surface S′. Hence, the obliquity of the surface can cause an enhancement of the skin dose because

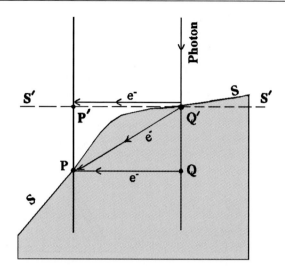

Fig. 15.7. Diagram to explain the enhancement of skin dose caused by obliquity of incidence of a high-energy photon beam. Lines marked e⁻ define the path of the secondary electrons produced by photon interactions

of partial secondary-electron build-up. The additional build-up caused by obliquity moves the depth of the peak dose closer to the skin. Proper assessment of the dose in the build-up region remains a challenging problem [19]. This is because it is subject not only to the partial build-up effects that we just discussed, but also to the influence of secondary electrons from the beam-limiting diaphragms, trays, shielding blocks, and other accessories in the path of the beam [20–25]. A note of caution should be sounded that many computer algorithms used for dose distribution calculations do not allow for these effects in sufficient detail to give an accurate dose assessment in the build-up regions.

15.6
Planning of Dose Distributions

15.6.1
Zones to be Considered

In every beam of a multiple-beam arrangement, the following zones can be identified (see Figure 15.8):

A build-up zone (BZ) at the skin entrance
An entrance zone (ENZ) after the initial build-up, but prior to intersection with other beams
A target zone (TZ), where the beam crosses the target volume treated and where it may overlap with other beams
The exit zone (EXZ) beyond the target volume and before the beam exits from the patient
The penumbra zone (PZ) at the beam edges
The annular zones (AZ) that form the regions not directly irradiated by any beam

These various zones have been identified in Figure 15.8 for a simple case of a combination of two oblique beams. During the planning of multiple-beam treatments,

Fig. 15.8. A combination of two oblique beams. BZ, ENZ, TZ, EXZ, PZ, and AZ identify build-up zone, entrance zone, target zone, exit zone, penumbra zone, and annular zone, respectively

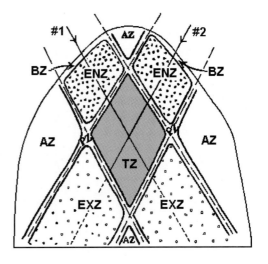

it is necessary to determine where the various zones will fall in relation to the tissues to be treated or protected. The direction of a beam should be such that the entrance and exit paths minimize the dose to normal tissues that have critical or limited tolerance. Short entrance and exit routes are preferable to long ones. After it has passed through the build-up zone, any beam delivers a gradually decreasing dose as it goes from its entrance zone through its target zone to its exit zone. Multiple beams should divide the entrance and exit doses suitably and ensure that the tolerance doses of normal tissues along the paths of the beams are not exceeded. Ideally, the beams should be located so that any highly radiosensitive organ will fall in an annular zone. The combined beams should give a concentrated, uniform dose to a planned target volume.

The ICRU in Reports 50 and 62, provides guidelines for prescribing, recording, and reporting in photon beam therapy [26, 27]. It defines three distinct volumes, respectively called the gross tumor volume (GTV), clinical target volume (CTV), and planning target volume (PTV). The GTV covers the known extent of the tumor, as can be determined by all available methods such as palpation, direct visualization, or diagnostic imaging. The CTV is a larger volume surrounding the GTV that is designated to receive the radiation dose. The CTV is defined with a margin around the GTV to cover possible microscopic tumor extensions and subclinical disease. The PTV is an even larger volume that surrounds the CTV with added internal margins (IMs) and setup margins (SMs). The role of IM is to allow for possible change of shape, movement of anatomic position, and variation in anatomy. Any geometric uncertainties during daily patient setup are allowed for in the SM.

15.6.2
Examining a Dose Distribution

The dose distribution for the arrangement of two oblique beams is shown in Figure 15.9a for X-ray beams of 4 MV energy. The entrance zones and exit zones receive about 70% and 40% of the target dose, respectively. This may or may not satisfy the requirement of not exceeding the tolerance of tissues in the entrance and exit zones in a specific clinical situation. However, in the target zone (i. e., the zone where the beams overlap), an uneven dose distribution is observed, with the dose received ranging from 110% on one side to 70–80% on the opposite side. This may not be acceptable if we desire that the target dose should be uniform within ±10%. The reason for this nonuniformity can be understood if it is realized that the part of the target zone receiving the higher dose of 110% is at a shallow depth for both beams, and that the zone receiving 70 to 80% in the target volume is at a greater depth for both beams. The uniformity can be improved if the photon fluence reaching the region of 110% is reduced and that in the region of 70% is increased. The use of wedge-shaped, fluence-modifying filters, called 'wedge filters,' in the manner illustrated in Figure 15.9b can help. Figures 15.10a and b show dose distributions for the same beam arrangement for ^{60}Co beams. Wedge filters of different designs and performance are usually available in a clinic for various treatment situations.

15.7
Principles of the Use of Wedge Filters

15.7.1
Wedge Angle

Figure 15.11 shows a single-beam dose distribution with a wedge filter. The isodose curves are inclined with respect to the central axis. The 50% isodose curve forms an angle θ with respect to the perpendicular to the central axis. The angle θ, which is called the 'wedge angle,' is a measure of the tilt of the isodose line from its normal horizontal course (i. e., when there is no wedge). There have been various definitions of the wedge angle. This angle can be defined in terms of the tilt of an isodose curve at a particular dose level (say, 50%) or at a specified depth (such as 10 cm). The wedge angle is a characteristic of the dose distribution that results when the wedge is inserted in the beam. It is important to note that the wedge angle is not the physical measure of the angle of the narrow end of the wedge itself.

It will be noticed from Figure 15.11 that the angles of higher-percentage isodose curves are more than θ. On the other hand, the angles of the lower-percentage isodose curves are less than θ. Thus, the value of θ stated for any wedge is merely a value that indicates the differences among the many wedges that a clinic has on hand. Wedge filters for wedge angles of 15°, 30°, 45°, and 60° are common. The design and use of wedge filters have been discussed in the literature [28–32]. The wedge is usually placed at a distance of 15 to 30 cm above the skin to reduce electron contamination (see Sections 9.3.5, 11.3, and 13.4). In modern times, wedge-like dose distributions are generated by therapy machines which use collimator jaws that are capable of independent motion. While one of the two jaws stays stationary, a computer-controlled motion of the second jaw produces an intensity gradient across the beam. Different programmed motions can provide different 'wedge angles' of a 'dynamic wedge' without insertion of any physical wedge [33–36].

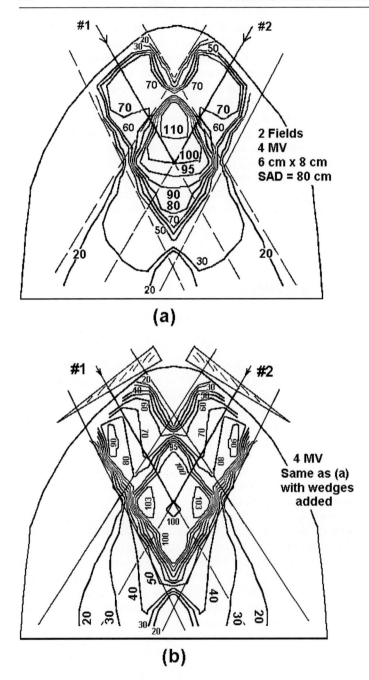

(a)

(b)

Fig. 15.9. Dose distributions for a combination of two oblique 4-MV X-ray beams (**a**) without wedges and (**b**) with wedges

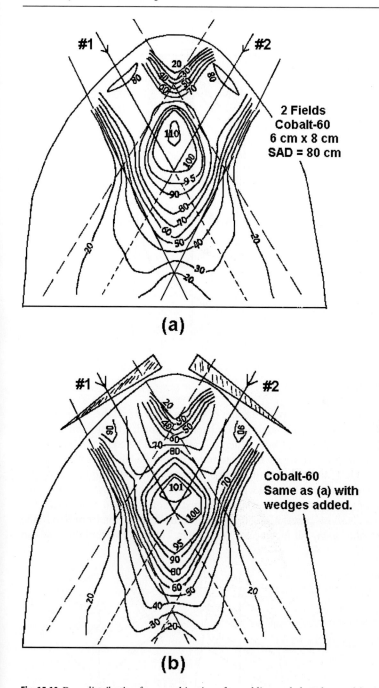

Fig. 15.10. Dose distribution for a combination of two oblique cobalt-60 beams (**a**) without wedges and (**b**) with wedges

Fig. 15.11. Single-beam dose distribution with a wedge. Angle θ is defined as the wedge angle

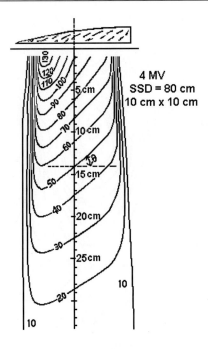

15.7.2
Wedged Oblique Pair

Figures 15.12a and b illustrate a wedged beam of wedge angle θ and the 'hinge angle' φ at which two wedged beams with angle θ have been combined, with the thick ends of the wedges facing toward the junction. When φ is selected to be equal to $(180° − 2θ)$, the isodose curves for the two wedge beams tend to run parallel to the vertical line AC that bisects the angle φ, and a near-uniform dose can result in the region of overlap of the two beams. This is seen in Figure 15.13, in which two wedged beams are combined at a hinge angle of $(180° − 2θ)$ and overlap over the diamond-shaped area ABCD. The line AC falls on an isodose curve. Along diagonal BD, in the direction from B to D, the dose falls off for one beam, but increases for the other. The decrease and increase can

Fig. 15.12. Illustration of (a) the wedge angle of a single wedged beam and (b) the appropriate hinge angle φ for combining two wedge fields with thick ends of the wedges toward the beam-bisecting line

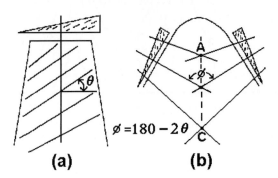

Fig. 15.13. Composite dose distribution at the region of overlap of two wedged beams with the thick ends of the wedges adjacent to each other. Compensating field gradients occur between points B and D when the beams are combined at the appropriate hinge angle. Then bisector AC falls on an isodose curve

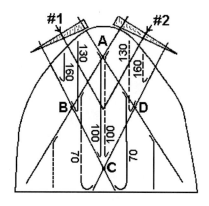

compensate each other to improve the uniformity of the dose along line BD. In an ideal situation, in which the isodose curves are equally spaced and parallel, the entire area ABCD can receive a uniform dose. The hinge angle of $(180° − 2\theta)$ is the appropriate one for wedge angle θ.

Because the ideal of equally spaced and parallel isodose curves does not occur in reality, it is difficult to achieve perfect uniformity. In addition, the dose fall-off in the penumbral zones of the beams cannot be avoided. Figures 15.14a, b, and c show 30°, 45°, and 60° wedge pairs combined at their respective appropriate (i. e., $180 − 2\theta$) hinge angles of 120°, 90°, and 60°, respectively. It is to be noted that, in the entrance zone, the wedge fields may produce hot spots toward the thin end of the wedge, as can be seen in Figures 15.9b and 15.10b.

15.7.3
Three-Field Techniques with Wedges

Apart from being used in wedge-pair geometries, wedges can be used in certain three-beam geometries. Figure 15.15a shows two 30° wedged fields, 1 and 2, combined at a hinge angle of 140°, which is larger than the hinge angle of 120° (i. e., $180° − 2\theta$) that is appropriate for using two 30° wedged beams. A dose gradient is observed along a line bisecting the hinge angle in the target zone. The delivery of a part of the dose by a third beam, 3 in Figure 15.15b, removes this gradient and makes for better dose uniformity.

Figure 15.16a shows a combination of two parallel opposed beams and a third beam normal to them. Beams 2 and 3 are lateral beams from the left and right sides of the patient, and beam 1 is incident from the front. The dose distribution is uniform within the target volume along the axes of beams 2 and 3. This is because beams 1 and 2 oppose each other and their gradients balance each other. However, the fall-off of dose along the axis of beam 1 causes a dose gradient from 110% to 90% across the target volume in the direction perpendicular to the central axis of beams 2 and 3. The inclusion of wedge filters in beams 2 and 3 (Figure 15.16b) compensates for the gradient caused by beam 1. It will be noticed that hot spots of 105% appear toward the thin end of the wedge in the entrance zones of beams 2 and 3.

This technique, sometimes referred to as 'three-field box,' requires optimization of the dose that is administered by each beam and of the wedges to be used.

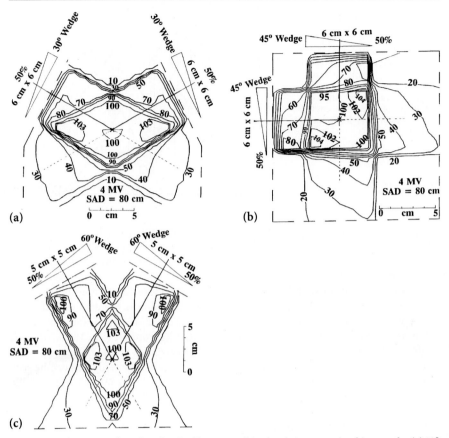

Fig. 15.14. Isodose curves for pairs of wedged beams combined at their appropriate hinge angles (a) 30° wedges, (b) 45° wedges, (c) 60° wedges

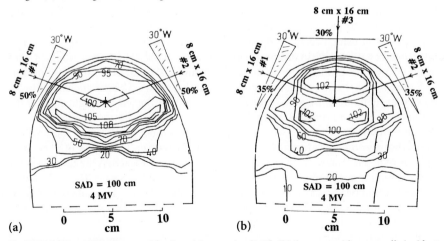

Fig. 15.15. (a) Two 30° wedges combined at a hinge angle of 140°; (b) the same, with a normally incident beam added along the bisecting line

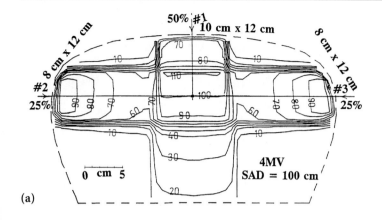

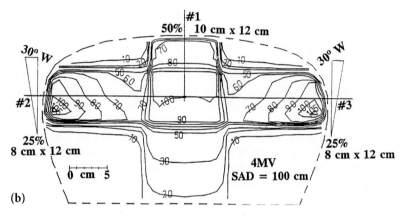

Fig. 15.16. (a) A three-field technique with bilateral opposing beams and an anterior beam perpendicular to them. (b) The same technique, with wedges added in the lateral beams as shown

15.8
Irraditions with Parallel Opposed Beams

15.8.1
On a Body Section of Medium Thickness

A combination of two opposing beams is a very simple and commonly used technique in radiation oncology. Figure 15.17 shows the central-axis dose profile for one set of opposing beams for different beam energies and a body thickness of 20 cm. Equal doses are delivered by the two beams at the patient's midline; hence, we refer to these as 'equally weighted.' In a clinical context, this resembles the treatment of a body section by an anterior (i. e., from the front) beam and an opposing posterior (i. e., from the back) beam. Figure 15.18 illustrates the isodose distributions obtained with opposing beams for different energies and treatment SADs. With such a technique, one can deliver a nearly uniform dose in the central region of the patient, with the

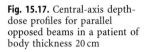
Fig. 15.17. Central-axis depth-dose profiles for parallel opposed beams in a patient of body thickness 20 cm

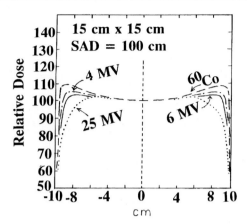

falling dose gradient of one beam compensating for the rising gradient of the opposing beam. However, the phenomena of exponential attenuation and inverse-square fall-off of photon fluence are such that exact compensation cannot occur over an extended region. Therefore, high doses can result at points close to the beam entry. For example, in Figure 15.17, the profile for cobalt-60 shows high doses or 'horns' at points far removed from the patient's midline and close to the entry of the beams. The uniformity improves for higher energies because of the reduced attenuation and less rapid depth-dose fall-off.

An initial dose increase with depth is noticeable in the profiles of the high-energy beams (Figure 15.17). This is caused by the secondary-electron build-up. As we discussed in Section 13.12, the treatment distance also can influence the depth-dose fall-off, although less dramatically than does the energy. Figures 15.18a and b are both for cobalt-60, but are for two different SADs. Figures 15.18c and d are comparisons for two SADs at 4 MV. Figure 15.18e is for a 25-MV beam for a SSD of 100 cm.

The technique in which two beams in a parallel opposed beam arrangement deliver unequal doses at the patient's midline is given the name 'unequally weighted parallel opposed beams.' In the example shown in Figure 15.19, the beams are weighted 80% : 20% in favor of beam 1. The target volume is located off-center and closer to the entrance surface of beam 1. The weighting has been planned so that a minimum dose of 90% will be delivered to the designated target volume.

15.8.2
On a Thin Body Section

Figure 15.20 addresses a situation in which equally weighted opposing beams irradiate a thin body section measuring 10 cm. The build-up region of the high-energy beams results in underdosing of a major part of the body section. Figure 15.21 represents a clinical parallel to this, with equally weighted bilateral fields used for treatment of the whole brain with ^{60}Co, 4-MV and 25-MV beams. In such treatments, if it becomes necessary to ensure adequate dose delivery even at shallow depths, the large build-up zone of very high-energy beams can become a disadvantage. One approach with a high-energy beam could be to place a layer of tissue-equivalent 'bolus' mate-

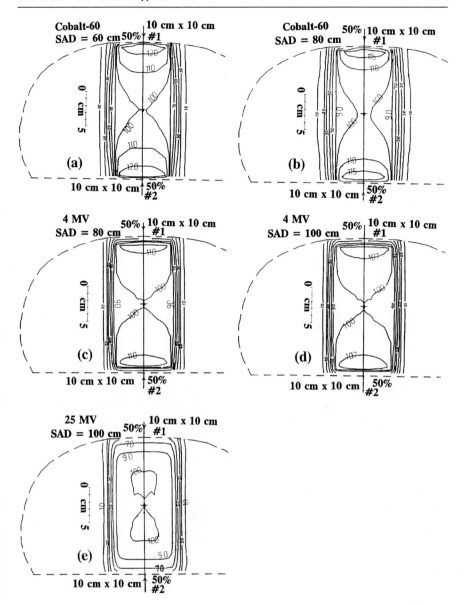

Fig. 15.18. Dose distribution for opposing beams from front and back on a 20 cm thick chest region of a patient: (a) and (b), for cobalt-60; (c) and (d), for 4 MV; and (e), for 25 MV

rials near or on the patient's skin and to provide secondary-electron build-up to the superficial regions [37, 38]. However, this procedure, called 'bolusing,' will increase the skin dose, and the skin-sparing advantage of high-energy beams will be compromised. Overall, lower-energy beams, such as ^{60}Co beams, are preferable for such situations.

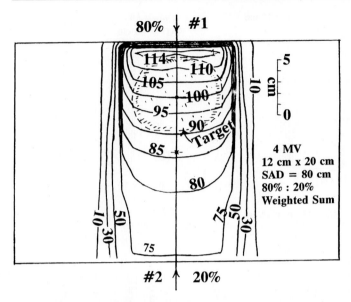

Fig. 15.19. Unequally weighted opposing beams for treatment of a target volume located anteriorly. The anterior beam delivers 80% of the target dose

Fig. 15.20. Central-axis depth-dose profiles for parallel op-posed beams in a body section of thickness 10 cm

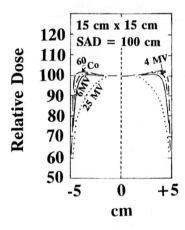

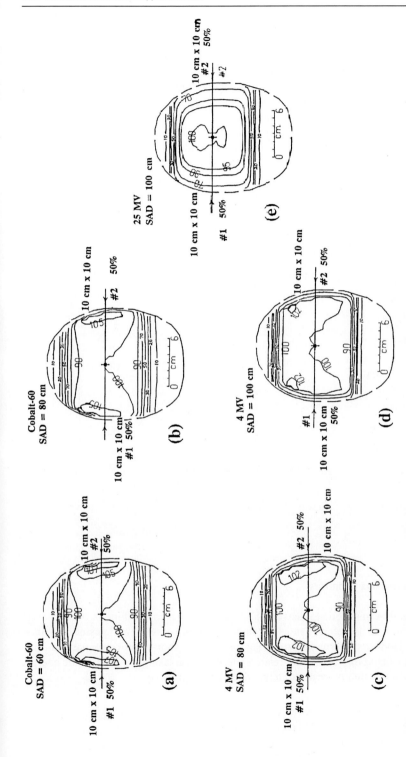

Fig. 15.21. Dose distribution for opposing beams irradiating a 14 cm thick section of the head of a patient: (a) and (b), for cobalt-60; (c) and (d) for 4 MV; and (e) for 25 MV

15.8.3
On a Thick Body Section

Figure 15.22 addresses the use of equally weighted opposing beams on a large body section of 50 cm thickness. The difference between high and low energies is very significant for this thickness. Thicknesses of such magnitude may be encountered when opposing lateral beams (from the right and left sides) are used on a very thick body section such as pelvis. Figure 15.23 presents the isodose curves for equally weighted bilateral beams of different energies and SADs, incident on a patient with an average body thickness of 34 cm. The lateral subcutaneous doses are reduced from 220% in Figure 15.23a to 112% in Figure 15.23e by gradual improvement of the depth-dose fall-off with the use of increasing SAD and energy.

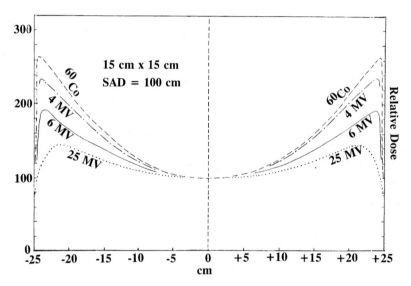

Fig. 15.22. Central-axis depth-dose profiles for parallel opposed beams in a body section of thickness 50 cm

15.8.4
In a Four-Field Box Geometry

Using lateral beams alone to deliver a high target dose is rarely done in practice. It is more common to use lateral beams in combination with anterior and posterior beams. Thus, the isodose patterns shown in Figure 15.24 for four-beam combinations (also called 'four-field box') reflect the relative merits of increasing the SAD or the energy, or both, in a way that more accurately reflects actual practice.

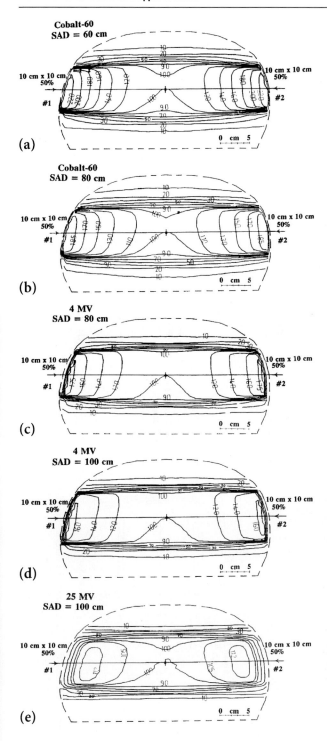

Fig. 15.23. Dose distributions for opposing beams from the sides, irradiating a 34 cm thick pelvic region of a patient: (a) and (b), for cobalt-60; (c) and (d) for 4 MV; and (e) for 25 MV

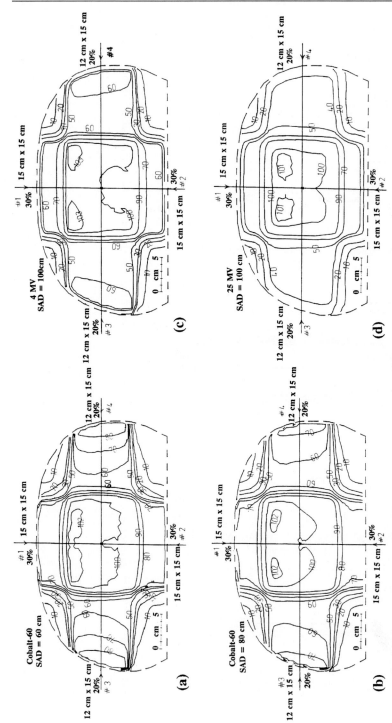

Fig. 15.24. Dose distributions for a rectangular four-field 'box' technique. Front and back beams together deliver 60% of the target dose of 100%. Beams from the sides deliver the remaining 40%. (a) Cobalt-60, SAD 60 cm; (b) cobalt-60, SAD 80 cm; (c) 4-MV X-rays, SAD 100 cm; (d) 25-MV X-rays, SAD 100 cm

15.8.5
On a Section of Uneven Body Thickness

In situations where the thickness of the patient changes significantly within the field, parallel opposed beams can give a dose gradient along the patient's midline. Figure 15.25a illustrates this for parallel opposed 6-MV beams irradiating the neck and chest region of a patient. The dose is seen to vary from 109% to 90% along the patient's midline from the thin side to the thick side. In Figure 15.25b, the uniformity is improved when a bolus or wax is used on the patient's surface to fill the thickness deficits and level the surface. Such bolusing on the skin is a disadvantage, as the secondary electrons from the bolus will enhance the skin dose and eliminate the build-up and skin-sparing advantage of high-energy photon beams. In an alternative approach, which is shown in Figure 15.25c, a specially designed filter called a 'tissue compensating filter' is placed at a distance above the surface to filter the radiation in such a way as to improve the dose uniformity. One can specially design the shape of the compensating filter by exactly taking into account the variation in the patient thickness across the field [39–43]. The compensating filter can be placed at a large distance (20 cm or more) from the skin, so

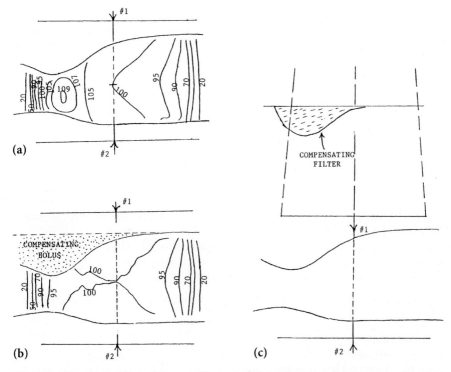

Fig. 15.25. (a) A pair of 6-MV parallel opposed beams irradiating the neck and chest regions of a patient, resulting in nonuniform delivery of dose along the patient's midline. (b) A compensating bolus has been placed on the patient's skin to level the surface and improve the dose uniformity. (c) A compensating filter is inserted in the beam

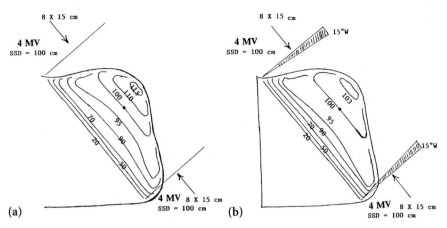

Fig. 15.26. Dose distributions obtained for tangentially opposing fields used for irradiation of breast and chest wall. (**a**) Without tissue compensation wedges, (**b**) with wedges used for tissue compensation

that the fluence of secondary electrons from the filter does not contribute significantly to the skin dose and thereby spoil the dose build-up and skin-sparing effect.

In situations where the change in patient thickness within the field is gradual, wedge filters can be used as compensating filters. Figures 15.26a and b illustrate the dose distributions without and with wedge compensation in a case of irradiation of the breast and chest wall by tangentially opposing beams.

15.9
Other Common Techniques

Figures 15.27 to 15.31 present the isodose distributions for some commonly employed techniques of irradiation. The techniques covered are

'Three-field-obliques,' with three beams in an oblique geometry (Figure 15.27)
'Four-field-obliques,' with four beams in an oblique combination (Figure 15.28)
'Full 360° rotation,' which uses an isocentric beam that makes a complete circle around the patient (Figure 15.29)
'Posterior skip arc,' with a moving beam that rotates around an isocenter, but skips an 80° arc segment at the posterior side of the patient (Figure 15.30)
'Bilateral arcs,' that is, two arcs on either side of the patient (Figure 15.31)

Each illustration provides four isodose patterns covering the following energies and SADs:

(a) Cobalt-60, SAD = 60 cm
(b) Cobalt-60, SAD = 80 cm
(c) 4-MV X-rays, SAD = 100 cm
(d) 25-MV X-rays, SAD = 100 cm

From (a) to (d), the above sequence upgrades the machine from an early cobalt machine to a high-energy accelerator through two interim stages. The reader is advised

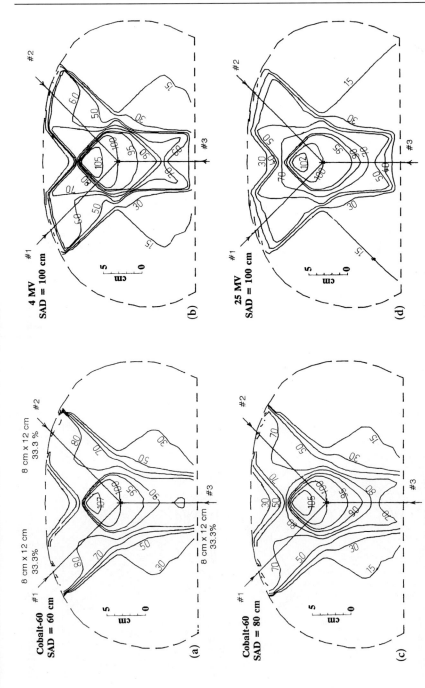

Fig. 15.27. Dose distributions for three-field oblique technique with an equal part of the 100% target dose delivered by each beam. (a) Cobalt-60, SAD 60 cm; (b) cobalt-60, SAD 80 cm; (c) 4-MV X-rays, SAD 100 cm; (d) 25-MV X-rays, SAD 100 cm

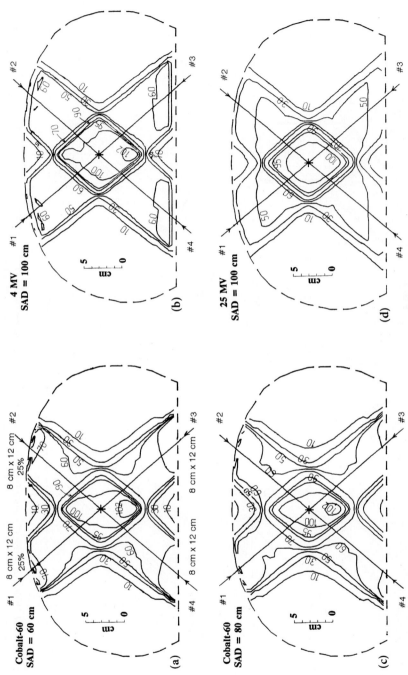

Fig. 15.28. Dose distributions for a combination of four oblique fields with equal amount of 100% target dose delivered by each beam. (a) Cobalt-60, SAD 60 cm; (b) cobalt-60, SAD 80 cm; (c) 4-MV X-rays, SAD 100 cm; (d) 25-MV X-rays, SAD 100 cm

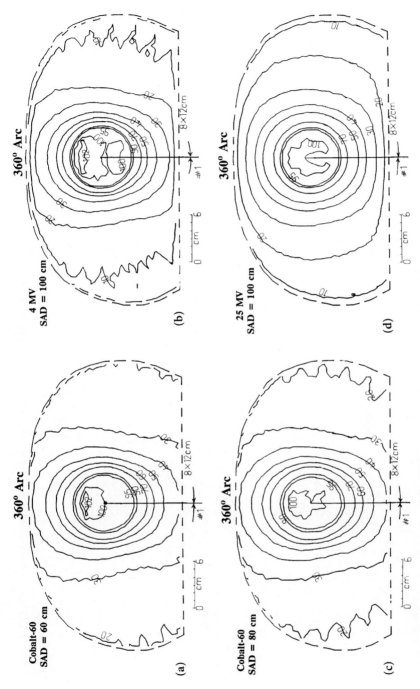

Fig. 15.29. Dose distributions for 360° rotation. (a) Cobalt-60, SAD 60 cm; (b) cobalt-60, SAD 80 cm; (c) 4-MV X-rays, SAD 100 cm; (d) 25-MV X-rays, SAD 100 cm

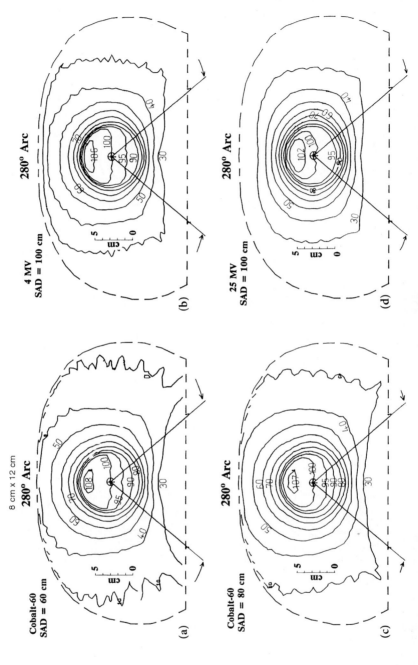

Fig. 15.30. Dose distribution for 'posterior skip arc' with a 280° moving beam. (a) Cobalt-60, SAD 60 cm; (b) cobalt-60, SAD 80 cm; (c) 4-MV X-rays, SAD 100 cm; (d) 25-MV X-rays, SAD 100 cm

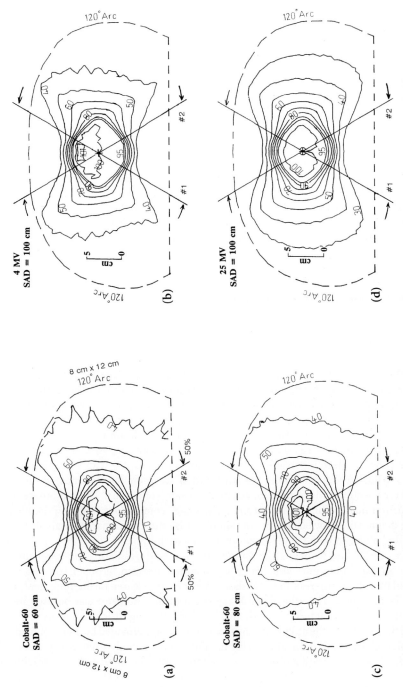

Fig. 15.31. Dose distribution for bilateral 120° arcs. (a) Cobalt-60, SAD 60 cm; (b) cobalt-60, SAD 80 cm; (c) 4-MV X-rays, SAD 100 cm; (d) 25-MV X-rays, SAD 100 cm

to observe the isodose patterns to discern (i) the shape of the target zones covered, (ii) the hot spots and cold spots in the target zone, (iii) the doses at the entrance and exit zones, (iv) the location of the annular zones, (v) the fall-off in the penumbral zones, and (vi) the dose increase in the build-up zones. In a given clinical situation, the selection or suitability of one dose distribution over another can be guided by the above factors. Atlases of multiple-beam and moving-beam dose distributions have been published for study and teaching purposes [44, 45].

Many radiotherapy clinics have treatment-planning computers that can calculate and display the dose distributions based on patient-specific and treatment-machine-specific data input. Such treatment-planning computers may rely on one or more of various available dose calculation approaches [46–48]. These methods include use of numerical data tables, empirical or semi-empirical analytical expressions, mathematical summation and interpolation algorithms, and Monte Carlo calculations. The data base used by any treatment planning system, and the reliability and limitations of its calculation approach, should be ascertained by a quality control process that is implemented by a qualified clinical physicist [49–52].

15.10
Treatment Planning: A Practical Case

15.10.1
Therapy Simulator

A radiotherapy simulator is a machine that uses a diagnostic X-ray tube as a radiation source and mimics, in all of its adjustments and motions, the radiotherapy machine to be used for the actual treatment [53–55]. Simulation is a process of developing, evaluating, and accepting a treatment strategy for a given patient situation. The planning phase of the treatment of a patient can require a considerable amount of time, and it is therefore not wise to use a treatment machine for planning purposes. The treatment machine is best utilized for treating as many patients as possible with strategies that are already finalized. A part of the planning and of accepting the treatment strategy is to take projection radiographs for particular beam conditions. The radiotherapy simulator is a major tool for this purpose. The image contrast obtainable in the film with the diagnostic X-ray beam from the simulator is different from that obtainable in a 'port film' obtained with the high-energy therapy beam.

Figures 15.32a and b show a simulation film of a field irradiating the vocal cord and the corresponding port film. The bony shadows are seen in better contrast in the simulation film, whereas the soft-tissue outlines are clearer in the high-energy therapy beam image. The kilovoltage X-ray beam of the simulator can be used for localizing the bony structures for dose distribution planning. It is prudent to verify whether the location of the different beams and the coverage provided by them conform to the plan chosen. Injection of contrast medium into the body cavities can aid in the localizing and verification process where appropriate. The simulated radiographic image in Figure 15.32a includes the images of horizontal and vertical pairs of wires which delineate the geometric edges of a rectangular field intended for treatment. The X-ray beam used for radiographing can be larger than the intended field of treatment

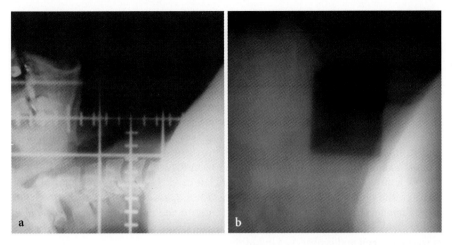

Fig. 15.32. (a) Simulation radiograph obtained with 80-kV X-rays. (b) A therapy port radiograph obained with 4-MV X-rays

to show a broader background. The radiograph also shows the image of a graduated cross hair at the two principal axes of the rectangular field. These gradations, which signify 1-cm spacings at the distance of the isocenter, are helpful in the evaluation or in suggesting changes.

Simulation radiographs involve much less exposure to the patient than does imaging with the therapy beam itself. Changes can be made in successive steps until the optimum beam coverage is achieved. With modern simulators, the beam delineation and orientation and patient positioning can be done under fluoroscopic observation. Any treatment beam should also be verified with a port film radiograph taken with the therapy beam, as illustrated in Figure 15.32b. A port film can combine two images on one film – the first obtained with a therapy beam of a size identical to that of the intended treatment beam and the second obtained with a larger beam covering the surrounding body structures as well.

In this section, we have so far discussed a conventional radiotherapy simulator that mimics a treatment machine and uses conventional films for radiographic imaging. The advent of computed tomography has made it possible to do the beam simulations based on CT scans of the patient [56]. A CT simulator employs a dedicated CT scanner in a radiotherapy department first to produce digital images of successive transverse sections of the patient covering the anatomic region of interest. Then the CT images are used with mathematical ray-tracing methods for construction of digital radiographs. Any beam with any size and orientation is simulated by defining the geometrical parameters of the beam and overlaying it on the CT scans. A digitally reconstructed radiograph (DRR) is created for the beam based on the CT scan. This is sometimes referred to as 'virtual simulation,' because it is not obtained by the use of a therapy-like x-ray beam. The resolution and details of the DRR can approach that of the film if the thickness and spacing of the CT images are very small. The use of CT images for tumor localization in beam's-eye view is discussed later in Section 15.11.

15.10.2
Localization for Treatment of the Esophagus

We now discuss the specific case of a patient with cancer of the esophagus. Figures 15.33a and b are AP (i. e., front to back) and lateral (i. e., side view) radiographic projections of a section of the patient taken with barium contrast medium in the esophagus. The contrast medium outlines the organ and helps the physician to identify the target volume of treatment which includes subclinical disease and the surrounding routes of spread. (The target volume for dose delivery may often include more than the known tumor volume.) Figures 15.34a and b are line drawings of the visible outlines from the radiographs in Figures 15.33a and b. In Figure 15.34a, the marks (A_R, A_L), (B_R, B_L), and (C_R, C_L) indicate the right and left extents of the target volume at three levels in the patient as indicated by the physician. Likewise, in Figure 15.34b, at the same three levels, the upper and lower (i. e., anterior and posterior) limits of the target volume have been identified as (A_U, A_D), (B_U, B_D), (C_U, C_D). The course of the spinal cord is also seen and is observed in both projections.

We would like to have available a transverse contour of the patient through point M_0 (Figure 15.34b), where M_0 is the center of the field on the body surface. The contour can usually be obtained by placing of a moldable plaster-of-paris cast on the patient's surface and waiting for it to harden. Then the cast is removed and placed on a sheet of paper (Figure 15.35). When the cast is on the patient, marks (e. g., M_0, M_1, and M_2 as shown in Figure 15.35) are made on it to identify the points of entry of the AP beam and the entrance and exit points of the lateral beam as simulated. The measured lateral and front-to-back thicknesses of the patient between these (and any other) fiducial marks

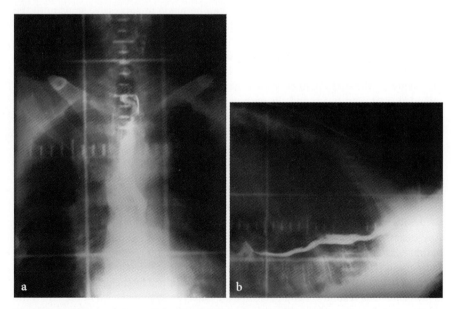

Fig. 15.33. The first simulation radiographs of a cancer patient with contrast medium in the esophagus. (**a**) AP projection, (**b**) lateral projection

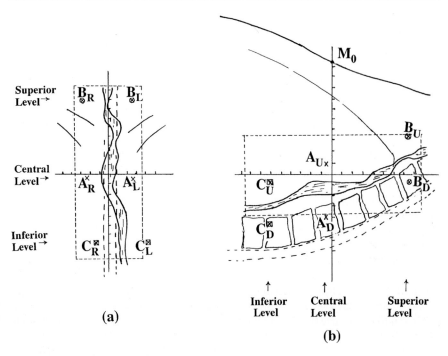

Fig. 15.34. Line drawings of the radiographs in Figure 15.33. (a) AP projection, (b) lateral projection

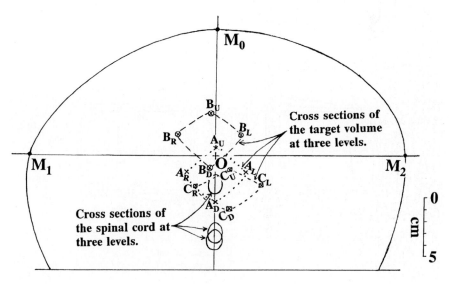

Fig. 15.35. Patient contour drawn with skin marks M, M_1, and M_2, and localization of the front-to-back (i. e., AP-PA) and left-to-right (i. e., lateral) extents of the target volume and spinal cord, as interpreted from Figure 15.32. x, $\otimes$ and H refer to A points, B points, and C points, respectively

are used for appropriate placement of the plaster-of-paris cast on a sheet of paper for tracing of the contour, as shown in Figure 15.35. The vertical line through M_0 and the horizontal line M_1M_2 intersect at O. The point O, which is the location of the isocenter at simulation, can be used as the origin of a rectangular (x, y) coordinate system.

As a next step, the positions of points (A_R, A_L) and (A_U, A_D) (from Figures 15.34a and b) should be localized with respect to the origin O in Figure 15.35. In the absence of full information (such as a CT scan may provide) in the transverse plane, the points A_R, A_L, A_U, and A_D have been localized in Figure 15.35 with the assumption that the lines A_RA_L and A_UA_D bisect one another. In the same manner, the points (B_R, B_L, B_U, B_D) and (C_R, C_L, C_U, C_D) have been localized. These give a perspective of the progression of the target volume along the length of the patient. In Figure 15.35, the points have been connected to indicate the areas to be covered in the irradiation. By a similar approach, the sections of spinal cord have been drawn at the three levels, because it is a critical organ with limited radiation tolerance.

15.10.3
Case-Specific Isodose Planning

Let us say that the physician desires to deliver a dose of 60 Gy to the target volume. He would like to use a technique that would (i) keep the dose to the spinal cord below 45 Gy and (ii) minimize the dose to the lungs. Figures 15.36, 15.37, and 15.38 illustrate the design of three different treatment plans, assuming that a 4-MV X-ray machine is available in the clinic. The first plan, in Figure 15.36, is a four-field box technique that delivers 66% of the target dose by AP-PA fields 1 and 2 and the remaining 34% by lateral fields 3 and 4. The second plan, in Figure 15.37, uses front-to-back fields 1

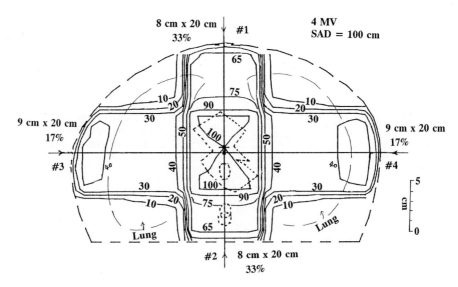

Fig. 15.36. A rectangular four-field box technique for treating the esophagus case of Figure 15.32. Front-to-back beam delivers 66% of the target dose and lateral opposing beams deliver the remaining 34%

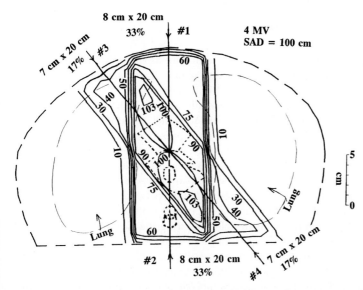

Fig. 15.37. A four-field technique for treating the esophagus case of Figure 15.32. Front-to-back beams deliver 66% of the target dose, and oblique opposing beams deliver the remaining 34%

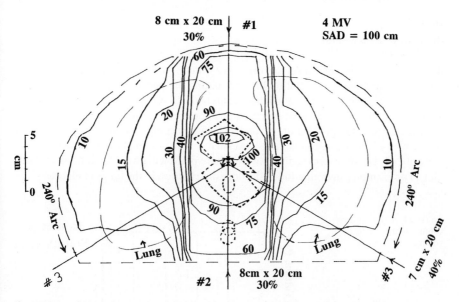

Fig. 15.38. A technique that combines front-to-back beams for delivery of 60% of the dose, with a 240° arc technique to deliver the remaining 40%, for treating the esophagus case of Figure 15.33

and 2 to deliver 66% of the target dose and employs opposing oblique fields 3 and 4 for the remaining 34%. The third plan, in Figure 15.38, uses front-to-back fields 1 and 2 to deliver 60% of the total dose and a 240° arc to add the remaining 40%.

15.10.4
Comparative Evaluation of the Plans

Uniformity of dose within the target volume is accomplished in all three plans. This is to be expected, because they were designed to achieve this as a minimum objective. The total dose delivered with any plan, however, can be limited by the tolerance dose of the other organs that are irradiated incidentally. Therefore, let us first look at the plans from the point of view of the spinal cord tolerance. All three plans have been designed so as to deliver not more than 75% of the prescribed target dose of 60 Gy to the mid- and lower segments of the spinal cord. However, the upper segment of the spinal cord is much closer to the isocenter and is seen to receive the same dose as the target dose. Here, we need to remember that the plan we see is two-dimensional and does not display all of the details along the length of the patient. At simulation, we can observe the fields along their lengths. The protection of the upper spinal cord can be taken care of by shaping of the field with blocks during the stages of simulation and verification of the beams.

The three plans differ with regard to protecting the lungs and minimizing pulmonary damage. The plans of Figures 15.36 and 15.38 are both poor in this respect compared to that in Figure 15.37. It appears that the plan of Figure 15.37 is the most acceptable overall. A more quantitative comparison for this purpose can be made with the use of dose-volume plots.

15.10.5
Use of Dose-Volume Plots

A graphic plot of the fraction of any organ (or volume) that receives more than various assigned dose levels is a useful tool for evaluating the performance of different dose distributions. Such plots are called dose-volume plots. A typical dose-volume plot for a target volume to be irradiated may have an appearance as shown in Figure 15.39, for any plan designed to give a uniform dose. The figure compares the plot for ideal dose uniformity within the target volume with what can be obtained in real situations. For any critically sensitive organ, different treatment plans will give different dose-volume plots. For example, an evaluation of the dose distribution in the lungs in Figures 15.36,

Fig. 15.39. A typical dose-volume plot for a target volume

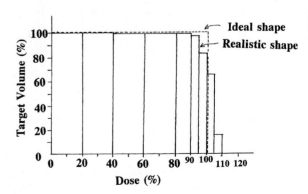

Fig. 15.40. Dose-volume plots for lung. The three curves labeled **A**, **B**, and **C** are for the plans of Figures 15.36, 15.37, and 15.38, respectively

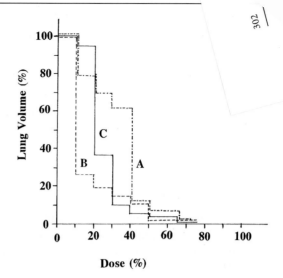

15.37, and 15.38 resulted in the dose-volume plots shown in Figure 15.40. Thus, the relative merits of these three plans from the point of view of sparing the lung volume are compared side by side. If a cut-off level of 20% dose is used for lung tolerance, the plot labeled B, applicable to the plan in Figure 15.37, is seen to irradiate a minimum lung volume above this dose, compared to the two others labeled A and C. This again affirms the selection of the plan of Figure 15.37.

Dose-volume plots are sometimes also called dose-volume histograms (DVHs). Use of DVHs to compare treatment plans has become possible in recent years because of the availability of 3-D treatment-planning systems. The interpretation of DVH can be complex [57–59]. Using them requires an understanding of the degree of adverse reaction possible when different partial volumes of an organ at risk are irradiated to different doses. In this context, the ICRU speaks about a serial organ, parallel organ, and serial-parallel organ [27]. A serial organ (like a spinal cord) should not receive a dose exceeding its tolerance anywhere within it. If that happens, its function can break down. On the other hand, a partial damage of a parallel organ (like lung) may not inhibit the functioning of its undamaged sections. Although such partial damage can lower the level of performance of the organ, a total failure does not happen. Some organs (like heart or kidney) can be expected to display a combination of both behaviors. These are called serial-parallel organs.

15.10.6
Integral Dose (Σ)

Ideally, one would like to irradiate the target volume only, with no dose delivered elsewhere. After assuring that the target dose is uniform, we can look among several techniques for one that results in minimum energy absorbed in the whole body. Integral dose (Σ) was defined as an index by Mayneord for such a comparative evaluation [60]. If a volume of tissue having mass M receives an average dose D_{Av}, Σ is given by

$$\Sigma = \text{mass} \times \text{average dose} = M \times D_{Av}$$

EXAMPLE 15.2

A cylindrical body section has a diameter of 20 cm and a length of 15 cm. The density of tissue is $1.0\,g\,cm^{-3}$. In a treatment plan adopted for irradiation, the average dose to the volume is assessed to be 1200 cGy. Calculate the integral dose.

Radius of cylinder (r) $= 20/2 = 10$ cm; Length (L) $= 15$ cm; volume (V) $= \pi r^2 L = 3.1416 \times 10^2 \times 15 = 4712\,cm^3$

$$\text{Mass of volume} = 4712\,cm^3 \times 1.0\,g\,cm^{-3} = 4.712\,kg$$

$$\text{integral dose} = \text{average dose} \times \text{mass receiving the dose}$$
$$= 1200\,cGy \times 4.712\,kg = 4.712\,kg \times 1200 \times 10^{-2}\,J\,kg^{-1}$$
$$= 56.5\,J$$

In general, different volumes may be enclosed between different isodose surfaces plotted in a plan. If so, Σ is given by the following sum:

$$\Sigma = {}_i\Sigma\,\rho\,|V_{i+1} - V_i|\,(D_{i+1} + D_i)/2$$

where V_i = volume enclosed within isodose level i; D_i = dose corresponding to isodose level i; and ρ = density of the medium.

From the two-dimensional isodose curves, it is possible only to obtain area A_i enclosed by an isodose curve for dose D_i. In a simplistic way, if the same distribution is assumed to be valid in all transverse planes along the field length L, the following approximation results:

$$V_i = A_i \times L$$

and

$$\Sigma = {}_i\Sigma\rho L|A_{i+1} - A_i|(D_{i+1} + D_i)/2$$
$$= {}_i\Sigma\rho L\Delta A_i(D_{i+1} + D_i)/2$$

where ΔA_i is the annular area enclosed between isodose levels i and i+1. Figures 15.41a, b, and c are plots of the annular areas between different isodose curves of Figures 15.36, 15.37, and 15.38. The average doses estimated for the three planes are 21%, 17%, and 16%, respectively. These numbers are directly proportional to the Σ values for the three plans. However, these diagrams and numbers are not particularly useful for making any decision. This is because Σ is a sum that does not distinguish between different organs and their individual tolerances. Σ increases with the thickness of the patient through which the beam passes. For example, in the case of a centrally located target site, Σ will be larger for a technique that uses lateral beams than for another technique that employs AP–PA beams. However, the overall dose distribution, rather than Σ, should influence how much dose can be given in each beam orientation. As in our example in Section 15.10.3, the tolerance of an organ (such as the spinal cord) can be a more significant factor for limiting the AP–PA component than is any fear of a possible increase in Σ by use of any other beam directions.

Fig. 15.41. Plots of the percent area of the patient's cross section enclosed between different isodose levels. Diagrams (a), (b), and (c) are for the dose distributions in Figures 15.36, 15.37, and 15.38, respectively

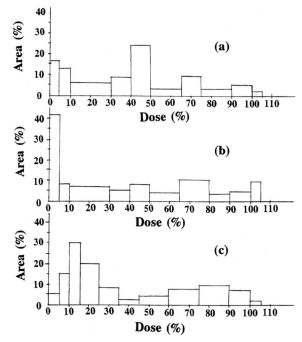

15.10.7
Simulating the Accepted Plan

The geometric aspects of the paper plan of Figure 15.37 should now be implemented on the patient. Beams 1 and 2 have the isocenter at O, which is the same isocenter that was used during the first simulation. This isocenter can be identified within the patient by means of the skin marks M_0, M_1, and M_2 (see Figure 15.35), which are retained by the patient. To implement the treatment plan in which the two oblique beams 3 and 4 are used, we need to simulate these beams. In general, these beams may have their isocenter at a point I different from O. Setting the isocenter at I can be done through the following steps:

(i) Identify the offsets a and b (Figure 15.42a) from isocenter I with respect to O.
(ii) Set up beam 1 with the isocenter at O, as was done during the initial localizing simulation.
(iii) The patient is moved in the left-right direction through a distance **a** to have the beam axis go through the isocenter I (see Figure 15.42b).
(iv) The patient is then moved in the front-back direction through a distance **b** so that the isocenter coincides with I.
(v) The beam is swung to assume the oblique direction of beam 3 (Figure 15.42c), and a simulation radiograph is obtained.
(vi) The same procedure is repeated for beam 4.

Fig. 15.42. Diagrams (a), (b), and (c) show the steps by which the isocenter is placed at point I of the plan in Figure 15.36. In (a), the patient is set up so as to have the isocenter at point O used during initial simulation. The patient is then moved by offset distances **a** and **b** in (b) and (c)

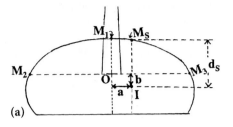

(a)

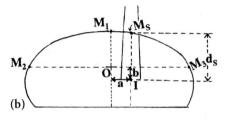

(b)

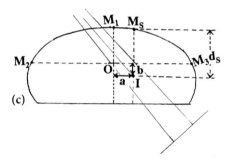

(c)

Figure 15.43 shows the simulation radiographs for oblique beam 3. Figure 15.44 is a line drawing of the contents of Figure 15.43. In the plan of Figure 15.37, the oblique beams were designed to treat the target volume without irradiating the spinal cord in the mid-transverse section of the fields. In Figures 15.43 and 15.44, it is seen that the field edges (as indicated by the shadow of field-delineating wires) fall far from the spinal cord in the lower sections of the field. However, the spinal cord courses within the field at one corner. For protection of this part of the spinal cord, a shielding block is added. With the block included, the entire field length of beam 3 conforms to the geometric criteria (concerning the field edge) that made the paper plan of Figure 15.37 acceptable. A similar block can be designed for oblique field 4 after that field is simulated. With such specially shaped oblique fields, the patient can be treated.

We refer the reader to References 61, 62, and 63 for several other practical aspects of photon beam treatment planning.

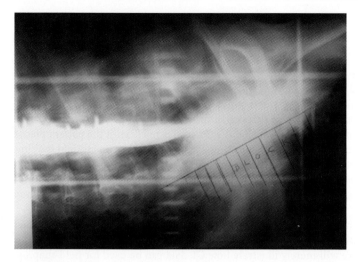

Fig. 15.43. Simulation radiograph of oblique field no. 3 of Figure 15.36. A block is shown shielding the cord where it falls within the collimated rectangular field

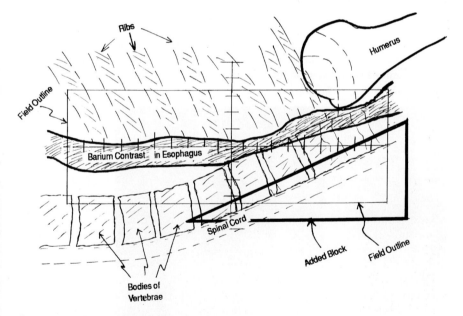

Fig. 15.44. Line drawing of the radiograph in Figure 15.43

15.11
Use of CT Data

15.11.1
CT Transverse Cuts

Computed-tomography (CT) scanners provide detailed anatomic and diagnostic information in successive transverse sections of the patient. The CT images can be used directly for treatment planning, provided the CT scan is made with the patient placed in a position identical to the treatment position. In the positioning, one should use similar patient supports with the same positions of arm, shoulder, neck, etc. to maintain identical relative positions between different anatomical regions. With any change of position, the organ delineations can differ between the CT and the treatment position of the patient.

Many advances are being made in the transfer and processing of CT images for direct 3D planning in radiotherapy [1–9]. It is not within the scope of this text to discuss this subject in detail. We will merely illustrate how CT data can be used for field shaping, using just one example.

15.11.2
CT for Field Shaping

We use the example of a lung tumor for which the physician has already simulated an anterior field, as shown in Figure 15.45. This radiograph does reveal the presence of the tumor, but not in the same detail and clarity as provided by a CT scan. Figure 15.46 shows some examples of CT images of the patient. We can interpret the CT

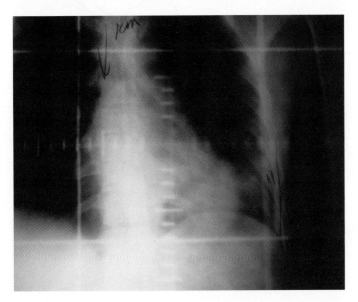

Fig. 15.45. The first (tentative) simulation radiograph of an AP field setup for a patient with a lung lesion

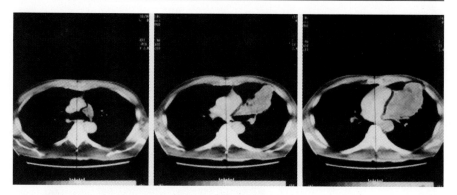

Fig. 15.46. Examples of CT images of the patient with a lung lesion. The tumor outlines have been drawn

tumor outlines and project them on the simulation radiograph. The tumor outline in Figure 15.45 has been drawn based on the CT images by a projection procedure that is described next. Figure 15.47 gives the line drawing representation of the same CT images. These drawings highlight the tumor, the vertebral body, the sternum, and the outer body contour in each section. A minified line drawing of the film view is shown in Figure 15.47e, which shows the apex of the lung, the bronchial carina, and the diaphragm, along with bony structures. The scale in the middle marks the levels of the different CT images from 3 to 21. These have been localized by identification of the levels of a few salient anatomic landmarks, such as the apex of the lung, the bronchial carina, and the diaphragm. In Figures 15.47a to d, rays through the edges

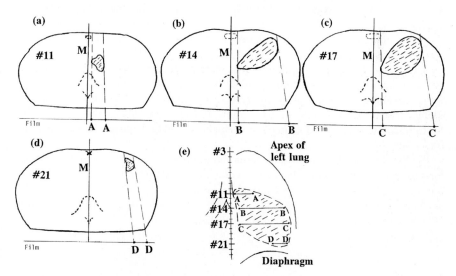

Fig. 15.47. (a) to (d) Line drawings of the CT images of Figure 15.46, showing the salient structures. The rays projecting the right-left extent of the tumor onto the plane of the simulation radiograph are also illustrated schematically. (e) Line drawing of the AP radiograph of Figure 15.45, including the projection of the tumor volume from CT images

Fig. 15.48. Port film image
of a shaped field including a
block and the tumor volume
projected from CT

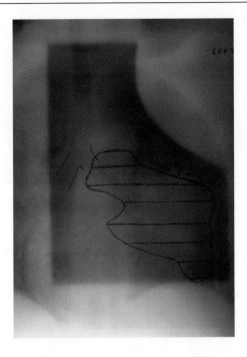

of the tumor have been drawn that project points AA, BB, CC, and DD at the level
of the film. The distance of these points from the midline M of the patient is first
measured on the CT image. Then these points are relocated in the film, as illustrated
in Figure 15.47e. The scale of the CT image is usually small compared to the scale of
the actual patient. On the other hand, because of the beam divergence, the simulation
radiograph shows the patient anatomy on a magnified scale. Thus, both the scale of the
CT image and that of the simulation radiograph should be taken into account in the
projection of the extent of the CT image of the tumor on the simulation radiograph.
Such a 'beam's-eye' projection of any structure seen in CT on the film plane is very
useful for shaping the treatment field. Figure 15.48 is a port film of the field showing
the tumor volume projected from CT and a block placed to shape the field accepted for
treatment.

Here we have dealt with a simple situation of projecting a tumor volume from CT
for a vertical beam of simple geometry irradiating a patient from front to back. With
the use of computer graphic workstations and geometrical coordinate transformation
algorithms, one can project the beam's-eye view of a tumor or any other organ from
CT for any arbitrary beam orientation [1–9]. This is the basis of modern 3D planning
systems, and CT simulation.

15.12
Treatment of Adjacent Sites

15.12.1
Problem of Concern

In radiotherapy practice, situations may be encountered in which it becomes necessary to treat a site adjacent to a site either treated previously or under current treatment. If both sites are being treated concurrently, the reason for the split may be that the maximum field size provided by the treatment machine is inadequate to include both sites in a single beam. When separate fields are used, it is important to take into account the overlap or gaps between the edges of the adjacent fields. Ignoring this can result in overdosage because of superposition of the beam edges or underdosage because of gaps between them at the interface [64, 65] The gradual fall-off of dose caused by a beam with a penumbra is a blessing in these situations, as it can diffuse the severity of the effects of mismatches, gaps, or overlaps.

The junction problem has been studied and reported for various situations. Different approaches have been used for overcoming the problem. These include such methods as the use of a separation between the adjacent beam edges on the skin, angular rotation of the beam to orient its edges, adopting half-beam blocking and using the nondiverging central axis of the adjacent beams to coincide, using penumbra spreaders, and moving the junction during phases of treatment [66–76]. In the next sections, we discuss the general aspects of this problem.

15.12.2
Both Sites Treated from One Direction

A very simple situation is shown in Figure 15.49a, where two beams irradiate adjacent sites. Fields 1 and 2 have their field lengths L_1 and L_2 specified at their respective SAD_1 and SAD_2 of treatment. The skin is at level d above the junction between the two fields. The divergences of the beams are such that a separation (or skin gap) S between the edges of the fields is needed at the skin level so that the edges intersect at the depth d. The field lengths L_1' and L_2' of the two fields at the skin surface are

$$L_1' = L_1 \times \frac{(SAD_1 - d)}{SAD_1} = L_1 - L_1 \times \frac{d}{SAD_1}$$

$$L_2' = L_2 \times \frac{(SAD_2 - d)}{SAD_2} = L_2 - L_2 \times \frac{d}{SAD_2}$$

The skin gap S is related to L_1, L_2, L_1' and L_2' by

$$2S = (L_1 + L_2) - (L_1' + L_2') = \left[\frac{L_1}{SAD_1} + \frac{L_2}{SAD_2} \right] d$$

Hence, the skin gap

$$S = \frac{1}{2} \left[\frac{L_1}{SAD_1} + \frac{L_2}{SAD_2} \right] d$$

Fig. 15.49. (a) Diverging edges of two adjacent fields of lengths L_1 and L_2 set up at distances SAD_1 and SAD_2. (b) The dose distribution for two adjacent beams with 4-MV X-rays positioned for a skin gap of 1.2 cm to match the diverging edges at 5 cm depth. (c) Dose distribution for the same beams when the skin gap is increased to 2 cm

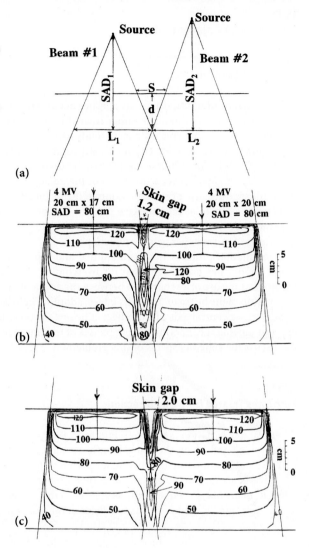

In the above calculation attention is given to the distances from the source at which L_1 and L_2 are specified. In the above description, L_1 is specified at distance SSD_1 and L_2 at distance SSD_2. Hence, the ratios (L_1/SSD_1) and (L_2/SSD_2) govern the rate of divergence of the beam. In general, S can be derived by the concept,

$$S = [1/2] \times [\text{Rate of Divergence of Beam 1} + \text{Rate of Divergence of Beam 2}]$$
$$\times [\text{Depth of match level from skin}]$$

That is,

$$S = [1/2] \times [\{L_1/\text{Distance (from source) where } L_1 \text{ is specified}\} \\ + (L_2/\text{Distance (from source) where } L_2 \text{ is specified}\}] \\ \times [\text{Depth of match level from skin}]$$

In a simpler context, both L_1 and L_2 may be measured at one and the same SSD or SAD. If, let us say, $SAD_1 = SAD_2 = SAD$, then

$$S = \frac{d(L_1 + L_2)}{2 \times SAD}$$

EXAMPLE 15.3

Two adjacent fields have lengths of 17 cm and 20 cm as specified at an SAD of 80 cm. Calculate the skin gap needed for matching of the field edges at 5 cm depth.

In this example,

$$L_1 = 17\,\text{cm}; \quad L_2 = 20\,\text{cm}, \quad SAD = 80\,\text{cm}; \quad d = 5\,\text{cm}$$
$$S = \frac{S(L_1 + L_2)}{2 \times SAD} = \frac{5(17 + 20)}{2 \times 80} \approx 1.2\,\text{cm}$$

Figure 15.49b shows the isodose curves for this example for 4 MV beams. The prescription dose of 100% has been taken at a depth of 5 cm for both sites. It is seen that, at the overlap between the fields, the dose rises to 120%. An increase of the skin gap to 2.0 cm (see Figure 15.49c) reduces the dose at the overlap to 90%, but at the cost of underdosing the tissue just below the skin gap.

15.12.3
Adjacent Parallel Opposed Fields

The beam divergence calculation that gave the skin gap S is equally applicable to situations in which adjacent sites are treated by parallel opposed beams. For such beams, the dose prescription is usually made at the midplane of the patient. The beam edges can also be matched at the patient's midplane.

Figures 15.50a to d consider the use of different skin gaps for two adjacent sites treated by fields of lengths 12 cm and 15 cm at an SAD of 80 cm. In Figure 15.50a, no skin gap is used, and the field edges are matched on the skin. It is seen that an overdose of up to 170% occurs at the junction. The skin gap which would match the field edges at the midplane without overlap is calculated in the next example.

EXAMPLE 15.4

The patient's thickness at the junction is 18 cm.

$$L_1 = 12\,\text{cm}, \quad L_2 = 15\,\text{cm}, \quad d = 18/2 = 9\,\text{cm}, \quad SAD = 80\,\text{cm}$$
$$\text{Skin gap } S = \frac{d(L_1 + L_2)}{2 \times SAD} = \frac{9(12 + 15)}{2 \times 80} \approx 1.5\,\text{cm}$$

The dose distribution obtained with the above 1.5-cm skin gap is shown in Figure 15.50b. There are cold spots at shallow depths under the skin gap. Figure 15.50c

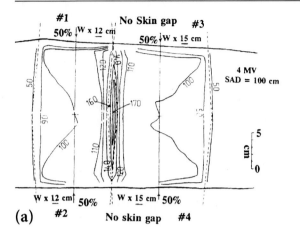

(a)

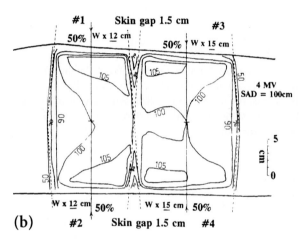

(b)

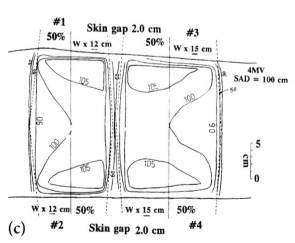

(c)

Fig. 15.50a–f. Dose distribution for adjacent sites treated with 4-MV X-ray beams. (a) to (d) Both sites treated by opposing beams: (a) with edges matched on the skin, leaving no skin gap; (b) with a calculated 1.5-cm skin gap to match the edges of the beams at the patient's midline; (c) with a 2-cm skin gap; (d) with a 1.5-cm calculated gap and 'feathering' in three steps, with moving of the junction from a-a′ to b-b′ to c-c′. (e) and (f) The left site is treated by opposing beams with 100% dose at the midline. The right site is treated by a beam from one side only, with 100% dose at 5 cm depth. (e) A calculated skin gap of 1.0 cm is used which matches the edges of the new beam with the previously treated beam at 5 cm depth. (f) A skin gap of 1.5 cm to match the edges of all three beams at the midline

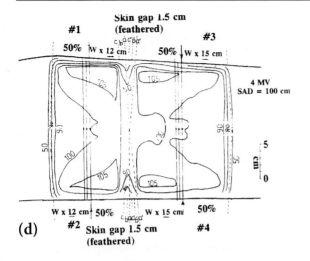

(d)

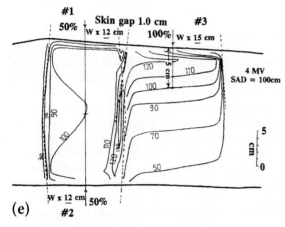

(e)

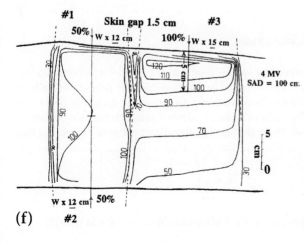

(f)

Fig. 15.50d–f.

n gap of 2.0 cm, which results in a 60% cold spot at the junc-
ot enough merely to use a skin gap and accept the cold spots.
use to remove the extent of underdosing below the skin gap
hs of the adjacent fields and to move or 'feather' the junction
reatment. This can be done only when both sites are treated con-
of feathering is illustrated in Figure 15.50d, where the position of
nges from a-a′ to b-b′ and to c-c′ during three successive segments
he greater the number of segments, the less can be the inadequacy
of an‚   ‚r the severity of a resulting hot spot. Feathering once a week can be
a clinically pr‚‚ticable procedure. Feathering can also diffuse the consequence of any
random errors in daily positioning and setup.

15.12.4
Matching Opposed Beams with a Single Beam

In Figures 15.50e and f, we consider a site previously treated by parallel opposed beams,
with the dose prescribed to the midline. Let us say that an adjacent site is now to be
treated by a beam from only one side of the patient and that the dose is prescribed at a
depth of 5 cm. We assume that the dose prescribed for the current treatment is the same
as that delivered at the previously treated site. First, let us match the new field edge at
5 cm depth with the previously treated beam from its own side only (i. e., ignoring the
second beam that irradiated the patient from the opposite side). This suggests a skin gap
of 1.0 cm. Figure 15.50e shows the resulting dose distribution. There is a considerable
overlap with the (ignored) beam from the opposite side at the junction, resulting in hot
spots of up to 140%. If the opposing beam is not to be ignored, the matching should
be done at the patient's midline. This needs a larger skin gap of 1.5 cm. Figure 15.50f
shows the dose distribution with the 1.5-cm skin gap. This avoids the overlap and the
high doses, but regions under the skin gap at shallow depths become underdosed. Such
trade-offs of hot spots and cold spots are unavoidable when adjacent sites are treated
with different fields. The physician's clinical insight and discretion should govern how
much dose to prescribe, where to position the junction, what level of a high or low dose
to accept, and what skin gap to use.

15.12.5
Angle Match Between Orthogonal Beams

In Figure 15.51, beam no. 1 treats the spinal column at the back of a patient. Beams 2
and 3 are laterally incident, parallel opposed beams that treat the patient's brain from
the sides. The continuous edges of beams 2 and 3 represent the beam outlines in the
patient's lateral midplane. The outlines shown by dashed lines are the field outlines at
the level of the surface of head where the beams enter. These are smaller because they
are at a distance closer to the source. The diverging angle of the edge of beam 1 is given
by

$$\tan \theta = \frac{0.5 \times L}{SAD}$$

where L is the field length of beam 1 at the SAD. Hence, $\theta = \tan^{-1}[(0.5L)/SAD]$.

Fig. 15.51. Angular matching
of orthogonal beams. Beam
no. 1 treats the patient from
the back. Beams 2 and 3 treat
the patient from the sides.
(a) Outlines of beams 2 and
3 are rotated to match the
diverging edge of beam 1 at
the patient's lateral midline.
(b) The diverging edges of
beams 2 and 3 are shown in
the plane perpendicular to the
central axis of beam 1. Angle
ϕ can be compensated for by a
couch rotation

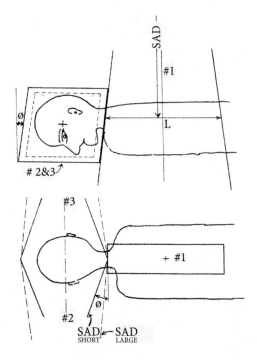

A rotation of the collimator by θ, for beams 2 and 3, will match their field outline at
the midplane with the edge of beam 1. The dashed edge (at the surface of entrance) also
can next be matched by a rotation of the patient's couch around a vertical axis through
an angle ϕ. In clinical practice, the light-beam localizer can be used for verifying that
the calculated angles do give the expected matches between the adjacent field edges on
the surface of the patient.

15.13
3D-CRT, SRT, IMRT

Delivery of a very high radiation dose to a well-defined target volume, without exceeding the tolerance of any other normal organ or tissue in the body has been a
major challenge for radiotherapy in general, and external-beam therapy in particular.
Much success of radiotherapy in the past could be attributed to striving for a constant
improvement in the above aspect. In an effort to increase the dose delivered to the
target, the physics of radiotherapy has made much progress. Irradiation of the skin
and subcutaneous tissues is unavoidable in external-beam therapy. Historically, the
most limiting case was the use of single kilovoltage x-ray beams. Through various progressive steps of combining multiple x-ray beams at angles with wedge filters, use of
cobalt-60 beams with a skin-sparing dose buildup, employment of machines capable of
isocentric rotation to distribute the subcutaneous dose, adopting even higher-energy
accelerator-produced X-ray beams in the 6-MV to 25-MV range, it has been possible to increase the dose delivered to tumors from 20–30 Gy to 65–68 Gy. We already

discussed in this chapter the need to plan judiciously both the orientation and the amount of radiation dose delivered by the individual beams in multiple beam arrangements that cross-fire toward the target. Of late, there have been discussions about the use of further improvements in technology to escalate the dose delivery to the range of 70–80 Gy. New terms such as 3D CRT (three-dimensional conformal radiotherapy), SRT (stereotactic radiotherapy), IMRT (intensity-modulated radiotherapy), and, tomotherapy, have come into vogue to refer to such recent technical advances. Although these terms and technologies are new, the concepts that they endeavor to extend are old. It is not within the scope of this text to deal with upcoming trends, except to mention them briefly. Interested readers are advised to study the references cited critically.

In '3D CRT', multiple beam arrangements are configured to irradiate the target, as was also done in conventional treatments [77–82]. The shape of each beam cross-section is planned to cover the target volume and block the normal tissues in the beam's-eye views, hence the name 'conformal.' To achieve this, a patient's digital CT scan images are transferred to computerized-graphic workstations, and the outlines of target volumes and organs to be protected are delineated. Unconventional or complex beam directions can be included and the beam's-eye views projected along with the DRR of the patient anatomy. The conventional wisdom that any chosen beam direction should lend itself to blocking of the normal organs without blocking of the tumor does still hold true (see Sect. 15.6.1). The beam shaping can be done with facility by multi-leaf collimators (MLCs), but properly shaped blocks of low-melting alloy can be used as well. '3D CRT' can be thought of as an improvement of some early techniques that went by the name of conformation therapy [83–85]. Old techniques used film-based radiographic images, analogue method of transfers tomography, and shaping of field cross-sections with conventional blocks, as compared to the much superior digital image processing and MLC employed in '3D CRT.'

SRT also is a category of conformal therapy that uses beams of very small cross sections (<1–$2\,cm^2$) to irradiate small lesions, especially in the brain [86]. For SRT therapy, linear accelerators can be used with special collimator attachments that produce the tiny beams. A 'gamma knife' is another specially designed treatment machine that uses about 200 single cobalt-60 sources for stereotactic irradiation. The sources are set up in a hemispherical array in a source head [87]. Each radiation source can provide a collimated narrow beam, giving the possibility of several beams converging to a focal point of irradiation in the patient. Because of the smallness of the volume treated, special efforts are needed in SRT for both localizing the volume and focusing the beams.

In IMRT, a modular intensity (that is, fluence) pattern is created within the cross section of each beam [88–90]. The distinction between IMRT and '3D CRT' is that, in the latter, any region within a beam cross-section is merely blocked or left open. The intensity modules within an IMRT beam are created by configuring of different MLC arrangements and delivery through them of different monitor units. (It is relevant to note that the wedge filters and compensating filters accomplish a similar function of causing an intensity variation) [91–94]. The size of the rectangular intensity modules is dictated by the width of the leaves of the MLC. Each module is, in fact, a narrow pencil beam. The smaller the width of the leaves, the finer can be the size of the modules. Like conventional treatments, IMRT treatments also essentially rely on dividing the total dose to be delivered in an appropriate manner among many incident beams. IMRT also depends strongly on the strategy of cross-firing beams from several, appropriately chosen, directions (as discussed in Sect. 15.6.1). However, each beam in IMRT is made up of a multitude of 'sub-beams' (or 'beam-lets'). The treatment is done by computer-controlled MLC changes. Both dynamic MLC changes and step-by-step MLC changes during dose delivery have been used [95–98].

With so many beams and variables to be selected, a reliance on mathematical formulations for optimizing both the shape of these sub-beams and the amount of radiation fluence delivered by them becomes essential. Different constraints based mathematical optimization methods have been adopted [99–104]. Such methods have been used in operations research and industrial engineering and have gradually been adopted for radiotherapy [105, 106]. In general, they permit dose limits to be set for the points that cover the sensitive organs and maximize the dose and uniformity of dose among points in the target volume. This is equivalent to setting upper and lower limits for the dose D_i (see Section 15.5.2 and 15.5.3) at various points in the patient, to obtain several constrained algebraic sums. Use of such mathematically constrained optimization methods is being referred to as 'inverse' planning. This is unlike 'forward' planning, in which a user starts with an already chosen beam combination and strives to improve it, by his experience or insight, in a trial-and-error process.

Many times any mathematical optimization may also start with a tentative initial plan and improve it by a back-and-forth iterative, corrective process to reach an optimum plan based on either random or gradient search methods. The true merit of such an optimized plan will depend on the correctness of the assumptions behind the formulations. Such formulations cover dose calculation algorithms, cost functions and constraints governing the dose response of normal tissues and structures, the definition and the extent of the target volumes, and the degree of non-uniformity of the dose acceptable there. All optimizations are subject to the limits inherent in the physics of penetration and propagation of the radiation beam. If the mathematical conditions set are physically impossible unrealistic solutions with negative fluence values may be obtained. (This is like needing to incorporate negative values of G_i in the linear sums for D_i in Sect. 15.5.2 and 15.5.3). If this happens, the impractical conditions will need to be relaxed, and compromises made for obtaining realistic solutions.

The intensity-modulated beams depend on blocking of some chosen modules while delivering radiation through other selected open modules. The open and closed modules change as more and more irradiation is done. The process continues in repetitive irradiations until the intensity sought in each module is attained. Hence, the number of monitor units needed per treatment increases to 3–10 times the value used in conventional treatments for delivering the same daily fractional dose. Thus, IMRT uses the treatment time and monitor units inefficiently. The total monitor units used increase the leakage radiation through the source-head per treatment. This has implications of not only increasing the whole-body dose to the patient, but also the room shielding requirements [107–109]. Furthermore, 6-MV x-rays are thought of as optimum for IMRT as beams of higher energies can cause a greater neutron fluence that is of radiation safety concern [110].

Tomotherapy can be regarded as a variation of IMRT done with a rotating fan beam with slits. It irradiates one thin planar transverse section of the patient at a time and spirals along the patient's axis to irradiate a 3D volume [111].

15.14
Concluding Remarks

The Physics of radiotherapy has always addressed the need to confine the high-dose region to a target volume and spare the damage to normal tissues. In the past, different techniques and solutions have been found for different contexts of tumors, body sites, and anatomy. These include electron therapy, intra-operative radiotherapy, and brachytherapy. The treatment planning should be considered as a convergent process, with newer techniques and innovations adding the new terms toward reaching an ultimate converging solution. Adding a sophisticated computer-driven technology to deliver a mathematically optimized treatment can warrant a greater vigil to test the reliability of both its hardware and software performance. Such quality assurance may call for a very time-consuming evaluation and verification of dose delivery from patient to patient and treatment to treatment [112]. Studies are under way to see whether such superior technical innovations can also translate into superior clinical outcome and be cost-effective [89, 113–117]. There are several questions to be answered for which the critical faculty of physicists may be called for [118].

Glossary of Acronyms
(Used in Chapter 15)

AZ	Annular zone	PTV	Planning target volume
BZ	Buildup zone	PZ	Penumbra zone
CT	Computed-tomography	SAD	Source to axis distance
CTV	Clinical target volume	SSD	Source to skin distance
DRR	Digitally reconstructed radiograph	SM	Setup margin
DVH	Dose-volume histogram	SRT	Stereotactic Radiotherapy
ENZ	Entrance zone	TAR	Tissue-air ratio
EXZ	Exit zone	TMR	Tissue maximum ratio
GTV	Gross tumor volume	TZ	Target zone
IM	Internal margin	3D	Three-dimensional
IMRT	Intensity-modulated radiotherapy	3D CRT	Three-dimensional conformal
MLC	Multi-leaf collimators		radiotherapy
PDD	Percent depth dose	2D	Two-dimensional

References

1. Tepper, J.E., and Chaney, E.C. (Eds.), Three-Dimensional Treatment Planning, Seminars in Oncology, Vol 2 (No. 4), W.B. Saunders, Philadelphia, 1992.
2. Goitein, M., and Mark, A., Multi-dimensional treatment planning. I. Delineation of anatomy, Int. J. Radiat. Oncol. Biol. Phys., Vol 9, p777–787, 1983.
3. Goitein, M., Abrams, D., Rowell, H., Pollari, H., and Wiles, J., Multi-dimensional treatment planning. II. Beam's-eye-view, back projection, and projection through CT sections, Int. J. Radiat. Oncol. Biol. Phys., Vol 9, pp789–797.
4. Mohan, R., Barest, G., Brewster, L.J., Chui, C.S., Kutcher, G.J., Laughlin, J.S., and Fuks, Z., A comprehensive three-dimensional radiation treatment planning system, Int. J. Radiat. Oncol. Biol. Phys., Vol 15, pp481–495, 1988.
5. Rosenman, J., Sherouse, G.W., Fuchs, H., Pizer, S.M., Skinner, A.L., Mosher, C., Novins, K., and Tepper, J.E., Three-dimensional display techniques in radiation therapy treatment planning, Int. J. Radiat. Oncol. Biol. Phys., Vol 16, pp263–269, 1989.

6. Jacky, J., 3-D radiation therapy treatment planning: Overview and assessment, Am. J. Clin. Oncol., Vol 13, pp331–343, 1990.
7. Nishida, T., Nagata, Y., Takahashi, M., Abe, M., Yamaoka, N., Ishihara, H., Kubo, Y., Ohta, H., and Kazusa, C., CT simulator, a new 3-D planning simulating system for radiotherapy: I. Description of system, Int. J. Radiat. Oncol. Biol. Phys., Vol 18, pp499–504, 1990.
8. McShan, D.L., Frass, B.A., and Lichter, A.S., Full integration of the beam's eye view concept into computerized treatment planning, Int. J. Radiat. Oncol. Biol. Phys., Vol 18, pp1485–1494, 1990.
9. Ling, C.L., Rodgers, C.C., and Morton, R.J. (Eds.), Computed Tomography in Radiotherapy, Raven Press, Washington, D.C., 1982.
10. Tsien, K.C., and Cohen, M., Isodose Charts and Tables for Medium Energy X-Rays, Butterworths, London, 1962.
11. Webster, E.W., and Tsien, K.C., Atlas of Dose Distributions, Vol I, Single-field Isodose Charts, International Atomic Energy Agency, Vienna, Austria, 1965.
12. Munro, P., Rawlinson, J.A., and Fenster, A., Therapy imaging: Source sizes of radiotherapy beams, Med. Phys., Vol 15, pp517–524, 1988.
13. ICRU, International Commission on Radiological Units and Measurements, Determination of absorbed dose in a patient irradiated by beams of x or gamma rays in radiotherapy procedures, ICRU Report 24, International Commission on Radiological Units and Measurements, Washington, D.C., 1976.
14. Bush, R.S., and Johns, H.E., The measurement of build-up on curved surfaces exposed to cobalt-60 and cesium-137 beams, Am. J. Roentgenol., Vol 87, pp89–93, 1962.
15. Jackson, W., Surface effects of high-energy X-rays at oblique incidence, Br. J. Radiol., Vol 44, pp109–115, 1971.
16. Orton, C.G., and Seibert, J.B., Depth dose in skin for obliquely incident cobalt-60 radiation, Br. J. Radiol., Vol 45, pp271–275, 1972.
17. Hughes, H.A., Measurements of superficial absorbed dose with 2 MV X-rays used at glancing angles, Br. J. Radiol., Vol 32, pp255–258, 1959.
18. Gagnon, W.F., and Peterson, M.D., Comparison of skin doses to large fields using tangential beams from cobalt-60 gamma rays and 4 MV X-rays, Radiology, Vol 127, pp785–788, 1978.
19. Klein, E.C., and Purdy, J.A., Entrance and exit dose regions for a Clinac-2100, Int. J. Radiat. Oncol. Biol. Phys., Vol 27, pp429–435, 1993.
20. Khan, F.M., Use of electron filter to reduce skin dose in cobalt-60 teletherapy, Am. J. Roentgenol., Vol 111, pp180–181, 1971.
21. Saylor, W.L., and Quillin, R.M., Methods for enhancement of skin sparing in cobalt-60 teletherapy, Am. J. Roentgenol., Vol 111, pp174–179, 1971.
22. Khan, F.M., Moore, V.C., and Levitt, S.H., Effect of various atomic number absorbers on skin dose for 10 MV X-rays, Radiology, Vol 109, pp209–212, 1973.
23. Rao, P.S., Pillai, K., and Gregg, E.C., Effect of shadow trays on surface dose and build-up for megavoltage radiation, Am. J. Roentgenol., Vol 117, pp168–174, 1973.
24. Leung, P.M.K., and Johns, H.E., Use of electron filters to improve the build-up characteristics of large fields from cobalt-60, Med. Phys., Vol 4, pp441–444, 1977.
25. Gagnon, W.F., and Horton, W.L., Physical factors affecting absorbed dose to the skin from cobalt-60 gamma rays and 25 MV X-rays, Med. Phys., Vol 6, pp285–290, 1979.
26. ICRU, Report 50, Prescribing, Recording, and Reporting Photon Beam Therapy, International Commission on Radiological Units and Measurements, Bethesda, MD, USA, 1993.
27. ICRU, Report 62, Prescribing, Recording, and Reporting Photon Beam Therapy (Supplement to ICRU Report 50), International Commission on Radiological Units and Measurements, Bethesda, MD, USA, 1999.
28. Tranter, F.W., Design of wedge filters for use with 4 MeV linear accelerator, Br. J. Radiol., Vol 30, pp329–330, 1957.
29. Cohen, M., Burns, J.E., and Sear, R., Physical aspects of cobalt-60 therapy using wedge filters. I. Physical investigation, Acta Radiol., Vol 53, pp401–413, 1960.
30. Cohen, M., Burns, J.E., and Sear, R., Physical aspects of cobalt-60 therapy using wedge filters. II. Dosimetric considerations, Acta Radiol., Vol 53, pp486–504, 1960.
31. van de Geijn, J.A., A simple wedge filter technique for cobalt 60 teletherapy, Br. J. Radiol., Vol 35, pp710–712, 1962.
32. Aron, B.S., and Scappicchio, M., Design of universal wedge filter system for a cobalt 60 unit, Am. J. Roentgenol., Vol 96, pp70–74, 1966.
33. Kijewski, PK., Chin, L.M., Bjarngard, B.E., Wedge-shaped dose distributions by computer-controlled collimator motion, Med. Phys., Vol. 5, pp426–429, 1978.
34. Leavitt, D.D., Martin, M., Moeller, J.H., and Lee, W.L., Dynamic wedge field techniques through computer-controlled collimator motion and dose delivery, Med. Phys., Vol. 17, pp87–91, 1991.

35. Klein, E.E., Low, D.A., Meigooni, A.S., and Purdy, J.A., Dosimetry and clinical implementation of dynamic wedge, Int. J. Radiat. Oncol. Biol. Phys., Vol. 31, pp583–591, 1995.
36. Zhu, X.R., Gillin, M.T., Jursinic, P.A., Lopez, F., Grimm, D.F., and Rownd, J.J., Comparison of dosimetric characteristics of Siemens virtual and physical wedges, Med. Phys., Vol. 27, pp2267–2277, 2000.
37. Doppke, K., Novack, D.H., and Wang, C.C., Physical considerations in the treatment of advanced carcinomas of the larynx and pyriform sinuses using 10 MV X-rays, Int. J. Radiat. Oncol. Biol. Phys., Vol 6, pp1251–1255, 1980.
38. Binder, W., and Karcher, K.H., 'Super-stuff' als Bolus in der Strahlentherapie, Strahlentherapie, Vol 153, pp754–757, 1977.
39. Ellis, F., Hall, E.J., and Oliver, R., A compensator for variations in tissue thickness for high energy beam, Br. J. Radiol., Vol 32, pp421–422, 1959.
40. Khan, F.M., Moore, V.C., and Burns, D.J., The construction of compensators for cobalt teletherapy, Radiology, Vol 96, pp187–192, 1970.
41. Sewchand, W., Bautro, N., and Scott, R.M., Basic data of tissue equivalent compensators for 4 MV X-rays, Int. J. Radiat. Oncol. Biol. Phys., Vol 6, pp327–332, 1980.
42. Khan, F.M., Williamson, J.F., Sewchand, W., and Kim, T.H., Basic data for dosage calculation and compensation, Int. J. Radiat. Oncol. Biol. Phys., Vol 6, pp745–751, 1980.
43. Leung, P.M.K., Van Dyk, J., and Robins, J., A method for large irregular field compensation, Br. J. Radiol., Vol 47, pp805–810, 1974.
44. Cohen, M., and Martin, S.J., Atlas of Dose Distributions, Vol II, Multiple-Field Isodose Charts, International Atomic Energy Agency, Vienna, Austria, 1966.
45. Tsien, K.C., Cunningham, J.R., Wright, D.J., Jones, D.E.A., and Pfalzner, P.F., Atlas of Dose Distributions, Vol III, Moving-Field Isodose Charts, International Atomic Energy Agency, Vienna, Austria, 1967.
46. ICRU, Use of Computers in External Beam Radiotherapy Procedures with High Energy Photons and Electrons, ICRU Report 42, International Commission on Radiological Units and Measurements, Betheda, Maryland, USA, 1987.
47. Ahnesjo, A, and Asprdakis, M.M., Dose calculations for external photon beams in radiotherapy, Phys. Med. Biol., Vol. 44, pp R99–R155, 1999.
48. Jayaraman, S., An analytical beam model for computer based cobalt-60 treatment planning, Strahlentherapie, Vol. 157, pp459–469, 1981.
49. Rosenow, U., Qualitätskontrolle in der Bestrahlungsplanung, Z. Med. Phys., Vol. 1, pp59–67, 1991.
50. IPEMB, A guide to commissioning and quality control of treatment planning systems, IBEMP Report 68, Institution of Physics and Engineering in Medicine and Biology, York, England, 1996.
51. Van Dyk, J., Barnett, R.B., Cygler, J.E., and Shragge, P.C., Commissioning and quality assurance of treatment planning computers, Int. J. Rad. Onc. Biol. Phys. 26, pp261–273, 1993.
52. AAPM, Radiation Therapy Committee Task Group 53, Quality Assurance of Clinical Radiotherapy Treatment Planning, Med. Phys., Vol. 25, pp1773–1829, 1998.
53. Bomford, C.K., Dawes, P.J.D.K., Lillicrap, S.C., and Young, D.J., Treatment Simulators, Brit. J. Radiol. Supplement 23, British Inst. of Radiology, London, 1989.
54. McCullough, E.C., and Earl, J.D., The selection, acceptance testing, and quality control of radiotherapy treatment simulators, Radiology, Vol 131, pp221–230, 1979.
55. Karzmark, C.J., and Rust, D.C., Radiotherapy simulators and automation, Radiology, Vol 105, pp157–161, 1972.
56. Coia, L, Shultheiss, T., and Hanks, G., A practical guide to CT-simulation, Advanced Medical Publishing, Madison, Wisconsin, USA, 1995.
57. Withers, H.R., Taylor, J.M.G, and Maciejewski, B., Treatment volume and tissue tolerance, Int. J. Radiat. Oncol. Biol. Phys., Vol. 59, pp751–759, 1988
58. Kallman, P., Agren, A., and Brahme, A., Tumor and normal tissue responses to fractionated non uniform dose delivery, Int. J. Radiat. Oncol. Biol. Phys., Vol. 62, pp249–262, 1992.
59. Jayaraman, S., Asbell, S.O., Dose volume histograms can be interpreted in different ways, Letter to Editor, Cancer Investigation, Vol. 15, pp611–613, 1997.
60. Mayneord, W.V., The measurement of radiation for medical purposes, Nature, Vol 149, p600–601, 1942.
61. Rozenfeld, M., Treatment planning with external beams. Introduction and historical overview, Radiographics, Vol 8, pp557–571, 1988.
62. Hendrickson, F.R., Radiation treatment planning. The physician's role, Radiographics, Vol 8, pp987–991, 1988.
63. Jayaraman, S., Pathways and pitfalls in treatment planning with external beams: The role of the clinical physicist, Radiographics, Vol 8, pp1147–1170, 1988.
64. Hopfan, S., Reid, A., Simpson, L., and Ager, P.J., Clinical complications arising from overlapping of adjacent radiation fields, Int. J. Radiat. Oncol. Biol. Phys., Vol 2, pp801–808, 1977.

65. Agarwal, S.K., Marks, R.D., and Constable, W.C., Adjacent field separation for homogeneous dosage at a given depth for the 8 MV (Mevatron 8) linear accelerator, Am. J. Roentgenol., Vol 114, pp623–630, 1972.
66. Armstrong, D.J., The matching of adjacent fields in radiotherapy, Radiology, Vol 108, pp419–422, 1973.
67. Williamson, T.J., A technique for matching orthogonal megavoltage fields, Int. J. Radiat. Oncol. Biol. Phys., Vol 5, pp111–116, 1979.
68. Hale, J., Davis, L.W., and Bloch, P., Portal separation for pairs of parallel opposed portals at 2 MV and 6 MV, Am. J. Roentgenol., Vol 114, pp172–175, 1972.
69. Frass, B.A., Tepper, J.E., Glatstein, E. et al., Clinical use of a match line wedge for adjacent megavoltage radiation field matching, Int. J. Radiat. Oncol. Biol. Phys., Vol 9, pp209–216, 1983.
70. Svensson, G.K., Bjarngard, B.E., Chen, G.T.Y. et al., Superficial doses in treatment of breast with tangential fields using 4 MV X-rays, Int. J. Radiat. Oncol. Biol. Phys., Vol 2, pp705–710, 1977.
71. Burkoritz, A., Deutsch, M., and Slayton, R., Orthogonal fields, Variation in dose vs. gap size for treatment of the central nervous system, Radiology, Vol 126, pp795–798, 1978.
72. Gillin, M.T., and Kline, R.W., Field separation between lateral and anterior fields on a 6 MV linear accelerator, Int. J. Radiat. Oncol. Biol. Phys., Vol 6, pp233–237, 1980.
73. Dupont, J.C., Rosenwald, J.C., and Beauvais, H., Convolution calculations of dose in the build-up regions of high energy photon beams obliquely incident, Med. Phys., Vol 21, pp1391–1400, 1994.
74. Siddon, R.L., Tonnesen, G.L., and Svensson, G.K., Three field techniques for breast treatment using a rotatable half-beam block, Int. J. Radiat. Oncol. Biol. Phys., Vol 7, pp1473–1477, 1981.
75. Johnson, P.M., and Kepka, A., A double junction technique for total central nervous system irradiation with a 4 MV accelerator, Radiology, Vol 145, pp467–471, 1982.
76. Van Dyk, J., Jenkins, R.D.T., Leung, P.M.K. et al., Medulloblastoma treatment technique and irradiation dosimetry, Int. J. Radiat. Oncol. Biol. Phys., Vol 2, pp993–1005, 1977.
77. Powlis, W.D., Smith, A.R., Cheng, J.M., Galvin, F., Villari, F., Bloch, P., and Kligerman, M., "Initiation of multi-leaf collimator for conformal radiation therapy, Int. J. rad. Oncol. Biol. Phys., Vol. 25, pp171–179, 1993.
78. Webb, S, The Physics of three dimensional radiation Therapy: conformal therapy, radiosurgery and treatment planning, Institute of Physics Publishing, Bristol, UK, 1993.
79. Webb S, The physics of conformal radiotherapy, Institute of Physics Publishing, Bristol, UK, 1997.
80. Purdy, J.A., Starkschall, G., (Ed.), A practical guide to 3-D planning and conformal radiotherapy, Advanced Medical Publishing, Madison, Wisconsin, USA, 1999.
81. Tubiana, M., and Eschwege, F., Conformal radiotherapy and intensity modulated radiotherapy, Acta Oncol., Vol. 39, pp555–567, 2000.
82. Purdy, J.A., Grant III, W., Palta, J.R., Butler, E.B., and Perez, C.A., (Ed.) 3-D conformal and intensity modulated radiation therapy: Physics and clinical applications, Advanced Medical Publishing, Madison, Wisconsin, 2001.
83. Takahashi, S., Conformation radiotherapy: Rotation techniques as applied to radiography and radiotherapy of cancer, Acta Radiol., Suppl. Vol. 242, pp1–142, 1965.
84. Morita, K, and Kawabe, Y., Late effects on the eye of conformation radiotherapy of the paranasal sinuses and nasal cavity, Radiology, Vol. 130, pp227–232, 1979.
85. Morita, K., Cancer of the cervix, In Medical Radiology: Diagnostic imaging and radiation oncology. Radiation Oncology of Gynecological Cancer, Ed: Vahrson, H.W., Springer Verlag, Heidelberg, 1997.
86. Kondiziolka, D., (Ed), Radiosurgery, Vol. 4., Proceedings of 5th international stereotactic radiosurgery Society meeting, Las Vegas, Nev., June 10–13, 2001, S. Karger AG, Basel, 2002.
87. Flickinger, J.C., and Bloomer, W.D., Physics of gamma knife approach on convergent beams in stereotactic radiosurgery, Int. J. Radiat. Oncol. Biol. Phys., Vol. 18, pp941–949, 1990.
88. Sternick,E.S., (Ed.), The theory and practice of intensity-modulated radiation therapy, Advanced Medical Publishing, Madison, Wisconsin, USA, 1998.
89. IMRT Collaborative Working Group, Intensity modulated radiotherapy, Current status and issues of interest, Int. J. Radiat. Oncol. Biol. Phys., Vol. 51, pp880–914, 2001.
90. Webb, S., Intensity modulated radiation therapy, Institute of Physics Publishing, Bristol, UK, 2001.
91. Galvin, J.M., Chen, X.G., Smith, R.M., Combining multi-leaf field to modulate fluence distributions, Int. J. Radiat. Oncol. Biol. Phys., Vol. 27, pp697–705, 1993.
92. Bortfield, T.R., Kahler, D., Waldron, T.J., and Boyer, A.L., X-ray field compensation with multileaf collimators, Int. J. Radiat. Oncol. Biol. Phys., Vol. 28, pp72-3-730, 1994.
93. Hansen, V.N., Evans, P.M., Shentall, G.S., Helyer, S.J., Yarnold, J.R., Swindell, W. Dosimetric evaluation of compensation in radiotherapy of the breast: MLC intensity modulation and physical compensators. Radiother. Oncol. 42, pp249–256, 1997.
94. Mageras, G.S., Mohan, R., Burman, C., Barest, G.D., and Kutcher, G.J., Compensators for three dimensional treatment planning, Med. Phys., Vol. 18, pp133–140, 1991.

95. Yu, C, X., Symons, M.J., Du, M.N., Martinez, A. A., Wong, W.J., A method for implementing dynamic photon beam intensity modulation using independent jaws and a multileaf collimator, Phys. Med. Biol., Vol. 40, pp769–787, 1995.

96. Xia, P., and Verhey, L., Multileaf collimator leaf-sequencing algorithm for intensity modulated beams with multiple static segments, Med. Phys., Vol. 25, pp1424–1434, 1998.

97. Frass, B.A., Kessler, M.L., McShan, D.L., et al., Optimization and clinical use of multi-segment intensity modulated radiation therapy for high-dose conformal therapy, Semin. Radiat. Oncol., Vol. 9, pp60–77, 1999.

98. Webb, S., A new concept of multileaf collimator (the shuttling MLC) - an interpreter for high-efficiency IMRT, Phys. Med. Biol., Vol.45, pp3343–3358, 2000.

99. Brahme, A., Optimization of stationary and moving beam radiation therapy techniques, Radio-ther. Oncol., Vol. 12, pp129–140, 1988.

100. Lind, B.K., Properties of an algorithm for solving the inverse problem in radiation therapy, Inverse Problems, Vol. 6, pp415–426, 1990.

101. Shepard, D.M., Olivera, G.H., Reckwerdt, P.J., and Mackie, T.R., Iterative approaches to dose optimization in tomotherapy, Vol. 45, pp69–90, 2000.

102. Morril, S.M., Lane, R.G., Jacobson, G, and Rosen, I., Treatment planning optimization using constrained simulated annealing, Phys. Med. Biol., Vol. 36, pp1341–61, 1991.

103. Wu, Q., Mohan, R., Algorithms and functionality of an intensity modulated radiotherapy optimization system, Med. Phys., Vol. 27, pp701–711, 2000.

104. Brahme, A., Treatment optimization using physical and radiobiological objective functions, In Smith, A.R., (Ed.) Radiationtherapy Physics, Springer-Verlag, Berlin, 1995.

105. Winston, W.L., Operations Research Applications and Algorithms, Wadsworth Publishing, Belmont, Califormnia, 1991.

106. Jayaraman, S, Shaping of isodose curves in intracavitary irradiation using afterloading methods-A feasibility study involving mathematical simulation by computer, Radiology, Vol. 120, pp435–438, 1976.

107. Followill, D., Geis, P., Boyer, A., Estimates of whole-body dose equivalent produced by beam intensity conformal therapy, Int. J. Radiat. Oncol. Biol. Phys., Vol. 38, pp667–672, 1997.

108. Verellen, D., and Vanhavere, F., Risk assessment of radiation-induced malignancies based on whole-body equivalent dose estimates for IMRT treatment in the head and neck region, Radiother. Oncol., Vol. 53, pp199–203, 1999.

109. Mutic, S., Low, D.A., Klein, E.E., Dempsey, J.F., and Purdy, J.A., Room shielding for intensity modulated radiationtherapy treatment facilities, Int. J. Radiat. Oncol. Biol. Phys., Vol. 50, pp239–246, 2001.

110. Rawlinson, J.A., Islam, M.K., and Galbraith, D.M., Dose to radiation therapists from activation at high-energy accelerators used for conventional and intensity modulated radiation therapy, Med. Phys., Vol. 29, pp598–608, 2002.

111. Mackie, T.R., Holmes, T., Swerdloff, S., Reckwerdt, P., Deasy, J.O., Yang, J., Paliwal, B., Kinsella, T., Tomotherapy: a new concept for the delivery of dynamic conformal radiotherapy. Med. Phys. 20, 1709–19, 1993.

112. Xing, L., Curran, B., Hill, R., Holmes, R., Ma, L., Forster, K.M., and Boyer, A. L., Dosimetric verification of a commercial inverse treatment planning system, Phys. Med. Biol., Vol. 44, pp463–478, 1999.

113. Xia, P., Fu, K.K., Wong, G.W., Akazawa, C., Verhey, L.J., Comparison of treatment plans involving intensity modulated radiotherapy for nasopharyngeal carcinoma, Int. J. Radiat. Oncol. Biol. Phys., Vol. 48, pp329–337, 2000.

114. Chao, K.S., Low, D.A., Perez, C.A., et al., Intensity modulated radiationtherapy in head and neck cancers: The Mallincrodt experience, Int. J. Cancer, Vol. 90, pp92–103, 2000.

115. Lee, N., Xia, P., Quivey, J.M., Sultanem, K., Poon, I., Akazawa, C., Akazawa, P., Weinberg, V., Fu, K.K., Intensity modulated radiation therapy in the treatment of nasopharrygeal carcinoma: An update of the UCSF experience, Int J Radiat. Oncol. Biol. Phys., Vol. 53, pp12–22, 2002.

116. Nutting, C., Dearnaley, D.P., and Webb, S., Intensity-modulated radiation therapy: A clinical review, Br. J. Radiol., Vol. 73, pp459–469, 2000.

117. Grant W., III and Woo, S. Y., Clinical and financial issues for intensity-modulated radiation therapy delivery, Semin. Radiat. Oncol., Vol. 9, pp99–107, 1999.

118. Schultz, R.J., and Kagan, A.R., On the role of intensity-modulated radiation therapy in radiation oncology, Med. Phys., Vol. 29, pp1473–1482, 2002.

CHAPTER 16

Physical Aspects of Electron Beam Therapy

16.1
Electron Transport

For the clinical applications of electron beams, the physical behavior of electrons has to be well understood. In this chapter, we discuss the fundamental features of electron transport and the ways in which they influence the dose distribution patterns. Electrons are more complex than photons in their transport behavior. The dose distribution for electron beams can be well documented for standard conditions of a beam incident on a unit-density medium with a flat surface. For nonstandard situations that may be encountered in actual clinical contexts, the interpretation and prediction of electron beam dose distributions pose many challenges.

In Chapter 4, we discussed the collision and radiation energy losses suffered by charged particles. The electrons in a clinical electron beam also undergo such energy losses. Apart from losing their energies, the electrons change their direction of motion in the electric fields of the nucleus and of the atomic orbital electrons in the target material [1–5]. These changes are caused by electron-nuclear scattering and electron-electron scattering. In electron-nuclear scattering with a high-Z nucleus, the large charge of the nucleus deflects the electron trajectory considerably. However, the energy loss suffered is negligible because the mass of the nucleus is much greater than that of the electron. The electron-nuclear scattering probability is proportional to Z^2/E, where E is the electron energy and Z is the nuclear charge.

Electron-electron scattering contributes not only to deflection of the path of the electron, but also to energy loss. The electron-electron scattering probability for any atom is approximately proportional to Z, which equals the number of electrons per atom. In high-Z materials, nuclear scattering predominates over scattering by electrons. The details of the scattering of electrons are explained well only by relativistic wave mechanics. Explanations based on principles of classical mechanics fail in the range of nuclear dimensions, which are of the order of 10^{-13} cm. In electron beam therapy, there are two regions in which an understanding of multiple scattering of electrons is of importance. One of these is the region between the electron source and the surface of the patient's body, and the other is the region within the body.

16.2
Electron Beam from Machine to Patient

The energetic electron beam emerging through the vacuum window of an accelerator is a very thin pencil beam and is not suitable for use on a patient. There are two established methods by which the electron fluence of the pencil beam can be spread

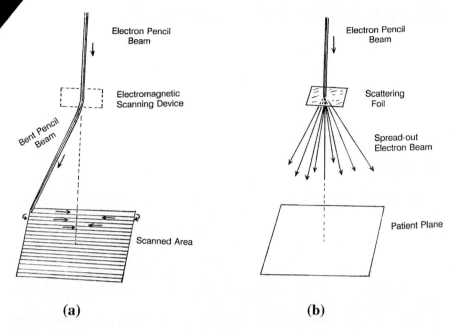

Fig. 16.1. Schematic diagrams of spreading of an electron pencil beam to cover a clinically useful area. (a) Use of electromagnetically steered scanning. (b) Use of a scattering foil

over a larger area. In one approach (illustrated in Figure 16.1a), an electromagnetic steering device is used which scans the pencil beam over a large area [6]. In the other approach (illustrated in Figure 16.1b), the electrons are spread over a large area by multiple scattering in foils made of a high-Z material that is interposed in the pencil beam [5, 7]. The thickness of the foils and the Z of its material together influence the number of multiple scattering events that can occur within it and the extent of spread of the beam. The foil also produces bremsstrahlung and contributes a photon component to the electron beam. The foil can be optimized to produce the desired angular spread with a very low bremsstrahlung component. Most commercially available electron beam machines are designed to give a choice of preselectable electron energies and at least one photon energy. Different scattering foils may be used for different electron energies.

Figure 16.2 illustrates an electron beam delivery system that incorporates two scattering foils: a primary scattering foil that spreads the electron beam and a secondary scattering foil that functions as a beam-flattening filter [7]. The broadened electron beam needs first to pass through the primary collimator, which is used for photons and electrons. The primary collimator is usually placed well above the level of the skin of the patient because it is a part of the treatment head. Because the electrons that strike the primary collimator are scattered further, a rather diffuse beam edge results. The electron beam edges can be sharply defined only if the collimation is extended toward the skin of the patient by attachment of trimmers, as shown in Figure 16.2. Without trimmers, the field projected by the light beam localizer through the primary photon

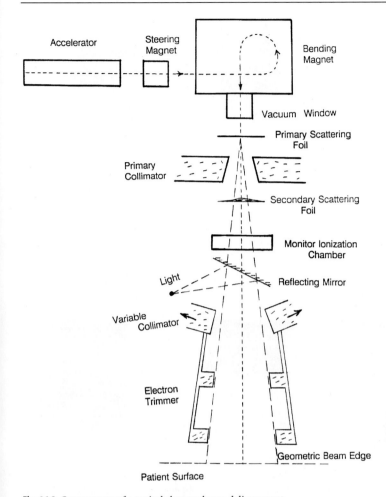

Fig. 16.2. Components of a typical electron beam delivery port

(variable) collimator will give a very misleading impression of the true electron field [8]. Usually, the primary collimating aperture and the trimmers for the electron beams are optimally designed to give an electron beam of uniform fluence, conforming to the light beam indication at the level of the patient's skin. The reflecting mirror shown in Figure 16.2 is retracted away from the beam during patient irradiation.

16.3
Electron Beam After Entering the Patient

Figure 16.3 is a photographic image of an electron beam of 22 MeV energy, alongside a 25-MV X-ray beam, as they enter and penetrate the body. The images were obtained by sandwiching of a film between polystyrene blocks and irradiation of the film. It will be observed that the electron beam penetrates to a finite depth with a clear-cut range.

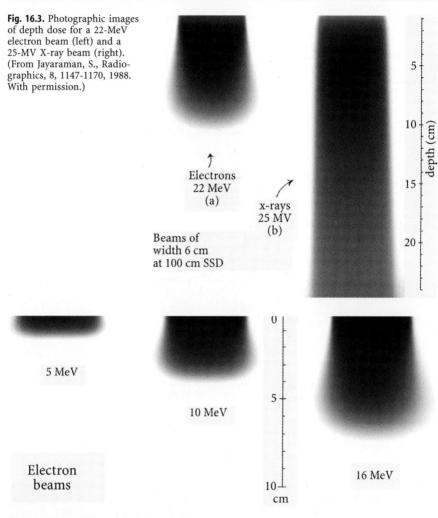

Fig. 16.3. Photographic images of depth dose for a 22-MeV electron beam (left) and a 25-MV X-ray beam (right). (From Jayaraman, S., Radiographics, 8, 1147-1170, 1988. With permission.)

Electrons
22 MeV
(a)

x-rays
25 MV
(b)

Beams of
width 6 cm
at 100 cm SSD

5 MeV

10 MeV

Electron
beams

16 MeV

Fig. 16.4. Photographic images of penetration of electron beams of different energies. (From Jayaraman, S., Radiographics, 8, 1147–1170, 1988. With permission.)

The photon beam, on the other hand, proceeds with no indication of any finite range. The range of penetration of the electron beam is a function of the electron energy. Figure 16.4 shows the film blackening for electron beams of different energies.

The dose distribution in an electron beam is influenced by the following:

(a) The energy loss interactions suffered by the incident primary electrons
(b) The extent of production of secondary electrons
(c) The change in direction and the dispersion of the electrons
(d) The bremsstrahlung contamination in the beam
(e) The beam divergence contributing to the inverse-square fall-off of the electron fluence.

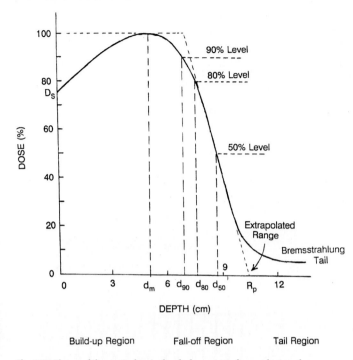

Fig. 16.5. Shape of the central-axis depth dose curve for an electron beam

The characteristics of the electrons, which undergo changes in their directions of travel and lose energy along their paths by ionization and excitation until all their energies are spent, influence the dose distributions resulting from electron beams.

The central-axis dose profile of a typical electron beam of 21 MeV energy is shown in Figure 16.5. The curve is made up of three segments: an initial increase, a fall-off, and a flat tail. The dose is D_S at the surface and increases to a peak value D_m at the depth d_m. The convention for normalization is to take this peak dose as 100%. Beyond depth dm, the dose falls off slowly at first, then quite rapidly in a straight line. Extrapolation of the straight-line segment to zero dose defines the maximum electron range R_p. This is referred to as the extrapolated range. The relatively flat tail in the depth-dose curve that is beyond the extrapolated range is attributable to the bremsstrahlung component in the beam.

The reason for the surface dose build-up of a photon beam was discussed in Section 11.3. It is caused by the build-up of the secondary-electron fluence. We explained that the dose delivered to a layer is approximately proportional to the number of electrons crossing that layer. In the case of electron beams also, secondary electrons are set in motion by the primary electrons. However, the dose build-up due to the increase in the number of secondary-electron tracks is marginal and is dominant only in the initial shallow depths.

A more significant effect than this is a dose build-up that occurs in electron beams as a direct result of their angular scattering and dispersion. This is illustrated in

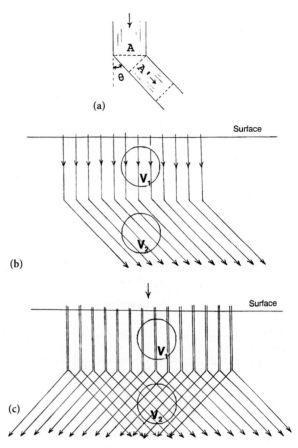

-up of electron angular disper-rons incident deflected by through area), which is smaller than A. (b) Multiple electron tracks deflected by angle θ pass through volumes V_1 and V_2 of identical dimensions. (c) Electrons are shown deflected to the right and left with equal probability

Figures 16.6a to c. The electrons, as they enter the patient, are essentially parallel and normal to the body surface. Figure 16.6a shows an electron beam incident on an area A, and deflected through an angle θ, which then passes through an area A'. The fact that A' is smaller than A, but the number of electron tracks has remained the same, means that the fluence and the dose have increased. This same phenomenon is illustrated in a different way in Figure 16.6b, where a series of electron tracks are deflected through an angle θ. Volumes V_1 and V_2 are identical in size. Being crossed by the inclined tracks, V_2 sees more fluence than does V_1, which is in the initial beam. The dose to V_2, thus, will be greater than that to V_1.

In the above discussion, the assumption that all electrons are deflected through the same angle θ with respect to the incident direction and travel parallel to each other does not correspond to reality. We made such a simple assumption merely to explain how angular deflection can contribute to a build-up of fluence and dose. In reality, neither do all electrons undergo the same angle of deflection, nor do they continue to travel parallel to each other.

To add just one further degree of complexity, in Figure 16.6c, we consider two possible directions of deflection for the electrons, to the left as well as to the right, with the same probability. The number of incident electrons has been doubled (con. to that in Figure 16.6b). The fluence in V_2 is greater than that in V_1. A lateral tronic equilibrium is created because, whereas some electrons are deflected away from reaching V_2, some others come into V_2 from the opposite side and compensate for the loss. (Overall, the flux in V_2 in Figure 16.6c is twice that in Figure 16.6b, because of the twofold increase in the number of incident electrons.) Figure 16.6c also shows how the beam broadens with depth due to angular dispersion.

With increasing depth, the electron-electron and electron-nuclear scattering cause the moving electrons to have progressively larger angles with the initial beam direction. The extent of the surface dose build-up changes as a function of the electron energy. Low-energy electrons undergo deflections by larger angles, and thus the surface dose build-up is greater at lower than at higher energies. One typical accelerator gave skin doses of 74%, 82%, and 93% of the peak dose for electron beams of 5 MeV, 10 MeV, and 16 MeV with a field of 10 cm × 10 cm cross section.

The fall-off part of the electron beam depth dose curve is caused by the finite range of travel of the primary electrons. The fall-off is steep, but gradual, indicating that different electrons penetrate to different depths. This is called 'range straggling.' An electron that suffers minimum angular scattering and travels mostly in a straight line will have the maximum depth of penetration. At any chosen depth, there will be a distribution of electron energies. This is because, even if all of the electrons incident on a material have the same initial energy, their energy losses occur in individual interactions. The statistical variations in the number of these interactions and the energy losses that occur in them cause a spread in electron energies. This is referred to as 'energy straggling.' The extrapolated range R_p is also called the 'practical range' of the electrons (Figure 16.5). The depth d_{50}, where the dose is 50% of the maximum dose, is the '50% range.'

We pointed out that the tail part of the depth dose curve is due to the bremsstrahlung component in the beam. The bremsstrahlung yield (see Chapter 4) increases with the energy of the electrons and the Z of the scattering foils. In practical situations, the bremsstrahlung tail may contribute a dose that is 0.5 to 5% of the maximum dose.

Because electrons are indistinguishable from one another, in an electron-electron interaction the electron with the higher energy is considered to be the primary electron and the lower-energy electron is regarded as the secondary electron.

16.4
Electron Beam Depth Dose Date

Central-axis depth dose curves for broad (compared to the range of the electrons) electron beams of different energies are shown in Figure 16.7. For routine clinical selection of electron beam energies, it is useful to have the depth dose features presented in the form shown in Table 16.1. 'Gradient' refers to the decrease in dose per unit depth. The features listed are strongly machine-dependent because the electron energy spectrum incident on the patient is greatly influenced by the design of the machine. The stated initial energy is a typical value specified by the manufacturer. The values of the characteristics as tabulated converge and become stable for broad beams. However, for narrow beams of dimensions comparable to the electron range, the absence of lateral electronic equilibrium can cause a considerable reduction in the depth dose values (see

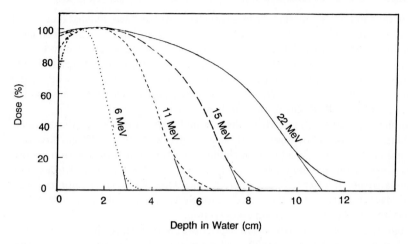

Fig. 16.7. Central-axis depth dose curves for broad electron beams of different energies

Sections 16.5 and 16.8). For any given electron beam, the depth dose characteristics tend to stabilize and become unique for large fields. Stated in terms of the extrapolated range R_p, the stability occurs for field diameters of $1.5\,R_p$ at 3.2 MeV, $1.0\,R_p$ at 8 MeV, and $0.6\,R_p$ at 15 MeV and above [9]. For broad beams in water, the following approximations hold, when the electron beam energy E is expressed in MeV:

$$R_p \approx E/2\,\text{cm}$$
$$D_{80\%} \approx E/3\,\text{cm}$$

The above expressions are not exact, but can provide some guidelines for treatment planning.

16.5
Planning a Simple Electron Beam Treatment

Electron beam treatments are generally designed for irradiation of the superficial regions of tissue up to a chosen depth. For example, let us say that the superficial lymph nodes in a patient's neck extend to an assessed maximum depth of 3 cm. It is decided to treat them with electrons in such a way that the deepest aspect of the nodes receives at least 90% of the peak dose. From Table 16.1, it can be seen that a 10-MeV electron beam can achieve this objective. The surface dose will be 82% of the peak dose, which helps to assure some degree of skin sparing. The skin sparing can be improved, when needed, by delivery of a part of the dose by a photon beam of 4 MV or from cobalt-60. At lower electron energies, the surface dose falls and a nonuniform dose distribution results from the surface to the depth of the peak dose. For this reason also, a part of the total dose might preferably be delivered by a photon beam. For very high-energy electron beams, the surface dose is nearly the same as the peak dose, and there is practically no advantage of a dose build-up. The difference between the depth of the 80% dose and that of the 10% dose is an indication of the excess tissue

Table 16.1. Typical Electron Beam Data for Broad Beams

Beam Energy (MeV)	Surface Dose (% of Peak Dose)	Depth (cm)					Practical Range (cm)
		d_m	d_{90}	d_{80}	d_{50}	d_{10}	R_p
5	74	0.9	1.2	1.4	1.7	2.2	2.3
7	76	1.6	2.0	2.2	2.7	3.3	3.4
10	82	2.4	3.1	3.4	3.9	4.8	4.9
13	88	3.2	4.0	4.3	5.1	6.1	6.4
16	93	3.4	5.1	5.6	6.5	8.0	8.0
19	94	2.6–3.6	5.9	6.7	7.8	9.5	9.5
22	96	2.6–3.6	6.5	7.6	9.3	11.3	11.4
25	96	2.6–3.6	6.5	8.0	10.1	12.4	12.4

irradiated on the exit side of the beam. This difference increases from 1.4 cm at 10 MeV to 4.4 cm at 25 MeV. This, together with the fact that there is very little skin sparing at higher electron energies, makes energies above 16 MeV less useful clinically than lower energies.

16.6
Electron Beam Depth Dose and Field Size

When the field sizes are large compared to the range of the electrons and the distance of their lateral spread, the depth dose characteristics stabilize and become unique for a given energy. The data given in Table 16.1 are limiting values for such large or 'infinite' beam sizes. For small field sizes, the depth dose values drop off considerably. Figure 16.8 shows the depth dose for 10-MeV electrons for a small field of 1 cm × 1 cm and for a larger field of 5 cm × 5 cm. The superficial dose build-up is reduced for small fields,

Fig. 16.8. Dependence of depth dose on field size for two narrow electron beams

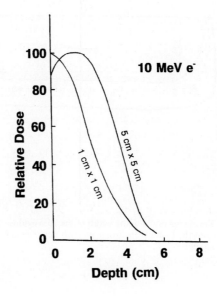

because of the lack of lateral scatter. Such a deficiency of laterally scattered electrons occurs at the field edges even for large fields and has to be allowed for in planning of the field dimensions to cover the target volume. To ensure that the deeper aspects of the edges of the target volume are within the 90% isodose curve, the field size at the surface should be more generous than a size that will merely include the target cross section at the surface inside 90%. This is particularly important at high electron energies. Figures 16.9a and b illustrate this. Thus, very small electron fields may not be suitable with regard to both depth dose and lateral dose.

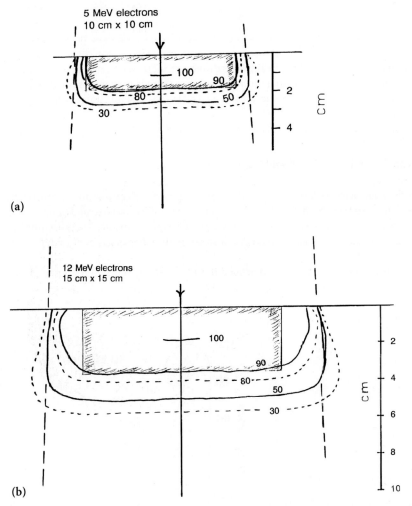

Fig. 16.9. Narrowing down of the width of the 90% isodose curve with increasing depth for (**a**) 5-MeV electrons and (**b**) 12-MeV electrons and two field sizes. The superficial target volumes are shown as shaded rectangles

16.7
Electron Pencil Beam

Figure 16.10 shows the dispersion of electrons in an incident pencil beam. The figure is a cloud chamber image of a finite number of electrons. There are sparse and dense regions, which will become more alike when the number of electrons becomes very large and the pencil beam disperses into a balloon-shaped volume. In general, the behavior of electron beams can be understood if one thinks of the beam as consisting of several narrow pencil beams that are dispersed in the shape of a balloon.

Many successful theoretical calculation models for predicting the dose distribution in electron beams rely on the dispersion and diffusion of thin electron pencil beams by multiple scattering. Many articles have been published on this subject; a few [10–28] are listed at the end of this chapter for interested readers. Some of these models allow for the scattering effect of edges and inhomogeneities. It is advisable to validate the dose distributions predicted by any model for specific experimental situations before it is adopted for clinical decision-making [29]. It is not within the scope of this text to cover these theoretical approaches. However, we will use the pencil beam and ballooning phenomenon to discuss the behavior of electron beams in a few special situations.

Fig. 16.10. Cloud chamber image showing the dispersion of an electron pencil beam. (Figure courtesy of Rolf Wideroe.)

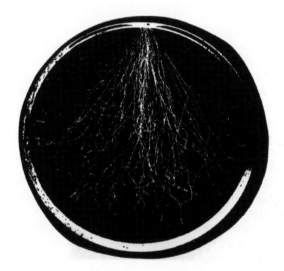

16.8
Oblique Incidence and Depth Dose

The central-axis depth dose of an electron beam changes with the obliquity of the incident beam with respect to the surface of incidence [30, 31]. The standard isodose patterns measured for normal incidence cannot be used for a beam incident on a

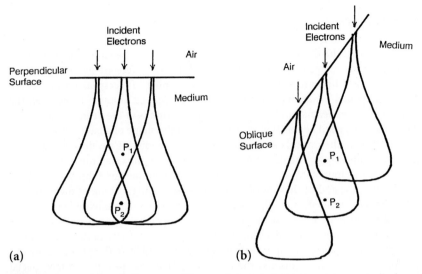

Fig. 16.11. Superposition of adjacent pencil beams of electrons incident on (a) a perpendicular surface and (b) an oblique surface

curved surface without remeasurement or corrections [32–34]. In Figure 16.11a, three pencil beams are shown incident normally on a surface. The three ballooning beams have not yet augmented each other at the shallow depth of point P_1, but they do overlap at the depth of P_2. This should be compared with the oblique incidence illustrated in Figure 16.11b. Here, the pencil beam on the right strikes the surface at a location closer to the source than do the other pencil beams shown, and the interactions spread the electrons to reach point P_1. However, because of the limited range, the pencil beam on the right does not penetrate to point P_2. Thus, whereas for point P_1 the pencil beam on the right does augment the dose, for point P_2 it does not. In obliquely incident beams, the maximum dose thus moves upward to shallow depths. The depth dose at larger depths becomes less than that for normal incidence. Figure 16.12 compares the central-axis depth dose for an obliquely incident beam with that for a normally incident beam.

The isodose patterns become distorted when the beam is used on a non-flat surface. In Figure 16.13, the surface S is curved. Curve I traces a constant depth from the surface, with the depth chosen to be at 80% depth dose for a normal beam. It will be noticed that the isodose curves have moved closer to the surface where the obliquity is high.

Fig. 16.12. Comparison of the central-axis depth-dose curves for 10-MeV electrons at normal incidence and incidence at 45° with respect to the entrance surface

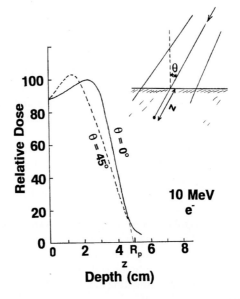

Fig. 16.13. Isodose distribution for a single electron beam incident on a curved surface

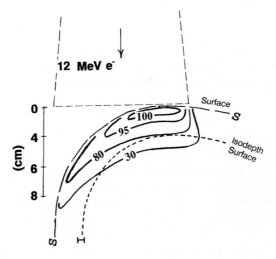

16.9
Electron Beams: Some Practical Consideration

16.9.1
Electron Beam Output Factors

The dose output of any electron beam is measured at the depth of the peak dose according to the American Association of Physicists in Medicine (AAPM) Task Group 21 protocol [35]. Because electron beam treatments are usually done with fixed source-to-skin distance (SSD) techniques, the calculation of the monitor units (Mu) can be based on Equation (13-20):

$$\dot{D}_P = CPOR \cdot NPOF(A_{dm}) \cdot [PDD(SSD, A_m, d)/100]$$

It is convenient to adjust the sensitivity of the monitoring ionization chamber to obtain a calibrated peak output rate (CPOR) of 1 cGy Mu^{-1} for a chosen standard field size A_{St} (usually 10 cm × 10 cm) and for the standard SSD used. The output factors for any other field size A can be stated as a normalized peak output rate, NPOR(A), as was done for photon beams.

The output factors for electron beams can vary over a wide range as the field changes from a small to a large size. The output of an electron beam can be very sensitive to the position of the photon-collimating diaphragms and the scattered electron fluence from them. We already explained how the field outline at the skin level is defined by the electron penumbra trimmers that extend close to the patient [36, 37]. Usually, the size of the photon collimator opening to go with any particular electron cone (or trimmers) is so designed by the manufacturers as to minimize the variation in the output factors between different cones. The interlocks of the machine may automatically select a particular aperture of photon collimation on attachment of a specific cone. Arbitrary changes of photon-collimating diaphragms can cause a large variation in output, by a much as a factor of 2 [38].

EXAMPLE 16.1

An electron beam treatment is to be done with 13-MeV electrons, with a field size of 7 cm × 7 cm at SSD = 100 cm. The calibrated peak output rate (CPOR) for a 10 cm × 10 cm field is 1.0 cGy Mu^{-1}, and the normalized peak output factors (NPOF) are as follows:

Field Size (A_o)	NPOF (A_o)
5 cm × 5 cm	0.93
6 cm × 6 cm	0.97
8 cm × 8 cm	0.99
10 cm × 10 cm	1.00
12 cm × 12 cm	1.01
15 cm × 15 cm	1.01

It is desired to deliver a dose of 180 cGy at the level of the 90% depth dose. What should be the Mu and what is the maximum dose per treatment?

     CPOR = 1.0 cGy Mu^{-1}

     NPOF for field size 7 cm × 7 cm = 0.98 (from the table above)

     PDD = 90% (as prescribed)

     Dose to be delivered = 180 cGy

Based on expression (13-20),

$$\begin{aligned} \text{Dose rate} &= \text{CPOR} \times \text{NPOF} \times \text{PDD}/100 \\ &= 1.0\,\text{cGy Mu}^{-1} \times 0.98 \times (90/100) = 0.882\,\text{cGy Mu}^{-1} \end{aligned}$$

Mu to deliver $180\,cGy = 180/0.882 = 204\,Mu$

Maximum dose corresponding to PDD $= 100\%$ is $180\,cGy \times (100/90) = 200\,cGy$

The selection of a PDD of 90% for dose prescription in the above example is somewhat arbitrary. A more scientific approach could be to prescribe the dose at d_m (PDD $= 100\%$) after appropriately selecting an electron energy to provide the needed depth coverage.

16.9.2
Output Factors for Non-Square Fields

For dosimetry of rectangular fields of photon beams, we used the empirical approximation of an equivalent square field. This approach does not work equally well for electron fields. This is because, as we know, the electron beam output is much influenced by the scattered fluence from the beam-defining devices and the air.

It has been determined empirically that the output factor for a rectangular electron field of width W_0 and length L_0 can be derived from the output factors for square fields of sides W_0 and L_0 by the relation [39–41]

$$NPOR(W_0 \times L_0) = [NPOR(W_0 \times W_0) \times NPOR(L_0 \times L_0)]^{1/2}$$

In irregularly shaped fields produced by placement of shields in the path of the beam, the output rates can be very sensitive to the scattered fluence from the shield itself, depending upon the position of the shield. Any interpretive or approximate method used for deriving the output rate for irregularly shaped fields should be established for routine use only after verification by measurements [42–44].

16.9.3
Field Shaping and Selective Shielding

Electron beams are used for treatment of superficial lesions, which the physician can often palpate and outline on the skin. Lead cutouts can be used for shaping of the electron beam portal to the outline drawn. The lead shielding used should be of sufficient thickness to stop the electrons completely [43, 45–47]. A lead shield of inadequate thickness may slow down the energy of the electrons without stopping them. Under such conditions, the scattering events in the high-Z shielding material can actually increase the electron fluence in the region behind the shield and cause up to 30% enhancement of the dose [46]. Figure 16.14a shows an experimental setup that irradiates a photographic film with an electron beam within which different parts have been subjected to different thicknesses of lead shielding. Figure 16.14b shows the image obtained on the film in this setup. It should be noticed that the area under the inadequately thin lead shield on the left part of the image is darker than the unshielded area in the middle of the beam. The area below the thick lead shield on the right side appears light, indicating that it is well shielded. The lead thickness used should be optimal, because over-cautious use of a generous thickness will make the shield unduly heavy and difficult to use [48].

There can be an inclination to place a shield behind the target volume in an accessible body cavity, to protect any organ in the exit path of an electron beam. However,

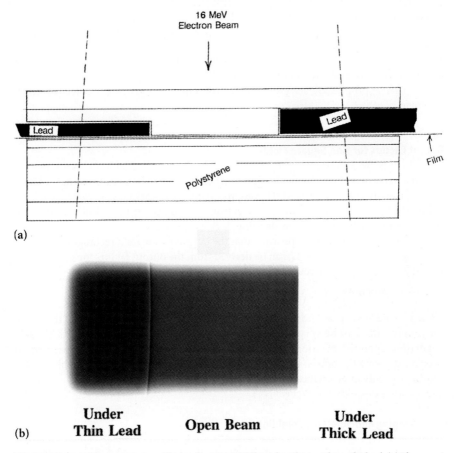

Fig. 16.14. Dose enhancement caused by inadequate shielding of an electron beam by lead. (a) Placement of the film and the shield in the phantom during irradiation. (b) Film image obtained, showing the variation in the darkening behind inadequate shielding (on the left side), no shielding (in the middle), and adequate shielding (on right side)

this can have an adverse effect of producing dose enhancement in the region above the shield because of the electrons that are back-scattered by the shield [28, 46, 49–51]. For example, one might want to shield the floor of the mouth while irradiating the tongue by placement of a lead sheet under the tongue. Although the lead layer may be of sufficient thickness to protect the floor of the mouth, the electrons back-scattered from the lead can adversely enhance the dose to the tongue above. Figure 16.15a shows an experimental setup in which a film is irradiated by an electron beam and a part of the beam behind the film is shielded by lead. Figure 16.15b shows the image registered by the film. It can be observed that the area on the left side of the film that lay above the lead shield is darker than the right side. The higher the atomic number Z of the shielding material used, the greater is the back-scattered fluence and the consequent dose enhancement. For 6.4-MeV electrons, it has been reported that lead, copper, and

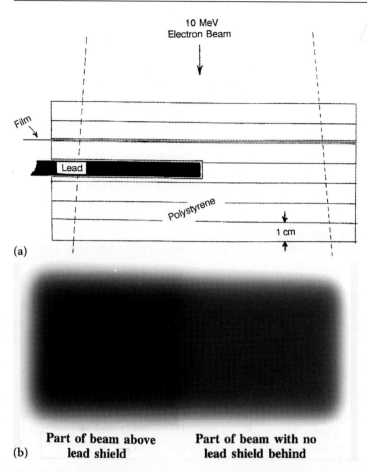

Fig. 16.15. Upstream dose enhancement caused in an electron beam by a high-Z shield placed behind the region treated. (a) Placement of the film and the shield in the phantom during irradiation. (b) Film image obtained, showing the increased darkening on the left side that lay above the shield

aluminum shields enhanced the dose upstream by about 73%, 33%, and 15%, respectively [49]. Furthermore, the average energy of the back-scattered electrons increases with the atomic number Z of the back-scattering material [52]. For higher values of Z, the dose enhancement becomes observable farther above the shield. Such a dose enhancement by back-scattered electrons from an internal shield is not unique to electron beams. It also applies to shields inserted in beams of kilovoltage X-rays [53] (which may also be used for treatment of superficial lesions [see Section 16.11]) and high-energy photons [54]. One can avoid the undesirable effect of the dose enhancement by covering the internal shield by a layer of a low-Z material of thickness equal to or larger than the range of the back-scattered electrons to absorb them. Without such a preventive measure, the dose enhancement can be significant enough to cause adverse clinical reactions.

16.9.4
Effective SSD

At times, it is not possible to set up the patient at the normal SSD, which we will refer to here as SSD_N. This could happen because of interference of a protruding body part (such as the shoulder) with the electron trimmers. An additional air gap **g** may need to be accepted, giving an extended SSD, $SSD_{ext}(= SSD_N + \textbf{g})$. The influence of scatter from the collimators and trimmers above the patient in an electron beam makes the focus of electron emission apparently diffuse and uncertain. The output factors measured at the normal SSD cannot be converted to provide the output factors for the SSD_{ext} by a simple inverse-square factor based on distance. However, inverse-square corrections can be applied by determination of an effective SSD, which we will refer to here as SSD_{eff}, because the fall-off of the fluence with distance in an electron beam occurs as if there were an effective point of electron emission [55, 56]. If $(OR)_N$ (in cGy Mu^{-1}) is the peak output rate at the depth d_m, with SSD $= SSD_N$, the peak output rate, $(OR)_{ext}$, at the depth d_m, with SSD $= SSD_{ext}$, can be derived by a relation of the form

$$(OR)_{ext} = (OR)_N \left[\frac{(SSD_{eff} + d_m)}{SSD_{eff} + \textbf{g} + d_m)} \right]^2$$

The value of SSD_{eff} should be determined experimentally by actual measurement of the output rates for different values of the gap **g**. A plot of the square root of the ratio $[(OR)_N/(OR)_{ext}]$ vs. **g** has a slope equal to $[1/(SSD_{eff} + d_m)]$, as shown in Figure 16.16. The method for deriving the output at the extended SSD should be used with caution and should be limited to small values of **g**, up to about 10 cm. The SSD_{eff} is a function of electron energy, field size, and the actual scatter geometry, which can vary from machine to machine. For small field sizes, the SSD_{eff} is much shorter than the SSD indicated during setup. In one case, as the field size changed from 6 cm $\times$ 6 cm to 25 cm $\times$ 25 cm, the SSD_{eff} changed from 70 cm to 95 cm, whereas the actual setup indicated an SSD of 100 cm.

EXAMPLE 16.2

A 10-MeV electron beam has an output rate of 0.98 cGy Mu^{-1} at the depth of the peak dose when used at the normal setup with $SSD_N = 100$ cm. For one patient, it becomes necessary to use an extended SSD_{ext} of 105 cm. The beam is known to have an SSD_{eff} of 80 cm. Compare the two output rates obtained by use of SSD_{eff} and SSD_N for estimating the inverse-square divergence. Use $d_m = 2.5$ cm.

In this case, $\textbf{g} = 5$ cm; $d_m = 2.5$ cm; $SSD_{eff} = 80$ cm; and output at $SSD_N = 0.98$ cGy Mu^{-1}.

(i) Inverse-square correction for $SSD_{eff} = 80$ cm:

$$\left[\frac{(SSD_{eff} + d_m)}{(SSD_{eff} + \textbf{g} + d_m)} \right]^2 = \left[\frac{80 + 2.5}{80 + 5 + 2.5} \right]^2 = 0.889$$

Estimated output rate for SSD of 105 cm $= 0.98$ cGy Mu$^{-1} \times 0.889 = 0.871$ cGy Mu^{-1}.

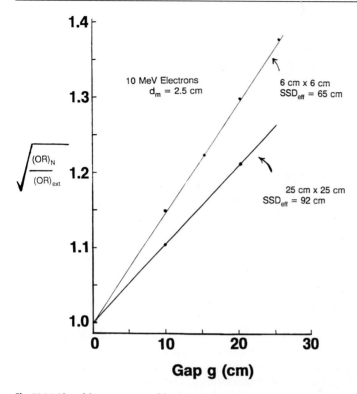

Fig. 16.16. Plot of the square root of the ratio of electron beam output rates with distance g for derivation of SSD_{eff}. The gap g is the distance between the SSD used for the measurements and SSD_N

(ii) Inverse-square correction for the normal $SSD_N = 100$ cm:

$$\left[\frac{(SSD_N + d_m)}{(SSD_N + g + d_m)} \right]^2 = \left[\frac{100 + 2.5}{100 + 5 + 2.5} \right]^2 = 0.909$$

Estimated output rate for SSD of 105 cm = 0.98 cGy Mu$^{-1} \times 0.909 = 0.891$ cGy Mu^{-1}.

Note that, even for a small value of **g** of 5 cm, the two calculated outputs differ by about 2% in the above example.

16.9.5
Agreement of Light Field and Radiation Field

The projection of the collimating aperture by the localization light beam generally indicates a beam cross section that appears as if the beam emerged from a point. However, we just discussed that the electron fluence falls off with distance as if the source were at an effective SSD. These two facts together mean that the assumption that the light beam outline can represent the radiation beam outline cannot be taken for granted as readily for electrons as for photons. Figures 16.17a, b, and c show the

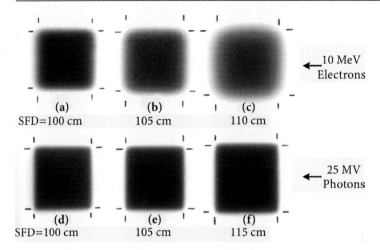

Fig. 16.17. Agreement of light field and radiation field, as obtained on a photographic film at the normal treatment distance, and with the distance 5 cm and 10 cm larger than normal. (a), (b), and (c) are for a 10-MeV electron beam; (d), (e), and (f) are for a 25-MV photon beam. The corners of the light field are indicated by lines made with a ballpoint pen on the emulsion

photographic images of the cross section of an electron beam at the standard SSD used and at two other distances applicable for two values of the air gap g. The extension of the light field edges is indicated by straight lines outside the beam. It can be seen that the beam edges become diffuse with increasing g. On the other hand, the edges for photon beams, as illustrated in Figure 16.17d, e, and f, follow the light beam indication closely. For electron beams, if the patient is set up at an extended distance, the light beam outline seen on the patient's surface cannot be taken to represent the outline of the beam. Furthermore, if any lead shield or block is placed far above the patient, the shadow of the light field cannot truly indicate a shielded region. The blocking or field shaping should be done close to the patient's body surface to be effective.

16.10
Influence of Inhomogeneities

The dose at any point in an electron beam is not only dependent upon the path traversed by the ray connecting that point to an apparent or virtual source position. Structures (or inhomogeneities) in the regions lateral to the ray and above the point of dose calculation can also affect the fluence reaching the point. The influence of any structure can depend in a complicated way on its shape and size, the electron density, and the scattering power as governed by the atomic number. This phenomenon was known and studied already during the early years of the practice of electron therapy [57–61]. More recently, this subject has been addressed with several theoretical models [15, 19, 21, 24, 62, 63].

Here, we endeavor to explain the phenomenon brought about by the inhomogeneities by using the conditions shown in Figure 16.18. Figure 16.18a shows a uniform water-equivalent medium within which a volume is replaced by air in Figure 16.18b

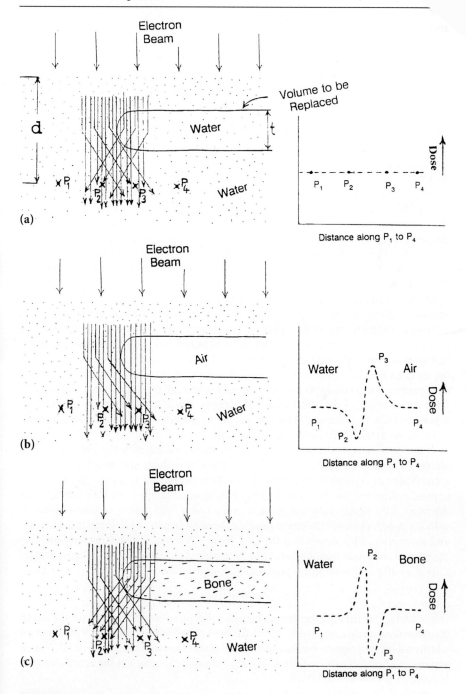

Fig. 16.18. Dispersion of electrons by the edge of an inhomogeneity. (a) A uniform water-equivalent medium with a volume as marked. This volume is replaced by air in (b) and by bone in (c). The expected dose profiles through points P_1, P_2, P_3, and P_4 are shown on the right

n Figure 16.18c. Four points, P_1, P_2, P_3, and P_4, have been chosen at the
d, from the surface. Figure 16.18a shows how the medium overlying P_2
rons onto P_3 and vice versa. The scattered amount from above P_2 to P_3
sa is the same, because the media above P_2 and P_3 are identical. The fluence
the dose) at P_2 and P_3 is the same also.

In ... re 16.18b, the amount of scatter in the medium above P_2 is the same as before,
but the air above P_3 does not deflect as many electrons that reach P_2. The reduced
number of interactions in air also lets more electrons reach P_3. As a consequence, the
dose at P_3 will be increased at the expense of the dose at P_2. The change in the scattering
behavior with the change in medium does not influence the dose at P_1, because it is
located too far laterally from the edge of the inhomogeneity. The dose at P_1 will thus be
the same as that in Figure 16.18a. Point P_4 is likewise located too far laterally from the
edge of the inhomogeneity to be influenced by the edge scatter. However (assuming that
the density of air is almost zero), the dose at P_4, which is located directly underneath
the air cavity, will correspond to an effective depth of $(d - t)$. The dose at P_3 is higher
than that at P_4 because P_3 receives more scatter from the high-density medium above
P_2. The cross-beam dose profile expected to be obtained below the transition interface
is shown on the right side of Figure 16.18b.

In Figure 16.18c, the air is replaced by bone. In bone, due to its high density, the
scattering events are more numerous than those in water. The dose at P_2 increases
because of the increased amount of scatter from bone, and the dose at P_3 consequently
is reduced. The dose profile expected to be obtained below the transition interface
is shown on the right side of Figure 16.18c. Thus, the inhomogeneities in electron
beams can cause hot spots and cold spots downstream from any transition edge. The
dose pattern is difficult to predict and quantify (although this is possible theoretically)
[19]. An example of the effect of a high-density (lead) inhomogeneity is shown in
Figure 16.14. The dense and light regions below the edge of the lead in the film are
attributable to the phenomenon described above.

If the point of calculation is considerably displaced laterally (i.e., at least by an
electron range) from any transition edge, one can evaluate the dose by estimating
a coefficient of equivalent thickness (CET). This is referred to as the 'infinite-limit'
approximation and can be applied to point P_4 in our example. The CET is defined as
the ratio of the linear thickness of water to the linear thickness of an inhomogeneity,
with the two thicknesses chosen to produce the same degrees of electron transmission
and absorption. This means that the CET for any material is given approximately by
the ratio of the linear stopping power of the material to that of water. In Figure 16.18c,
P_4 is at an effective water-equivalent depth, d_{eff}, given by

$$d_{eff} = \left[d + t(CET_{bone} - 1) \right]$$

where CET_{bone} is the CET for bone. The percent depth dose (PDD) read for the depth
d_{eff} from the standard depth dose tables cannot be used as such for point P_4 without an
additional inverse-square distance correction. This is because the standard PDD value
applies to a point at a distance $(SSD_N + d_{eff})$ from the source, but the actual distance
of point P_4 is $(SSD_N + d)$. Thus,

$$PDD \text{ at } P_4 = (PDD \text{ read for } d_{eff}) \times \left[\frac{SSD_N + d_{eff}}{SSD_N + d} \right]^2$$

In general, the value of the CET can vary with depth and beam energy. The above expression does not address the details of the perturbations caused by the presence of an inhomogeneity. Calculation models based on pencil beam dispersion by multiple coulomb scattering are better suited to solution of the problem [15, 19, 21, 24, 26, 62, 63]. By modern computed tomography (CT), the theoretical models can directly utilize the detailed patient anatomy provided by the pixel-to-pixel variation of the CT numbers [15, 26].

16.11
Comparison of Kilovoltage X-Ray and Electron Beams

It is interesting to compare the relative merits of electron beams and kilovoltage X-ray beams for treatment of superficial lesions. Figure 16.19 compares the doses delivered by electron beams of three different energies with that for a 250-kV X-ray beam (2.5 mm Cu HVT). For a selected maximum target depth of 3 cm, it is seen that the 10-MeV electron beam and the X-ray beam provide dose distributions that are nonuniform to the same degree within the target volume. However, the X-ray beam delivers a much higher exit dose beyond the target depth. In addition, we recall (from our discussions in Chapters 11 and 14), that a 1.5 to 4 times higher dose can result in bone compared to soft tissue with low-energy X-rays. The mass stopping power (and hence the energy absorbed per unit mass) is not too different between bone and soft tissue for electrons. For 10-MeV electrons, the mass stopping power of soft tissue and bone is 1.974 and 1.835 MeV cm^2 g^{-1}, respectively. This implies that an 8% higher dose will be delivered to soft tissue than to bone if both are irradiated with the same electron fluence.

Some advantages of X-ray beams over electron beams in certain situations have also been noted [64, 65]. These advantages include a higher skin dose, gradual fall-off of the dose on the exit side to cover uncertain tumor extensions, the possibility of using very small field sizes without compromising the coverage, the adequacy of

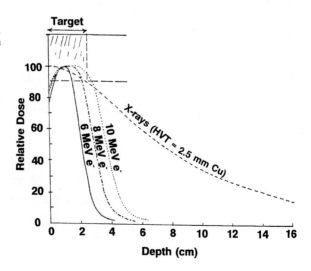

Fig. 16.19. Depth dose curves for electron beams of 6, 8, and 10 MeV energies and a 2.5-mm HVT kilovoltage X-ray beam for treatment of a 3-cm thick superficial target volume

thinner lead cutouts (of only a few millimeters) for field shaping, thinner inserted lead shields for protection of tissues on the exit side of the beam, a smaller thickness (only a few millimeters) of plastic needed on any inserted lead shielding to absorb the back-scattered electrons for prevention of dose enhancement to tissues overlying the shield, and a lower overall cost of the radiation generator.

16.12
Total-Skin Electron Treatment

In certain clinical situations, a radiation dose may need to be delivered to the superficial cutaneous tissues of the entire body. The need to cover the entire body will require a very large beam cross section, with good uniformity of electron energy and fluence within it. Such large field sizes are possible only at very large treatment distances, making use of the entire treatment room.

In a different approach, a beam collimated to produce a narrow strip of radiation beam has been used for scanning across the patient [66]. The techniques and dosimetry of carrying out total-skin electron irradiation can be very involved. The reader should study the comprehensive reviews listed in References 67 and 68.

Figure 16.20a shows a geometry in which oblique beam orientations are employed to provide large coverage. Two different oblique orientations are shown, and these

Fig. 16.20. Total-skin electron beam irradiation. (a) Beams at ±20° inclinations with the patient at a very large distance and an acrylic scatterer in the beam. (b) Six different patient orientations are used for diffusion of nonuniformity

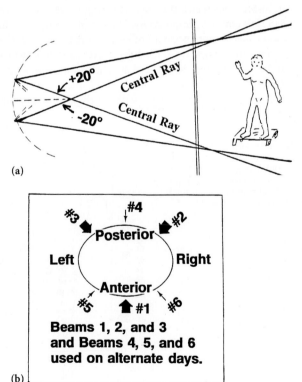

(a)

(b)

can be used alternately, making the total fluence uniform. The uniformity of electron fluence within the field is improved further by placement of a plastic sheet, which acts as a scatterer of electrons between the source and the patient, so as to diffuse the beam and improve the uniformity. However, it also degrades the beam energy.

The depth dose characteristics of the electron beam as documented for the usual treatment distance cannot be applied to the total-skin irradiation setup. The presence of the lucite scatterer, together with the beam obliquity with respect to the patient's surface, can annul the dose build-up at the skin. In fact, the selection of the beam energy, and of the thickness and position of the scatterer, should be done with the objective of producing acceptable dose uniformity and depth dose. It is necessary to diffuse the self-shielding and shadowing effects of one part of the body on another to avoid cold spots. Some have used a pedestal and rotation of the patient during the treatment. One technique [69], developed at Stanford, uses six different orientations of the patient, as illustrated in Figure 16.20b, with three beams used each day. The patient's extremities should be extended and exposed at different orientations as well. It might be necessary to boost the dose to selected body parts, such as the armpits and feet, in a follow-up treatment. Selective shielding of the eyes or other sensitive areas can be employed.

16.13
Intraoperative Electron Therapy

In intraoperative radiotherapy (IORT), the radiation beam is directed through a surgical opening for treatment of an internal target site [70–78]. The normally overlying body tissues are thus spared from exposure to radiation. A large single dose of radiation is usually delivered by an electron beam. Here we attempt to give only a very brief overview.

IORT requires a special collimating system (Figure 16.21), which usually consists of (i) a large cylindrical collimator made of stainless steel that is attached to the front face of the machine, and (ii) interchangeable applicators or 'cones' of cylindrical or elliptical cross section, made of metal or transparent plastic. (Some IORT systems do not use rigid fastening to the machine.) The cylindrical steel collimator shown in Figure 16.21 can incorporate a viewing mechanism with a mirror for obervation of the tumor site during setup. The applicators have a wall thickness of 3 to 5 mm and are 20 to 40 cm long. Because most of the electrons travel in straight lines, the leakage through the walls is negligible. The diameters of the applicators range from 3.0 cm to 12 cm. On the beam exit end, the applicator can have either a flat or a beveled end. The output rate and the depth dose distributions of all IORT applicators should be measured individually and should be available prior to their use.

Compact treatment machines that produce only electron beams (and no X-ray beams) and that are designed especially for intraoperative radiotherapy have come into use [78–81]. These machines, because they produce only electron beams, can have less source-head shielding. Hence, they are not very heavy. They can be rolled into the surgical suite when needed. Although no specially shielded vault is necessary as for X-ray therapy machines, the electron beams do produce penetrating bremsstrahlung X-rays. For that reason, these machines have to be used with proper radiation safety precautions. They should be used in selected surgical suites with attention paid to

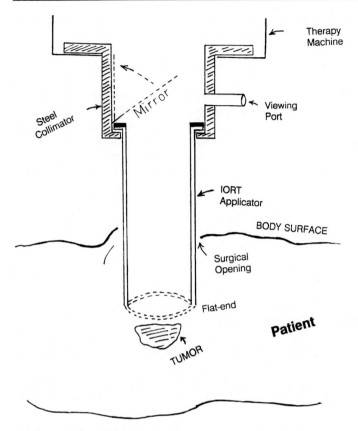

Fig. 16.21. Schematic diagram of an electron beam irradiating a deep-seated tumor intraoperatively. An applicator is inserted through a surgical incision

concepts such as distance, directions of beam usage, and workload, that are discussed in Chapter 19.

16.14
Electron Arc Therapy

Electron arc therapy can be used for treatment of a large superficial layer of a target volume on a curved body surface. However, the planning for arc treatment with electrons is more complex than that with photons [82–90]. We will discuss it only briefly, mainly to indicate its complexity. Users wishing to practice arc therapy should do a more detailed study based on the references cited.

Patients are not perfect cylinders. The output rate of an arc changes with the radius of curvature of the surface irradiated. If the surface curvature changes gradually along the longitudinal axis of the patient, there will be a corresponding change in the dose delivered by the arc. By use of custom-designed secondary collimators that produce a field of trapezoidal shape, the uniformity of the dose can be improved.

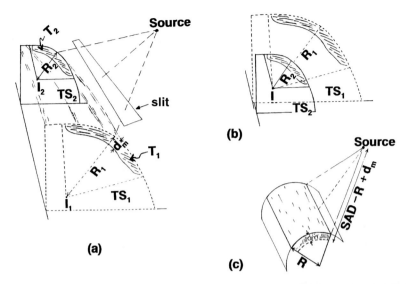

Fig. 16.22. Planning of electron arc therapy. (a) Illustration of changing body size along the length of the patient. Points I_1 and I_2 have been identified as centers of circles of radii R_1 and R_2 that nearly approximate the surfaces in body sections TS_1 and TS_2. The field is shaped by a slit. (b) The body is aligned by couch rotation and patient tilt so that centers I_1 and I_2 coincide with the axis of rotation of the beam, I. (c) A cylindrical surface treated with an arc

Figure 16.22a shows two transverse sections, TS_1 and TS_2, which may be located in two different planes of a patient's body. The target volumes in these two sections with different radii are identified as T_1 and T_2. The points I_1 and I_2 in the two sections are such that circles drawn with these points as the origins nearly match the body outlines at the two levels. The radii of curvature are R_1 and R_2 for the two sections. The beam can rotate around only one axis. This requires manipulation of the patient support system (i. e., couch rotation and a patient tilt) to bring points I_1 and I_2 into line and in alignment with the isocentric axis of rotation I of the treatment apparatus. The expected result is shown in Figure 16.22b, where the two sections have been overlaid so that I_1 coincides with I_2 at I. The arc of the beam should span a larger area than needed to cover the target surface. The edges of the arc can be custom-trimmed by placement of lead shields on the skin. The field width chosen should be sufficiently small to have minimum obliquity and surface curvature within itself in all directions, but large enough to give a good output rate. A field width of about 5 cm may achieve this in many actual situations. The peak output rate for the arc is sensitive to the field width. For a chosen field width, with an increase in the angle of arc, an equilibrium output rate is reached in the central region covered by the arc. The output rate for the arc is determined by placement of the single-electron-beam isodose curve along several adjacent radii and integrating of the doses. This can be done manually or by computer. Uniformity of dose delivery is achieved by designing the shape of the trapezoidal secondary collimator to suit the body shape, as explained next.

The electron fluence is spread out in two directions: in the plane of rotation and perpendicular to it (Figure 16.22a and b). Hence, the dose delivered by the arc is influenced by the radius of curvature R of the treated body section in two ways. First, in the plane of rotation, because the arc length is proportional to R, the fluence dilution is greater for a larger radius. The peak dose is therefore proportional to $1/(R - d_m)$. Thus, a large R means a low dose rate. Next, when we look at a cylindrical surface in the direction perpendicular to the plane of rotation, a large radius presents the surface closer to the electron source than does a small radius (Figure 16.22c). In this perpendicular direction, the spread of the beam is proportional to the distance $(SAD - R + d_m)$, and the fluence is inversely proportional to that distance. Combining both, we obtain

$$\text{Dose} \propto \frac{1.0}{(R - d_m) \times (SAD - R + d_m)}$$

If the peak doses are D_1 and D_2 in sections TS_1 and TS_2, from the above reasoning, we obtain the ratio

$$\frac{D_1}{D_2} = \frac{(R_2 - d_m) \times (SAD - R_2 + d_m)}{(R_1 - d_m) \times (SAD - R_1 + d_m)}$$

Because the output increases with the field width, the difference between D_1 and D_2 can be improved if one uses different field widths for the two sections. In fact, a slit that produces a field of trapezoidal cross section, as shown in Figure 16.22a, can be designed to narrow the field width progressively from large to small body sections.

The depth dose characteristics of an arc are different from those of a fixed beam of the same electron energy. The cross-firing in the arcs reduces the skin dose and increases the depth of the peak dose.

In an alternate approach to arc therapy, the arc is replaced by several adjacent stationary beams [91–94]. This is also referred to as 'pseudo-arc technique.' In the implementation of this technique, care should be exercised to avoid cold or hot spots at the junction between adjacent beams.

16.15
Adjacent Electron Fields

It is desirable to keep in mind the behavior of the isodose curves along the edges of electron beams when several such beams are juxtaposed. In electron beams, the isodose curves of high denominations (above 70%) curve from the beam edge inward to become narrower with increasing depth. However, the lower-denomination isodose curves (below 30%) expand in width and balloon outward with increasing depth. The fact that electron beam isodose curves do not follow the geometric edge of the beam causes special problems when adjacent electron fields are to be matched with skin gaps or appropriate relative beam orientations [95–97]. Generally, it is desirable to encompass the entire surface region to be treated by a single electron beam of large cross section. However, situations can occur where it may be advantageous to split the target volume and treat it with two different beams.

Figure 16.23a illustrates two adjacent sites treated with 7-MeV and 16-MeV electron beams. Here, the split is used to tailor the energy of the two beams to suit the difference in depth of the target volume. The beams are shown positioned with the light fields of the two beams (which, by definition, are also the 50% dose with respect to the central-axis dose) abutting on the body surface. The combined isodose distribution for this

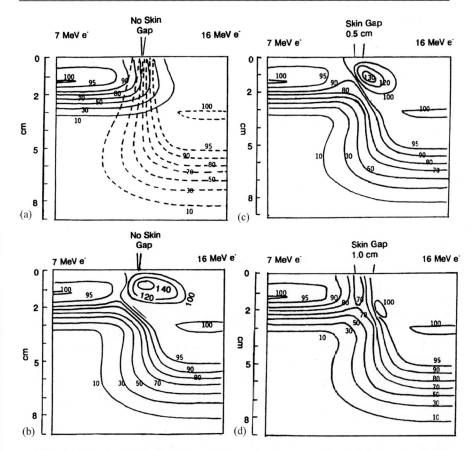

Fig. 16.23. Illustration of treatment of adjacent sites with electron fields of different energies. (**a**) Isodose curves of individual beams shown juxtaposed, with no skin gap between the geometric edges. (**b**), (**c**), and (**d**) show combined isodose curves for no skin gap, 5-mm skin gap, and 1.0-cm skin gap, respectively

situation is one of 'no skin gap,' as shown in Figure 16.23b. Figures 16.23c and d give the dose distributions when 0.5-cm and 1.0-cm skin gaps are used.

Some investigators have reported about attaching 'penumbra producers' or 'beam spoilers' at the end of electron cones to improve the match. These methods perturb the beam energy and its penumbra so as to modify the isodose curves at the matching edge [98–103].

A similar problem of beam placement can occur whenever an electron beam is juxtaposed to a site treated by photon beams. Because photon beams are often used as parallel opposed beams, there can be an exiting and an entering photon beam at the surface of match. Situations such as these may call for a careful trade-off between hot and cold spots.

References

1. Moliere, G., Theorie der Streuung schneller geladener Teilchen II, Mehrfach- und Vielfachstreu-ung, Z. Naturforsch., Vol 3a, p78–97, 1948.
2. Bethe, H.A., Rose, M.E., and Smith, L.P., The multiple scattering of electrons, Proc. Am. Philos. Soc., Vol 78, p573–585, 1938.
3. Heitler, W., The Quantum Theory of Radiation, Third Edition, p414, Oxford University Press, London, 1954.
4. Scott, W.T., The theory of small-angle multiple scattering of fast charged particles, Rev. Mod. Phys., Vol 35, p2–313, 1963.
5. Lanzl, L.H., Fundamental interactions of electrons with water, p21–24, in Proceedings of the Symposium on Electron Dosimetry and Arc Therapy, Paliwal, B. (Ed.), American Institute of Physics, New York, 1982.
6. Lanzl, L.H., Electron pencil beam scanning and its application in radiation therapy, p55–66, in Frontiers of Radiation Therapy, Oncology, Vol 2, Karger, Basel, 1968.
7. Mandour, M.A., and Harder, D., Systematic optimization of the double scatterer system for electron beam field flattening, Strahlentherapie, Vol 154, p328–322, 1978.
8. Lax, I., and Brahme, A., On the collimation of high energy electron beams, Acta Radiol. Oncol., Vol 19, p199–207, 1980.
9. Markus, B., Energie-Bestimmung schneller Elektronen auf Tiefendosiskurven, Strahlentherapie, Vol 116, p280–286, 1961.
10. Perry, D.J., and Holt, J.G., A model for calculating the effects of small inhomogeneities on electron beam dose distributions, Med. Phys., Vol 7, p207–215, 1980.
11. Hogstrom, K.R., and Mills, M.D., Electron beam dose calculations, Phys. Med. Biol., Vol 26, p445–459, 1981.
12. Werner, B.L., Khan, F.M., and Diebel, F.C., Model for calculating electron beam scattering in treatment planning, Med. Phys., Vol 9, p180–187, 1982.
13. Jette, D., Pagnamenta, A., Lanzl, L.H., and Rozenfeld, M., The application of multiple scattering theory to therapeutic electron dosimetry, Med. Phys., Vol 10, p141–146, 1983.
14. Storchi, P.R.M., and Huizenga, H., On a numerical approach of the pencil beam model, Phys. Med. Biol., Vol 30, p467–473, 1985.
15. Kirsner, S.M., Hogstrom, K.R., Kurup, R.G., and Moyers, M.F., Dosimetric evaluation in heterogeneous tissue of anterior electron beam irradiation for treatment of retinoblastoma, Med. Phys., Vol 14, p772–779, 1987.
16. Lax, I., Brahme, A., and Andreo, P., Electron beam dose planning using Gaussian beams, Acta Radiol. Suppl., 364, Vol 36, p49–59, 1983.
17. McParland, B.J., Cunningham, J.R., and Woo, M.K., The optimization of pencil beam widths for use in an electron pencil beam algorithm, Med. Phys., Vol 14, p489–497, 1988.
18. Jette, D., Electron dose calculation using multiple-scattering theory. A Gaussian multiple-scattering theory, Med. Phys., Vol 15, p123–137, 1988.
19. Jette, D., Lanzl, L.H., Pagnamenta, A., Rozenfeld, M., Bernard, D., Kao, M., and Sabbas, A.M., Electron dose calculation using multiple scattering theory: Thin planar inhomogeneities, Med. Phys., Vol 16, p712–725, 1989.
20. Huizenga, H., and Storchi, P.R.M., Numerical calculations of energy deposition of broad high energy electron beams, Phys. Med. Biol., Vol 34, p1371–1396, 1989; Corrigendum, Phys. Med. Biol., Vol 35, 1445, 1990.
21. Jette, D., Electron dose calculation using multiple-scattering theory: Localized inhomogeneities – a new theory, Med. Phys., Vol 18, p123–132, 1991.
22. McLellan, J., Sandison, G.A., Papiez, L., and Huda, W., A restricted angular scattering model for electron penetration in dense media, Med. Phys., Vol 18, p1–6, 1991.
23. Shiu, A.S., and Hogstrom, K.R., Pencil beam redefinition algorithm for electron dose distributions, Med. Phys., Vol 18, p7–18, 1991.
24. Jette, D., and Walker, S., Electron beam dose calculation using multiple scattering theory: Evaluation of a new model for inhomogeneities, Med. Phys., Vol 19, p1241–1254, 1992.
25. Petti, P.L., Differential pencil beam dose calculation for charged particles, Med. Phys., Vol 19, p137–149, 1992.
26. Al-Beteri, A.A., and Raeside, D.E., Optimal electron beam treatment planning for retinoblastoma using a new three-dimensional Monte Carlo based treatment planning system, Med. Phys., Vol 19, p125–135, 1992.
27. Ma, C.M., and Jiang, S.B., Monte Carlo modeling of electron beams from medical accelerator, Phys. Med. Biol., Vol.44, pp R157–189, 1999.
28. Morawska-Kaczynska, M., and Huizenga, H., Numerical calculations of energy deposition by broad high-energy electron beams, Phys. Med. Biol., Vol 37, p2103–2106, 1992.

29. Shiu, A.S. et al., Verification data for electron beam dose algorithms, Med. Phys., Vol 19, p623–636, 1992.
30. McKenzie, A.L., Air-gap correction in electron treatment planning, Phys. Med. Biol., Vol 24, p628–635, 1979.
31. Ekstrand, K.E., and Dixon, R.L., Obliquely incident electron beams, Med. Phys., Vol 9, p276–278, 1982.
32. Biggs, P.J., The effect of beam angulation on central axis depth dose for 4-29 MeV electrons, Phys. Med. Biol., Vol 29, p1089–1096, 1984.
33. Khan, F.M., Deibel, F.C., and Soleimani-Meigooni, A., Obliquity correction for electron beams, Med. Phys., Vol 12, p749–753, 1985.
34. Ulin, K., and Sternick, E.S., An isodose shift technique for obliquely incident electron beams, Med. Phys., Vol. 16, p905–910, 1989.
35. Task Group 21, Radiation Therapy Committee, American Association of Physicists in Medicine, A protocol for the determination of absorbed dose from high-energy photon and electron beams, Med. Phys., Vol 10, p741–771, 1983.
36. Biggs, P.J., Boyer, A.L., and Doppke, K.P., Electron dosimetry of irregular fields on the Clinac-18, Int. J. Radiat. Oncol. Biol. Phys., Vol 5, p433–440, 1979.
37. Purdy, J.M., Choi, M.C., and Feldman, A., Lipowitz metal shielding thickness for dose reduction of 6-20 MeV electrons, Med. Phys., Vol 7, p251–253, 1980.
38. Lightstone, A.W., Videla., N., and Mason, D.L.D., Exceptional increases in electron cone output as the backup diaphragms are opened, Med. Phys., Vol. 24, pp 133–134, 1997.
39. Mills, M.D., Hogstrom, K.R., and Almond, P.R., Prediction of electron beam output factors, Med. Phys., Vol 9, p60–68, 1982.
40. McParland, B.J., A parametrization of the electron beam output factors for a 25 MeV linear accelerator, Med. Phys., Vol 14, p666–669, 1987.
41. McParland, B.J., A method of calculating output factors for arbitrarily shaped electron fields, Med. Phys., Vol 16, p88–93, 1989.
42. McParland, B.J., An analysis of equivalent fields for electron beam central axis dose calculation, Med. Phys., Vol 19, p901–906, 1992.
43. Choi, M.C., Purdy, J.A., Gerbi, B.J., Abrath, F.G., and Glasgow, G.P., Variation in output factors caused by secondary blocking for 7-16 MeV electron beams, Med. Phys., Vol 6, p137–139, 1979.
44. Khan, F.M.,and Higgins, P.D., Calculation of depth dose and dose per monitor unit for irregularly shaped electron fields, Phys. Med. Biol., Vol. 44, pp N77–N80, 1999.
45. Giarattano, J.C., Duerkes, R.J., and Almond, P.R., Lead shielding thickness for dose reduction of 7-20 MeV electrons, Med. Phys., Vol 2, p336–337, 1975.
46. Khan, F.M., Moore, V.C., and Levitt, S.H., Field shaping in electron therapy, Br. J. Radiol., Vol 49, p883–886, 1976.
47. Khan, F.M., Werner, B.L., and Deibel, F.C., Lead shielding for electrons, Med. Phys., Vol 8, p712–713, 1981.
48. Asbell, S.O., Sill, J., Lightfoot, D.A., and Brady, N.L., Individualized eye shield for use in electron beam therapy as well as low energy photon irradiation, Int. J. Radiat. Oncol. Biol. Phys., Vol 6, p519–521, 1980.
49. Saunders, J.E., and Peters, V.G., Backscattering from metals in superficial therapy with high energy electrons, Br. J. Radiol., Vol 47, p467–470, 1974.
50. Gagnon, W.F., and Cundiff, J.H., Dose enhancement from back-scattered radiation at tissue metal interfaces irradiated with high energy electrons, Br. J. Radiol., Vol 53, p466–470, 1980.
51. Klavenhagen, S.C., Lambert, G.D., and Arbari, A., Backscattering in electron therapy for energies between 3 and 35 MeV, Phys. Med. Biol., Vol 27, p363–373, 1982.
52. Frank, H., Zur Vielfachstreuung und R$_\check{}$cksdiffusion schneller Elektronen nach Durchgang durch dicke Schichten, Z. Naturforsch., Vol 14a, p247–261, 1959.
53. Bjarngard, B.E., McCall, R.C., and Berstein, I.A., Lithium fluoride teflon thermoluminescent dosimeters, p308–316, in Proceedings of First International Conference on Luminescence Dosimetry, Stanford, Attix, F.H. (Ed.), Conference no. 650637, U.S. Atomic Energy Commission, Washington, D.C., 1967.
54. Dutreix, J., and Bernard, M., Dosimetry at interface for high-energy x and ? rays, Br. J. Radiol., Vol 39, p205–210, 1966.
55. Khan, F.M., Sewchand, W., and Levitt, S.H., Effect of air space on depth dose in electron beam therapy, Radiology, Vol 126, p249–252, 1978.
56. Jamshedi, A., Kuchnir, F.J., and Reft, C.S., Determination of the source position for the electron beams from a high energy linear accelerator, Med. Phys., Vol 13, p942–948, 1986.
57. Laughlin, J.S., High-energy electron treatment planning for inhomogeneities, Br. J. Radiol., Vol 38, p143–147, 1965.

58. Boone, M.L.M., Jardine, J.H., Wright, A.E., and Tapley, N., High-energy electron dose perturbations in the regions of tissue heterogeneity. I. In vivo dosimetry, Radiology, Vol 88, p1136–1145, 1967.
59. Almond, P.R., Wright, A.E., and Boone, M.L.M., High-energy electron dose perturbations in regions of tissue heterogeneity. II. Physical models of tissue heterogeneities, Radiology, Vol 88, p1146–1153, 1967.
60. Pohlit, W., Calculated and measured dose distributions in inhomogeneous materials and in patients, Ann. N.Y. Acad. Sci., Vol 161, p189–197, 1969.
61. Brenner, M., Karjalainen, P., Rytila, A., and Jungar, H., The effects of inhomogeneities on dose distribution of high-energy electrons, Ann. N.Y. Acad. Sci., Vol 161, p189–197, 1969.
62. Shrott, K.R., Ross, C.K., Bielajew, A.F., and Rogers, D.W.O., Electron beam dose distributions near standard inhomogeneities, Phys. Med. Biol., Vol 31, p235–249, 1986.
63. Hogstrom, K.R., Dosimetry of electron heterogeneities, p532–561, in Radiation Oncology Physics – 1986, Medical Physics Monograph 15, Keriakes, J.G., Elson, H.R., and Born, C.G. (Eds.), American Institute of Physics, New York, 1987.
64. Amdur, R.J., Kalbaugh, K.J., Ewald, L.M., Parsons, J.T., Mendenhall, W.M., Bova, F.J., and Million, R.R., Radiation therapy of skin cancer near the eye: Kilovoltage X-rays versus electrons, Int. J. Radiat. Oncol. Biol. Phys., Vol 23, p769–779, 1992.
65. Lovett, R.D., Perez, C.A., Shapiro, S.J., and Garcia, D.M., External irradiation of epithelial skin cancers, Int. J. Radiat. Oncol. Biol. Phys., Vol 19, p235–242, 1990.
66. Williams, P.C., Hunter, R.D., and Jackson, S.M., Whole body electron therapy in mycosis fungoides – a successful translational technique achieved by modification of an established linear accelerator, Br. J. Radiol., Vol 52, p302–307, 1979.
67. AAPM Task Group 30, AAPM Monograph 23, Total Skin Electron Therapy and Dosimetry, American Association of Physicists in Medicine, Radiation Therapy Committee, Report of Task Group 30, American Institute of Physics, New York, 1988.
68. Almond, P.R., Total skin electron irradiation and dosimetry, p296–332, in Radiation Oncology Physics – 1986, Medical Physics Monograph 15, Keriakes, J.G., Elson, H.R., and Born, C.G., (Eds.), American Institute of Physics, New York, 1987.
69. Page, V., Garner, A., and Karzmark, C.J., Patient dosimetry in electron treatment of large superficial lesions, Radiology, Vol 94, p635–641, 1970.
70. Goldson, A.L., Preliminary clinical experience with intraoperative radiotherapy, J. Natl. Med. Assoc., Vol 70, p493–495, 1978.
71. Biggs, P.J., Epp, E.R., Ling, C.L., Novack, D.H., and Michaels, H.B., Dosimetry, field shaping and other considerations for intraoperative electron therapy, Int. J. Radiat. Oncol. Biol. Phys., Vol 7, p875–884, 1981.
72. McCullough, E.C., and Anderson, J.A., The dosimetric properties of an applicator system for intraoperative electron-beam therapy utilizing a Clinac-18 accelerator, Med. Phys., Vol 9, p261–268, 1982.
73. McCullogh, E.C., and Biggs, P.J., Intraoperative electron therapy, p333–347, in Radiation Oncology Physics – 1986, Medical Physics Monograph 15, Keriakes, J.G., Elson, H.R., and Born, C.G., (Eds.), American Institute of Physics, New York, 1987.
74. Hogstrom, K.R., Boyer, A.L., Shiu, A.S., Ocharn, G., Kirsher, S.M., Krispel, F., and Rich, T., Design of metallic electron beam cones for an intraoperative therapy linear accelerator, Int. J. Radiat. Oncol. Biol. Phys., Vol 18, p1227–1332, 1991.
75. Nelson, C.E., Cook, R., and Rafkel, S., The dosimetric properties of an intraoperative radiation therapy applicator system, Med. Phys., Vol 16, p794–799, 1989.
76. Palta, J.R., Biggs, P.J., Hazle, J.D., Huq, M.S., Dahl, R.A., Ochran, T.G., Soen, J., Dobelbower, Jr., R.R., and McCullough, E.C., Intraoperative electron beam therapy: technique, dosimetry, and dose specification: Report of Task Force 48, Radiation Therapy Committee, American Association of Physicists in Medicine, Int. J. Radiat. Oncol. Biol. Phys., Vol. 33, pp725–746, 1995.
77. Dobblebower, R.R. and Abe, M. (Eds.), Intraoperative Radiation Therapy, CRC Press, Boca Raton, Florida, 1989.
78. Calvo, F.A., Hoekstra, H.J., and Lehnert, T., Intraoperative radiotherapy: 20 years of clinical experience, technological development and consolidation of results (Review), European J. Surg. Oncol., Vol. 26, Spplement A, pp S1–S4, 2000.
79. Valentini, V., Balducci, M., Morganti, A.G., De Giorgi, U., and Fiorentini, G., Intraoperative radiotherapy: current thinking, European J. of Surg. Oncol., Vol. 28, pp180–185, 2001
80. Mills, M.D., Fajardo, L. C., Wilson, D. L., Daves, J. L. and Spanos, W.J., Commissioning of a mobile electron accelerator for intraoperative radiotherapy, J. Appl. Clin. Med. Phys., Vol. 2., pp121–130, 2001.

81. Meurk, M.L., Goer, D.A., Spalek, G., and Cook, T., The Mobetron: A new concept for IORT, pp 65-70, in Intraoperative Radiotherapy in the Treatment of Cancer, (ED: Vaeth, J.M.), Karger, Basel, 1997.

82. Leavitt, D.D., Peacock, L.M., Gibbs, F.A., and Stewart, J.R., Electron arc therapy: Physical measurements and treatment planning techniques, Int. J. Radiat. Oncol. Biol. Phys., Vol 11, p985–999, 1985.

83. Hogstrom, K.R., and Leavitt, D., Dosimetry of arc electron therapy, p265–295, in Radiation Oncology Physics – 1986, Medical Physics Monograph 15, Keriakes, J.G., Elson, H.R., and Born, C.G., (Eds.), American Institute of Physics, New York, 1987.

84. Khan, F.M., Calibration and treatment planning of electron beam arc therapy, p249–266, in Electron Dosimetry and Arc Therapy, Proceedings of Symposium, Paliwal, B. (Ed.), American Institute of Physics, New York, 1982.

85. Levitt, D.D., Stewart, J.R., Moeller, J.H., and Early, L., Optimization of electron arc therapy by multi-vane collimator control, Int. J. Radiat. Oncol. Biol. Phys., Vol 16, p489–496, 1989.

86. Lam, K.S., Lam, W.C., O'Neill, M.J., and Zinreich, E., Electron arc therapy: Beam data requirements and treatment planning, Clin. Radiol., Vol 38, p379–383, 1987.

87. Pla, M., Podgorsak, E.B., Pla, C., and Freeman, C.R., Determination of secondary collimator shape in electron arc therapy, Phys. Med. Biol., Vol 38, p999–1006, 1993.

88. Pla, M., Pla, C., and Podgorsak, E.B., The influence of beam parameters on percentage depth dose in electron arc therapy, Med. Phys., Vol 15, p49–55, 1988.

89. Pla, M., Podgorsak, E.B., Freeman, C.R., Souhami, L., and Guerra, J., Physical aspects of the angle β concept in electron arc therapy, Int. J. Radiat. Oncol. Biol. Phys., Vol 20, p1331–1339, 1991.

90. Olivares-Pla, M., Podgorsak, E.B., and Pla, C., Electron arc dose distributions as a function of beam energy, Med. Phys., Vol. 24, pp127–132, 1997

91. Boyer, A.L., Fullerton, G.D., and Mira, J.G., An electron beam pseudoarc technique for irradiation of large areas of chest wall and other curved surfaces, Int. J. Radiat. Oncol. Biol. Phys., Vol 8, p1969-1974, 1982.

92. McKenzie, M.R., Freeman, C.R., Pla, M., Guerra, J., Souhami, L., Pla, C., and Podgorsak, E.B., Clinical experience with pseudoarc therapy, Br. J. Radiol., Vol 66, p234–240, 1993.

93. Boyer, A.L., Fullerton, G.D., Mira, J.G., and Mok, E.C., An electron beam pseudo arc technique, p267–293, in Electron Dosimetry and Arc Therapy, Proceedings of Symposium, Paliwal, B. (Ed.), American Institute of Physics, New York, 1982.

94. Pla, M., Podgorsak, E.B., and Pla, C., Electron dose rate and photon contamination in electron arc therapy, Med. Phys., Vol 16, p692–697, 1989.

95. Bagne, F., Adjacent fields of high-energy X-rays and electrons, Phys. Med. Biol., Vol 23, p1186–1191, 1978.

96. Bhaduri, D., Choi, M.C., Weaver, J., and Agarwal, S.K., Matching of electron fields on flat surfaces, J. Am. Assoc. Med. Dosim., Vol 9, p12–16, 1984.

97. Frass, B.A., Tepper, J.E., Glatstein, E., and van de Geijn, J.A., Clinical use of a matchline wedge for adjacent megavoltage radiation field line matching, Int. J. Radiat. Oncol. Biol. Phys., Vol 9, p209–216, 1983.

98. Kalend, A., Zwicker, R.D., Wu, A., and Sternick, E.S., A beam edge modifier for abutting electron fields, Med. Phys., Vol 12, p793–798, 1985.

99. Kurup, R.G., Wang, S., and Glasgow, G.P., Field matching of electron beams using plastic wedge penumbra generators, Phys. Med. Biol., Vol 37, p145–153, 1992.

100. Kurup, R.G., Glasgow, G.P., and Leybovich, L.B., Design of electron beam wedges for increasing penumbra abutting fields, Phys. Med. Biol., Vol 38, p667–674, 1993.

101. McKenzie, A.L., A simple method for matching electron beams in radiotherapy, Phys. Med. Biol., Vol. 43, pp3465–3478, 1998.

102. Lachance, B., Tremblay, D., and Pouliot, J., A new penumbra generator for electron fields matching, Med. Phys., Vol. 24, pp485–495, 1997.

103. Papiez, E., Dunscombe, P.B., and Malakar, K., Matching photon and electron fields in the treatment of head and neck tumors, Med. Phys., Vol 19, p335–341, 1992.

Additional Reading

1. Task Group 25, Radiation Therapy Committee, American Association of Physicists in Medicine, Clinical Electron Beam Dosimetry, Med. Phys., Vol 18, p73–109, 1991.

2. ICRU Report 35, Radiation Dosimetry: Electron Beams with Energies Between 1 and 50 MeV, International Commission on Radiological Units and Measurements, Bethesda, Maryland, 1984.

3. Klavenhagen, S.C., Physics of Electron Beam Therapy, HPA Medical Physics Handbook 13, Adam Hilger, Bristol, 1985.
4. Keriakes, J.G., Elson, H.R., and Born, C.G. (Eds.), Radiation Oncology Physics – 1986, Medical Physics Monograph 15, American Institute of Physics, New York, 1987.
5. Vaeth, J.M., and Meyer, J.L. (Eds.), The Role of High Energy Electrons in the Treatment of Cancer, Karger, Basel, 1991.
6. Jayaraman, S., Pathways and pitfalls in treatment planning with external beams: the role of the clinical physicist, Radiographics, Vol 8, p.1147–1170, 1988.

CHAPTER 17

Physics of the Use of Small Sealed Sources in Brachytherapy

17.1
Brachytherapy

Brachytherapy is a method of radiation treatment in which discrete radiation sources are placed in close proximity to or within the tissues to be treated. The prefix 'brachy' means 'short-range' in Greek. The word 'endocurie therapy' also has been in use ('endo' = within). Most of these treatments are performed with photons; in a few situations, beta particles and neutrons are used. The brachytherapy sources may be in the form of radioactive seeds or linear capsules. These sources generally contain a small amount of radioactive material within a metallic capsule having a wall of 0.1 to 1 mm thickness. The container keeps the radioactive material from entering the patient's tissues or body fluids during its use. It also prevents contamination of the surroundings with radioactivity during source storage and handling.

In early brachytherapy practice [1], naturally occurring radium encapsulated in platinum was used as the source of radiation. Martin and Martin [2], in 1959, documented pictorially the regression of several tumors treated with gamma rays emanating from radium needles. Radium, however, has the major disadvantage that its decay product, radon, is a gas. Thus, any breach in a radium container can result in leakage of radon gas into the atmosphere. The diffusing radon can spread, decay further into its own radioactive daughter products, and contribute to widespread radioactive contamination [3]. All radium sources need to be tested frequently for radon leaks.

Since artificially produced radionuclide sources became available, they have been favored as substitutes for radium [4–6] In general, all brachytherapy sources should be tested to ensure the integrity of their encapsulation and thus to avoid the spread of radioactivity [7, 8]. In some localities, regulations stipulate the frequency with which sealed sources should be tested for leakage.

Some beta sources are also used in brachytherapy for treatment of superficial lesions [9–12]. However, most common brachytherapy applications make use of the dose delivered by the penetrating photons emitted from radioactive sources. Another purpose served by the capsule, apart from helping to contain the radioactive material, is that it is thick enough to absorb any short-range beta particles emitted by the source. The useful radiation fluence is made up mostly of gamma rays, and also of characteristic X-rays emitted incidental to the atomic and nuclear transitions. In addition, there is a contribution by characteristic X-rays and bremsstrahlung produced in the source capsule. However, these usually form a negligible component. Table 17.1 lists the characteristics of several radionuclides for use in brachytherapy. In this chapter, we discuss the dosimetry of the gamma ray sealed sources used in brachytherapy and

Table 17.1. Physical Properties of Radionuclide Sources Used in Brachytherapy

Element	Source isotope	Beta(s) (E_β)max (keV)	Energy Range of Photons (keV)	Mean Photon Energy (keV)	Half-Life T_h	HVT in Lead (mm)	TVT in Lead (mm)	Exposure Rate Constant (Γ_x) $\mu C\,kg^{-1}\,cm^2\,MBq^{-1}\,h^{-1}$ [$R\,cm^2\,mCi^{-1}\,h^{-1}$]	Air-kerma Rate Constant (Γ_{ak}) $\mu Gy\,cm^2\,MBq^{-1}\,h^{-1}$	Dose Rate (Λ) $cGy\,h^{-1}$ $cGy\,cm^2\,h^{-1}$
Photon Sources										
Radium	226Ra	17–3260	47–2440	830	≈1600 years	14	42	58.2 [8.35][b]	1971	1.10
Radon	222Rn	17–3260	47–2440	830	3.8 d	14	42	58.2 [8.35]	1971	1.10
Gold	198Au	29–1370	412–1088	416	2.7 d	3	11	16.3 [2.34]	552	1.13
Cobalt	60Co	313	1170, 1330	1250	5.26 years	11	46	90.5 [12.98]	3064	1.11
Cesium	137Cs	514, 1170	662	662	30 years	6	22	22.9 [3.28]	774	1.11
Tantalum	182Ta	180–514	43–1453	670	115 d	12	39	54.0 [7.75]	1829	1.13
Iridium	192Ir	240–670	136–1062	380	74 d	3	12	32.7 [4.69]	1107	1.12
Iodine	125I	None	27–35	29	59.6 d	0.025	0.1	10.11 [1.45]	342	0.90
Palladium	103Pd	None	20–23	21	17 d	0.008	0.03	10.32 [1.48]	349	0.74
Americium	241Am	None	60	60	432 years	0.125	0.4	0.850 [0.122]	28.8	–
Samarium	145Sm	None	38–61	41	340 d	0.06	0.2	6.17 [0.885]	209	–
Ytterbium	169Yb	None	49–308	93	32 d	0.2	0.7	12.55 [1.8]	425	1.19
Beta Sources										
Strontium	90Sr & 90Y	540 & 2270	None	None	28.9 years & 64 h					
Phosphorous	32P	1710	None	None	14.3 d					
Ruthenium	106Ru & 107Rh	39 & 3540	None & 500 (in 21% of decay and other photons of energies up to 1550 in very low intensities)	None	368 d & 40 sec					

Note: Data subject to continuous revisions and update. The above values are assembled by the authors based on various references 6, 27 to 31 (including Jani, S.K., Handbook of Dosimetry Data for Radiotherapy, CRC Press, Boca Raton, Florida, 1993, and their own calculations and estimates).
[a] Estimated for an ideal point source with isotropic emission. Actual sources may have a range of values.
[b] Applicable for radium sources filtered by 0.5 mm Pt. Assumes 0.988 mCi/mg Ra.

the problem of planning the dose distribution in brachytherapy for controlled delivery of the radiation dose.

17.2
Categories of Applications

Brachytherapy can be classified broadly into three categories: *surface, interstitial,* and *intra-cavitary* applications.

In *surface* applications, a block of wax, dental compound, or any near-tissue-equivalent plastic material is molded to form a layer of uniform thickness. The molded layer is placed on a body surface that bears a superficial lesion to be irradiated, as shown in Figure 17.1. An outline is drawn with a margin around the lesion, identifying the 'target area' for the treatment. The sources are distributed on the top surface of the mold over a 'source area.' The thickness of the mold, h, is referred to as the treatment distance.

For practical treatments, on many occasions, **h** is chosen to be 0.5 cm; at other times, it may be an integral multiple of 0.5 cm. The value of **h** influences the dose fall-off with depth within the lesion. The smaller the value of **h**, the steeper the dose fall-off with depth from the skin. Surface application is not suitable for lesions deeper than a few millimeters.

For thick lesions, an *interstitial* application, in which the sources are implanted or embedded directly in the lesion, is favored. Such an application is called an implant. The simplest of these is a single-plane implant, in which sources are spread over an area in one plane within the slab of tissue to be treated. It is obvious that the dose rate will be high in the implant plane (i. e., the source plane) and fall off at distances away from it. It has traditionally been assumed that sources implanted in a plane can adequately irradiate tissues located up to 0.5 cm away from it, as illustrated in Figure 17.2a. Thus,

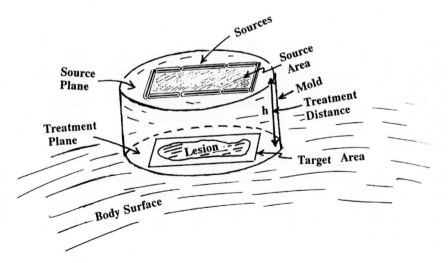

Fig. 17.1. A surface application with discrete sources arranged on top of a mold

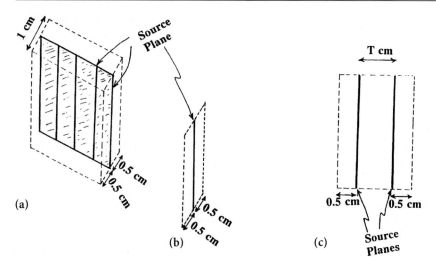

Fig. 17.2. Size of the target volumes for planar implants. (a) A single-plane implant in a three-dimensional view. (b) End-on view of a single-plane implant. (c) End-on view of a two-plane implant with an interplanar spacing T

the target volume for a single-plane implant is regarded to be a slab of tissue of 1 cm thickness extending up to 0.5 cm on either side of the implant plane.

For treatment of lesions thicker than 1 cm, a two-plane implant of sources in two parallel planes can be considered. With the assumption that any plane implant can treat up to a distance of 0.5 cm, implants in two planes separated by T cm can irradiate a target volume of thickness (T + 1) cm, as illustrated in Figure 17.2c. If the two source planes are 1.0 cm apart, the target thickess will be 2 cm. With a separation of 1.0 to 2.0 cm between the two source planes, a two-plane implant can treat a slab of 2.0 to 3.0 cm thickness.

Use of two-plane separations of more than 1.5 cm can create low-dose regions midway between the source planes. For larger thicknesses, the use of more than two planes of sources may be appropriate. The implant is then called a volume implant. The implanted volume can be of any chosen shape – rectangular, cylindrical, spherical, or ellipsoidal – so as to cover the lesion and the target volume.

If sources are implanted for a specified duration of irradiation and then removed, the implant is a temporary implant. The term 'removable implant' is also sometimes used. In some instances, short-lived radionuclide sources may be implanted and left permanently in the body to decay. Such an implant is called a permanent implant.

In *intracavitary* insertions, the sources are positioned in accessible body cavities to irradiate lesions located there. Tumors that grow around the uterine and vaginal cavities have been successfully irradiated by intracavitary insertions of radioactive sources. Lesions in esophageal and bronchial passages have also been treated by insertion of tubes and placement of sources. These techniques are sometimes referred to as 'intraluminal' therapy.

In the early practice of brachytherapy, radium needles were pushed directly into tissues as implants. For intracavitary insertions, catheters and applicators loaded with radioactive sources were inserted into the patient. Thus, the applicators were 'preloaded' with the sources prior to insertion into the patient. Because the procedure involved handling of applicators that already contained the radioactive sources, the personnel was exposed to radiation even during the time of insertion and positioning of the sources in the cavities. In contrast, in modern practice, afterloading techniques have become common [13–20]. In these techniques, empty guides or catheters, without radioactive sources, are first inserted and positioned in the patient. Thus, in the early part of the procedure of handling the catheters, radiation exposure to personnel is avoided. After making sure that the catheters are properly positioned, one can promptly load the radioactive sources into them. The simplest approach is manual insertion of the sources, which are held with a handle.

Sophisticated remote-handling apparatus has also become available for source insertion and retrieval. These devices steer the sources into the catheters and retrieve them after a preassigned period of irradiation. With such remote-handling techniques it is possible and safe to use sources of very high activities and employ a high-dose-rate (HDR). Such HDR techniques deliver a large radiation dose in a very short period of only a few minutes. This is in contrast to the conventional low-dose-rate (LDR) techniques that employ dose rates in the range of 10–100 cGy h^{-1} with the treatment time lasting for 1–7 days. In relation to cell damage, repair, division and multiplication, the radiobiological implications of HDR and LDR treatments are known to be very different. A dose of 60 Gy delivered in a few days using sources with low activities (of 100 to 1000 MBq) can have a drastically different biological effect than the same dose delivered in a few minutes using sources of very high activities (of 100 to 1000 GBq). The radiation safety aspects to personnel and surroundings are also quite different for the two situations. But the physical principles that govern the radiation dose distributions and delivery are same for both. Hence no distinction is made in this chapter between HDR and LDR brachytherapy.

17.3
Source Strength of Brachytherapy Sources

17.3.1
Need for Specification of Source Strength

An institution may possess several sources that are identical in physical size, construction, and the radionuclide contained, but each of the individual sources may give different fluence yields, i. e., the sources may be of different strengths. This is analogous to having electric bulbs of different wattages providing distinct luminescence yields. Each brachytherapy source has a specified source strength that is used for the calculation of dose rate. The source strength is generally specified in a certificate issued by the source supplier. It is possible to state the source strength in terms of one of several interrelated physical quantities. These quantities are radium-equivalent mass, absolute activity, apparent activity, and air-kerma yield rate. The numerical relationships of the source strengths as specified by these quantities for brachytherapy sources in common use are given in Reference 21. It is currently recommended that the physical quantity to be preferred for specifying the source strength is the air-kerma yield rate [22].*

---

* Also called reference air-kerma rate.

The unit in which the source strength is specified should be traceable to the standards maintained by the national and international standardization laboratories.

17.3.2
Specification by Radium-Equivalent Mass

In the early practice of brachytherapy, radium* was the predominant source in use. The radium sources were assayed in terms of the actual mass of radium contained (in milligrams). The standard radium sources were contained in 0.5 mm thick platinum (with 10% iridium) capsules. The radium source strength was specified in milligrams and was intended to be used together with a radium exposure rate constant $\Gamma_x = 8.25\,R\,cm^2\,mg^{-1}\,h^{-1}$ (i. e., equivalent to $\Gamma_{ak} = 8.25 \times 0.873 = 7.20\,cGy\,cm^2\,mg^{-1}\,h^{-1}$; see Section 11.9), which applied specifically to radium sources in containers having a 0.5-mm platinum wall thickness.

Using the mass for specification of source strength was possible with radium, because all of the radium nuclides without exception are radioactive. However, in artificially produced radioactive materials, only a certain percentage of the target nuclides are activated and become radioactive (see Section 5.4). Thus, the mass is not a direct measure of the radioactivity contained. However, if the exposure rate (or air-kerma rate) from such a non-radium source is compared with that from a radium source of known mass, its strength (i. e., radioactivity) in terms of radium-equivalent mass can be assessed.

A reentrant ionization chamber, shown schematically in Figure 17.3, is a device that is useful for rapid verification of the source strength in hospital settings. The chamber has a well-type receptacle for the source. The ion-collection volume of the chamber surrounds the source in almost all directions, except in the direction toward the opening of the well.

Let us say that a standard radium source of strength S_{stmg} mg is placed in the receptacle and a reading of the ionization current, R_{st}, is obtained. Next, the source is replaced by the non-radium source to be assayed in the same geometry, and a reading, R, is obtained. The milligram radium equivalent (mgRaeq), S_{mg} (0.5 mm PtIr), of the assayed source is

$$S_{mg} = \frac{R}{R_{st}} S_{stmg}\ mgRaeq\ (in\ a\ 0.5\text{-}mm\ PtIr\ capsule) \qquad (17\text{-}1)$$

The value S_{mg} stated in mgRaeq units (in a 0.5-mm PtIr capsule) can be used together with the radium exposure rate constant $(\Gamma_x)_{Ra} = 8.25\,R\,cm^2\,mg^{-1}\,h^{-1}$ to yield the exposure rate, $\dot{X}_{air}$ at a distance r from the source in air, as follows:**

$$\dot{X}_{air} = \frac{(\Gamma_x)_{Ra} \cdot S_{mg}}{r^2} \qquad (17\text{-}2)$$

A similar equation can be used with the air-kerma rate constant for radium, $(\Gamma_{ak})_{Ra} = 7.70\,cGy\,cm^2\,mg^{-1}\,h^{-1}$, to give the kerma rate in air, $\dot{k}_{air}$, at a distance r

---

* Radium in medicine typically means ^{226}Ra.

** A dot placed over any quantity such as, $\dot{X}_{air}$ or $\dot{k}_{air}$ indicates the time rate of change of that quantity.

Fig. 17.3. A reentrant ionization chamber useful for source
strength intercomparisons

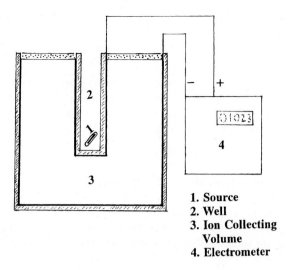

1. **Source**
2. **Well**
3. **Ion Collecting
   Volume**
4. **Electrometer**

from the source by the relation

$$\dot{k}_{air} = \frac{(\Gamma_{ak})_{Ra} \cdot S_{mg}}{r^2} \qquad (17\text{-}3)$$

The use of a reentrant chamber as described above, however, has some limitations
[23, 24].

17.3.3
Specification by Activity

The most fundamental physical quantity that specifies the strength of a source is its
absolute disintegration rate (i. e., activity), S_{act}. For example, S_{act} may be stated to be
100 MBq. If it is a point source having a capsule that filters the radiation by a factor
A_{enc}, then the air-kerma rate, $\dot{k}_{air}$, at a distance r from the source is given by

$$\dot{k}_{air} = \frac{\Gamma_{ak} S_{act} A_{enc}}{r^2} \qquad (17\text{-}4)$$

where Γ_{ak} is the air-kerma rate constant for the radionuclide composing the source (see
Section 11.9). Although the activity S_{act} is fundamental in its nature, specification in
terms of it can cause discrepancies in dosimetry and hence is not recommended. This
is because, in practice, the activity is often derived indirectly, based on an exposure or
air-kerma rate measurement. The vendor may report the value of S_{ak} to the user in a
certificate, but may actually have measured $\dot{k}_{air}$ and derived the value of S_{act} through
Equation (17-4) by assuming certain values for Γ_{ak} and A_{enc}. The user, in turn, cannot
use the reported value of S_{act} for practical dosimetry without assigning values for Γ_{ak}
and A_{enc}. The method or the references by which he selects these values may disagree
with those which the source vendor adopted, thus leaving room for a discrepancy
between $\dot{k}_{air}$ as derived by the vendor and that derived by a user. A part of this problem

is solved if the vendor derives and reports to the user an apparent activity, S_{app}, given by

$$S_{app} = (S_{act} \cdot A_{enc}) = \frac{r^2 \dot{k}_{air}}{\Gamma_{ak}} \tag{17-5}$$

Using S_{app} (instead of S_{act}) allows the user to depend on the published references for Γ_{ak} only. However, Γ_{ak} values have been calculated and reported differently for many radionuclides by various investigators. Thus, the possibility for an inconsistency in the selection of Γ_{ak} and the derivation of $\dot{k}_{air}$ remains.

17.3.4
Specification by Air-Kerma Rate Yield

The source strength can be specified in terms of the kerma rate, $\dot{k}_{air}$, in air at a particular distance r from the source, with the source in free space [22]. The air-kerma rate yielded by the source value can be expressed as normalized at a unit distance of 1 cm or 1 m from the source. That is, the air-kerma strength, S_{ak}, of a source is defined to be such that

$$\dot{k}_{air} = \frac{S_{ak}}{r^2} \tag{17-6}$$

or

$$S_{ak} = \dot{k}_{air} r^2 \tag{17-7}$$

S_{ak} can be expressed in units of μGy m^2 h^{-1} (or cGy cm^2 h^{-1} which are equivalent).* In writing the above equations, we have assumed that the source is a point isotropic source giving the same $\dot{k}_{air}$ at a distance r in all directions. Linear sources have non-isotropic emissions. For these, a source strength S_{ak} can be based on the convention that the value of $\dot{k}_{air}$ is measured at a point along the mid-perpendicular line of the source at a distance very much larger than the active length of the source. It is apparent from (17-4) and (17-7) that

$$S_{ak} = \Gamma_{ak} S_{act} A_{enc} \tag{17-8}$$

17.3.5
Specification by Water-Kerma Rate Yield

The source strength can be specified also in terms of the kerma rate, $\dot{k}_{water}$, yielded in water at a stated distance r from the source, with the source in free space. Again, the value can be presented as normalized at a unit distance of 1 cm or 1 m from the source. That is, the water-kerma strength, S_{wk}, of a source is given by

$$S_{wk} = \dot{k}_{water} r^2 \tag{17-9}$$

S_{wk} and S_{ak} are related by

$$\frac{S_{wk}}{S_{ak}} = \frac{[\mu_{tr}/\rho]_{water}}{[\mu_{tr}/\rho]_{air}} \tag{17-10}$$

---

* S_{ak} is also referred to as 'reference air-kerma rate'. Some literature refer to one unit of μGy m^2 h^{-1} ($\approx$ cGy cm^2 h^{-1}) as 1 U. See also Section 11.10 in Chapter 11.

17.4
Source Strength and Time Product

17.4.1
Significance

The dose delivered in any particular brachytherapy application increases in direct proportion to both the source strength employed and the duration of irradiation. The dose delivered to the patient can be controlled by either or both of these. For delivery of a given dose, sources of low strength can be used over a long treatment time, or sources of high strength can be employed for a correspondingly shorter time. Thus, the product of source strength and time of irradiation can serve as a single index of treatment. Brachytherapy dosage tables have been published giving the value of this index for the delivery of a stated dose for different source arrays, with the stated dose conforming to a particular definition or system. The systems or approaches are explained in Section 17.9.

17.4.2
Milligram Hours of Treatment

The dosage tables published for radium sources in the past used milligram hours (mgh) as the treatment index. In general, if a source of strength S_{mg} is used for T hours, the mgh is $S_{mg} \times T$. If an array of **m** sources with source strengths $(S_{mg})_1, (S_{mg})_2, \ldots, (S_{mg})_m$ is used over an irradiation period T, the total mgh is the following sum:

$$\left[(S_{mg})_1 + (S_{mg})_2 + \ldots + (S_{mg})_m\right] \times T \text{ mgh}$$

17.4.3
Air-Kerma Yield of Treatment

If the source strength is evaluated in air-kerma rate yield in $cGy\,cm^2\,h^{-1}$, the product of source strength and time becomes $cGy\,cm^2$. We will call this the air-kerma yield of treatment. It is an overall index of both the source strength employed and the time of irradiation. In general, if a source of strength S_{ak} ($cGy\,cm^2\,h^{-1}$) is used for T hours of irradiation, the corresponding air-kerma yield of treatment is

$$(S_{ak}\,cGy\,cm^2\,h^{-1} \times T\,h) = (S_{ak} \times T)\,cGy\,cm^2$$

If it is an array of **m** sources with source strengths $(S_{ak})_1, (S_{ak})_2, \ldots, (S_{ak})_m$, used over an irradiation period T, the corresponding air-kerma yield is the following sum:

$$[(S_{ak})_1 + (S_{ak})_2 + \ldots + (S_{ak})_m] \times T\,cGy\,cm^2$$

EXAMPLE 17.1

Early tables of radium dosage presented the data as milligram hours required to deliver an exposure of 1000 R. A radium exposure rate constant of $\Gamma_x = 8.40\,R\,cm^2\,mg^{-1}\,h^{-1}$ was used. All calculations were done in air, ignoring tissue attenuation, scatter, and filtration in the capsule. It has been determined that the milligram hours will increase, on the average, by a factor of 1.015 if these effects are allowed for [25]. Derive the factor by which the milligram hours for 1000 R can be converted to air-kerma yield (cGy cm^2) for delivery of a dose of 1 cGy to water. (Given: $1\,R = 2.58 \times 10^{-4}\,C\,kg^{-1}$, $W = 33.85\,J\,C^{-1}$, $(f_{xd})_{water} = 0.965\,cGy\,R^{-1}$ for radium gamma rays.)

The exposure yield calculated for 1 mgh of radium irradiation was

$$\Gamma_x \times 1\,mgh = 8.40\,R\,cm^2\,mg^{-1}\,h^{-1} \times 1\,mgh = 8.40\,R\,cm^2$$

The corresponding air-kerma yield is

$$8.40\,R\,cm^2 \times 2.58 \times 10^{-4}\,C\,kg^{-1}\,R^{-1} \times 33.85\,J\,C^{-1}$$
$$= 8.4 \times 8.733 \times 10^{-3}\,J\,kg^{-1}\,cm^2$$
$$= 7.336\,cGy\,cm^2$$

In addition, an exposure of 1000 R is equivalent to a dose of

$$1000\,R \times (f_{xd})_{water} = 1000\,R \times 0.965\,cGy\,R^{-1} = 965\,cGy$$

Furthermore, to allow for attenuation and scatter in tissue and filtration in the capsule, the milligram hours should be increased by 1.015. Hence, M mgh for delivery of 1000 R in the early data becomes:

$$M\,mgh \times 1.015 \times (7.336\,cGy\,cm^2/mgh) \times (1/965\,cGy)$$
$$= [7.716 \times 10^{-3}\,M]\,cGy\,cm^2\ air\text{-}kerma\ yield\ for\ delivery\ of\ 1\ cGy\ in\ water$$

In more recent times, dosage tables giving milligram hours for 1000 cGy have been published for Γ_x of 8.25 R cm^2 mg^{-1} h^{-1}, $(f_{xd})_{tissue}$ of 0.957 cGy R^{-1}. These, unlike the tables of earlier years, did allow for tissue attenuation and filtration. For such cases, M mgh for 1000 cGy will convert to

$$(M\,mgh/1000\,cGy) \times 8.25\,R\,cm^2\,mg^{-1}\,h^{-1} \times 2.58 \times 10^{-4}\,C\,kg^{-1}\,R^{-1}$$
$$\times\ 33.85\,J\,C^{-1} \times [0.957\,cGy\,R^{-1}/0.965\,cGy\,R^{-1}]$$
$$= [7.145 \times 10^{-3}\,M]\,cGy\,cm^2\ for\ delivery\ of\ 1\ cGy\ in\ water$$

17.5
Dosimetry of a Point Source in Water

17.5.1
Theoretical Approach

A theoretical formula can be developed for the dosimetry of an ideal point source which (i) has a radioactive volume of near-zero dimensions and (ii) emits radiation isotropically. Such an ideal source S that has a source strength S_{ak} and has an encapsulation is shown located in air in Figure 17.4a and in water in Figure 17.4b. In the latter case, the attenuation and scatter in water make the situation comparable to that in a patient. Point P is at distance r from the source. The dose rate, $(\dot{D}_P)_{in\ air}$, to a mass of water large enough to provide charged-particle equilibrium (see Section 11.7.2) surrounded

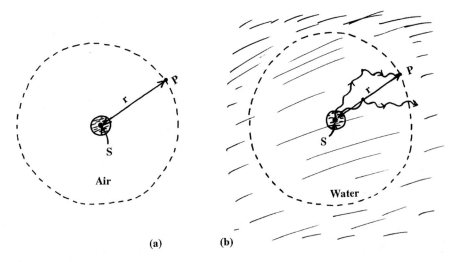

Fig. 17.4. An encapsulated point source (a) in air under minimum attenuation and scatter conditions, (b) in water with attenuation loss and scatter gain

Table 17.2. Air-Kerma To Water Dose Conversion Factors

Photon Energy (keV)	Factor $(f_{akmd})_{water}$ [a]
30	1.007
50	1.030
100	1.094
600	1.111
800	1.111
1000	1.104
1500	1.102

[a] Given by the ratio $\dfrac{[\bar{\mu}_{ab}/\rho]_{water}}{[\bar{\mu}_{tr}/\rho]_{air}}$

by air at P is

$$(\dot{D}_P)_{in\ air} = \dot{k}_{air} \cdot (f_{akmd})_{water} = (S_{ak}/r^2) \cdot (f_{akmd})_{water} \qquad (17\text{-}11)$$

where $(f_{akmd})_{water}$ is the air-kerma to medium-dose conversion factor, the medium being water. Values of $(f_{akmd})_{water}$ at different photon energies are given in Table 17.2.

To derive the dose rate in water, $(\dot{D}_P)_{in\ water}$, at point P at distance r from the source, we modify the calculated $(\dot{D}_P)_{in\ air}$ to allow for attenuation and scatter in water. We will refer to this factor as the water perturbation correction (WPC).* The WPC is a function of the distance r from the source and is defined by the ratio

$$WPC(r) = \frac{\text{dose (to water) at distance r in water}}{\text{dose (to water) at distance r in air}} = \frac{(\dot{D}_P)_{in\ water}}{(\dot{D}_P)_{in\ air}}$$

---

* Some literature refer to WPC as tissue-attenuation and buildup correction.

Thus, the dose rate, $(\dot{D}_P)_{in\ water}$, at P when the source is immersed in water is

$$(\dot{D}_P)_{in\ water} = \dot{k}_{air} \cdot (f_{akmd})_{water} \cdot WPC(r) = \frac{S_{ak}}{r^2} \cdot (f_{akmd})_{water} \cdot WPC(r) \qquad (17\text{-}12)$$

The values of WPC(r) have been studied by different investigators with both theoretical and experimental methods. The values given in Table 17.3 are indicative of the trend and relative magnitudes of the perturbation corrections (as compiled by the authors of this book based on published results) [26] for various isotopes in common use. Among the sources listed in Table 17.3, all except ^{103}Pd emit photons of high energy (several hundred kiloelectron volts). We can explain why the WPC for these high-energy emitters remains so close to unity, particularly at distances within 3 cm of the source. Water is a denser medium than air. Hence, there is a reduction in the primary photon fluence reaching point P in water compared to air due to attenuation along the ray SP in Figure 17.4. However, in the denser medium of water, more scattering events also occur all around compared to air. Thus, the scattered photon fluence reaching point P is greater in water than in air. Overall, in water at distances close to the source, the reduction in the primary fluence through attenuation is nearly balanced by the increased scatter fluence. At large distances from the source, the WPC values are significantly below unity. For ^{125}I and ^{103}Pd, which emit photons of particularly low energies (in the 20- to 30-keV range), the Compton scatter events are fewer, and consequently the WPC values are very low even at short distances. Overall, at close distances of interest in brachytherapy, the geometric inverse-square fall-off of intensity becomes a more significant factor than the WPC. This is because the bulk of the dose delivered to any point is likely to be contributed by the sources located near that point.

It is to be noted that WPC(r) is related to the buildup factor B(μr) (discussed in Sections 11.10.2 and 7.10.2) through the relation WPC(r) $\approx [e^{-\mu r} B(\mu r)]$, with μ being the attenuation coefficient in water.

A point-source approximation may be valid for the dosimetry of many radioactive-seed implants. The isodose surfaces from an ideal point source are concentric spheres which almost follow the inverse-square law at distances close to the source. The water perturbation corrections cause a deviation from strict adherence to the inverse-square law. Such deviations become significant at distances of several centimeters from the source.

Table 17.3. Water Perturbation Corrections (WPC) for Different Radionuclides Used in Brachytherapy

Source	Distance from Source (cm)									
Nuclide	0.5	1.0	2.0	3.0	4.0	5.0	6.0	8.0	10.0	
^{226}Ra	0.999	0.994	0.985	0.972	0.957	0.945	0.915	0.894	0.860	*
^{137}Cs	1.004	1.000	0.989	0.978	0.966	0.952	0.936	0.913	0.856	*
^{192}Ir	0.994	1.017	1.018	1.017	1.013	1.006	0.997	0.968	0.925	**
^{60}Co	0.991	0.986	0.974	0.958	0.940	0.919	0.897	0.852	0.813	*
^{198}Au	1.027	1.023	1.017	1.012	1.006	0.997	0.987	0.954	0.901	*
^{103}Pd	0.974	0.725	0.391	0.209	0.113	0.065	0.038	–	–	**

* Average of several published values based on Meisberger et al. [26]
** From Meigooni, A.S. et al. [31]

If $\dot{D}(r_0)$ and $\dot{D}(r)$ are the dose rates at a reference distance r_0 close to the source and at a distance r, respectively, a radial function $g(r)$ is defined by the ratio*

$$g(r) = \frac{\dot{D}(r)r^2}{\dot{D}(r_0)r_0^2} \qquad (17\text{-}13)$$

The value of $g(r)$ is a measure of the lack of conformity to the inverse-square fall-off caused by absorption and scatter in the medium. Thus, $g(r)$ is a measure of the penetration of radiation in tissue (or water). The functions $g(r)$ and $WPC(r)$ are related by

$$g(r) = [WPC(r)/WPC(r_0)]$$

The reference distance r_0 is usually 1.0 cm. Values of $g(r)$ for several source nuclides are given in Table 17.4.

Table 17.4. Values of $g(r)$ for Different Radioisotope Sources

Source Nuclide	Distance from source r (cm)							
	1.0	2.0	3.0	4.0	5.0	6.0	8.0	10.0
^{137}Cs	1.00	0.99	0.98	0.97	0.96	0.95	0.91	0.88
^{192}Ir	1.00	1.03	1.00	0.97	0.97	0.97	0.94	0.87
^{198}Au	1.00	1.01	1.01	1.01	1.01	1.01	0.98	0.95
^{125}I*	1.00	0.85	0.655	0.50	0.36	0.275	0.18	–
^{103}Pd	1.00	0.54	0.29	0.16	0.09	0.05	–	–
^{145}Sm	1.00	1.02	0.97	0.92	0.87	0.78	0.61	0.44
^{169}Yb	1.00	1.10	1.18	1.21	1.23	1.23	1.17	1.10

* Values presented here are average for two different source models.
Reproduced from Jani, S.K., p161, Handbook of Dosimetry Data for Radiotherapy, CRC Press, Boca Raton, Florida, 1993.

17.5.2
AAPM and ICWG Empirical Approach for Dosimetry of Radioactive Seeds

Radioactive seeds used in practice may have a finite length of 2 to 3 mm. In addition, the radioactive seeds available commercially are not quite isotropic in their physical construction or radiation emission [27–31]. These facts were recognized by an Interstitial Collaborative Working Group (ICWG) that was sponsored by the U.S. National Cancer Institute and a task group appointed by the American Association of Physicists in Medicine (AAPM) [6, 27, 28]. They outlined an empirical dose calculation approach, which we describe next.

In general, one may want to calculate the dose rate $\dot{D}(r, \phi)$ at a point P which is on a radial line at an angle ϕ with respect to the perpendicular to the source and at a distance r from its center, as shown in Figure 17.5. A reference point R is located at $r_0 = 1$ cm and $\phi = 0$, and the dose rate at R per unit air-kerma strength is Λ. Λ,

---

* Some literature refer to $g(r)$ as 'radial dose function'.

Fig. 17.5. Radial distance r and polar angle ϕ defining the location of point P with respect to the center and axis of a source. R is a reference point on the mid-perpendicular line of the source

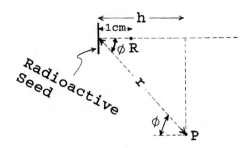

called the "dose rate constant," is a characteristic value for a source of a particular design or construction. Its value is to be determined by an experimental measurement on a reference source that has a known source strength, $(S_{ak})_{ref}$, and is of identical construction and design. That is,

$$\Lambda = \left[\dot{D}(r_0 = 1\,\text{cm},\ \phi = 0)/(S_{ak})_{ref}\right] \qquad (17\text{-}14)$$

For another source that has an air-kerma strength S_{ak}, the dose rate at R is

$$\dot{D}(r_0 = 1\,\text{cm},\ \phi = 0) = \Lambda S_{ak} \qquad (17\text{-}15)$$

The dose rate, $\dot{D}(r, \phi)$, at any other point such as P at location (r, ϕ) can be calculated by the relation

$$\dot{D}(r, \phi) = \Lambda \times S_{ak} \times \frac{G(r, \phi)}{G(r_0 = 1\,\text{cm},\ \phi = 0)} \times g(R) \times F(r, \phi) \qquad (17\text{-}16)$$

where $G(r, \phi)$ is the geometric term $(= 1/r^2)$ that accounts for inverse-square fall-off (as would apply for an ideal point source); $g(r)$ is the radial function that allows for photon absorption and scatter in water along the direction $\phi = 0$; and $F(r, \phi)$ is a dimensionless factor that is included as a correction for anisotropy and is normalized to be 1.0 at the angle $\phi = 0$.

For an ideal point-isotropic source, for a point at 1 cm distance from the source, and for all values of ϕ, we can substitute in (17-16):

$$r = 1\,\text{cm};\ g(r) = 1;$$
$$\frac{G(r, \phi)}{G(r_0 = 1\,\text{cm},\ \phi = 0)} = 1;\ \text{and}\ F(r, \phi) = 1$$

Hence, the dose rate at this point is

$$\dot{D}(r = 1\,\text{cm},\ \phi = 0) = \Lambda \times S_{ak}$$

From (17-11), we obtain

$$\dot{D}(r = 1\,\text{cm},\ \phi = 0) = S_{ak} \times (f_{akmd})_{water} \times \text{WPC}(r = 1.0\,\text{cm})$$

A comparison of the above two expressions gives the relation

$$\Lambda = (f_{akmd})_{water} \times \text{WPC}(r = 1.0\,\text{cm})$$

The values of $g(r)$ and $F(r, \phi)$ can be obtained by the following expressions:

$$g(r) = \frac{\dot{D}(r, \phi = 0)\, G(r_0 = 1\,\text{cm}, \phi = 0)}{\dot{D}(r_0 = 1\,\text{cm}, \phi = 0)\, G(r, \phi = 0)} \qquad (17\text{-}17)$$

$$F(r, \phi) = \frac{\dot{D}(r, \phi)\, G(r, 0)}{\dot{D}(r, 0)\, G(r, \phi)} \qquad (17\text{-}18)$$

Values of $g(r)$ and $F(r, \phi)$ have been derived from experimentally observed dose distributions for some radioactive seeds [6, 27, 28, 32]. Readers having a deeper interest in dosimetry may also concurrently review the discussion about Λ in Section 11.10 of Chapter 11.

17.6
Dosimetry of a Linear Source

17.6.1
Encapsulated Source in Air

We first address the simple situation of the dose delivered by a finite line source situated in air. The symbols for the physical dimensions of a typical sealed linear source, as shown in Figure 17.6a, are the following:

L_a, length of the inner radioactive region
L_t, total external length of capsule

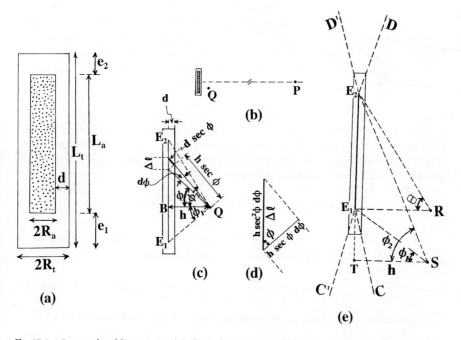

Fig. 17.6. 6 Encapsulated line source: (a) physical parameters; (b) locations of a distant point P and a proximal point Q with respect to the source; (c) source geometry; (d) an element of the active length of the source; (e) demarcation of different zones around the source

e_1 and e_2, length of inactive regions at either end
R_a, radius of the inner radioactive region
R_t, total radius of the external dimension
$d = (R_t - R_a)$, the thickness of the capsule

Let us consider a linear source having a strength S_{ak} as specified by its air-kerma rate yield. The point P is located in a region perpendicular to the source (Figure 17.6b) and at a distance large compared to the active length, L_a, of the source. For the dosimetry of this point at a large distance from the source, we can regard the source as a point source, and expression (17-11) can be used. Furthermore, all of the rays can be assumed to emerge normal to the source and undergo an attenuation, A_{normal}, in the capsule that is given by

$$A_{normal} = e^{-\mu_{eff} d} \qquad (17\text{-}19)$$

where μ_{eff} is an effective attenuation coefficient for the encapsulating material.

For the dosimetry of a point such as Q (Figure 17.6b) in the closer vicinity of the source, we need to recognize the linear spread of the source activity and the emergence of the rays in directions oblique to the source axis. The oblique rays are subject to more than the normal attenuation, A_{normal}, in the capsule. We can consider the linear source as being made up of a series of point sources. We define linear source strength (i. e., the source strength per unit length of the source), ρ_{ak}, as given by

$$\rho_{ak} = \frac{S_{ak}}{L_a \cdot A_{normal}} \qquad (17\text{-}20)$$

In Figure 17.5c, we have simplified the source to be an ideally thin linear source by reducing its active radius to zero. B is a point at the base of the perpendicular from Q to the source. The end points E_1 and E_2 of the active length of the source subtend angles ϕ_1 and ϕ_2, respectively, with line BQ. The elemental source length, $\Delta\ell$, between angles ϕ and $\phi + \Delta\phi$ as shown in Figure 17.6d is given by

$$\Delta\ell = h \sec^2\phi \Delta\phi \qquad (17\text{-}21)$$

Point Q is at a distance of $h \sec\phi$ from this source, and the ray passes through a thickness $d \sec\phi$ of encapsulating material. If we regard the element $\Delta\ell$ as a point source of strength $\rho_{ak}\Delta\ell$, the dose rate contributed by it to a small mass of water in air (see Section 11.7.2) at Q, $(\Delta\dot{D}_Q)_{in\ air}$, is given by

$$(\Delta\dot{D}_Q)_{in\ air} = \frac{\rho_{ak}\Delta\ell(f_{akmd})_{water}}{(h\sec\phi)^2} e^{-(\mu_{eff}d)\sec\phi} \qquad (17\text{-}22)$$

The exponential term allows for the attenuation along the oblique path through the source capsule. Substituting for $\Delta\ell$ and simplifying, we obtain

$$(\Delta\dot{D}_Q)_{in\ air} = \frac{\rho_{ak}(f_{akmd})_{water}}{h} e^{-(\mu_{eff}d)\sec\phi}\Delta\phi \qquad (17\text{-}23)$$

The total dose rate, $(\dot{D}_Q)_{in\ air}$, is obtained by summation from angle ϕ_1 to ϕ_2:

$$(\dot{D}_Q)_{in\ air} = \frac{\rho_{ak}(f_{akmd})_{water}}{h} \int_{-\phi_1}^{\phi_2} e^{-(\mu_{eff}d)\sec\phi} d\phi \qquad (17\text{-}24)$$

A limiting case of the above integral results when $\phi_1 = 0$ and the calculation is for a point such as R in Figure 17.6e, which is at the same level as the lower active end of the linear source. In this case, if θ is the total angle subtended by the source at R, the dose rate to water in air at R, $(\dot{D}_R)_{\text{in air}}$, is given by

$$(\dot{D}_R)_{\text{in air}} = \frac{\rho_{ak}(f_{akmd})_{\text{water}}}{h} \int_0^{\theta} e^{-(\mu_{\text{eff}}d)\sec\phi}\,d\theta \qquad (17\text{-}25)$$

Denoting the integral term by $I(\mu_{\text{eff}}d, \theta)$, we obtain

$$(\dot{D}_R)_{\text{in air}} = \frac{\rho_{ak}(f_{akmd})_{\text{water}}}{h} I(\mu_{\text{eff}}d, \theta) \qquad (17\text{-}26)$$

The integral I is called Sievert's integral and has to be evaluated numerically. Values of this integral for various values of θ and the product $(\mu_{\text{eff}}d)$ were published by Sievert [33]. The dose rate at point Q in Figure 17.6c can be evaluated if one knows the values of the two integrals $I(\mu_{\text{eff}}d, \phi_1)$ and $I(\mu_{\text{eff}}d, \phi_2)$, because expression (17-22) for $(\dot{D}_Q)_{\text{in air}}$ can be rewritten as

$$(\dot{D}_Q)_{\text{in air}} = \frac{\rho_{ak}(f_{akmd})_{\text{water}}}{h}\left[I(\mu_{\text{eff}}d, \phi_2) + I(\mu_{\text{eff}}d, \phi_1)\right] \qquad (17\text{-}27)$$

Similarly, the dose rate at a point such as S in Figure 17.6e, lying beyond the active region of the source, can be derived as the difference of two Sievert's integrals for angles ϕ_2 and ϕ_1:

$$(\dot{D}_S)_{\text{in air}} = \frac{\rho_{ak}(f_{akmd})_{\text{water}}}{h}\left[I(\mu_{\text{eff}}d, \phi_2) - I(\mu_{\text{eff}}d, \phi_1)\right] \qquad (17\text{-}28)$$

In the above expression, the first integral overestimates the dose because the angle ϕ_2 applies to a source length TE_2. The second integral corrects this by subtracting the contribution from the nonactive length TE_1.

The exponent of the exponential term in the Sievert's integral assumes that all of the rays from the source to the point of dose calculation emerge through the cylindrical surface of the capsule. This can be universally valid if the source capsule is of infinite length, extending far beyond its active ends. For actual sources (Figure 17.6e), if the point of calculation falls between lines C and C' (or D and D') in the paraxial end region of the source, some rays will emerge through the end faces of the source. For such points, the Sievert integral will overestimate the attenuation and underestimate the dose. The calculations can be improved if, for rays such as those that emerge through the bottom end of the source, the term $e^{-(\mu_{\text{eff}}d)\sec\phi}$ in the integrand of expression (17-24) is replaced by $e^{-\mu e_1}$ to correspond to the attenuation through the bottom end e_1 in Figure 17.6a during the numerical integration.

17.6.2
Unencapsulated Source in Air

For a bare source without any encapsulation, $\mu_{\text{eff}}d = 0$, and the integral I reduces to

$$I(\mu_{\text{eff}}d, \phi) = \phi \qquad (17\text{-}29)$$

With $\mu_{eff}d = 0$, expressions (17-26), (17-27), and (17-28) reduce to the following:

$$(\dot{D}_Q)_{in\ air} = \frac{\rho_{ak}(f_{akmd})_{water}}{h}[\phi_2 + \phi_1] \tag{17-30}$$

$$(\dot{D}_S)_{in\ air} = \frac{\rho_{ak}(f_{akmd})_{water}}{h}[\phi_2 - \phi_1] \tag{17-31}$$

$$(\dot{D}_R)_{in\ air} = \frac{\rho_{ak}(f_{akmd})_{water}}{h}[\theta] \tag{17-32}$$

In Figure 17.6c, if point Q lies on the mid-perpendicular line of the source, ϕ_1 and ϕ_2 will be equal. Under that condition, if the distance h is very short, the angles gradually will approximate their mathematical limits of $\pi/2$ and $-\pi/2$ (i. e., right angles). Then,

$$(\dot{D}_Q)_{in\ air} = \frac{\rho_{ak}(f_{akmd})_{water}}{h}[\pi/2 - (-\pi/2)] = \frac{\pi\rho_{ak}(f_{akmd})_{water}}{h} \tag{17-33}$$

Thus, for elongated sources, at distances very close to the source, the air-kerma rate opposite the midregion of the active length of the source and parallel to the source will be uniform, and it will fall off inversely with the distance h. This limiting behavior of inverse distance fall-off may apply in clinical situations in which a very long radioactive wire is used in body cavities such as an esophagus, a bronchial branch, or a cardiovascular vessel, for irradiation of tissues proximal to the wire.

EXAMPLE 17.2

The dose to the esophagus of a patient who was already irradiated with external beams needs to be boosted by brachytherapy. This is done by intraluminal insertion of a 12 cm long radioactive wire along the esophageal axis. It is known that the spinal cord, which already received 4000 cGy during the external-beam therapy, will be at a distance of 1.0 cm from the wire. What is the maximum dose that can be delivered at a distance of 0.5 cm from the wire without exceeding a total spinal cord tolerance dose of 4500 cGy?

Spinal cord tolerance dose = 4500 cGy.

Dose already delivered (by external beam) = 4000 cGy.

Hence, the dose that can be added in the current treatment is 4500 − 4000 cGy = 500 cGy.

Let us assume (i) that the source is very long compared to the distances of dose calculations and hence the limiting assumption of an inverse distance fall-off can be adopted, and (ii) that no tissue fluence corrections are needed, i. e., WPC = 1.0. The ratio of the dose rates is given by

$$\frac{\text{Dose rate at 0.5 cm}}{\text{Dose rate at 1 cm}} = \frac{1.0\ cm}{0.5\ cm} = 2.0$$

We calculated that, at most, 500 cGy can be delivered at 1.0 cm. The dose at 0.5 cm then would be 2 × 500 cGy = 1000 cGy. (A calculation using the more exact geometric expression of (17-30) gives a dose rate ratio of 2.11 and a maximum deliverable dose of 2.11 × 500 = 1055 cGy.)

17.6.3
Linear Source in Water

Up to now, we have addressed the situation of a linear source in air, ignoring the attenuation and scatter corrections in water. The elemental source $\Delta\ell$, is at a distance $h\sec\phi$ from the point of dose calculation. For calculation of the dose in water, the water perturbation correction (WPC) for this distance, WPC($h\sec\phi$), should be incorporated in the integrand of expression (17-24):

$$(\dot{D}_Q)_{\text{in water}} = \frac{\rho_{ak}(f_{akmd})_{\text{water}}}{h} \int_{\phi_1}^{\phi_2} e^{-(\mu_{\text{eff}}d)\sec\phi}\, \text{WPC}(h\sec\phi)\, d\phi \qquad (17\text{-}34)$$

17.6.4
Dose Distribution for Linear Sources

Figure 17.7 presents a comparison between calculated and experimentally measured isodose curves for a linear cobalt-60 source [34]. The experimental results were obtained with thermoluminescent dosimeters in a solid tissue-equivalent medium. The

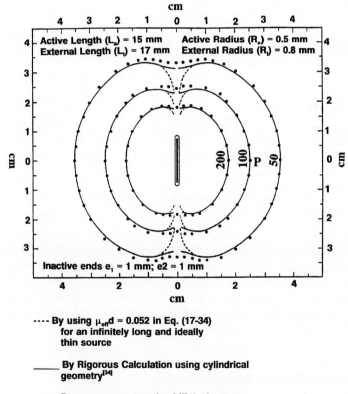

---- By using $\mu_{\text{eff}}d$ = 0.052 in Eq. (17-34)
for an infinitely long and ideally
thin source

_____ By Rigorous Calculation using cylindrical
geometry[34]

• By measurements using LiF dosimeters

Fig. 17.7. Calculated and experimentally determined isodose curves for a linear cobalt-60 source

Table 17.5. Air-Kerma Yield (cGy cm^2) Needed to Deliver 10 cGy in Water at Points in the Vicinity of Cesium Line Sources

Perpendicular Distance from the Source (cm)	Distance from Center of Source Along Source Axis (cm)									
	0.0	0.5	1.0	1.5	2.0	2.5	3.0	3.5	4.0	5.0
Cesium-137; Active Length 1.4 cm; Wall Thickness 1.0 mm Stainless Steel										
0.5	3.393	4.094	8.500	19.50	36.76	60.17	89.96	126.2	169.3	276.8
1.0	10.49	11.91	17.10	27.50	43.58	65.35	93.00	126.6	166.5	266.5
1.5	22.04	23.84	29.64	40.19	56.01	77.22	104.1	136.8	175.5	271.6
2.0	38.28	40.29	46.50	57.37	73.26	94.35	120.9	153.3	191.0	285.7
2.5	59.32	61.47	67.96	79.19	95.23	116.5	142.9	175.1	212.6	306.5
3.0	85.33	87.53	94.23	105.7	122.1	143.4	170.1	202.3	239.7	333.8
3.5	116.3	118.6	125.5	137.1	153.9	175.5	202.3	235.0	272.6	366.3
4.0	152.6	154.9	162.0	173.8	190.5	212.6	239.7	272.6	310.5	403.5
4.5	194.1	196.2	203.5	215.8	232.7	255.1	282.3	316.0	353.6	449.2
5.0	241.3	243.8	250.6	263.6	280.1	302.7	330.7	364.4	403.5	499.5
Cesium-137; Active Length 3.0 cm; Wall Thickness 0.5 mm Stainless Steel										
0.5	5.541	5.681	6.361	9.584	21.19	41.38	68.28	101.5	141.2	241.3
1.0	14.08	14.61	16.65	22.00	33.22	51.53	76.47	107.6	144.9	238.1
1.5	26.48	27.44	30.71	37.49	49.33	67.13	91.22	121.5	157.7	248.0
2.0	43.26	44.57	48.79	56.69	69.28	87.32	111.1	140.9	176.4	266.5
2.5	64.70	66.26	71.21	79.98	93.37	111.8	135.8	165.3	200.6	290.3
3.0	90.99	92.76	98.25	107.7	121.7	140.6	165.0	194.6	230.4	318.9
3.5	122.3	124.2	130.1	140.3	154.9	174.2	199.0	228.9	264.5	353.6
4.0	158.7	160.9	167.3	177.7	193.0	212.6	238.1	268.5	305.2	394.6
4.5	200.6	202.9	209.5	220.4	235.7	256.9	282.3	313.3	350.1	443.6
5.0	248.0	250.6	256.9	268.5	284.6	305.2	332.2	362.6	401.3	492.6
Cesium-137; Active Length 4.5 cm; Wall Thickness 0.5 mm Stainless Steel										
0.5	7.675	7.733	7.944	8.528	10.64	20.25	42.31	73.26	111.3	208.8
1.0	18.04	18.28	19.15	21.19	26.03	36.89	56.37	84.13	119.2	209.5
1.5	31.83	32.35	34.09	37.75	44.67	56.82	75.90	102.2	135.8	222.5
2.0	49.64	50.41	53.06	58.16	66.75	80.16	99.48	125.5	158.0	242.9
2.5	71.78	72.88	76.31	82.57	92.64	107.1	127.1	153.3	185.5	269.5
3.0	98.65	99.90	104.1	111.4	122.5	138.2	143.1	185.5	217.8	301.4
3.5	137.9	131.8	136.6	144.9	157.0	173.4	195.2	221.8	255.1	338.5
4.0	167.3	168.9	174.2	183.1	196.2	213.2	235.7	263.6	297.6	382.0
4.5	209.5	211.3	216.4	226.0	239.7	257.9	281.2	310.5	343.4	384.0
5.0	256.9	258.8	264.5	274.7	289.2	307.9	332.2	360.7	396.8	482.6

Uses conversion 1 cGy/mgh $\approx$ 71.45 cGy cm^2 air-kerma for 10 cGy (see Section 17.4.3).
Based on data from Krishnaswamy, V., Radiology, Vol 105, p181–184, 1972.

agreement between measurement and calculation is good in regions perpendicular to the active length of the source, but there are disagreements in the paraxial end regions of the source. Fortunately, in many clinical situations, structures of dosimetric importance lie in the regions in which the agreement is acceptable. Dose rate tables for linear sources have been published by several authors [35–38]. Table 17.5 provides the dosimetry data for a few typical Cs^{137} sources.

17.6.5
AAPM and ICWG Approach for Linear Source Dosimetry

The geometric factor G(r, ϕ) in the ICWG approach (described in Section 17.5.2) applied to a point source. For linear sources, the dosimetry approach of the AAPM Task

Group and ICWG suggest a modified geometric factor that is based on expressions (17-30) to (17-32) [6, 27, 28]. For example, for point S of Figure 17.6e, based on expression (17-31), it is given by

$$G(r, \phi) = [\phi_2 - \phi_1]/[L_a h] \qquad (17-35)$$

17.7
A Simple Line Source Treatment

Table 17.6 is a linear-source dosage table that was originally derived for radium sources. The table gives the equivalent air-kerma yield for delivery of 10 cGy in tissue at different distances from the source along its mid-perpendicular line for sources of different lengths. The sources are assumed to be bare (i. e., unencapsulated). The table is useful for planning of treatments with a single linear source, as illustrated in the following example.

EXAMPLE 17.3

It is desired to treat an obstructive bronchial lesion with local irradiation by insertion of a straight 7 cm long radioactive wire. The plan is to deliver a dose of 2000 cGy at 0.5 cm from the axis of the airway in 48 h. Calculate (i) the source strength required and (ii) the dose delivered in the central region at 1.0 cm from the source.

Let us say that the source strength is S_{ak} and the treatment time is τ.

Table 17.6. Linear Source Dosage Table: Air-Kerma Yield (cGy cm^2) for Delivery of 10 cGy (in Water)

Active Length (cm)	Perpendicular Distance from the Source (cm)						
	0.5	0.75	1.00	1.50	2.00	2.50	3.00
0.0	2.31	5.09	9.18	20.67	36.71	57.38	82.61
0.5	2.55	5.40	9.33	20.98	36.87	57.62	82.76
1.0	2.93	5.94	9.80	21.37	37.33	58.08	83.45
1.5	3.63	6.63	10.64	22.14	38.33	58.93	84.46
2.0	4.24	7.56	11.80	23.22	39.57	60.16	85.92
2.5	4.94	8.64	12.96	24.68	41.26	61.70	87.70
3.0	5.71	9.64	14.19	26.46	43.04	63.55	89.70
3.5	6.48	10.80	15.66	28.38	44.97	65.79	91.94
4.0	7.25	11.80	16.97	30.23	47.13	68.34	94.25
5.0	8.95	14.11	19.98	34.17	52.06	73.81	99.81
6.0	10.64	16.51	22.91	38.41	57.23	79.83	106.3
7.0	12.26	18.82	25.99	42.65	62.63	86.23	113.4
8.0	13.88	21.13	29.31	47.20	68.41	92.86	120.9
9.0	15.43	23.68	32.47	51.75	74.28	99.65	128.7
10.0	17.05	25.99	35.71	56.38	80.37	106.7	136.8
12.0	20.29	30.93	42.11	65.79	92.25	121.3	153.8
14.0	23.60	35.94	48.67	75.28	104.5	136.4	171.2
16.0	26.92	41.03	55.15	84.84	117.1	151.9	189.1
18.0	30.39	45.97	61.86	94.41	129.8	167.4	207.2
20.0	33.71	51.06	68.41	104.3	142.6	182.9	226.0

Original data giving mgh for 1000 R from Meredith, W.J., Radium Dosage – The Manchester System, Williams & Wilkins, Baltimore, MD, 1967, have been converted as shown in Example 17.1 in text (Section 17.4.3).

(i) From Table 17.6, a source of 7 cm active length will deliver 10 cGy at 0.5 cm, if the air-kerma yield $S_{ak} \times \tau$ equals 12.26 cGy cm^2. For delivery of 2000 cGy, the required air-kerma yield is

$$S_{ak} \times \tau = [12.26 \, \text{cGy cm}^2/10 \, \text{cGy}] \times 2000 \, \text{cGy} = 2452 \, \text{cGy cm}^2$$

Because $\tau = 48$ h, the source strength S_{ak} needed is

$$S_{ak} = 2452 \, \text{cGy cm}^2/48 \, \text{h} = 51.1 \, \text{cGy cm}^2 \, \text{h}^{-1}$$

(ii) From Table 17.6, we obtain a value of 25.99 cGy cm^2 for a central point 1 cm away from a 7 cm long source. The dose delivered at 1 cm for 2452 cGy cm^2 is

$$[10 \, \text{cGy}/25.99 \, \text{cGy cm}^2] \times 2452 \, \text{cGy cm}^2 = 943 \, \text{cGy}$$

Sometimes a string of point sources can be used as a substitute for a linear source. Point sources loaded in a nylon tube can give flexibility for passage through curved airways. The dose distribution possible with multiple point sources spaced 1 cm apart is illustrated in Figure 17.8.

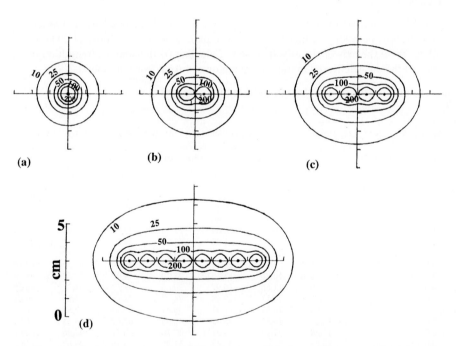

Fig. 17.8. Radioactive seeds used as dose building blocks: (a) a single seed, (b) two seeds, (c) four seeds, (d) eight seeds. All isodose curves are normalized to 100% in the central region at a distance 5 mm away from the source

EXAMPLE 17.4

It is decided to treat the case in the previous example by use of radioactive seeds loaded at 1-cm spacing in a nylon ribbon. The seeds available are of strength 5.8 cGy cm^2 h^{-1}.

Calculate the treatment time, assuming that it is possible to approximate a line source by a series of point sources.

The 7-cm radioactive length needed can be made up of 8 seeds at 1-cm spacing. The total source strength of 8 seeds $= 8 \times 5.8\,\mathrm{cGy\,cm^2\,h^{-1}} = 46.4\,\mathrm{cGy\,cm^2\,h^{-1}}$. Total $\mathrm{cGy\,cm^2}$ of treatment (from Example 17.3) $= 2452\,\mathrm{cGy\,cm^2}$. Time of treatment $= 2452\,\mathrm{cGy\,cm^2}/46.4\,\mathrm{cGy\,cm^2\,h^{-1}} = 52.8\,\mathrm{h}$. The treatment time has been changed from the initial plan of 48 h to 52.8 h to accommodate the source strength available for use.

It is worthwhile to mention here that only marginal changes in the treatment duration can be accepted. Any major change in the treatment time can have a bearing on the radiobiological response and the treatment outcome.

17.8
Forming Multiple Source Arrays

17.8.1
Sources as Dose Building Blocks

Brachytherapy is a local irradiation technique in which the irradiation takes place just around the sources. We can regard the sources as 'dose building blocks.' The sources can be arranged to make a geometric pattern to spread the dose delivered and to fashion the dose distribution. Figure 17.8 demonstrates the use of adjacent point sources for producing source arrays that give line source-like dose distributions. In the same manner, several line sources can be used with suitable spacing between them to produce a planar source array. Having several planes of sources can create a volume source array. In clinical situations, the source arrays should be planned and positioned appropriately in relation to the tissues targeted for irradiation.

17.8.2
Uniform vs. Differentially Distributed Arrays

When sources are spread over an area or volume, the two characteristics of the array that need to be planned are the spatial distribution and the source strength distribution. With regard to spacing of the sources, the practice has been to keep it simple by adopting a uniform spacing between sources. With regard to the distribution of source strengths, two different approaches, a uniform distribution and a differential distribution, have been used.

In the first approach, the sources are such that the total source strength can be spread out uniformly over the area or volume. This can be accomplished by use of either point sources of identical strengths or linear sources of the same linear strengths. Such a uniform source strength distribution is known to result in a nonuniform dose distribution, giving a higher dose in the central regions of the source array than at the periphery.

In the second approach, that of using a differential source strength distribution, the area or volume that is implanted is visualized to be made up of a central 'core' zone and a peripheral 'rind' zone. The strength of the sources used in the core zone is less than that used in the rind zone; that is, the source strength is located preferentially in the periphery. Such a differential distribution of source strengths in favor of the periphery can produce a more uniform dose. The differences in the dose distributions as obtained by the two approaches are elucidated in a series of examples that follow.

Figures 17.9a and b show orthogonal planar views of a single-plane implant that has five parallel line sources of 6-cm active length with a 1-cm spacing between the sources. All sources are of the same strength. Four different planes, A, B, C, and D, have been selected for examination of the dose distribution. Planes A and B are parallel to the source plane. Plane A contains the sources and plane B is 0.5 cm away from plane A. Planes C and D are perpendicular to the sources. Plane C passes through the central part of the implant and plane D is at 1 cm inward from the ends of the line sources. The isodose distributions shown in Figures 17.9c, d, e, and f are, respectively, applicable to planes A, B, C, and D. The isodose curves are normalized, with the dose received at the center of plane B (which is located 0.5 cm away from the implanted plane) taken as 100%.

The isodose pattern in Figure 17.9c shows high-dose regions of 150% or more. Such high-dose regions appear as discrete volumes surrounding individual sources. The 100% isodose curve covers a contiguous volume that circumscribes adjacent sources. In Figure 17.9e, the dose falls off rapidly with distance from 100% at 0.5 cm to about 60% at 1.0 cm, in the direction perpendicular to the plane of the implant. Figure 17.9d shows that the dose delivered is 100% at the center and falls off to 60-80% at the periphery and in the corners. This is also reflected in Figure 17.9f, which represents the peripheral zone near the source ends.

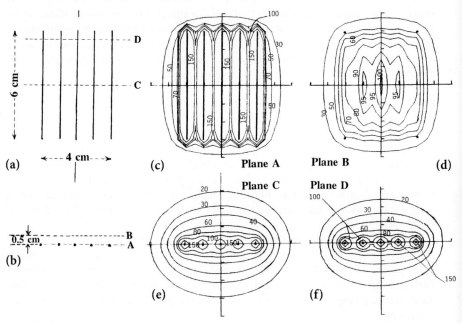

Fig. 17.9. An array of five parallel linear sources of 6 cm active length, evenly spaced 1 cm apart. All sources are of the same linear source strength. (a) Side view showing planes C and D perpendicular to the sources. (b) End-on view showing plane A containing the sources and plane B at 0.5 cm away from it. (c), (d), (e), and (f) give isodose curves in planes A, B, C, and D, respectively. Isodose curves are normalized to 100% at the center of plane B

Figure 17.10 shows the dose distribution in a plane 0.5 cm away from the implanted plane for four possible variations in source arrangements. The source arrays considered are presented in the figure. Figure 17.10a is identical to Figure 17.9d, with the five parallel line sources all having the same strength. In Figure 17.10b, the linear source strengths of the two sources at the periphery are 1.5 times that of the three sources in the middle region. This gives a more uniform dose distribution. Doses in the range of 90 to 95% are seen in the lateral edge regions. This configuration of sources and source strengths is far more uniform than the distribution in Figure 17.10a, but has not improved the doses received in the end regions.

Figure 17.10c shows sources of one uniform source strength, but has two perpendicular line sources added which 'cross' the ends. The crossing of the ends removes the fall-off of dose in the end regions, but the low doses in the lateral regions remain. An all-over improvement in dose uniformity is seen in Figure 17.10d, which makes use of both crossed ends and sources of a higher linear source strength in the periphery.

Figure 17.11 illustrates the dose distributions obtained for a two-plane implant that uses linear sources of the same uniform linear strength with uncrossed ends. The isodose curves displayed in Figures 17.11c, d, e, and f are for the four planes identified as A, B, C, and D in Figures 17.11a and b. Figure 17.12 is a two-plane array of the same geometric configuration as in Figure 17.11, but uses peripheral sources that have 11/2 times the linear source strength of the central sources.

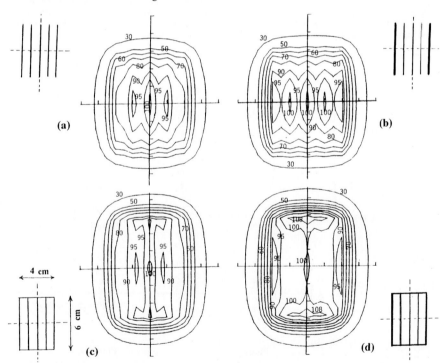

Fig. 17.10. Isodose distribution in the plane 0.5 cm away from the plane of the implant for four different linear source arrrays occupying a 4 cm wide, 6 cm long area. In (a) and (b), all sources are of the same linear strength. In (c) and (d), the linear strength of the peripheral sources is 1.5 times the linear strength of the inner sources. In (c) and (d), the ends are crossed

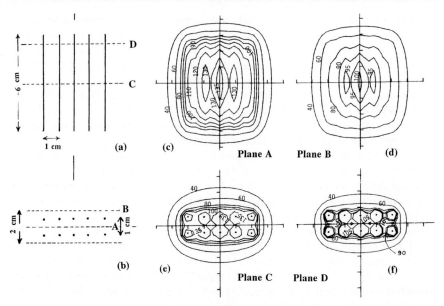

Fig. 17.11. A two-plane implant having five parallel linear sources of 6 cm active length, evenly spaced 1 cm apart in each plane, with an interplanar separation of 1 cm. All sources are of the same linear source strength. (**a**) Side view showing planes C and D perpendicular to the sources. (**b**) End-on view showing plane A midway between the source planes and plane B 0.5 cm away from a source plane. (**c**), (**d**), (**e**), and (**f**) give isodose curves in planes A, B, C, and D, respectively. Isodose curves are normalized to 100% at the center of plane B

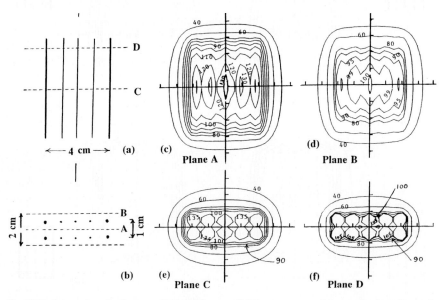

Fig. 17.12. A two-plane implant consisting of five parallel linear sources of 6 cm active length, evenly spaced 1 cm apart in each plane and with an interplanar separation of 1 cm. The peripheral sources have 1.5 times the linear strength of the inner sources. (**a**) Side view showing planes C and D perpendicular to the sources. (**b**) End-on view showing plane A midway between the source planes and plane B 0.5 cm away from the sources. (**c**), (**d**), (**e**), and (**f**) give isodose curves in planes A, B, C, and D, respectively. Isodose curves are normalized to 100% at the center of plane B

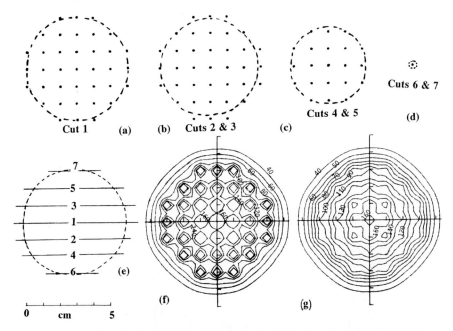

Fig. 17.13. A near-spherical volume implant of radioactive seeds of uniform strength. (a), (b), (c), and (d) show the array of seeds as visualized in cuts 1-7 through the sphere as indicated in (e). (f) Isodose curves in cut 1 containing the sources, and (g) isodose curves in a plane between cuts 1 and 2. 100% dose has been chosen to be midway between cuts 1 and 2 and between the peripheral sources

Figure 17.13 shows a radioactive-seed implant of a spherical volume. The source array as seen in seven different cuts through the sphere is presented in Figures 17.13a to d. The isodose curves are shown for a plane through the center of the sphere bearing the radioactive sources (Figure 17.13f) and for an adjacent parallel plane 0.5 cm away and falling half-way between the source planes (Figure 17.13g). The former shows the high-value isodose curves of 160% encircling 13 implanted seeds. The latter shows the gradual fall-off of the dose from the center (160%) to the periphery (80 to 90%) and only one seed encircled by the 160% isodose curve.

Figure 17.14 is a variation of the same volume implant, but it uses, on the periphery of the sphere, seeds of strength 1.5 times that of those at the center, as is illustrated for one central cut in Figure 17.14a. The isodose curves are displayed for a central plane carrying the sources (Figure 17.14b and a plane midway between the source planes (Figure 17.14c). In both of these planes the uniformity of dose delivery is much better than that in Figure 17.13. The fall-off of dose outside the implanted volume is rapid in either case.

Figure 17.15 addresses the situation of a cylindrical mold used for irradiation of the surface of a cylindrical body part. Figures 17.15a and b show twelve linear sources that have been placed at angular intervals of 30° on the surface of a cylindrical plastic applicator of 1 cm thickness. All sources have the same strength. Isodose curves are shown for a mid-plane perpendicular to the sources (Figure 17.15c) and a plane parallel to the sources through the axis of the cylinder (Figure 17.15d). The 100% dose level is

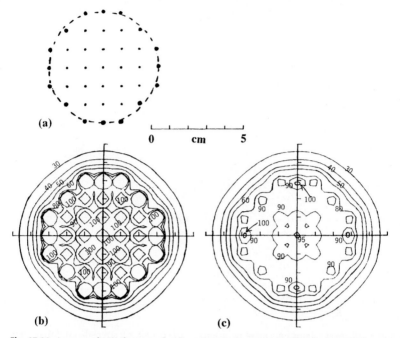

Fig. 17.14. A near-spherical array of radioactive seeds geometrically identical to that shown in Figure 17.13, but with the strength of the seeds on the surface increased to 3/2 times that of those inside. (a) The array of seeds as seen in cut 1 (see Figure 17.13). (b) Isodose curves in cut 1. (c) Isodose curves between cuts 1 and 2 (see Figure 17.13). 100% dose has been chosen to be midway between cuts 1 and 2 and between the peripheral sources

assigned to the inner surface of the mold at 1 cm depth from the outer surface. It will be noticed that the middle region of the surface receives a uniform dose, with some fall-off near the source ends. The central region of the body part irradiated receives 80%. As we move along the cylinder axis away from the center, the dose falls off to 60–50%.

For more illustrations of brachytherapy dose distributions, the reader is advised to refer to published atlases [39, 40].

17.9
Systems for Brachytherapy

17.9.1
What are Systems or Approaches?

Brachytherapy irradiations result in a rather nonuniform dose delivery compared to the uniformity levels possible in external-beam therapy. In any implant, the doses to tissues close to the sources are bound to be very high. The dose falls off with distance from the sources, and the surface of an implanted target volume may receive a lower dose than does its core. Planning of practical treatments in brachytherapy can involve the following three stages:

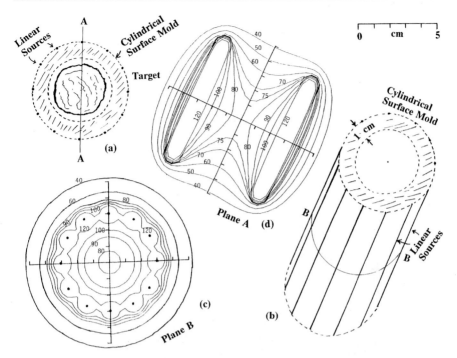

Fig. 17.15. A linear source array on the surface of a cylindrical mold of 1 cm thickness. (a) Cut view perpendicular to the cylinder axis. (b) Overall view of the mold and the linear sources. (c) Isodose curves in the central plane B, shown in (b), perpendicular to the sources. (d) Isodose curves in plane A, shown in (a), containing the cylindrical axis and passing through a pair of sources. The 100% value is the dose between the sources on the inner surface of the mold

(a) Identification and delimiting of the tumor extent and the target volume
(b) Planning of the source array in terms of the number of sources to be used, their relative strengths, and their positions to produce an acceptable dose distribution
(c) Assessment of a 'reference dose rate' and the duration of treatment for delivery of a stated or prescribed radiation dose

There are different practices for, or approaches to, the above steps. These are also referred to as different brachytherapy systems.

17.9.2
Quimby Approach

The approach called the 'Quimby system' conceived of uniformly distributed arrays of sources of the same strength and provided tables of data for calculation of the reference dose rate for such arrays [41, 42]. We already saw, through examples, how a uniform distribution of source strength results in poor uniformity of dose delivery, and how certain nonuniform distributions of source strength result in a more uniform dose

Table 17.7. Dosage Table for Single-Plane Array of Uniformly Distributed Sources: Air-kerma Yield ($cGy\ cm^2$) to Deliver 10 cGy in Water

Distance (cm)	Circular Areas Diameter (cm)					
	1.0	2.0	3.0	4.0	5.0	6.0
0.5	3.40	5.79	7.95	13.1	16.9	23.1
1.0	10.5	13.6	17.0	23.1	28.5	35.0
1.5	21.8	25.0	30.9	36.7	43.4	52.5
2.0	38.3	41.8	46.8	54.0	61.3	70.8
2.5	56.7	61.3	66.7	73.7	89.1	97.6
3.0	84.1	88.7	94.1	101.9	110.5	120.7

Distance (cm)	Square Areas Side of Square (cm)					
	1.0	2.0	3.0	4.0	5.0	6.0
0.5	3.55	6.17	8.87	15.2	19.3	27.0
1.0	10.9	14.5	18.4	25.2	31.2	34.9
1.5	22.8	26.6	32.0	39.4	46.3	56.7
2.0	38.6	44.0	49.7	57.6	66.0	77.2
2.5	56.3	61.3	69.1	77.9	88.0	105.7
3.0	84.1	88.7	98.0	107.3	117.3	128.9

Distance (cm)	Rectangular Areas Length of Sides (cm)					
	1×1.5	2×3	3×4	4×6	6×9	8×12
0.5	3.94	7.95	11.0	22.1	44.0	73.7
1.0	11.4	16.5	21.1	32.9	56.0	85.6
1.5	23.0	28.5	36.0	48.1	72.9	104.6
2.0	39.0	45.5	55.2	67.1	95.7	128.9
2.5	55.6	64.8	76.4	88.0	117.3	154.3
3.0	85.6	91.8	103.2	117.3	148.9	192.9

Uses the conversion 1 mgh for 1000 R $\approx 7.716 \times 10^{-2}\ cGy\ cm^2$ air kerma yield for 10 cGy (see Section 17.4.3). Reference points for dosage are at different distances perpendicular to the source plane opposite the center of the source array.

Based on data from Glasser, O., Quimby, E.H., Taylor, L., and Weatherwax, J.L., Physical Foundations of Radiology, Paul Hoeber, New York, 1952.

delivery. For *planar* source arrays, Quimby adopted the dose delivered at the central point at different distances from the source plane as the reference dose. Figures 17.16a and b illustrate a Quimby-type rectangular planar implant made with evenly spaced line sources of the same linear activity. For *volume* implants, Quimby's tables adopted the minimum dose in the region between the sources on the surface of the implant as the reference dose. This dose is called the minimum peripheral dose (MPD). Tables 17.7 and 17.8 give data for calculation of the reference doses for planar and volume implants by the Quimby approach.

Table 17.8. Volume Implant Dosage Table: Quimby System* Air-Kerma Yield to Deliver 10 cGy Minimum Peripheral Dose

Volume (cm^3)	Air-Kerma Yield (cGy cm^2)	Diameter of Sphere (cm)	Air-Kerma Yield (cGy cm^2)
5	15.4	1.0	3.09
10	24.7	1.5	7.72
15	30.1	2.0	13.9
20	34.0	2.5	21.6
30	41.7	3.0	30.1
40	47.8	3.5	36.7
60	57.9	4.0	44.4
80	67.1	4.5	52.1
100	77.2	5.0	61.0
125	86.4	6.0	82.6
150	96.5	7.0	108.0
175	107.3		
200	115.7		
250	129.6		
300	138.9		

* Uses the conversion 1 mgh for 1000 R $\approx$ 7.716 $\times$ 10^{-2} cGy cm^2 air-kerma yield for 10 cGy (see Section 17.4.3).

Based on data from Glasser, O., Quimby, E.H., Taylor, L.S., and Weatherwax, J.L., Physical Foundations of Radiology, 2nd Edition, Paul B. Hoeber, New York, 1952.

Fig. 17.16. (a) End-on and (b) side views of a Quimby-type single-plane implant. Sources are evenly spaced and are of uniform activity, with the implanted area matching the target cross section as shown by dashed lines

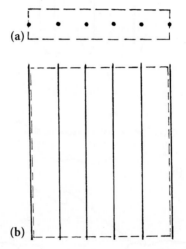

17.9.3
Paris Approach

The approach called the 'Paris system' [43–45] addresses the use of linear radioactive wires of uniform linear strength. Wires of ^{192}Ir are cut to desired lengths and are implanted with a chosen uniform spacing between them. The source ends are left uncrossed. To avoid any underdosing of the end regions of the target volume because of the uncrossed ends, the system specifies that the length of the implanted wires extend beyond the target volume by 10 to 20%. The spacing between the source lines can be flexible, falling in the range of 0.5 to 2.2 cm, with the larger spacing intended for larger volumes and for wires of 10 cm or more in length. An indication of the mean thickness, t, of the target volume for a single-plane implant can be derived as 60% of the spacing, e, employed between the source lines. This means that if e = 1.0 cm, then t ≈ 0.6 cm, and if e = 1.5 cm, then t ≈ 0.9 cm.

Figures 17.17a and b illustrate the relationship of the source array to the target volume and the reference isodose curve in the Paris approach. In the Paris practice, basic dose points (shown by x marks) that are in the central part of the array midway between adjacent source lines are identified. The dose rates at these points are the minimal dose rates in the region between the sources. The numerical average of the dose rates at these points is evaluated and is referred to as the basic dose rate. In the Paris

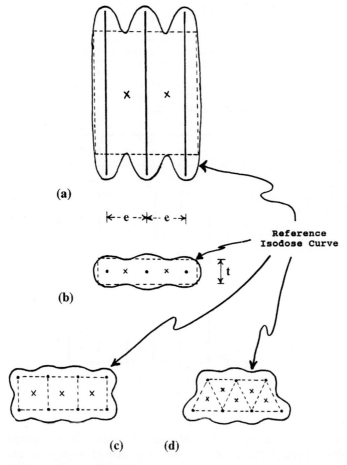

Fig. 17.17. (a) Side and (b) end views of a Paris-type single-plane implant. The source wires are evenly spaced and are of equal linear strength. The implanted area is 20% larger than the target cross section marked by the dashed lines. (c) A rectangular configuration of source wires in a two-plane implant. (d) A triangular configuration of source wires. Cross marks, x, indicate the reference points where the basic doses are evaluated. Dots mark the source locations in (b), (c), and (d). The reference isodose curve, taken to be 85% of the basic dose, is shown in each plane

approach, the stated dose and the duration of treatment are based on a reference dose rate that is chosen to be 85% of the basic dose rate. The target volume is, accordingly, the volume covered by the isodose surface for this 85% dose.

In brachytherapy with implanted sources, it is inevitable that the tissues adjoining any source will receive the highest dose. However, these very high doses seem to be well tolerated because the volumes of tissue they cover are not contiguous, but are distributed around the various discrete sources. The basic dose value obtained between two adjacent sources has the significance of representing the maximum dose level at which the isodose volume becomes contiguous to go around both sources. For dose levels that exceed the basic dose, the isodose volumes become discrete volumes that surround the individual sources.

For two-plane or volume implants, the wires are located at corners of either rectangles or equilateral triangles, as shown in Figures 17.17c and d. For these, the dose rates at the central points (as indicated by crosses) within the triangles or rectangles in the midplane of the implant need to be evaluated and averaged to yield the basic dose rate.

17.9.4
Approach of Memorial Hospital in New York

The approach to the design of source arrays and evaluation of the dose delivered as developed at Memorial Hospital, New York, is referred to as the New York or Memorial system. This system adopts the use of sources of uniform activity in a uniform spacing. Laughlin et al. [46], in 1963, published dosage tables for planar and volume implants of seeds of uniform strength spaced 1 cm apart. For single-plane implants, their reference dose was the minimum peripheral dose, defined as the dose at a point opposite the corner of the implanted area in a plane 0.5 cm away from the plane of the implant. For volume implants, they defined a minimum peripheral dose (MPD), a centerline peripheral dose (CPD), and a maximum reference dose. MPD represented the dose obtained half-way between adjacent seeds near a corner of an array. CPD referred to the dose half-way between adjacent seeds in the central region of the surface of an array. The maximum reference dose was the dose obtained between adjacent seeds in the central core of the implant.

The dosage tables for planar and volume implants as derived by the Memorial group are modified and presented in Tables 17.9 and 17.10, respectively. Revised tables for planar implants have been published more recently by Anderson et al. [47] for the New York system. These data, presented in Table 17.11, apply to an array of parallel nylon ribbons carrying radioactive seeds spaced 1 cm apart. The point for the reference dose has been defined to be the point lying midway between the two edge ribbons at 1.5 seed spacings inward along the ribbons from the source ends.

For permanent volume implants of ^{125}I seeds, the New York approach is based on the average dimensions (rather than the volume) of the target region to be implanted. The system specifies the total initial source strength to be implanted [48–50] as a function of the average dimension. This method is called the dimension-averaging method. It results in delivery of increasing doses to increasing volumes [51]. Nomograms for planning the number of seeds and the strength of seeds by the New York approach have been published [52, 53].

Table 17.9. Planar Implant Dosage Table: Air-Kerma Yield to Deliver 10 cGy to Designated Reference Points for Planar Point Source Arrays

Area (cm^2)	Reference Point		Ratio of central to Peripheral Dose
	Peripheral Point (cGy cm^2)	Central Point (cGy cm^2)	
1	6.84	6.05	1.13
2	8.36	6.77	1.23
3	9.94	7.71	1.29
4	11.9	8.93	1.33
5	13.6	9.94	1.37
6	15.2	11.0	1.39
7	17.0	12.0	1.42
8	18.4	12.8	1.44
9	20.2	13.9	1.45
10	21.6	14.7	1.47
12	24.6	16.4	1.50
14	27.4	18.0	1.52
16	30.2	19.6	1.54
18	32.7	21.0	1.56
20	35.2	22.4	1.57
25	41.1	25.5	1.61
30	46.8	28.7	1.63
35	52.9	31.8	1.66
40	58.5	34.9	1.68
45	64.3	38.0	1.69
50	70.1	41.0	1.71

Note: Modified Memorial System. The sources are of uniform strength spaced 1 cm apart. The peripheral and the central reference points lie in a plane 5 mm away from the source plane opposite the interspace between corner sources and the central sources, respectively. Values are based on data from Laughlin, J.S., Siler, W.M., Holodney, E.I. et al., Am. J. Roentgenol., Vol 89, p470–490, 1963. Uses a conversion 1 mgh for 1000 rad $\approx 7.205 \times 10^{-2}$ cGy cm^2 for 10 cGy (see Section 17.4.3).

17.9.5
Manchester Approach of Paterson and Parker

Paterson and Parker [54–56] evolved very sophisticated and comprehensive source distribution rules and dosage tables for brachytherapy practice. In their approach, which is called the Manchester system, they considered arrays of different possible geometries and provided guidelines for the spacings between the sources, the source strengths to be used, and dosage tables for calculation of the treatment time [54–57]. A spacing of 1 cm between sources for a single-plane implant was suggested. They recommended a nonuniform distribution of source strengths to obtain improved dose uniformity. The principle was to concentrate the source strengths more in the peripheral regions of the array than at the center. For example, they recommended that, for a rectangular array (see Figure 17.18a and b), if ρ is the linear source strength of four line sources forming the periphery, the linear source strength for the sources in the central region should be $2\rho/3$. If there were only one central line, the recommended linear source strength would be $\rho/2$. Such nonuniform loading reduced the disparity between the central dose and the peripheral dose. This also demanded the use of sources of different strengths at the center and at the periphery. Thus, a complicated inventory of

Table 17.10. Volume Implant Dosage Table: Air-Kerma Yield (cGy cm^2) to Deliver 10 cGy in Water at Selected Reference Points

Volume (cm^3)	cGy cm^2 to Deliver 10 Gy			Central Dose Expressed as Multiple of	
	At Corner of Surface[a]	At Center of Surface[b]	At Center of Array[c]	Corner Surface Dose	Central Surface Dose
1	6.84	6.84	6.05	1.13	1.13
5	13.3	11.9	10.4	1.27	1.14
10	18.3	15.4	13.3	1.37	1.16
15	23.2	18.9	16.2	1.43	1.17
20	27.2	21.7	18.4	1.48	1.18
25	31.2	24.4	20.5	1.52	1.19
30	34.0	26.4	22.0	1.55	1.20
40	40.3	30.5	25.2	1.60	1.21
50	46.1	34.4	28.1	1.64	1.23
60	51.8	39.2	31.0	1.67	1.24
80	62.3	45.0	36.0	1.73	1.25
100	72.0	51.5	40.7	1.77	1.27
120	81.4	57.6	45.0	1.81	1.28
140	89.3	63.0	49.0	1.83	1.29
160	98.3	68.6	53.0	1.86	1.30
180	106.3	73.5	56.6	1.88	1.30
200	113.5	78.5	59.8	1.90	1.31
250	132.6	90.1	68.1	1.95	1.32
300	149.9	100.9	75.6	1.98	1.34
350	166.4	111.7	83.2	2.00	1.34
400	183.0	121.8	90.4	2.20	1.35

Note: Modified Memorial System. Arrays are made of point sources of uniform strength spaced 1 cm apart.

[a] At a point between seeds at the corner of the surface of the array.
[b] At a point between seeds on the central region of the surface of the array.
[c] At a point between seeds in the central region of the array of sources.

Based on data from Laughlin, J.S., Siler, W.M., Holodny, E.I. et al., Am. J. Roentgenol., Vol 89, p470–490, 1963. Uses a conversion 1 mgh for 1000 rad $\approx 7.205 \times 10^{-2}$ cGy cm^2 air-kerma yield for 10 cGy (see Section 17.4.3).

Table 17.11.
Planar Implant Dosage Table for Iridium-192 Seeds:
Air-Kerma Yield to Deliver 10 cGy at the Reference Point

Area (cm^2)	Air-Kerma Yield for 10 cGy (cGy cm^2)
10	17.2
20	28.7
30	38.7
40	48.8
50	58.1
60	66.7
80	83.9
100	100.4
120	116.2
140	131.9
160	147.1
180	162.1
200	176.4
250	211.6
300	246.1
350	278.0
400	311.4

Note: Values derived from mgh for 1000 cGy from Anderson, L., Hilaris, B.S., and Wagner, L.K., Endocurietherapy/Hyperthermic Oncology, Vol 1, p9–15, 1985, assuming that 1 mg Raeq of iridium-192 yields × 7.174 CGy cm^2 h^{-1} air-kerma. Sources are in nylon ribbons implanted in parallel lines with 1 cm of inter-seed and inter-ribbon spacing. The reference point is in a plane 5 mm away from the source plane and is removed from the corner seed of the array by 5 mm perpendicular to the ribbons and 15 mm along the ribbons.

Fig. 17.18. (a) End and (b) side views of a Manchester-type single-plane implant. Sources are distributed along the periphery and evenly in the central region, with the linear strength higher in the periphery. The implanted area matches the target cross section indicated by the dashed lines

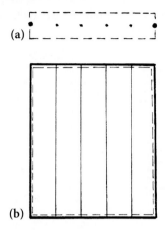

sources consisting of varying linear strengths was needed. (This is unlike the philosophy in the Paris and Quimby systems of using sources of uniform linear strength to keep the inventory simple, even if it does not give the best possible uniformity of dose distribution.) The reference dose in the Manchester system is an effective minimum dose called net minimum dose (NMD), defined to be 10% higher than the actual minimum dose. Tables 17.12, 17.13, and 17.14 are dosage tables for surface molds,

Table 17.12. Dosage Table for Planar Molds with Source Arrays Conforming to the Manchester System: Air-Kerma Yield (cGy cm^2) for Delivering 10 cGy to Water

Area (cm^2)	Treatment Distance (cm)					
	0.5	1.0	1.5	2.0	3.0	5.0
1	5.25	13.19	–	–	–	–
2	7.48	16.43	28.93	46.14	92.30	240.48
3	9.26	19.06				
4	10.88	21.45	35.64	53.85	100.68	250.20
5	12.42	23.61				
6	13.66	25.69	41.35	60.31	108.40	259.22
8	15.89	29.63	46.21	50.91	115.73	267.86
10	18.13	33.41	50.53	71.21	122.67	276.20
15	23.30	42.12	60.87	83.55	138.21	295.79
20	28.39	49.45	70.21	94.51	152.68	314.77
30	37.80	61.33	88.11	114.72	178.99	349.80
40	46.52	72.06	103.84	133.62	202.13	381.28
50	54.39	82.70	117.42	151.06	184.93	410.98
60	61.72	93.04	129.77	168.19	243.79	438.98
80	75.68	113.41	151.68	197.66	282.14	489.90
100	89.11	132.39	172.66	222.96	317.86	536.60
150	148.46	177.68	225.30	277.97	–	–
200	145.04	217.56	274.65	330.82	–	–
300	192.49	289.08	367.23	434.35	–	–
400	237.62	356.43	450.56	529.56	–	–

Values have been derived from original data from Meredith, W.J., Radium Dosage – The Manchester System, Williams & Wilkins, Baltimore, MD, 1967, assuming that 1 mgh for 1000 R $\approx 7.716 \times 10^{-2}$ cGy cm^2 air-kerma yield for 10 cGy. See Example 17.1 in text.

Table 17.13.
Single-Plane Implant Dosage Table (Manchester System):
Air-Kerma Yield (cGy cm^2) for Delivering 10 cGy to Water

Area (cm^2)	(cGy cm^2) for 10 cGy
0	2.31
2	7.48
3	9.26
4	10.88
5	12.42
6	13.66
8	15.89
10	18.13
15	23.26
20	28.39
30	37.80
40	46.52
50	54.39
60	61.72
80	75.68
100	89.11
150	118.4
200	145.0
300	192.5
400	237.6

Values are derived from original data from Meredith, W.J., Radium Dosage – The Manchester System, Williams & Wilkins, Baltimore, MD, 1967, assuming 1 mgh for 1000 R $\approx 7.716 \times 10^{-2}$ cGy cm^2 air-kerma yield for 10 cGy. See Example 17.1 in text.

Table 17.14.
Volume Implant Dosage Table (Manchester System):
Air-Kerma Yield for 10 cGy Reference Dose to Water

Volume (cm^3)	(cGy cm^2) for 10 cGy
1	2.63
2	4.17
3	5.47
4	6.63
5	7.69
10	12.2
15	16.0
20	19.4
25	22.5
30	25.4
40	30.8
50	35.7
60	40.3
70	44.7
80	48.8
90	52.8
100	56.7
125	64.4
150	74.3
200	90.0
250	104
300	118
350	131
400	143

Values are derived from data from Table E in Meredith, W.J., Radium Dosage – The Manchester System, Williams & Wilkins, Baltimore, MD, 1967. Uses a conversion 1 mgh for 1000 R $\approx 7.716 \times 10^{-2}$ cGy cm^2 air-kerma yield for 10 cGy. See Example 17.1 in text.

single-plane implants, and volume implants when the sources are arranged according to the Manchester distribution rules.

An overview of the Manchester system can enrich our understanding of the physics of brachytherapy. Many insights provided by the Manchester system are useful for the day-to-day practice of brachytherapy, even if the system may not be fully adhered to. For this reason, in Section 17.10, we provide a brief review of the distribution rules of the Manchester system, recommending to the reader References 54 and 57 for a more detailed study.

17.9.6
Pitfalls of Mixing Systems or Approaches

Apart from the systems discussed above, various other approaches have been outlined (for example, References 58 to 64) for planning the source arrays and determining the treatment time. It is to be noted that the relationship of the source arrays with respect to the target volume, the nonuniformity of the dose distribution accepted for treatment, and the basis of the stated dose are all subject to variation, based on the system or approach used. Some articles have compared the differences in these respects between various approaches [65–69].

It is worth reiterating that the doses prescribed and delivered in brachytherapy are based on past clinical experience. Much caution should be exercised before one assumes that clinical results obtained with doses stated for any one system of practice can be adopted *in toto* for a practice that follows another system. It would be better to follow the same system or approach in planning, monitoring, and administration of the current treatment as was used for past treatments on which a prescription is based. This also means that the clinical results reported as having been obtained with stated doses in one institution practicing one particular system cannot be compared with the doses and results in another institution practicing another system, without taking into account the differences in the systems. Through inter-institutional and international study groups, the radiation oncology community should develop a universal system for the practice of brachytherapy that becomes acceptable to all institutions in the future. ICRU has recently published a report to promote this cause [70].

It is also worthwhile to mention that the data tables for radium should be used with caution for planning of treatment with other radioisotope sources. This is because the dose rate depends not only on the air-kerma rate, but also on the values of $(f_{akmd})_{water}$ and WPC(r), both of which can vary for different sources. Fortunately, the variations of $(f_{akmd})_{water}$ and WPC(r) are not too significant among ^{226}Ra, ^{60}Co, ^{137}Cs, ^{192}Ir, and ^{198}Au, because all emit photons of sufficiently high energies. However, for ^{125}I and ^{103}Pd sources, which emit low-energy photons, only data tables especially generated for them should be used.

17.10
Manchester (Paterson and Parker) Distribution Rules

17.10.1
Surface Applications

In surface applications, the sources are placed on top of a mold of thickness **h** placed on the surface area to be treated, which can be of any shape (circular, rectangular, or irregular). Paterson and Parker recommended ways of distributing the radioactive material to obtain $\pm 10\%$ uniformity of dose in the treated area. The reference dose was selected to be 10% above the minimum dose observed in the treated area. For rectangles, the low doses in the corner regions were disregarded. Thus, the reference dose became much like a single representative dose, valid within $\pm 10\%$, stated for the entire area. Table 17.12 gives 'area tables,' which list the air-kerma yield that corresponds to delivery of a 10-cGy reference dose, when Paterson and Parker's distribution rules are followed. The data in the table are applicable to both circular and rectangular areas, if the source arrays conform to the recommended distribution rules.

Circular Areas: Distribution Rules

Let us assume that the treated area is a circle of diameter **D** and **h** is the distance between the source plane and the target plane. For very small circles with $\mathbf{D} < 3\,\mathbf{h}$, the rule recommends that the radioactive material be placed uniformly around the periphery of the circle to provide $\pm 10\%$ uniformity of dose in the treated area (Figure 17.19a). For $3 < \mathbf{D/h} < 6$, the recommendation is to have, in addition to the peripheral circle, a central source having 5% of the total radioactive strength (Figure 17.19b). For still larger **D/h** values, two concentric circles of sources and a center source are recommended (Figure 17.19c), with the center source having 3% of the total radioactive strength. The distribution of the radioactive strength between the inner circle and the outer circle is to be a function of **D/h**, as given in Table 17.15.

Table 17.15. Circular Areas: Source Strength Distribution

D/h	< 3	> 3 < 6	> 6 < 7.5	> 7.5 < 10	> 10
Peripheral circle	100%	95%	80%	75%	70%
Center spot	0%	5%	3%	3%	3%
Inner circle	0%	0%	17%	22%	27%

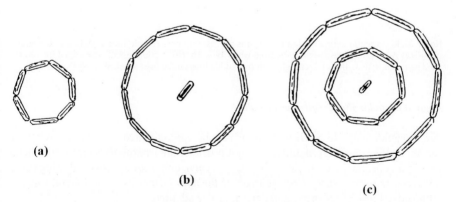

(a)

(b)

(c)

Fig. 17.19. (a) Small circle with sources forming the periphery. (b) A larger circle with peripheral sources and a central source. (c) A still larger circle with pheripheral sources, a central source, and an inner ring of sources

Rectangular Areas: Distribution Rules

For rectangular areas, the approach illustrated in Figure 17.20 is to be followed. For areas of small width, the periphery alone is lined with radioactive sources. As the width increases, any underdosing of the central region of the target volume is avoided by addition of lines parallel to the long side of the rectangle at a spacing not exceeding **2h** (where **h** is the distance between the source and target planes.) If L is the length and W the width of the rectangle, for **W < 2h**, only the peripheral sources are needed (Figure 17.20a). If W exceeds 2h, a central line source is added (Figure 17.20b). If **W** exceeds **4h**, a second, parallel line source is added (Figure 17.20c). Every additional increment of W by 2h warrants addition of a line. If the linear source strength for the peripheral sources is ρ, a single added line should have a linear source strength of $\rho/2$. If there are multiple added lines, the recommended linear source strength for them is $2\rho/3$.

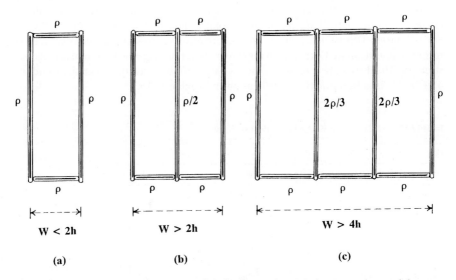

Fig. 17.20. Rectangular arrays of area W × L; h is the distance between the source plane and the target plane. (a) A peripheral rectangle to be used when W < 2h. (b) Rectangle with one added line, to be used when 2h < W < 4h. (c) Rectangle with two added lines, to be used when W > 4h

Areas of Irregular Shape: Distribution Rules

Any irregular shape to be treated can usually be approximated by either a circle or a rectangle. If such an approximation is not possible, the irregularly shaped periphery should first be lined with radioactive sources. Then, either the approach of using rings and a center source, as for circular areas, or the approach of using peripheral sources with added lines, as for rectangular areas, can be adopted.

17.10.2
Single-Plane Implants

Single-plane implants are utilized for treating a slab of target volume having a cross section that matches the area covered by the sources and a thickness extending up to 0.5 cm from the source plane to either of its sides. The same distribution rules as proposed for surface applications can be adopted for implants, with the reference dose rate also maintained to be the net minimum dose in the plane 0.5 cm away. This means that the spacing between adjacent lines in a rectangular array cannot exceed $2 \times h = 2 \times 0.5$ cm $= 1$ cm.

The distribution rules for implants have also been presented in another form in terms of the way in which the total source strength can be divided between the periphery and the central region of the implant. The recommendation presented in Table 17.16 is useful for planning of treatments with radioactive seeds. Table 17.14 gives the dosage data for Manchester-type single-plane implants.

Table 17.16. Planar Implants: Distribution Rules

Area	< 25 cm^2	25–100 cm^2	> 100 cm^2
Peripheral fraction of total source strength	2/3	1/2	1/3

Thus far, we have assumed that it is always possible to line up the radioactive material along the periphery of the area to be treated. With some implants, this is not possible. For example, in the case of a rectangular tongue implant, the far side of the tongue may not be accessible for implanting, and thus the far side of the rectangle may remain uncrossed. In the Manchester system, the dose fall-off caused by an uncrossed end is presumed to cause the effective area treated to be 10% smaller than the implanted area. Therefore, if crossing an end is not possible in a practical situation, the length of the implant should extend 10% beyond the area that needs to be treated.

17.10.3
Two-Plane Implants

The distribution rules for single-plane implants are also recommended for two-plane implants. The data for two-plane implants are obtained by multiplication of the data in Table 17.13 for single-plane implants by the two-plane correction factors given in Table 17.17. Together with the correction factor, the reference dose is the net minimum dose in the plane 0.5 cm outward from either implanted plane (and not between the planes).

Table 17.17. Two-Plane Separation Factors

The data for single-plane implant in Table 17.14 are to be increased by this factor. The specified dose is on planes at 0.5 cm away from either implanted plane, and not on the plane between them.

Separation (cm)	Factor
1.5	1.25
2.0	1.4
2.5	1.5

17.10.4
Volume Implants

In a volume implant, the sources are implanted to cover an entire volume of tissue to be irradiated. An attempt can be made to encompass the tumor volume by one of several simple geometric shapes, such as a cylinder, cube, sphere, or ellipsoid. Paterson and Parker visualized any volume as consisting of two components, a rind and a core. The rind for the sphere is the surface or shell. For a cylinder, the rind consists of the curved surface and the two ends. For a cube, it is made up of the six faces. In all of these cases, the core is the whole volume enclosed within the surface. The amount of radioactivity implanted in the rind and the core should bear a suggested ratio. For this purpose, it is recommended that the total amount be divided into eight parts and then allocated as follows for the different shapes of the volumes implanted:

(a) Cylinder
   Belt, four parts
   Core, two parts
   Each end, one part
(b) Sphere
   Shell, six parts
   Core, two parts
(c) Cube
   Each side, one part
   Each end, one part
   Core, two parts

All of the above distributions adopt a surface-to-core ratio of 6 : 2 of radioactive material. The recommendation is to use sources at not more than 1.0- to 1.5-cm spacing and to spread them out as evenly as possible over the surfaces and within the volume.

Paterson and Parker provided a volume dosage table (Table 17.14) for dosage evaluations when their distribution rules are adopted. The stated reference dose is the 'net minimum dose,' which is defined to be 10% higher than the absolute minimum dose in the effective volume. The tabulated data apply directly to all shapes if the three dimensions, length, width, and height, are approximately equal for the volume implanted. However, if the volume is elongated, the source strength to be used should be increased by the elongation factors given in Table 17.18, according to the ratio of the longest to the shortest dimension.

Table 17.18. Elongation Correction Factors for Volumes

Ratio of Longest to Shortest Dimension	Correction Factor[a]
1.5	1.036
2.0	1.073
2.5	1.111
3.0	1.150

[a] Recommended multiplicative factor to increase the air-kerma yield to reference dose ratio in Manchester system [57].

17.11
Planning and Implementing a Practical Case

17.11.1
A Sample Target Volume

Let us say that a breast lesion having a cross-sectional area of 4.5 cm × 4.5 cm and a thickness of 0.8 cm is to be implanted. For covering of the entire lesion with some margins, a volume having a cross section of 5.0 cm × 5.0 cm and a thickness of 1 cm is designated as the target volume. The plan is to deliver a dose of 2000 cGy in 40 h.

17.11.2
Planning the Geometry of the Array

We can treat the lesion by a single-plane implant. Our plan is to use nylon ribbons carrying ^{192}Ir seeds at 1-cm spacing, with an inter-ribbon spacing of 1 cm, and to leave the ribbon ends uncrossed. We decide to follow the Paterson and Parker distribution rules. The rules state that any uncrossed end can cause a 10% reduction in the area treated. Hence, the active length of the implanted ribbons should extend beyond the intended target area by 10% if any end is left uncrossed. Thus, for covering a 5-cm length, an active length of 6 cm should be used. Figures 17.21a and b show the views of a proposed array of radioactive seeds in two mutually perpendicular planes. Six nylon ribbons are spaced at 1-cm intervals, covering a width of 5 cm. Each ribbon carries seven radioactive seeds, with 1-cm spacing between seeds to give an active length of 6 cm.

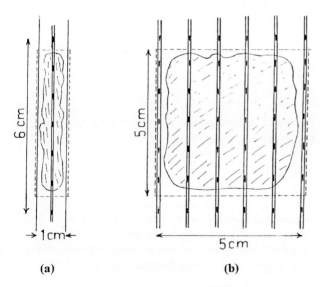

(a)   **(b)**

Fig. 17.21. (a) End and (b) side views of a single planar array of radioactive ^{192}Ir seeds in a nylon ribbon for treatment of a target volume having a 5 cm × 5 cm cross section

17.11.3
Determining the Source Strengths

In this case, we have the following information:

Length of implanted area = 6 cm
Width of implanted area = 5 cm
Length of target area = 5 cm (6 cm reduced by 2 × 10% for 2 uncrossed ends)
Width of the target area = 5 cm
Target area = 5 cm × 5 cm = 25 cm^2

From the Paterson and Parker single-plane implant dosage table (Table 17.13), it is noted that a total air-kerma of 33.1 cGy cm^2 can deliver a dose of 10 cGy. Accordingly, for a total of 2000 cGy to be delivered by the implant, the total air-kerma needed will be

$$(33.1 \text{ cGy cm}^2/10 \text{ cGy}) \times 2000 \text{ cGy} = 6620 \text{ cGy cm}^2$$

If this is to be delivered in a 40-h period, the total source strength to be employed will be

$$6620 \text{ cGy cm}^2/40 \text{ h} = 165.5 \text{ cGy cm}^2 \text{ h}^{-1}$$

The Paterson and Parker rules recommend the use of linear source strengths of ρ and of $2\rho/3$ in the peripheral and central source lines, respectively. This means that, if seeds of strength S_{ak} are used in the two peripheral ribbons, seeds of strength $2S_{ak}/3$ should be used in the four inner ribbons. Hence, the total strength of all seeds is

$$S_{ak} \times 7 \text{ seeds} \times 2 \text{ peripheral ribbons}$$
$$+ (2 S_{ak}/3) \times 7 \text{ seeds} \times 4 \text{ inner ribbons} = 165.5 \text{ cGy cm}^2 \text{ h}^{-1}$$

i. e.

$$32.7 S_{ak} = 165.5 \text{ cGy cm}^2 \text{ h}^{-1}$$

or

$$S_{ak} = 5.06 \text{ cGy cm}^2 \text{ h}^{-1} \text{ and } (2 S_{ak}/3) = 3.37 \text{ cGy cm}^2 \text{ h}^{-1}$$

This means that seeds of strengths 5.06 cGy cm^2 h^{-1} and 3.37 cGy cm^2 h^{-1} should be used in the peripheral and inner ribbons, respectively.

17.11.4
Procuring the Sources

The above sources are to be procured from a vendor. Let us say that, on contact with the vendor, it is found that these exact source strengths are not available, but seeds of 4.8 cGy cm^2 h^{-1} and 2.9 cGy cm^2 h^{-1} can be obtained as the closest approximations. If the available sources are used, the total source strength in the implant will be

$$4.8 \text{ cGy cm}^2 \text{ h}^{-1} \times 7 \text{ seeds} \times 2 \text{ peripheral ribbons}$$
$$+ 2.9 \text{ cGy cm}^2 \text{ h}^{-1} \times 7 \text{ seeds} \times 4 \text{ inner ribbons} = 148.4 \text{ cGy cm}^2 \text{ h}^{-1}$$

Because we have deviated from the distribution rules only marginally, we continue to use the information (derived in Section 17.11.3 based on data of Table 17.13) that 6620 cGy cm^2 can deliver a dose of 2000 cGy. Accordingly, the revised treatment time and dose rate will be

$$6620\,\mathrm{cGy\,cm^2}/148.4\,\mathrm{cGy\,cm^2\,h^{-1}} = 44.6\,\mathrm{h}$$

and

$$\mathrm{Dose\ rate} = 2000\,\mathrm{cGy}/44.6\,\mathrm{h} \approx 45\,\mathrm{cGy\,h^{-1}}$$

This value can be reascertained or fine-tuned on the basis of dosimetry calculations done with the aid of computers, after the plan is implemented on the patient.

17.11.5
Implanting the Sources

The treatment dose rate calculated above can be applied if, and only if, the spatial relationship between the sources as obtained in the patient conforms exactly to the planned array. In actual implants, such exact conformity may not be achieved. The spacings between the source ribbons can turn out to be uneven or nonparallel for practical reasons such as the need to avoid piercing of blood vessels, mechanical difficulties of passage, or inconvenient access. In the current-day practice of afterloading radiotherapy, it is usual to implant tubes or catheters first. The catheters can be loaded with dummy sources (nonradioactive sources that simulate the real sources) and radiographed. The radiotherapy simulator, with its isocentric rotation, can be used for radiography. The resulting radiographs showing the dummy seeds in the catheters can be used for judging the location of the target volume with respect to the catheters and the possible source positions. The number of seeds to be loaded in the different catheters can be altered or revised if needed. Detailed calculations can be done by computer in multiple planes through the implant and isodose curves plotted. Examination of the dose distribution can help to decide the actual treatment time. The afterloading catheters can then be loaded with radioactive sources according to the treatment plan. The sources are left in the patient for a predetermined period of irradiation.

17.11.6
Radiographic Localization of Sources

The aim of radiographic localization is to determine geometrically the spatial coordinates of the sources and any other identifiable point in the radiograph with respect to a reference origin. In the language of coordinate geometry, we would like to be able to decide the three-dimensional rectangular Cartesian coordinates (x, y, z) of any identifiable point in the radiograph. Because any radiograph is two-dimensional, it is necessary to have more than one radiograph to obtain the three-dimensional data sought. We will discuss here two common methods, tube-shift radiography and orthogonal radiography, for localization of implanted sources. Localization by orthogonal projections is known to provide better accuracy than do stereo projections [71].

Tube Shift Radiographic Localization

In this method, illustrated in Figure 17.22, a single film is exposed twice. A radio-opaque marker M has been placed on the patient support table and is maintained in a fixed geometry with respect to the patient. First, the film is exposed with the X-ray source at position S_1. Then either the X-ray source or the patient is moved so as to have the X-rays emerge from position S_2 relative to the patient, and another exposure is made. In the figure, the film is parallel to the (x, z) plane and is perpendicular to the y axis. The system of coordinates has its origin on the central ray for the first exposure at the level of the table top. The projection of a point P(x, y, z) on the film moves from P_1 to P_2 by a distance Δx_1 in the x direction. The displacements of point P_1 from the origin along the x and z directions are x_1 and z_1, respectively. The image of marker M has moved from M_1 to M_2 on the film. If SFD and STD are source-to-film distance and source-to-table-top distance, respectively, the following geometric relations hold true:

$$\frac{M_1M_2}{S_1S_2} = \frac{\text{vertical distance from film to table}}{\text{vertical distance from source to table}} = \frac{SFD - STD}{STD} = \frac{SFD}{STD} - 1$$

Hence,

$$STD = \frac{S_1S_2 \cdot SFD}{S_1S_2 + M_1M_2}$$

$$x = \frac{x_1(STD - y)}{SFD}; \ z = \frac{z_1(STD - y)}{SFD}$$

$$\frac{\Delta x_1}{S_1S_2} = \frac{\text{vertical distance from P to film}}{\text{vertical distance from source to P}} = \frac{SFD - STD + y}{STD - y}$$

Fig. 17.22. Illustration of the principle of single-film stereo radiography for localization of sources in an implant (see text for definition of symbols)

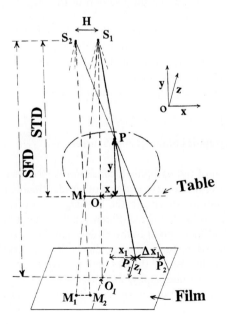

Hence,

$$y = \frac{[\Delta x_1 \cdot STD - S_1S_2(SFD - STD)]}{[\Delta x_1 + S_1S_2]}$$

If $y \ll STD$, the following approximations are possible for x and z:

$$x = x_1(STD/SFD) \quad \text{and} \quad z = z_1(STD/SFD)$$

Orthogonal Radiographic Localization

Figure 17.23 illustrates the principle of using orthogonal radiographic projections for three-dimensional localization of a point object in a patient. Two successive radiographs are taken as isocentric projections in mutually perpendicular directions, usually the front-to-back (AP) and right-to-left (lateral) projections. These can be obtained with the help of a radiotherapy treatment simulator. Ideally, there should be no motion of the patient between the two projections. The point P may represent a surgical clip, a point source, the end point of a line source, a bony landmark, or any other site that is uniquely identifiable in both radiographs. In Figure 17.23, the two positions of the X-ray source are S_1 and S_2. The central rays of the two projections strike the two radiographic images at points O_1 and O_2. The rectangular Cartesian coordinates of point P are (x, y, z) with respect to an origin O selected to be at the intersection of the

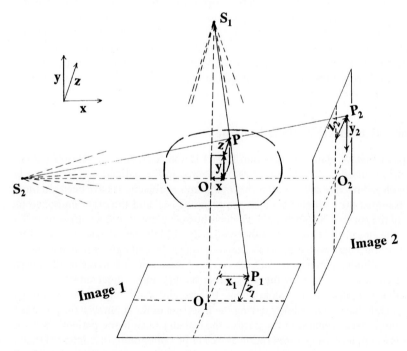

Fig. 17.23. Illustration of the principle of orthogonal radiography for localization of sources in an implant (see text for definition of symbols)

central rays S_1O_1 and S_2O_2. The x and y directions have been chosen to be parallel to S_2O_2 and S_1O_1. Image 1 is perpendicular to the y axis, and image 2 is perpendicular to the x axis. P_1 and P_2 are the observed images of point P in the two radiographs. It is noted that P_1 is at position (x_1, z_1) in image 1 and P_2 is at position (y_2, z_2) in image 2. The following simple geometric relationships hold:

$$x_1 = \frac{x \cdot S_1O_1}{S_1O - y} \quad z_1 = \frac{z \cdot S_1O_1}{S_1O - y}$$

$$y_2 = \frac{y \cdot S_2O_2}{S_2O + x} \quad z_2 = \frac{z \cdot S_2O_2}{S_2O + x}$$

In many practical situations, because the distances S_1O and S_2O are large (80 to 100 cm) compared to x, y, and z, the following approximations can be used:

$$x_1 = (MF_1) \cdot x \quad z_1 = (MF_1) \cdot z$$

$$y_2 = (MF_2) \cdot y \quad z_2 = (MF_2) \cdot z$$

where MF_1 and MF_2 are the magnification factors for the two images, given by

$$MF_1 = \frac{S_1O_1}{S_1O} \quad \text{and} \quad MF_2 = \frac{S_2O_2}{S_2O}$$

The values of the magnification factors can be determined as above if the relevant distances are known. Alternatively and more commonly, the location of the central ray and the magnification factor can both be inferred from the projection of a graduated cross hair in the therapy simulator. Furthermore, the fact that both images give information about the z coordinate (that is, z_1 and z_2) is useful for checking the mutual agreement between the two projections. In practice, some discrepancies in the z values as derived from the two radiographs can occur for several reasons, which include incorrect knowledge of the magnification factors, nonorthogonality, nonisocentricity, and patient motion.

17.11.7
Orthogonal Reconstruction -- A Practical Case

The implant that we planned in Section 17.11.1 is now to be carried out on a patient. Empty nylon tubes or catheters are first implanted in the patient, and these can be loaded with radioactive sources after the radiographic projections have been obtained. In our example, the catheters used have one end closed and the other end open for loading of the sources. Six such catheters have been implanted in the patient in such a way that the closed ends are toward the medial side and the open ends are toward the right side of the chest wall. Figures 17.24a and b show the orthogonal (AP and lateral) radiographs obtained after each catheter has been loaded with a string of 12 dummy seeds at 1-cm spacing, imitating the real sources. It is possible to determine the number of seeds that any catheter can accommodate by carefully observing how many dummy seeds go inside the patient's body during the insertion of the dummy string. The rest of the dummy seeds remain in the part of the catheter outside the patient's body, in air. In this example, by such observation as well as by radiography, it is inferred that, if the six catheters were each loaded with seven seeds, the coverage of the target volume would be adequate.

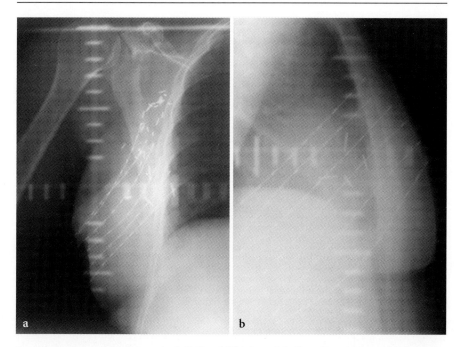

Fig. 17.24. Orthogonal (**a**) front-to-back (AP) and (**b**) left-to-right (lateral) projections of the catheters of a breast implant loaded with imitation seeds, as obtained with a radiotherapy simulator

Figures 17.25a and b are line tracings of the salient features in the orthogonal radiographs of Figure 17.24. They show the positions of the seeds to be loaded and the cross hair scale from the simulator indicating the magnification. The AP and lateral projections have been so positioned that the z coordinates of different seeds match after allowance is made for the difference in magnification between the two images. It can be observed that the positions of the cross hair scales representing the z = 0 level do not match exactly. This indicates apparent patient motion in the z (i.e., head-to-foot) direction between the two radiographs. This systematic error has been identified, and the z = 0 level in Figure 17.25b has been redefined to match the z = 0 level of Figure 17.25a.

17.11.8
Dosimetry Using Computer and Interpretation

The (x_1, z_1) and (y_2, z_2) coordinates of the different seeds from the two images (in Figure 17.25) are input to a computer, along with the information that the two peripheral catheters are loaded with seeds of 4.8 cGy cm^2 h^{-1} and the four central catheters with seeds of 2.9 cGy cm^2 h^{-1}, as has been planned. Here we use a computer program that offers the facility to transform the coordinate information, perform the dose calculations, and plot the dose distribution, in any plane through the implant. Figure 17.26 displays the isodose rate curves (in units of cGy h^{-1}) in two mutually perpendicular

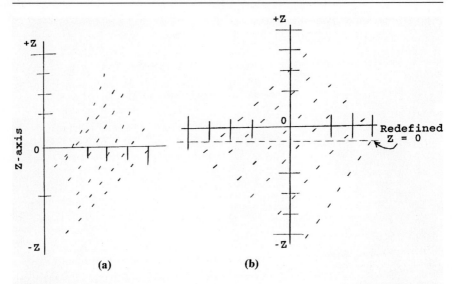

Fig. 17.25. Line tracings of the orthogonal radiographs of Figure 17.24, showing the positions of the seeds to be loaded and the cross hair image from the simulator

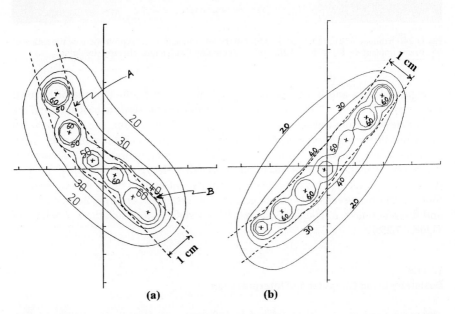

Fig. 17.26. Isodose rate curves in two central planes (**a** and **b**) in perpendicular directions through the breast implant, as obtained by computer dosimetry for nonuniform loading. The two outer catheters are loaded with sources having $4.8 \, \text{cGy cm}^2 \, \text{h}^{-1}$. The inner catheters carry sources of $2.9 \, \text{cGy cm}^2 \, \text{h}^{-1}$. The cross (x) marks are inferred positions of source ribbons

planes through the middle of the implant. These two planes have been chosen to be approximately perpendicular and parallel to the source ribbons.

The interpretation of these isodose curves requires both scientific and artistic intuition. It will be noticed that there are isodose curves of high denominations that encircle the apparent source positions. The source positions thus inferred have been identified by cross marks. We recall the convention that a single-plane implant treats a target of thickness of 1.0 cm extending up to 0.5 cm on either side of the source plane. Hence, the broken lines have been drawn on both sides of the source plane at 0.5 cm from it. In Figure 17.26a, the isodose rate curve for 40 cGy h^{-1} follows the dashed lines most closely, although a part of it falls within and some outside the dashed lines.

The next isodose rate levels plotted are for 50 cGy h^{-1} and 30 cGy h^{-1}. If we disregard the end regions of the implant and use visual interpolation, the surface dose rate appears to lie within 40 ± 5 cGy h^{-1}. This number should be compared with the 45 cGy h^{-1} that we estimated in Section 17.11.4 by using the area dosage tables. In this clinical example, the spacing between the catheters turned out to be uneven. The spacing is more than 1.0 cm on one side of the implant, less than 1.0 cm on the other side, and close to the intended 1.0 cm in the middle. The increased spacing results in a low dose at point **A** on the surface. At point **B**, the reduced spacing results in an increased dose rate.

We loaded the catheters with seeds of unequal strengths in the above case. However, let us say instead that the total strength of 148.4 cGy cm^2 h^{-1} used above is divided equally among the 42 seeds and that all catheters are loaded with seeds of identical strength of 3.53 cGy cm^2 h^{-1}. The dose distributions then change to those shown in Figures 17.27a and b for the same two planes through the implant. The reader is advised

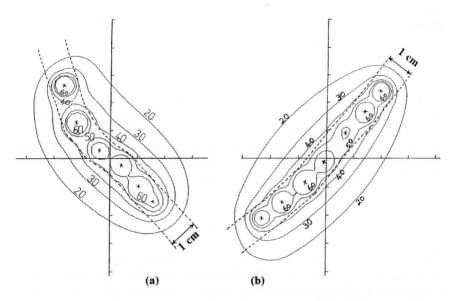

(a)   (b)

Fig. 17.27. Isodose rate curves in two central planes (**a** and **b**) in perpendicular directions through the breast implant, as obtained by computer dosimetry for uniform loading. All sources have a strength of 3.53 cGy cm^2 h^{-1}. The cross (x) marks are inferred positions of source ribbons

to compare the isodose pattern in Figure 17.27 with that in Figure 17.26 to understand the differences that result from the use of nonuniform and uniform source strengths.

EXAMPLE 17.5

Use the isodose rate curves of Figure 17.27a (i) to estimate the mean basic dose rate and (ii) to calculate the treatment time to deliver 2000 cGy if 85% of the mean basic dose rate is chosen as the reference dose rate.

By definition, the basic dose rate is the dose rate obtained at a point half-way between adjacent source lines in the central region of the implant. In Figure 17.27a, there are six catheters and five interspaces between them. If we adopt steps of 5 cGy h^{-1} for interpolation between the isodose curves, observation of the dose distribution in the five interspaces between the six source strings suggests that the dose rates at the midway points are 40, 45, 55, 60, and 75 cGy h^{-1}. Averaging these, the

$$\text{Mean basic dose rate} = (40 + 45 + 55 + 60 + 75)/5 \,\text{cGy h}^{-1}$$
$$= 55 \,\text{cGy h}^{-1}$$

$$85\% \text{ of mean basic dose rate} = 55 \times 0.85 \approx 47 \,\text{cGy h}^{-1}$$
$$\text{Treatment time to deliver 2000 cGy} = 2000/47 \approx 42.5 \,\text{h}$$

The above example resembles the dosimetry in the Paris system, although the Paris system addresses the use of continuous radioactive wires rather than seeds with spacings.

17.12
Permanent Implants

In permanent implants, the implanted sources are left in the patient to irradiate a lesion until they fully decay. The dose rate gradually decreases from a high value at the beginning of treatment to a negligible level in the natural radioactive decay process. The time of treatment is not a parameter controlled by the user, but is governed by the half-life of the source. The selection of the strength of the source for implantation thus becomes an important parameter for assuring the delivery of the preplanned dose. Most permanent implants are seed implants consisting of sources of 2 to 3 mm length. An interseed spacing of 1.0 cm or 0.5 cm can be adopted. Paying detailed attention to the number of planes to be implanted and the areas to be covered can help one to know in advance the size of the volume and the number of seeds that will be needed. ^{222}Rn, ^{198}Au, ^{125}I, and ^{103}Pd have been used for permanent implants.

EXAMPLE 17.6

A spherical volume (as illustrated in Figure 17.13) having a diameter of 7 cm is to be permanently implanted with seeds of radioactive gold, ^{198}Au. Calculate the initial source strength needed to deliver a total of 6000 cGy minimum peripheral dose. (Use an array of seeds with 1-cm spacing and the data in Table 17.10.)

First, we need to visualize the successive planes at 1-cm spacing throughout the volume to be implanted as filled with seeds spaced 1 cm apart. This has already been done in Figure 17.13. The total number of seeds spread over seven planes is 155. The volume of sphere of radius $(7.0\,\mathrm{cm}/2) = 3.5\,\mathrm{cm}$ is

$$V = (4/3)\pi(3.5)^3 \approx 180\,\mathrm{cm}^3$$

We assume that the data in Table 17.10 for radium can be used for ^{198}Au. (For ^{125}I and ^{103}Pd sources, which emit very low-energy photons, only data tables generated especially for them should be used.) From this table, the total air-kerma strength needed to deliver 10 cGy MPD for a volume of 180 cm^3 is 107.3 cGy cm^2. For 6000 cGy, we need

$$107.3\,\mathrm{cGy\,cm}^2 \times \frac{6000\,\mathrm{cGy}}{10\,\mathrm{cGy}} = 64380\,\mathrm{cGy\,cm}^2$$

^{198}Au decays with a half-life $T_h = 2.7$ days. Hence the effective duration of the treatment given is the mean life, T_m:

$$T_m = 1.44\,T_h = 1.44 \times 2.7\,\mathrm{d} \times 24\,\mathrm{h/d} = 93.3\,\mathrm{h}$$

$$\text{The total initial source strength needed} = \frac{64380\,\mathrm{cGy\,cm}^2}{93.3\,\mathrm{h}} \approx 690\,\mathrm{cGy\,cm}^2\,\mathrm{h}^{-1}$$

The needed intitial source strength per seed is

$$S_{ak} = \frac{690\,\mathrm{cGy\,cm}^2\,\mathrm{h}^{-1}}{155\,\mathrm{seeds}} \approx 4.45\,\mathrm{cGy\,cm}^2\,\mathrm{h}^{-1}/\mathrm{seed}$$

17.13
Intracavitary Irradiation

17.13.1
Vaginal Cylinder

Insertion of a plastic cylindrical applicator inside the vaginal canal and loading of the cylinder axis with a series of line sources in tandem is a commonly used intracavitary irradiation technique. Several cylinders of different diameters and lengths can be kept in stock, and the size that best fits a particular patient can be selected for use. The cylinder helps to keep the tissues irradiated at a fixed geometry with respect to the sources. It also displaces the tissues away from the sources and thereby avoids regions of very rapid dose fall-off in the immediate proximity of the sources. The sources can first be loaded in a nylon tube, and that tube can be afterloaded into the applicator.

Figures 17.28a and b illustrate the dose distributions obtained around a vaginal cylinder loaded with sources in two different arrangements. In both distributions, the 100% dose has been normalized to lie at the surface of the central part of the applicator. In Figure 17.28a, three linear sources of identical active length (2 cm) and linear strength are used. In Figure 17.28b, a dumb-bell-type source loading has been used, with a central source of 4 cm active length and two end sources of 1 cm active length. The end sources have a linear strength about three times that of the central source. Such a 'dumb-bell' arrangement gives isodose curves that are nearly parallel to

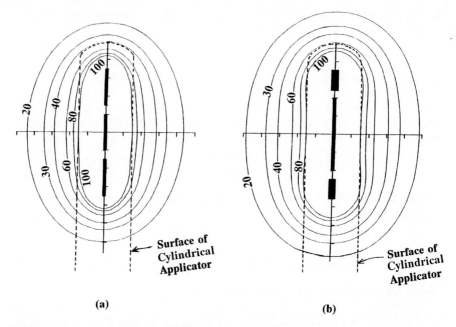

(a)   **(b)**

Fig. 17.28. Dose distributions for a vaginal cylinder loaded with linear sources along the cylinder axis (a) for three linear sources of identical length and source strength; (b) for a nonuniform 'dumb-bell'-type loading that uses a linear strength ratio of 3.3 : 1 between end sources and the central source. The 100% level is the dose on the surface of the cylinder in the central region

the surface of the applicator, indicating a uniform delivery of surface dose. The volume covered by the isodose curves is larger than that obtained with the use of uniform linear activity.

17.13.2
Pairs of Colpostats

In a different type of vaginal irradiation, a pair of applicators (called colpostats) is inserted to occupy the vaginal fornices. The source-carrying part of the applicator is specially designed to keep the irradiated tissue surface at a distance from the source and to make it conform to the shape of a cylinder or ovoid (a volume of oval cross section). For example, the applicators may have an external cylindrical surface of 3.0 cm length and a diameter of 2.0 cm. By addition of plastic caps of 2.5 mm or 5 mm thickness, the external diameter can be increased to 2.5 cm or 3.0 cm. Each applicator may be loaded with a linear source of about 1.4 cm active length and 2.0 cm external length. This size comes from the experience of using radium sources of similar dimensions in the past. In afterloading designs, a long access handle may be provided through which the linear source, which is held at the tip of a wire, can be inserted into the colpostat and removed. Some colpostats have been designed to incorporate lead shields in an appropriate manner to provide a 15% to 20% reduction in dose in the direction of radiosensitive normal organs, including the bladder and rectum [72–74].

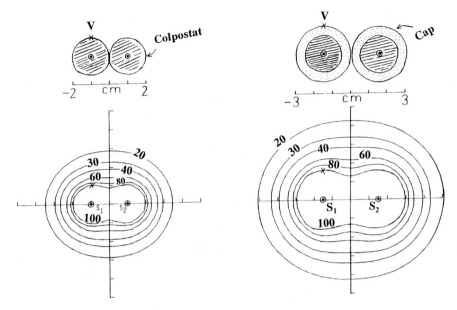

Fig. 17.29. Pairs of colpostats in the vaginal apex. (a) Small pair without caps, and (b) large pair with caps. The 100% dose is on the surface at point V

The isodose distribution for a pair of applicators with 2.0 cm external diameter is shown in Figure 17.29a. Figure 17.29b shows the distribution when caps of 0.5 cm thickness are added. It is necessary in such treatments not to exceed the tolerance of the normal tissues touching the surface of the applicators. For this purpose, the dose rate can be monitored at a point such as V on the vaginal cuff. It is obvious that, if one is to obtain the same dose rate at point V, the source strength to be used without caps will be less than that to be used when the caps are affixed. It is estimated that total strengths (as composed by both sources) amounting to 40–45 cGy cm² h⁻¹ and 80– 85 cGy cm² h⁻¹ can deliver a dose of 1000 cGy in about 24 h at V in the two situations of Figures 17.29a and b, respectively. (The reader is prompted to verify this by using data from Table 17.5 or Table 17.6, as an exercise).

17.13.3
Irradiations of Uterine Cervix

Figure 17.30 shows the long-established irradiation technique used for treatment of cancer of the cervix [72–74]. The cervix is the site where the uterine canal meets the vaginal canal. The cancer is known to originate at the cervix and invade the parametrium. A typical source arrangement that consists of a series of line sources, S_1, S_2, and S_3, in tandem along the uterine canal and a pair of colpostats in the vaginal canal is shown. Such intracavitary irradiation methods deliver an enormously high dose to the cancerous sites adjoining the sources. No accurate quantitative dosimetry is possible at these sites. However, the clinically established norms with respect to the source strengths to be used at these locations should be observed. It is usual that the

Fig. 17.30. Source arrangement used for intracavitary
irradiation of cancer of the
cervix. The uterine canal carries sources S_1, S_2, and S_3. A
pair of vaginal colpostats carry
sources S_4 and S_5. Points A
and B are reference points for
dosage control (see text)

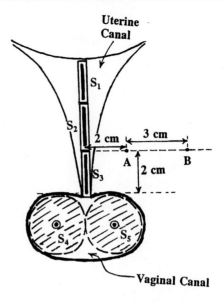

bottom end of the lowest source, S_3, in the uterine canal is positioned so as to be at the
cervix, where it delivers a high dose.

In the Manchester system [57, 75], a reference point, called point A, is chosen for
dosimetry purposes. Point **A**, shown in Figure 17.30, is meant to signify a cancerous site
that needs to be irradiated, but that is also in a region of limited radiation tolerance.
In this region, called the paracervical triangle, a major blood vessel to the uterus
crosses the ureter on its route from the kidneys to the bladder. For clinical dosimetry
purposes, the position of point A has often been defined in geometric terms (rather
than in anatomic terms) to be a point 2 cm lateral to the uterine canal and 2 cm above
the level of the cervix and vaginal vault.

Point B is another reference point, chosen to represent the lymph nodes near the
pelvic wall. It is defined to be at the same level as point **A**, but 5 cm away from the uterine
canal. Many physicians prescribe the dose as stated at point **A**, and they calculate the
dose rate there to determine the treatment duration. The dose at point **B** can be useful
for deciding whether the dose to the pelvic nodes is adequate or will need to be boosted
by an external beam.

The anatomy of the patient may determine the number of sources that can be lined
up in the uterine canal and the size of the colpostats that the vagina can accommodate. In the Manchester system, different combinations of source strengths and source
arrangements have been recommended not only for maintaining a constant dose rate
at point **A**, but also for keeping a balance between the dose to the vaginal mucosa and
that to point **A**.

In afterloading techniques, a long intrauterine tube is first inserted and positioned
along with the afterloadable vaginal colpostats. The sources are inserted after it is
ascertained that the applicators have been positioned acceptably. Dummy sources simulating the real ones can first be inserted and radiographs obtained with radio-opaque
contrast medium in the bladder and rectum to indicate their locations, because the

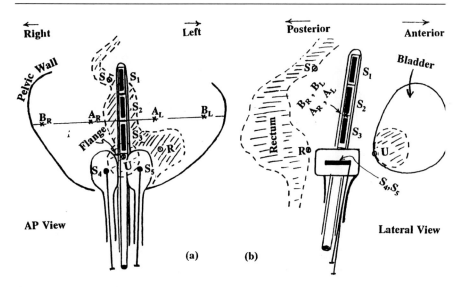

Fig. 17.31. Projections of a typical intracavitary insertion for treatment of cervical cancer, showing the locations of the various reference points and the contrast-delineated outlines of bladder and rectum. (a) AP view, (b) lateral view

bladder and rectum are known to be radiosensitive organs and their tolerance doses can limit the duration of intracavitary irradiation.

Figures 17.31a and b illustrate schematically the coronal and sagittal views of such an intrauterine application. The following reference points have been identified in the figures for dosimetric control:

Points A_L, A_R – Point **A** on the left and right sides of the uterine canal
Points B_L, B_R – Point **B** on the left and right sides of the uterine canal
Point **S** – A reference point for the sigmoid colon
Point **R** – A reference point for the rectum
Point **U** – A reference point for the urinary bladder

In Figure 17.31, the reference points **S**, **R**, and **U** are chosen at positions in close proximity to the radioactive sources. ICRU Report 38 provides many guidelines for dosimetry in intracavitary irradiation for gynecologic applications [77].

The dose distributions obtained in two perpendicular planes for a typical cervical cancer insertion are shown in Figures 17.32a and b. The two planes correspond to the midcoronal and midsagittal planes through the cervix. The orientations of the tubes in the vaginal colpostats are such that the isodose curves are narrower in the sagittal plane (thus sparing the bladder and rectum) than in the coronal plane (to encompass the usual route of spread of the disease).

Use of only a single line of sources along the uterine canal, such as in Figure 17.32, produces a rapid fall-off of dose from the uterine wall. Cancerous lesions of the body of the uterus may need delivery of a substantial dose to tissues extending to 1.0–2.0 cm from the uterine axis. The dose distribution becomes broader if the uterine cavity is packed with multiple sources. This is referred to as Heyman packing [76].

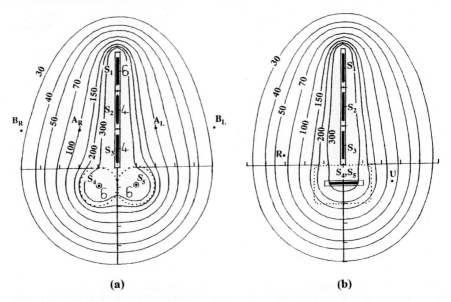

(a)   (b)

Fig. 17.32. Isodose curves in two perpendicular planes (a) and (b) for a typical intracavitary insertion. Sources S_1, S_2, S_3, S_4, and S_5 have relative source strengths of 6, 4, 4, 6, and 6, respectively. The 100% dose is taken to be the dose received at point A

References

1. Quimby, E.H., Fifty years of radium, Am. J. Roentgenol., Vol 60, p723–730, 1948.
2. Martin, C.L., and Martin, J.A., Low Intensity Radium Therapy, Little, Brown, Boston, 1959.
3. Wood, V.A. (Ed.), A collection of radium leak test articles, U.S. Dept. Health, Education and Welfare, MORP-68-1, Rockville, MD, March 1968.
4. International Atomic Energy Agency (IAEA), Physical Aspects of Radioisotope Brachytherapy, Technical Report Series No. 75, International Atomic Energy Agency, Vienna, 1967.
5. Trott, N.G. (Ed.), Radionuclides in Brachytherapy, Radium and After, Br. J. Radiol., Suppl. 21, British Institute of Radiology, London, 1988.
6. Nath, R., New directions in radionuclide sources for brachytherapy, Semin. Radiat. Oncol., Vol 3, pp279–289, 1993.
7. Hospital Physicists' Association, Guidance on Testing of Sealed Sources of Radioisotopes for Leakage and Surface Contamination, HPA Report Series No. 1, Hospital Physicists' Association, London, U.K., 1970.
8. International Organisation for Standardisation (ISO), Sealed Radioactive Sources – Leak Test Methods, Technical Report Series 4862, International Organisation for Standardisation, Geneva, Switzerland, 1979.
9. Lommartzsch, P.K., Beta irradiation of choroidal melanoma with 106Ru, 106Rh applicators, Arch. Ophthalmol., Vol 101, p713–717, 1983.
10. Freidel, H.L., Thomas, C.I., and Krohmer, J.S., An evaluation of the clinical use of a 90Sr beta ray applicator with a review of the underlying principles, Am. J. Roentgenol., Vol 71, p25–39, 1954.
11. Sinclair, W.K., and Trott, N.G., The construction and measurement of beta-ray applicators for use in ophthalmology, Br. J. Radiol., Vol 29, pp15–23, 1956.
12. Supe, S.J., and Cunningham, J.R., A physical study of a strontium-90 beta-ray applicator, Am. J. Roentgenol., Vol 89, pp570–574, 1963.
13. Henschke, U.K., Hilaris, B.S., and Mahan, G.D., Afterloading in interstitial and intracavitary radiotherapy, Am. J. Roentgenol., Vol. 90, pp386–395, 1963.
14. Paine, C.H., Modern afterloading methods for interstitial radiotherapy, Clin. Radiol., Vol 23, pp263–272, 1972.

15. Hillaris, B.S. (Ed.), Afterloading, 20 Years of Experience 1955–1975, Proceedings of the II International Symposium on Radiation Therapy, American Institute of Physics, Memorial Sloan-Kettening Cancer Center, New York, 1975.
16. Syed, A.M., and Feber, B.S., Technique of afterloading interstitial implants, Radiol. Clin., Vol 46, pp458–475, 1977.
17. Syed, A.M., Nisar, S., and Feber, B.S., Techniques of afterloading interstitial implants, in Renaissance of Interstitial Brachytherapy, Proceedings of the 12th Annual San Francisco Cancer Symposium, California, 1977, Frontiers of Radiation Therapy Oncology, Vol 12, Vaeth, J.M. (Ed.), S. Karger, Basel, 1978, pp119–135.
18. Delclos, L., Afterloading methods for interstitial gamma-ray therapy, Chapter 1, in Textbook of Radiotherapy, Fletcher, G.H. (Ed.), Lea & Febiger, Philadelphia, 1980, pp84-92.
19. Almond, P.R., Remote afterloading, Chapter 8, in Advances in Radiotherapy Treatment Planning, Wright, A.E., and Boyer, A.L. (Eds.), American Institute of Physics, New York, 1983, p601–619.
20. Delclos, L., Afterloading interstitial irradiation techniques, Chapter 11, p123-154, in Levitt and Tapley's Technological Basis of Radiation Therapy: Practical Clinical Applications, Levitt, S.L., Khan, F.M., and Potish, R.A. (Eds.), Lea & Febiger, Philadelphia, 1992.
21. Williamson, J.F., and Nath, R., Clinical implementation of Task Group 32 recommendations on brachytherapy source strength specification, Med. Phys., Vol 18, pp439–448, 1991.
22. American Association of Physicists in Medicine, AAPM Report 21, Specification of Brachytherapy Source Strength, Report of Task Group 32, American Institute of Physics, New York, 1987.
23. Williamson, J.F., Khan, F.M., Sharma, S.C., and Fullerton, G.D., Methods for routine calibration of brachytherapy sources, Radiology, Vol 142, pp511–515, 1982.
24. Williamson, J.F., Morin, R.L., and Khan, F.M., Dose calibrator response to brachytherapy sources: A Monte Carlo and analytic evaluation, Med. Phys., Vol 10, pp135–140, 1983.
25. Gibb, R., and Massey, J.B., Radium dosage; SI units and the Manchester system, Br. J. Radiol., Vol 53, pp1100–1101, 1980.
26. Meisberger, L.L., Keller, R.J., and Shalek, R.J., The effective attenuation in water of the gamma rays of gold-198, iridium-192, cesium-137, radium-226 and cobalt-60, Radiology, Vol 90, pp953–957, 1968.
27. Meli, J.A., Anderson, L.L., and Weaver, K.A., Dose distibution, pp21–34, in Interstitial Brachytherapy, Physical, Biological and Clinical Considerations, Interstitial Collaborative Working Group, Raven Press, New York, 1990.
28. Nath, R., Anderson, L.L., Luxton, G., Weaver, K.A., Williamson, J.F., and Meigooni, A.S., Dosimetry of interstitial brachytherapy sources: Recommendations of the AAPM Radiotherapy Committee, Task Group No. 43, Med. Phys., Vol 22, pp209–234, 1995.
29. Weaver, K.A., Anderson, L.L., and Meli, J.A., Source characteristics, pp3–13 in Interstitial Brachytherapy, Physical, Biological and Clinical Considerations, Interstitial Collaborative Working Group, Raven Press, New York, 1990.
30. Ling, C.C., Gromadzki, Z.C., Rustgi, S.N., and Cundiff, J.H., Directional dependence of radiation fluence from ^{192}Ir and ^{198}Au sources, Radiology, Vol 146, p791–792, 1983.
31. Meigooni, A.S., Sabnis, S., and Nath, R., Dosimetry of palladium-103 brachytherapy sources for permanent implants, Endocurietherapy/Hyperthermic Oncology, Vol 6, pp107–117, 1990.
32. Meigooni, A.S., and Nath, R., A comparison of radial dose functions for 103Pd, ^{125}I, ^{145}Sm, ^{241}Am, ^{169}Yb, ^{192}Ir, and ^{137}Cs brachytherapy sources, Int. J. Radiat. Oncol. Biol. Phys., Vol 22, pp1125–1130, 1992.
33. Sievert, R.M., Eine Methode zur Messung von Roentgen-, Radium- und Ultrastrahlung; uber die Anwendbarkeit derselben in der Physik und der Medizin, Acta Radiol. (Suppl. XIV), 1932.
34. Jayaraman, S., and Iyer, P.S., Dose distributions in paraxial regions of Cs-137 and Co-60 line sources, pp327–333, in Proceedings of Symposium on Biomedical Dosimetry, International Atomic Energy Agency, Vienna, Austria, 1975.
35. Quimby, E.H., Dosage tables for linear radium sources, Radiology, Vol 43, p572–577, 1944.
36. Young, M.E.J., and Batho, H.F., Dose tables for linear radium sources calculated by an electronic computer, Br. J. Radiol., Vol 37, pp38–44, 1964.
37. Krishnaswamy, V., Dose distribution about ^{137}Cs sources in tissue, Radiology, Vol 105, pp181–184, 1972.
38. Breitman, K.E., Dose rate tables for clinical ^{137}Cs sources sheathed in platinum, Br. J. Radiol., Vol 47, pp657–664, 1974.
39. Stovall, M., Lanzl, L.H., and Moos, W.S., Atlas of Radiation Dose Distribution, Brachytherapy Isodose Charts, Vol IV, Sealed Radium Sources, International Atomic Energy Agency, Vienna, Austria, 1972.
40. Hilaris, B.S., Nori, D., and Anderson, L.L., Atlas of Brachytherapy, MacMillan, New York, 1988.

41. Quimby, E.H., and Castro, V., The calculation of dosage in interstitial radium therapy, Am. J. Roentgenol., Vol 70, pp739–749, 1953.
42. Quimby, E.H., and Goodwin, P.N., Dosage calculations with radioactive materials, Chapter 13, in Physical Foundations of Radiology, 4th Ed., Harper & Row, New York, 1970.
43. Pierquin, B., Dutreix, A., Paine, C.H., Chassagne, D., Marinello, G., and Ash, D., The Paris system in interstitial radiation therapy, Acta Radiol. (Oncol. Radiat. Phys. Biol.), Vol 17, pp33–48, 1978.
44. Dutreix, A., and Marinello, G., The Paris system, pp25–42, in Modern Brachytherapy, Pierquin, B., Wilson, J.F., and Chassagne, D. (Eds.), Masson Publishers, New York, 1987.
45. Pierquin, B., Chassagne, D.J., Chahbazian, D.J., and Wilson, J.F., Dosimetry, Chapter 5, in Brachytherapy, Pierquin, B. (Ed.), W. H. Green, St. Louis, Missouri, 1978.
46. Laughlin, J.S., Siler, W.M., Holodny, E.J., and Ritter, F.W., A dose description system for interstitial radiation therapy, Am. J. Roentgenol., Vol 89, pp470–490, 1963.
47. Anderson, L.L., Wagner, L.K., and Schuer, T.H., Memorial methods of dose calculation for Ir-192, pp1–7, in Modern Interstitial and Intracavitary Radiation Cancer Management, George, F. III (Ed.), Masson, New York, 1981.
48. Henschke, U.K., and Ceve, P., Dimension averaging: A simple method for dosimetry of interstitial implants, Radiat. Biol. Ther., Vol 9, pp187-198, 1968.
49. Anderson, L.L., Kuan, H.M., and Ding, I.Y., Clinical dosimetry with I-125, pp9–15, in Modern Interstitial and Intracavitary Radiation Cancer Management, George, F. III (Ed.), Masson, New York, 1981.
50. Anderson, L.L., and Osian, A.D., Brachytherapy optimization and evaluation, Endocurietherapy/Hyperthermic Oncology, Vol 2, ppS25–S31, 1986.
51. Rao, U.V.G., Kan, P.T., and Howells, R., Interstitial volume implants with I-125 seeds, Int. J. Radiat. Oncol. Biol. Phys., Vol 7, pp431–438, 1981.
52. Anderson, L.L., Hilaris, B.S., and Wagner, L.K., A nomograph for planar implant planning, Endocurietherapy/Hyperthermic Oncology, Vol 1, pp9–15, 1985.
53. Anderson, L.L., Spacing nomograph for interstitial implants of I-125 seeds, Med. Phys., Vol 3, pp48–51, 1976.
54. Paterson, R., and Parker, H.M., A dosage system for gamma-ray therapy. I, Br. J. Radiol., Vol 7, pp592–632, 1934; reprinted Br. J. Radiol., Vol 68, No. 808, pH60–100, April 1995.
55. Paterson, R., and Parker, H.M., Dosage system for interstitial radium therapy, Br. J. Radiol., Vol 11, pp252–266, 1938.
56. Parker, H.M., A dosage system for interstitial radium therapy. II. Physical aspects, Br. J. Radiol., Vol 11, pp313–340, 1938.
57. Meredith, W.J. (Ed.), Radium Dosage – Manchester System, 2nd Ed., E & S Livingstone, Edinburgh, 1967.
58. Wu, A., Zwicker, R.D., and Sternick, E.S., Tumor dose specification of I-125 seed implants, Med. Phys., Vol 12, pp27–31, 1985.
59. Busch, M., Dosage in interstitial therapy with gamma emitters, Strahlentherapie, Vol 153, pp589–593, 1977.
60. Kwan, D., Kagan, A.R., Wollin, M. et al., A simple volume iridium implant dosimetry system, Endocurietherapy/Hyperthermic Oncology, Vol 3, pp183–191, 1987.
61. Casebow, M.P., Dosimetry tables for standard iridium-192 wire implants, Br. J. Radiol., Vol 57, pp515–518, 1984.
62. Neblett, D.L., Syed, N., and Puthawala, A.A., An interstitial implant technique evaluated by contiguous volume analysis, Endocurietherapy/Hyperthermic Oncology, Vol 1, pp213–222, 1985.
63. Olch, A., Kagan, A.R., Wollin, M. et al., A simple volume iridium implant dosimetry system, Endocurietherapy/Hyperthermic Oncology, Vol 3, pp183–191, 1987.
64. Murphy, D.J., and Doss, L.L., Small computer algorithms for comparing therapeutic performances of single-plane iridium implants, Med. Phys., Vol 11, pp193–196, 1984.
65. Olch, A., Kagan, A.R., Wollin, M. et al., Multi-institutional survey of techniques in volume iridium implants, Endocurietherapy/Hyperthermic Oncology, Vol 2, pp193–197, 1986.
66. Gillin, M.T., Kline, R.W., Wilson, J.F., and Cox, J.D., Single and double plane implants: Comparison of the Manchester system with the Paris system, Int. J. Radiat. Oncol. Biol. Phys., Vol 10, pp921–925, 1984.
67. Paul, J.M., Koch, R.F., Philip, P.C., and Khan, F.R., Uniformity of dose distribution in interstitial implants, Endocurietherapy/Hyperthermic Oncology, Vol 2, pp107–118, 1986.
68. Dutreix, A., Can we compare systems for interstitial therapy?, Radiother. Oncol., Vol 13, pp127-135, 1988.
69. Paul, J.M., Koch, R.F., and Philip, P.C., Uniform analysis of dose distribution in interstitial brachytherapy and dosimetry systems, Radiother. Oncol., Vol 13, pp105–125, 1988.

70. ICRU Report 58, Dose and volume specification for reporting interstitial therapy, (Ed: Chassagne, D., and Dutreix, A.), International Commission on Radiological Units and Measurements, Bethesda, Md., 1997.
71. Sharma, S.H., Williamson, J.F., and Cytacki, E., Dosimetric analysis of stereo and orthogonal reconstruction of interstitial implants, Int. J. Radiat. Oncol. Biol. Phys., Vol 8, p1803–1805, 1982.
72. Fletcher, G.H., Shalek, R.J., and Cole, A., Cervical radium applicators with screening in the direction of bladder and rectum, Radiology, Vol 60, pp77–84, 1953.
73. Fletcher, G.H., Hamberger, A.D., Wharton, J.T., Rutledge, F.N., and Delclos, L., Female pelvis, Chapter 11, pp720–808, in Textbook of Radiotherapy, Fletcher, G.H. (Ed.), 3rd Ed., Lea & Febiger, Philadelphia, 1980.
74. Delclos, L., Gynecologic cancers: Pelvic examination and treatment planning, Chapter 11, pp193–227, in Technological Basis of Radiation Therapy: Practical Clinical Applications, Levitt, S.L., and Tapley, N. duV. (Eds.), Lea & Febiger, Philadelphia, 1984.
75. Todd, M., and Meredith, W.J., Treatment of cancer of the cervix uteri – a revised Manchester method, Br. J. Radiol., Vol 26, pp252–257, 1953.
76. ICRU, Dose and Volume Specification for Reporting Intracavitary Therapy in Gynecology, Report 38, International Commission on Radiation Units and Measurements, Bethesda, MD, 1985.
77. Heyman, J., Reuterwall, O., and Benner, S., The Radiumhemmet experience with radiotherapy of corpus of the uterus, Acta Radiol., Vol 22, pp11–98, 1941.

Additional Reading

1. Anderson, L.L. et al. (Eds.), Interstitial Brachytherapy: Physical, Biological and Clinical Considerations, Interstitial Collaborative Working Group, Raven Press, New York, 1990.
2. Pierquin, B., Chassagne, D., Chahbazian, D.J., and Wilson, J.F., Brachytherapy, W.H. Green, St. Louis, Missouri, 1978.
3. Dutreix, A., Marinello, G., and Wambersie, A., Dosimetrie en Curietherapie, Masson, Paris, 1982.
4. Glasgow, G., Physics of brachytherapy, Chapter 10, pp213-251, in Principles and Practice of Radiation Oncology, Perez, C.A., and Brady, L.W. (Eds.), J.B. Lippincott, Philadelphia, 1987.
5. Meredith, W.J. (Ed.), Radium Dosage – Manchester System, 2nd Ed., E & S Livingstone, Edinburgh, 1967.
6. George, F. III (Ed.), Modern Interstitial and Intracavitary Radiation Cancer Management, Masson, New York, 1981.
7. Hilaris, B.S., Nori, D., and Anderson, L.L., Atlas of Brachytherapy, MacMillan, New York, 1988.
8. Hilaris, B.S. (Ed.), Handbook of Interstitial Brachytherapy, Publishing Sciences Group, Acton, Massachussetts, 1975.
9. International Atomic Energy Agency (IAEA), Physical Aspects of Radioisotope Brachytherapy, Technical Report Series No. 75, International Atomic Energy Agency, Vienna, 1967.
10. Shearer, D.R. (Ed.), Recent Advances in Brachytherapy Physics, Proceedings of a Workshop of the American Association of Physicists in Medicine, American Institute of Physics, New York, 1979.
11. Trott, N.G. (Ed.), Radionuclides in Brachytherapy, Radium and After, Br. J. Radiology, Supplement 21, British Institute of Radiology, London, U.K., 1988.
12. Harrison, L.B. (Guest Ed.) and Tepper, J.E. (Ed.), Brachytherapy, Semin. Radiat. Oncol., Vol 3, No. 4, 1993.
13. Aird, E.G.A., Jones, C.H., Joslin, C.A.F., Klevenhagen, S.C., Rossiter, M.J., Welsh, A.D., Wilkinson, J.M., Woods, M.J., and Wright, S.J., Recommendations for brachytherapy dosimetry, Report of a joint BIR/IPSM working party, British Institute of Radiology, London, 1993.
14. ICRU Report 58, Dose and volume specification for reporting interstitial therapy, (Ed: Chassagne, D., and Dutreix, A.), International Commission on Radiological Units and Measurements, Bethesda, Md., 1997.
15. Williamson, J.F., Thomadsen, B.R., Nath, R. (Eds.), Brachytherapy Physics, Lectures presented at 1994 Summer School of American Association of Physicists in Medicine, Medical Physics Publishing, Madison, Wisconsin, 1995.
16. Joslin, C.A.F., Flynn, A., Hall. E.J., (Eds.) Principles and practice of brachytherapy using afterloading systems, Hodder Arnold Publisher, London, 2001.

PART VII

Radiation Safety

CHAPTER 18

Radiation Safety Standards

18.1
Introduction

Ionizing radiation is a beneficial agent that contributes to improved health care. However, unnecessary exposure to ionizing radiation can be harmful [1, 2] and should be avoided. Because penetrating radiations cannot be contained entirely, some irradiation of staff members, visitors, and the public is bound to occur incidental to any use of radiation. All radiation work should be carried out in a preplanned and controlled manner so that the exposure to the workers and persons in and near sites of radiation use is kept as low as reasonably achievable (ALARA) and does not exceed the recommended limits. In the U.S., guidelines to ensure the radiation safety of radiation and non-radiation workers and members of the public are provided by the National Council on Radiation Protection and Measurements (NCRP) [3]. Recommendations are also provided by the International Commission on Radiation Protection (ICRP) [4, 5], the International Atomic Energy Agency [6], and the European Atomic Energy Community [7]. In some geographic regions, governmental regulatory agencies formulate the safety limits for radiation exposure and mandate that radiation users adhere to them. A radiotherapy department should plan and conduct its activities in such a manner that the safety recommendations (or regulations) are followed.

Scientific committees that are engaged in the process of setting guidelines for safe use of radiation face a rather formidable job. Whereas radiation damage is readily observable at high doses, at low dose levels the harm done is not easily discerned. The radiation risk (i. e., the probability of an adverse effect) at low dose levels needs to be estimated based on effects observed at high dose levels. The estimation process is laborious and is subject to many assumptions and uncertainties. This task involves the following steps: (i) consolidating all available epidemiologic data on populations exposed to radiation; (ii) comparing these with the epidemiologic information on an unexposed control population; (iii) observing any increased incidence of adverse effects in the exposed population compared to controls; (iv) assessing the radiation dose, received by the exposed population, to which an excess incidence can be attributed; (v) establishing a relationship between the radiation dose and excess risk; (vi) identifying the excess risk that society is willing to accept (as judged from the risks due to causes other than radiation that society is known to tolerate); and (vii) using that insight to identify the level of radiation exposure that can be recommended as acceptable, commensurate with the benefit that the radiation use offers to society.

Assessments of radiation risk have been made and reported on by several committees [8–16]. The risk evaluation is an ongoing process in which advantage is taken of all the latest information and the models of analysis available to the scientific community. Accordingly, the recommendations on dose limits have also undergone several revisions over the years [17].

It is our purpose in this chapter to describe the harmful effects of exposure to low levels of ionizing radiation, the various uncertainties of correlating the dose with the risk of damage, and the philosophy of radiation safety, and to outline the most recent recommendations on dose limits for safe use of ionizing radiations. This presentation mainly covers the 1993 recommendations of the NCRP [3]. The discussion also touches on the 1991 recommendations of the ICRP [4, 5] wherever appropriate.

18.2
Harmful Effects of Radiation

18.2.1
Acute Radiation Syndrome

By 'acute irradiation' we mean a single, large, one-time, whole-body irradiation. Partial-body irradiation, as done in radiotherapy of malignant conditions, is not considered here. The acute radiation syndrome is dependent on the dose received and on the time that has elapsed after irradiation. At dose levels of less than 25 cGy, no detectable acute effects occur. At doses up to 100 cGy, nausea and lack of appetite may result in a few people. Additionally, some reduction in counts of red and white blood cells, blood platelets, and lymphocytes can be observed on careful scrutiny. At 300 to 600 cGy, severe bone marrow damage can result, leading to serious hematologic symptoms, sometimes to irreversible gastrointestinal symptoms of nausea and diarrhea, and to epilation. Fatalities may occur. At doses higher than 600 cGy, damage to the central nervous system can set in. It has been assessed that an acute whole-body dose of 300 cGy of gamma rays delivered to a human population can result in the death of 50% of the population within 30 days after the irradiation [18]. This dose is referred to as lethal dose for 50% in 30 days ($LD_{50/30}$).

18.2.2
Stochastic Effects and Deterministic Effects

In one method of classification, radiation effects are classified as stochastic effects or deterministic effects. Stochastic effects are effects that occur in a random manner. Let us say that a large group of people is exposed to a given dose. Over a period of time, we can expect to see excess cancers in them compared to the incidence in the normal population. This excess number of cancers (i. e., radiation-induced cancers) will increase with the size of the exposed population and with the dose received. It is impossible to foretell who among those irradiated will suffer a radiation-induced cancer. Furthermore, neither can the severity of the disease to be suffered by anyone be predicted. Hence, cancer induction by radiation is a stochastic effect.

Deterministic effects, on the other hand, are predictable events, usually with a known threshold dose above which the effect is known to happen. Acute irradiation to high doses has many demonstrable dose thresholds for deterministic effects. Examples of these effects are eye lens opacification (cataract), blood changes, and reddening of the skin. (We already discussed in this text the need to plan any radiotherapy treatment optimally to cause tumor regression without exceeding the known tolerance of any nearby normal organs.) For stochastic effects, *the probability of occurrence* increases with dose, whereas for deterministic effects *the severity of the effect* increases with dose.

18.2.3
Somatic and Genetic Effects

In another method of classification, radiation effects can be categorized as somatic or genetic. Somatic effects refer to the harm that exposed individuals suffer during their lifetime. Radiation-induced cancers, opacification of the eye lens, sterility, and life shortening are examples of somatic effects. Genetic effects are radiation-induced mutations to an individual's genes and DNA, which can contribute to the birth of defective descendants. Genetic effects show up in the progeny of those irradiated and may include stillbirths, major congenital defects, alteration of the sex ratio, impaired physical development at an early age, and childhood cancers [13, 14, 18, 19]. Exposure of a human embryo to radiation in the uterus has been interpreted to cause stunted growth, mental retardation, and carcinogenic effects [20].

18.3
Evaluation of Dose for Radiation Protection

18.3.1
Inadequacy of Dose as an Index of Harm

In radiation protection, we try to keep within limits the harm that can result from radiation exposure. Operationally, all radiation work should be carried out in such a way that the radiation exposure to the staff and to the general public is well below recommended safe limits. For evaluation of the degree of safety and for checking of compliance with regulations, such recommendations on safe limits of exposure should be stated as numerical limits of an evaluable quantity. This quantity needs to be evaluated in such a way that it would act as a measure of the radiation risk [21]. Hence, it should allow for as many factors that influence the radiation harm as can be identified and accounted for.

Although a numerical assessment of the radiation dose (which is the radiation energy absorbed per unit mass) is the first major step for evaluating the damage, it is not sufficient by itself to serve as an index of harm for radiation protection purposes. For example, it is known that the risk varies for different types of radiation at the same dose. Furthermore, the risk differs depending upon whether the whole body, a part of the body, or only an individual organ is irradiated. The stochastic risk and the radiosensitivity of the different body organs differ also. Thus, it is necessary to derive an index that can be correlated with the harm that can result to an individual or population from a radiation dose. Equivalent dose and effective dose are such indices, that have been defined by the ICRP [3], the NCRP [4, 5], and the ICRU [22]. The dose-limiting recommendations for safe use of ionizing radiation are stated in terms of these indices.

18.3.2
Microscopic Energy Deposition

It is known from biological experiments that different types of radiations (such as gamma rays, neutrons, and alpha particles) produce different degrees of biological damage for an identical dose [23]. Thus, for radiation protection purposes, it is necessary to give some consideration or weight to the kind of radiation to which a person is exposed, in addition to the radiation dose. In Chapter 11, we defined the radiation dose as the energy absorbed per unit mass of the substance irradiated. Dose is a macroscopic quantity and averages the energy absorbed over a mass consisting of an aggregate of cells. If the mass is subdivided into its component microscopic cells and the energy absorbed in the individual cells is observed, then, because of statistical variations, there will be differences in the energy absorbed by individual cells. It might happen that, among three adjacent cells, one is traversed by one ionizing particle, the second is spared altogether, and the third is traversed by two particles. Accordingly, the three cells might suffer damage of different degrees, such as undergoing partial damage, no damage, or irreversible damage.

The pattern of microscopic energy deposition varies for different types of radiation, such as X-rays, alpha particles, or neutrons. Therefore, equal doses of different radiations can produce unequal degrees of biological damage. The physical parameter of linear energy transfer (LET), discussed in Chapter 6, influences the effectiveness of different radiations for the same radiation dose delivered. As a charged particle traverses a medium, it leaves a trail of ions along its own track and along the tracks of the secondary electrons that it sets in motion. The linear density of ionization (i. e., the number of ions per unit path length) is a function of the LET. In Chapter 6 (Figures 6.8a and b), we illustrated schematically the trails of ions along low- and high-LET tracks, respectively.

In Figures 18.1a and b, we show a macroscopic square-shaped area irradiated by low-LET and high-LET radiations, respectively. The total number of ionizing events in the two squares is the same, although the ionization densities along the tracks are different. Three cells, numbered 1, 2, and 3, have been identified. If, say, a minimum of two

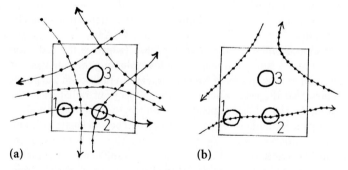

(a)   (b)

Fig. 18.1. A square volume of tissue with three distinct cells (identified as 1, 2, and 3) is traversed by ionizing tracks. Dots along tracks represent ionizing events. (a) Irradiation by six low-LET tracks, (b) irradiation by three high-LET tracks having twice the linear ionization density of those in (a). The total number of ionizing events within the square is the same in (a) and (b)

ionizing events within a cell is needed to cause permanent damage to its functioning, only cell 2 is killed with low LET in Figure 18.1a. However, both cells 1 and 2 are killed in Figure 18.1b for high LET. Thus, the probability of permanent damage increases with LET.

18.3.3
Relative Biological Effectiveness (RBE)

The relative biological effectiveness (RBE) is defined to serve as a measure of the biological effectiveness of any test radiation with respect to a reference radiation. If a dose D_g, given with a chosen type of radiation, produces a particular biological effect, and the same biological effect is produced by dose D_{ref} of a reference radiation, the RBE of the chosen radiation is given by the ratio

$$RBE = (D_{ref}/D_g) \qquad (18-1)$$

The reference radiation traditionally has been chosen as low-energy X-rays.

It will be noticed that no particular biological effect or endpoint is specified in the above definition of RBE. Because of this, it turns out that RBE is not a unique value for any given radiation. For example, the ratio may differ for skin erythema and for soft-tissue necrosis. It can also depend on the biological system chosen. Cells irradiated *in vitro* show a sensitivity different from that of cells *in vivo*. There are many other variables, such as dose rate, fractionation, temperature, oxygenation, spatial dose distribution, and volume of the sample, on which the RBE can depend. Table 18.1 gives the observed RBE values at minimal doses (denoted by RBE_M based on Table 4.1 of Reference 3) for fission neutrons and different biological endpoints. The lack of uniqueness of the RBE disqualifies it from serving as a ratio that can be applied to the dose as a weighting factor for different radiations for radiation protection purposes.

Table 18.1. Summary of RBE_M Values for Fission Neutrons vs. Gamma Rays[a]

Biological Endpoint	Range of Values of RBE_M
Chromosome aberrations, human lymphocytes in culture	34–53
Oncogenic transformation	3–80
Specific locus mutations in mice	5–70
Mutation endpoints in plant systems	–100
Life shortening in mice	10–46
Tumor induction in mice	16–59

[a] RBE_M is the limiting value of the relative biological effectiveness (RBE) at minimal dose levels. Table adapted from NCRP REPORT 116, 1993 [3].

18.3.4
Quality Factor and Dose Equivalent

In another approach to allowing for variations in the biological impact of different radiations for the same dose, the ICRU [24] defined the concepts of quality factor (denoted by Q) and dose equivalent (designated by H). The quality factor Q is a dimensionless weighting factor that is related to the physical parameter LET. This is unlike the RBE, which has a reference to a biological endpoint in its definition. The dose equivalent H is the dose delivered, D, times the quality factor, Q, recommended for the radiation; i. e.,

$$H = D \cdot Q \tag{18-2}$$

For distinguishing the dose equivalent from the dose, the dose equivalent is expressed in units of rem (an acronym for roentgen equivalent man) when the dose D is in rad. When D is expressed in Gy, the dose equivalent will be in sieverts (Sv).

Although Q is not related to any particular biological endpoint, the purpose in its use was to make it applicable to carcinogenic and mutagenic effects from the radiation protection point of view. Special consideration has been given to chromosome aberrations in human lymphocytes.

The values assigned to Q have undergone several revisions. Values of Q as a function of energy are given in the 1986 ICRU report for photons, neutrons, and alpha particles. The Q values for neutrons are known to change rapidly with neutron energy. Table 18.2 presents the quality factors as a function of LET as accepted by the NCRP [3] and ICRP [4].

Table 18.2. Quality Factor-LET Relationships

LET_∞ in Water (keV μm^{-1})	Q $(LET_\infty)^a$
<10	1
10 to 100	$0.32\,LET_\infty - 2.2$
>100	$300\,(LET_\infty) - 0.5$

^{a} Q should be rounded off to the nearest whole number and LET_∞ expressed in keV μm^{-1}.

Table adapted from NCRP Report 116, 1993 [3].

In general, a total dose D may be delivered with the LET spread over a spectrum of values. Let L denote the linear energy transfer (LET) (described in Volume 1, Chapter 6, Section 6.3.5). If D(L)dL is the dose in an LET interval L to (L + dL) and Q(L) is the corresponding quality factor, the effective quality factor $\bar{Q}$ can be evaluated by

$$\bar{Q} = \frac{1}{D} \int_0^\infty Q(L)D(L)\,dL \tag{18-3}$$

18.3.5
Weighting Factors for Different Radiations

The wide range of the observed RBE values at low doses prompted the question whether the detail and precision implied in the formal relationship of Q to LET can be valid for radiation protection purposes. The ICRP considered this issue in 1991 and suggested the use of a radiation weighting factor, W_R, rather than the quality factor $\bar{Q}$ to account for the biological effectiveness of different radiations at the same dose. Table 18.3 gives the radiation weighting factors as adapted by the NCRP (which closely follows the

Table 18.3. Radiation Weighting Factors, W_R

Type and Energy	W_R
X- and gamma rays, electrons,[a] positrons, muons	1
Neutrons, energy $<10\,\text{keV}$	5
$>10–100\,\text{keV}$	10
$>100\,\text{keV}^{-2}\,\text{MeV}$	20
$>2–20\,\text{MeV}$	10
$>20\,\text{MeV}$	5
Protons other than recoil protons, energy $>2\,\text{MeV}$	2[b]
Alpha particles, fission fragments, nonrelativistic heavy nuclei	20

Note: All values apply to radiation incident on the body or, if internal sources, emitted from the source.

[a] Excluding Auger electrons emitted from nuclei bound to DNA.

[b] For body irradiated by protons of >100 MeV energy, W_R of unity applies.

Adapted from NCRP Report 116, 1993 [3].

values recommended by the ICRP) for different radiations. The basis for these values is the observed RBE at low doses for biological endpoints of concern for radiation protection. For radiation types not included in Table 18.3, the ICRP and NCRP suggest that the value of W_R can be the same as the value of $\bar{Q}$ calculated from expression (18-3). It may be noted that the value of W_R to be applied for any neutron irradiation does significantly depend on the neutron energy spectrum [25].

18.3.6
Equivalent Dose

If a tissue or organ, T, receives an average dose, $D_{T,R}$, due to radiation, R, having a recommended weighting factor W_R, the equivalent dose, $H_{T,R}$, is evaluated by multiplication of $D_{T,R}$ by W_R. That is,

$$H_{T,R} = D_{T,R} \cdot W_R \qquad (18\text{-}4)$$

Equivalent dose and dose equivalent have different connotations. Dose equivalent is based on the absorbed dose at a *point* in tissue weighted by the quality factor Q, which, in turn, is related to the LET distribution at that point. Equivalent dose, on the other hand, uses not the point dose, but the average absorbed dose in the organ and weights it by the radiation weighting factor W_R.

If an organ T is irradiated by several types of radiation, the average organ dose, $D_{T,R}$, due to each radiation type R should first be evaluated. Then these averages should be multiplied by the respective radiation weighting factors, W_R, which will yield the equivalent doses, $H_{T,R}$, from each component. These equivalent doses should be summed up to give the total equivalent dose, H_T, to the organ. That is,

$$H_T = \sum_R D_{T,R} \cdot W_R \qquad (18\text{-}5)$$

The following example illustrates this.

EXAMPLE 18.1

A person receives 0.02 Gy (2 rad), 0.032 Gy (3.2 rad), and 0.015 Gy (1.5 rad) from X-rays, thermal neutrons, and alpha particles. Use the radiation weighting factors in Table 18.3 to evaluate the equivalent dose.

Radiation	Dose ($D_{T,R}$)	W_R (From Table 18.3)	Equivalent Dose $H_{T,R} = D_{T,R} \times W_R$
X-rays	0.02 Gy	1	0.02 Sv
Thermal neutrons	0.032 Gy	5	0.16 Sv
Alphas	0.015 Gy	20	0.30 Sv
Total	0.067 Gy (6.7 rad)		0.48 Sv (48 rem)

Total equivalent dose is 0.48 Sv (48 rem).

EXAMPLE 18.2

In the surroundings of a nuclear reactor, a person receives doses of 0.01 Gy from gamma radiation and 0.005 Gy from neutrons. The neutron energy is unknown. Estimate the equivalent dose in the best- and worst-case situations.

$$\text{Total equivalent dose} = \text{equivalent dose from gammas}$$
$$+ \text{equivalent dose from neutrons}$$

For the gamma component, $W_R = 1$. For the neutrons, in the best-case situation, we assume that the neutrons are all of low energy, with $W_R = 5$. Then

$$\text{Total equivalent dose} = 0.01\,\text{Gy} \times 1 + 0.005\,\text{Gy} \times 5 = 0.035\,\text{Sv}$$

In the worst-case situation, all of the neutron dose is from fast neutrons having $W_R = 20$. Then

$$\text{Total equivalent dose} = 0.01\,\text{Gy} \times 1 + 0.005\,\text{Gy} \times 20 = 0.11\,\text{Sv}$$

18.3.7
Weighting Factors for Different Body Tissues

Tissues or organs vary in their sensitivity to stochastic detriment, especially radiation-induced cancer [26, 27]. The ICRP, in 1977, considered making an allowance for this variation by using tissue weighting factors, W_T, for different organs in the body [28, 29]. Table 18.4 gives the W_T values recently adopted by the NCRP [3, 27] (as recommended by the ICRP [4, 5]) for 12 specific organs. W_T represents the proportionate detriment (stochastic) to a tissue T when the whole body is irradiated to an equivalent dose H_T. It will be noticed that the sum of W_T (for the 12 specified organs and the remainder) adds up to 1. The value of W_T specified for 'remainder' in Table 18.4 should be used in the way recommended in the footnote of the table.

18.3.8
Effective Dose

The effective dose, E, is the sum of the weighted equivalent doses for all irradiated tissues and organs. It is designed to serve as a single measure of effective detriment

Table 18.4. Tissue Weighting Factors (W_T) for Different Tissues and Organs

Organs	Bone surface Skin	Bladder Breast Liver Esophagus Thyroid Remainder[a,b]	Bone marrow Colon Lung Stomach	Gonads
W_T	0.01	0.05	0.12	0.20

[a] Remainder includes adrenals, brain, small intestine, large intestine, kidney, muscle, pancreas, spleen, thymus, and uterus as a group. It may also include any other tissues or organs selectively irradiated.

[b] If, in an exceptional case, one of the remainder tissues receives an equivalent dose greater than the highest dose to any of the 12 organs specifically identified in the table, a W_T of 0.025 is to be used for that tissue, together with a W_T of 0.025 applied to the average equivalent dose received by the other remainder tissues.

Table adapted from NCRP Report 116, 1993 [3].

and is given by

$$E = \sum_T H_T W_T = \sum_T W_T \sum_R D_{T,R} \cdot W_R \tag{18-6}$$

EXAMPLE 18.3

The film badge reading indicates that a staff member was exposed to low-energy X-rays and received a skin dose of 5.5 mGy and an average dose of 1.1 mGy to deep-seated organs. The gonads were completely shielded. Calculate the effective dose.

We tabulate the dose received, radiation weighting factor, equivalent dose, organ weighting factor, and effective dose to each individual organ, as shown below:

Organ(*)	Dose Received $D_{T,R}$ (mGy)	Radiation Weighting Factor W_R	Equivalent Dose $D_{T,R}W_R$ (mSv)	Organ(*) Weighting Factor W_T	Effective Dose $D_{T,R}W_RW_T$ (mSv)
Bone surface	1.1	1.0	1.1	0.01	0.011
Skin	5.5	1.0	5.5	0.01	0.055
Bladder	1.1	1.0	1.1	0.05	0.055
Breast	1.1	1.0	1.1	0.05	0.055
Liver	1.1	1.0	1.1	0.05	0.055
Esophagus	1.1	1.0	1.1	0.05	0.055
Thyroid	1.1	1.0	1.1	0.05	0.055
Remainder	1.1	1.0	1.1	0.05	0.055
Bone marrow	1.1	1.0	1.1	0.12	0.132
Colon	1.1	1.0	1.1	0.12	0.132
Lung	1.1	1.0	1.1	0.12	0.132
Stomach	1.1	1.0	1.1	0.12	0.132
Gonad	0.0	1.0	1.1	0.20	0.000

* As listed in Table 18.4

Total of column 5, $\Sigma W_T = 1.0$.
Total of column 6, $\Sigma D_{T,R}W_R W_T = 0.924$ mSv.

Thus, effective dose ≈ 0.92 mSv (92 mrem).

18.4
Uncertainties in Radiation Risk Assessment

18.4.1
Problem of Sample Size

In protecting radiation workers and the general public from exposures incidental to practical applications of radiation, we are concerned about the consequences of chronic low-level irradiations. To interpret the radiation risk for a human population, we need to rely on epidemiologic data on human populations exposed to radiation. The single largest group of exposed individuals from which much of our understanding has come is that of the survivors of the atomic bomb explosions in Japan. Another recent serious accident happened in 1986 at the Chernobyl nuclear power plant and exposed a population to large doses of ionizing radiation. The radiation effects on this population are also being studied [8].

The study of the effects of radiation on human populations is not easily accomplished. For a better understanding of this complex task, the reader is referred to the comprehensive reviews on this subject presented by a committee of experts [11, 12]. This section is restricted to a brief overview.

Almost all of the effects caused by radiation also occur from causes other than radiation. Basically, such a study needs two groups of people, one exposed to radiation and the other unexposed. The epidemiologic studies on the two populations should reveal an excess of defects, damage, or cancers in the irradiated compared to the unirradiated group. Thus, we are looking for 'excess effects' observable and attributable to radiation.

To distinguish the excess incidence from the normal background level of incidence in a statistically reliable manner, one needs large sample sizes. For example, let us say that about 250,000 solid cancers (excluding leukemia and bone cancers) are known to occur normally in a million persons and it is suspected that about 6,000 excess cancers of the same kind may be caused by a single exposure to 0.1 Gy (10 rad). For the comparison of the cancer incidence in an exposed group with that in an unexposed group to be statistically reliable, the exposed and unexposed groups should each consist of 60,000 people. However, it would be unethical to expose a human population only for the purpose of understanding the radiation risk.

Many radiation effects are demonstrable in animals. Animal experiments, in which large samples can be employed, are a possible option. However, experience has shown that not all radiation effects observed in animals can be proved in human subjects. Hence, epidemiologic studies have to be carried out with the limited sample sizes of already exposed human populations. It is a challenge to identify large groups of people who were incidentally exposed to radiation. Another problem is that, within a given group of people, one would need to allow for other factors such as smoking, alcoholism, sex, age, etc., that modify the effects of radiation. These further divide the existing sample size into smaller subsets. Furthermore, because low-level radiation effects occur over periods of several decades after irradiation, irradiated populations should be observed for many years.

18.4.2
Imperfect Knowledge of Radiation Dose

Because radioepidemiologic studies are retrospective studies on populations incidentally or accidentally irradiated, there is great difficulty in estimating the doses they
received. In this text, we have discussed methods for delivering a predetermined radiation dose in radiotherapy. We know that delivery of a therapeutic dose is not achieved
unless many parameters of irradiation are known exactly and a system for dose calculation together with appropriate data tables is established. If the dose determination
can be so difficult to achieve in a situation where controlled delivery of radiation is
the intent, it becomes a challenging task to calculate the dose received in a situation
where delivery of dose was not the intent, but was incidental. For example, the doses
received by the survivors of the atomic bomb explosions in Japan have been revised
and reassessed on an ongoing basis [30–34]. Accordingly, the risk estimates have also
changed.

18.4.3
Dose-Response Projection

The radiation hazard with which we are most concerned in setting radiation safety
limits for radiation workers is radiation-induced cancer, although genetic effects are
not to be ignored. Radioepidemiologic studies have detected excess cancers in various
groups of exposed populations.

One of the major questions confronted during the estimation of radiation risk
is, how can one extrapolate the excess cancer incidence observed in a population
exposed acutely to high doses and infer the possible rate of cancer induction at the
low levels of exposure that are encountered in occupational situations? That is, what
is the mathematical function that can relate the cancer incidence rate to the dose D?
Mathematically, this function can have the general form

$$F(D) = (\alpha_0 + \alpha_1 D + \alpha_1 D^2) \exp(-\beta_1 D - \beta_2 D^2) \qquad (18\text{-}7)$$

where $\alpha_0, \alpha_1, \alpha_2, \beta_1$, and β_2 are empirical parameters. The above expression is referred
to as a linear-quadratic model with cell killing and has the graphic form of curve
1 shown in Figure 18.2. At very high doses, the curve shows a reduction in cancer
incidence. This is attributable to the exponential term which indicates that cells, when
given high radiation doses, lose the capacity to become cancerous. Two simplified
versions of the above general expression are the linear quadratic model and the linear
model, which have the following forms:

$$F(D) = \alpha D + \beta D^2 \qquad (18\text{-}8)$$

and

$$F(D) = \alpha D \qquad (18\text{-}9)$$

The latter model gives higher risks at low doses compared to the former when the
effects observed at high doses are extrapolated to low doses, as is shown graphically
by curves 2 and 3 in Figure 18.2.

Fig. 18.2. Models of dose vs. cancer incidence. Curve 1: linear quadratic model with cell killing; curve 2: linear quadratic model; curve 3: linear model

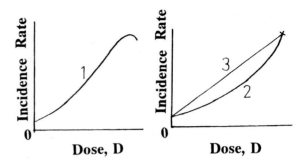

18.4.4
Lifetime Risk Projection

Cancer incidence rates vary with the age of the exposed population. The delivery of a radiation dose can cause an excess risk of cancer as a complex function of age at exposure and time after exposure. The radioepidemiologic analysis can be based on two different models of projecting the risk over the lifetime of an exposed population [11, 14]. These are absolute-risk and relative-risk models, as illustrated in Figure 18.3, in which curve 1 represents the normal rate of cancer incidence for a given population as a function of age. When a radiation dose, D, is received by the population at age t_X, the cancer incidence changes to curve 2 or 3 depending on the model of lifetime risk projection employed. Curve 2 applies for the absolute-risk model (also called additive-risk projection model). Curve 3 applies for the relative-risk model (also called multiplicative-risk projection model). Both curves show no observable number of excess cancers above the normal level for a latency period of ℓ years after age t_X. After that, curve 2 shows an excess risk that seems like an addition, [say, $F_A(D)$], over the normal risk (curve 1). The excess risk shown by curve 3 appears as a multiplier [say, $F_R(D)$] of the normal risk (curve 1).

Fig. 18.3. Projection of cancer incidence rate for an irradiated population. Curve 1 applies to a normal, unexposed population. Curves 2 and 3 represent absolute-risk and relative-risk models of lifetime risk projection, respectively. The radiation dose is received at age t_X, and ℓ is the latency period for cancer induction after irradiation

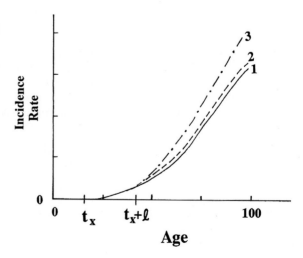

In a given population, there is a baseline rate of cancer incidence, $\lambda_0(t)$, at age t. In general, a radiation exposure to dose D(t) at age t may change the cancer incidence rate to $\lambda[T, D(t)]$ at an observation age T. Then, in the two models, the expressions for $\lambda[T, D(t)]$ are

$$\text{Absolute risk:}\quad \lambda[T, D(t)] = \lambda_0(t) + F_A[D(t)] \qquad (18\text{-}10)$$

$$\text{Relative risk:}\quad \lambda[T, D(t)] = \lambda_0(t)F_R[D(t)] \qquad (18\text{-}11)$$

For protracted exposures occurring over a lifetime, we can assume, in a simple model, that each increment of exposure contributes independently to the excess cancer rate. Then the excess cancer rate, $\Delta\lambda[T, D]$, that can represent the total lifetime risk when a radiation dose D(t) is received at age t is

$$\Delta\lambda[T, D] = \int_0^T \{\lambda[T, D(t)] - \lambda_0(t)\}\, dt \qquad (18\text{-}12)$$

In the absolute-risk hypothesis, the excess risk attributed to dose D is independent of the existing normal cancer risk. All populations, irrespective of their age, ethnic origin, or nationality, are assumed to have the same excess risk from dose D. However, in the relative-risk model, the excess cancers will be more numerous in the population that has a higher rate of normal cancer incidence, because the radiation dose plays the role of a catalyst that aggravates the already existing risk. For the relative-risk model, the expression for $\Delta\lambda[T, D]$ becomes

$$\Delta\lambda[T, D] = \int_0^T \{F_R[D(t)] - 1\}\,\lambda_0(t)\, dt \qquad (18\text{-}13)$$

To interpret the total risk to an actual living population for a given radiation exposure, one can employ standard life table techniques by using the mortality and cancer incidence data applicable to that population [35]. The fate of a population of a million newborn infants may be followed over a period of 100 years. For persons exposed to radiation at different ages, the probability of radiation-induced cancer at various time intervals can be evaluated after allowance is made for a latency period for cancer induction subsequent to the irradiation.

Our understanding of the subject of lifetime carcinogenic risk is gradually progressing. At this time, it seems that the absolute-risk model may apply to the incidence of leukemia and the relative-risk hypothesis to the induction of solid cancers.

18.4.5
Dose and Dose Rate Effectiveness Factor (DDREF)

The doses and dose rates at which persons are exposed incidental to the use of ionizing radiations are much lower than the high dose rates at which the populations used in epidemiologic studies were exposed. Hence, the risk factors evaluated in epidemiologic studies should be lowered by a dose and dose rate effectiveness factor (DDREF). (As an analogue, the damage caused by throwing of a heavy bowling ball cannot be matched by throws of hundreds of ping pong balls one at a time, even if all of their masses together equal the heavy mass of the bowling ball.) Based on experimental information and information on human subjects, the ICRP and the NCRP have adopted a DDREF of 2.0 in their recent reports [2, 3].

18.4.6
Assessed Radiation Risk

For radiation protection purposes, the ICRP estimated total detriment by adding to the risk of fatal cancer the risks of nonfatal cancers and severe genetic effects. The nominal values of the risk factors (as assessed by the ICRP and adopted by the NCRP) are given in Table 18.5 for an adult working population and a population of all ages, including children. The W_T values in Table 18.4 are based on the relative contributions of different body parts to the total detriment.

Table 18.5. Nominal Probability Coefficients for Stochastic Effects

Exposed Population	Detriment (10^{-2} Sv^{-1})			
	Fatal Cancers	Nonfatal Cancers	Severe Genetic Effects	Total Detriment
Adult workers	4.0	0.8	0.8	5.6
Whole population	5.0	1.0	1.3	7.3

Table adapted from NCRP Report 116 (1993) [3].

18.5
Radiation Safety Philosophy

18.5.1
Natural Background Radiation

In the development of a radiation protection philosophy for safe use of ionizing radiation, it is appropriate to keep in mind the fact that the manmade radiation sources used in radiologic applications are not the only cause of radiation exposure of the population. We do not live in a radiation-free world. A natural radiation background exists [36] and contributes to the equivalent doses listed in Table 18.6. This background consists in part of radiation coming from radioactive materials that are naturally present in the earth and in commonly used building materials. Such terrestrial emission depends

Table 18.6. Background Radiation Dose (Received by Body Soft Tissues)

Component	Total Dose Equivalent[a] Rate (mSv/year)
Cosmic rays	0.27
Cosmogenic	0.01
Terrestrial	0.28
Human body	0.35
Total	0.91

[a] Average values for U.S. population [36].

on the constituents of the terrain and varies from place to place. To this is added the radiation from outer space, called cosmic rays. The intensity of cosmic radiation is observed to vary with altitude and latitude. Cosmic ray-produced radionuclides (mainly ^{3}H, ^{14}C, ^{7}Be, and ^{22}Na) contribute the cosmogenic component in Table 18.6. In addition to the terrestrial and cosmic radiations, the human body contains radioactive atoms assimilated by ingestion and inhalation. A long-lived naturally occurring radionuclide, ^{40}K, is also a significant contributor. A small radiation component is added by the fallout from atomic weapons testing, the effluents from nuclear power plants, consumer products such as smoke detectors and watches with luminous dials that use radioactive materials, tobacco products, etc. Aircraft flying at high altitudes expose the passengers to cosmic ray intensities higher than those on the surface of the earth [37, 38]. During a 12-hour transcontinental flight from Tokyo to New York at a 12 km altitude, passengers can receive a dose equivalent of 70 μSv (7 mrem) to the whole body [37].

18.5.2
Medical Exposures

Medical exposures are exposures of patients for medical diagnosis or therapy. The medical procedures are carried out only when a physician prescribes them with the intention of providing a medical benefit to the exposed individual. Under such conditions, it is considered that the benefit from the radiation outweighs any risk. However, accumulation of medical exposures can gradually add to the genetic risk and stochastic risk to the population as a whole. Especially in order to control the genetic risk to progeny, all diagnostic medical procedures should be done in such a manner that the patient exposures remain optimally low without compromising the diagnostic reliability. All technologic advances should be applied for the purpose of reducing the exposure to patients and staff. Instances of procedures involving repeat radiation exposure (after a missed diagnosis) should be minimized.

18.5.3
Risk vs. Benefit Philosophy

The NCRP and ICRP provide recommendations on dose limits. For a more complete study of the subject, readers are referred to the original references [3–5] from which the safe exposure limits presented here were obtained.

As a matter of basic principle, no intentional exposure to radiation should occur unless there are benefits to be accrued either to an individual or to society. Any activity involving radiation should be planned and conducted in such a way that the exposures to individuals are optimally low, taking into consideration the economic and cost aspects [39–41]. This principle of optimization is called ALARA, as mentioned in the introduction to this chapter.

The aims in radiation protection are (i) to avoid the occurrence of deterministic effects and (ii) to limit the risk of stochastic effects. The control of deterministic effects is relatively straightforward; it should merely be ensured that, during the lifetime of an individual, the threshold doses above which these effects are known to occur are not exceeded. However, setting guidelines for the safe use of radiation to control the stochastic effects is not as straightforward. Derivation of the dose limits for restricting the stochastic detriment should be based on the perception of society regarding what can be considered an acceptable risk. A first step can be to look at the risks other than radiation which currently exist in society and which society perceives as acceptable.

In the implementation of a radiation safety program, the exposed populations are viewed as belonging to two distinct groups, radiation workers and the general public. The former are persons who are gainfully employed in an occupation that is related to a radiation application. The latter are those who themselves are not radiation workers, but who may work near or may visit a locale where radiation work is carried out. Whereas, for the former, working with radiation helps them to have an income and earn a livelihood, the latter have no such gain from radiation. Thus, it is appropriate to stipulate that the benefit-to-risk ratio for a certain level of radiation exposure is greater for the radiation workers than for the general public. Accordingly, the maximum exposure limits also should be set at different levels for the two groups.

The NCRP and ICRP have adopted an approach in which, first, the maximum exposure limits for radiation workers are set based on radiation risk estimates. Then the limits for the general public are set to be a fraction of those accepted for radiation workers.

Any occupation can have some associated risk. Let us say that the incidence of a radiation-induced cancer in a radiation worker is comparable to the occurrence of a fatal accident in any conventional industry. It is reasonable to stipulate that the chance for a radiation-induced cancer in a radiation worker should not be greater than that for a fatal incident to occur in (what NCRP refers to as) safe industries.

Although making such comparisons with other industries can place the acceptability of radiation risk in an overall perspective, there can be many areas of uncertainty. For example, in addition to fatal accidents, the other industries have incidents of non-fatal injuries with substantial morbidity. However, with the passage of time, initiation of safer practices in other industries can result in improved safety. In the same way, the detection and treatment of cancer are improving. It is also important to mention that cancer (whether caused by radiation or otherwise) apparently tends to be a disease of old age, whereas accidental death in industry has no such age bias. Consequently, the average number of livable years lost due to cancer and that due to an industrial accident are different at the ages of about 15 years and 40 years, respectively. Overall, a combination of observed effects and judgment needs to be employed for recommending the maximum limits of exposure acceptable for radiation workers.

18.6
Safety of Radiation Workers

18.6.1
Limits for Adult Workers

The current annual maximum dose limits for radiation workers are based on comparison of the fatal accident risk in safe industries with the assumed risk of radiation-induced fatal cancers, a fraction of the nonfatal cancers, and severe genetic effects. The annual rate of accidental deaths in industries is about 0.2 to 5 per year per 10,000 workers [21, 42]. Accordingly, in a worst-case situation, the total lifetime risk for an individual who works for 50 years in an unsafe industry is

$$(5/\text{year}) \times (50\,\text{years})(1/10,000) = 2.5 \times 10^{-2}$$

The dose limits to a radiation worker should be set such that the risk assessed for a radiation worker in a worst-case situation of his or her being exposed at the maximum suggested limit, year after year, throughout a working career, is nearly the same as the above number.

Radiation protection recommendations are intended for controlling both the annual risk and the cumulative risk to radiation workers. The NCRP and ICRP recommend that the occupational effective dose be limited to 50 mSv per year. The NCRP recommends that the accumulated effective dose not exceed the numerical limit given by 10 mSv multiplied by the individual's age, which implies a rate of 10 mSv per year. (The ICRP recommends a cumulative effective dose limit of 100 mSv in 5 years, which implies a rate of 20 mSv per year.) These limits apply to adult workers above the age of 18 years and are not intended to include exposures either for medical reasons or from natural background.

Many industries considered to be safe and not using radiation have fatal accident rates of one in 10,000 persons or less. Hence, it is only appropriate that industries which make use of radiation use it in such a way that the actual levels of exposures to individual workers stay well below the suggested maximum limits. The NCRP recommends that all new radiation facilities and practices be designed to limit the annual equivalent doses to individuals to a fraction of 10 mSv per year, so that the 5-year cumulative dose will also be well below the 50 mSv limit.

To control the deterministic effects, the NCRP observes that recommendations are required only for the crystalline lens of the eye, for the skin, and for the hands and feet. These limits (which are identical to the ICRP limits) for radiation workers are

Lens of the eye, 150 mSv/year

Skin, hands, and feet, 500 mSv/year

These limits recommended for stochastic risk are deemed to be adequate also for avoiding all possible deterministic effects. Table 18.7A summarizes the radiation safety limits for occupationally exposed populations.

Table 18.7A. Recommended Upper Limits of Exposure for Radiation Protection of Radiation Workers

Reference	Based on Stochastic Effects[a]	Based on Deterministic Effects[b]	Embryo-fetus[b]
NCRP-116 [3]	50 mSv annually and 10 mSv × age in years cumulative	150 mSv annually to lens of the eye and 500 mSv annually to skin, hands, and feet	0.5 mSv per month once pregnancy is known
ICRP-60 [4, 5]	50 mSv annually and 100 mSv in 5 years cumulative	150 mSv annually to lens of the eye and 500 mSv annually to skin, hands, and feet	2 mSv to woman's abdomen once pregnancy is known

[a] Stated in terms of effective dose.
[b] Stated in terms of equivalent dose.

18.6.2
Limits for Embryo or Fetus

For pregnant radiation workers, the NCRP recommends a monthly equivalent dose limit of 0.5 mSv to the embryo or fetus (excluding medical and natural background radiation) once the pregnancy is known.

18.6.3
Limits for Workers Under Age 18

Persons under the age of 18 years may occasionally be exposed to radiation during their education or training. In such situations, their work should be carried out with a high assurance of safety so that the following limits are met (excluding medical and natural background exposures):

> Annual (whole-body) effective dose, 1 mSv/year
>
> Lens of the eye, 15 mSv
>
> Skin, hands, and feet, 50 mSv.

18.6.4
Personnel Monitoring

All personnel who are occupationally exposed to radiation should wear a radiation monitoring device for measurement of the radiation exposures which they receive. The monitor should be worn continuously and evaluated at regular intervals. The measuring device should be of an appropriate type to be sensitive to the type of radiation to which the personnel are exposed and should cover the anticipated range of exposures. Photographic films, thermoluminescent dosimeters (TLDs), optically stimulated luminescent (OSL) dosimeters, and pocket condenser ionization chambers are common detectors used for personnel monitoring purposes (see Chapter 12). Film badges provide a permanent record of the exposure, but are less accurate than are thermoluminescent dosimeters. Pocket ionization chambers can give instant information on the exposure received and can offer an advantage when an immediate reading is necessary. The main measuring device is worn on the chest and is called a chest badge. It is meant to give an indication of the body dose. In addition, wrist badges and finger badges can be used during procedures (such as handling of sealed sources in brachytherapy) that can cause a high exposure to the wrist or finger. It is quite common to incorporate plastic, copper, or lead filters in the personnel dosimeters. Thus, multiple readings can be obtained under these filters. The material and thickness of filters can be chosen appropriately to provide discrimination of the dose contributions from penetrating X-rays and non-penetrating beta rays. Personnel monitoring is done with the purpose of ensuring that all operations are done to maintain ALARA. The radiation safety officer (RSO) of the institution is the person entrusted with the responsibilty of overseeing radiation safety on an ongoing basis. The RSO reports to the Radiation Safety Committee (RSC) of the institution. The RSC may typically be composed of radiation physicists, safety specialists, administrators, and representatives from different departments that use radiation. The RSO reviews the personnel exposures periodically to report to the

RSC on the status of safety. Any instance of high exposure to personnel can prompt the RSO and the RSC to discuss or investigate the case. This may result in the initiation of remedial steps either to improve the situation or to avoid a recurrence in the future. The details of the personnel monitoring program in an institution, such as the types of badges to be worn, the sites of monitoring, the frequency of evaluation of personnel exposure, and the levels of exposures that can be considered as acceptable ALARA, are all policy decisions to be made by the RSO and RSC based on the guidelines recommended by the NCRP and ICRP.

18.7
Safety of the General Public

For the protection of nonoccupationally exposed individuals and members of the public against stochastic effects in contexts of continuous (or frequent) radiation exposure, an annual effective dose of 1 mSv is recommended by the NCRP and also by the ICRP. This is 10% of the limit recommended for occupationally exposed persons. In addition, for situations that involve infrequent annual exposures, the NCRP suggests that a higher limit of 5 mSv may be observed, provided that such exposures are suffered only by 'a small group of people' and also not repeatedly by any one particular group. (The ICRP allows the annual limit of 1 mSv to be exceeded, if necessary, provided the average over 5 years does not exceed 1 mSv.)

Based on deterministic effects, the NCRP recommends an annual equivalent dose limit of 50 mSv to the lens of the eye, the skin, and the extremities, whereas the ICRP recommends an annual limit of 15 mSv for the lens of the eye and 50 mSv for skin and extremities. Table 18.7B summarizes the radiation safety limits for the nonoccupational population and the general public.

Table 18.7B. Recommended Upper Limits of Exposure for Radiation Protection of General Public

Reference	Based on Stochastic Effects[a]	Based on Deterministic Effects[b]
NCRP-116 [3]	1 mSv annually for continuous exposure and 5 mSv annually for infrequent exposure, cumulative	50 mSv annually to lens of eye, skin, and extremities
ICRP-60 [4, 5]	1 mSv annually and, if needed, higher values, provided that the annual average over 5 years does not exceed 1 mSv	15 mSv annually to lens of the eye and 50 mSv annually to skin, hands, and feet

[a] Stated in terms of effective dose.
[b] Stated in terms of equivalent dose.

References

1. ICRP, International Commission on Radiological Protection, Risks associated with ionizing radiations, Ann. ICRP, Vol 22, No. 1, Pergamon, New York, 1991.
2. ICRP, International Commission on Radiological Protection, Non-stochastic effects of radiation, ICRP Publication 41, Pergamon, Oxford, 1984.
3. NCRP, National Council on Radiation Protection and Measurements, Limitations of exposure to ionizing radiation, NCRP Report 116, National Council on Radiation Protection and Measurements, Bethesda, Maryland, 1993.
4. ICRP, International Commission on Radiological Protection, Recommendations of the ICRP, ICRP-60, Ann. ICRP, Vol 21, No. 1–3, Pergamon, Oxford, 1991.
5. ICRP, International Commission on Radiological Protection, Recommendations of the International Commission on Radiological Protection: User's Edition, Pergamon, Oxford, 1992.
6. IAEA, International Atomic Energy Agency, International Basic Safety Standards for Protection against Ionizing Radiation (Ed: IAEA Staff), International Atomic Energy Agency, Vienna, Austria, 1996.
7. European Atomic Energy Community, Radiation Protection 93: Standing Conference on Health and Safety in the Nuclear Age: Proceedings of the third meeting informing the public on European Safety Standards, Luxembourg, Nov 26–27, 1996 (Ed: European Commission Staff), The European Union's Publisher, 1997.
8. UNSCEAR, United Nations Scientific Committee on the Effects of Atomic Radiation, Sources, Effects, and Risks of Ionising Radiation, 2000 Report to the U.N. General Assembly, Vol.1. Sources, and Vol.2. Effects, United Nations Publications, New York, 2001.
9. UNSCEAR, United Nations Scientific Committee on the Effects of Atomic Radiation, Sources, Effects, and Risks of Ionising Radiation, 2001 Report to the U.N. General Assembly, Heriditary Effects of Radiation, United Nations Publications, New York, 2001.
10. Thompson, D., Mabuchi, K., Ron, E. et al., Solid Tumor Incidence in Atomic Bomb Survivors, 1958–87, RERF Technical Report 5-92, Radiation Effects Research Foundation, Hiroshima, Japan, 1992.
11. NRC, National Research Council, Committee on Biological Effects of Ionizing Radiation, BEIR V, Health effects of exposure to low levels of ionizing radiations, National Academy Press, Washington, D.C., 1990.
12. UNSCEAR, United Nations Scientific Committee on the Effects of Atomic Radiation, Sources, Effects, and Risks of Ionising Radiation, Report to the U.N. General Assembly, with annexes, United Nations Publications, New York, 1988.
13. UNSCEAR, United Nations Scientific Committee on the Effects of Atomic Radiation, Genetic and Somatic Effects of Ionising Radiation, Report to the U.N. General Assembly, with annexes, United Nations Publications, New York, 1986.
14. NRC, National Research Council, Committee on Biological Effects of Ionizing Radiation, BEIR III, The effects on population exposure to low levels of ionizing radiations, National Academy Press, Washington, D.C., 1980.
15. UNSCEAR, United Nations Scientific Committee on the Effects of Atomic Radiation, Sources, Effects of Ionising Radiation, Report to the U.N. General Assembly, with annexes, United Nations Publications, New York, 1977.
16. European Atomic Energy Community, Radiation Protection 125, Low Dose Ionizing Radiation and Cancer Risk, Proceedings of a scientific seminar held in Luxembourg, 9 November 2000, The European Union's Publisher, Luxembourg, 2001.
17. Kocher, D.C., Perspective on the historical development of radiation standards, Health Phys., Vol 61, p519–527, 1991.
18. Lushbaugh, C.C., Reflections on some recent progress in human radiobiology, p277-314, in Advances in Radiation Biology, Augenstein, L.G., Mason, R., and Zelle, M. (Eds.), Academic Press, New York, 1969.
19. Mole, R.H., Consequence of pre-natal radiation exposure for post-natal development: A review, Int. J. Radiat. Biol., Vol 42, p1–12, 1982.
20. Neal, J.V., Update on the genetic effects of ionizing radiation (Commentary), JAMA, Vol 266, p698-701, 1991.
21. ICRP, International Commission on Radiological Protection, Quantitative bases for developing a unified index of harm, ICRP Publication 45, Ann. ICRP, Vol 20 (1), 1985, Pergamon, Elmsford, New York.
22. ICRU, International Commission on Radiological Units and Measurements, Quantities and Units in Radiation Protection Dosimetry, ICRU Report 51, International Commission on Radiological Units and Measurements, Bethesda, Maryland, 1993.

23. NCRP, National Council on Radiation Protection and Measurements, Relative biological effectiveness of radiations of different quality, NCRP Report 104, National Council on Radiation Protection and Measurements, Bethesda, Maryland, 1990.
24. ICRU, International Commission on Radiological Units and Measurements, The quality factor in radiation protection, ICRU Report 40, International Commission on Radiological Units and Measurements, Bethesda, Maryland, 1986.
25. ICRU, Report 66, Determination of Operational Dose Equivalent Quantities for Neutrons (Ed: Inokuti, M.), Journal of the ICRU Vol. 1, No. 3, 2001.
26. Land, C.E., and Sinclair, W.K., The relative contribution of different organ sites to the total cancer mortality associated with low dose radiation exposure, p31–57, in Risks Associated with Ionizing Radiations, Ann. ICRP, Vol 22 (1), 1991.
27. NCRP, National Council on Radiation Protection and Measurements, Evaluation of risk estimates for radiation protection purposes, NCRP Report 115, National Council on Radiation Protection and Measurements, Bethesda, Maryland, 1993.
28. ICRP, International Commission on Radiological Protection, Recommendations of the ICRP, ICRP Publication 26, Ann. ICRP, Vol 1, No.3, 1977, Pergamon, Oxford.
29. McCollough, C.H., Schueler, B.A., Calculation of effective dose, Med. Phys., Vol. 27, pp828–837, 2000.
30. Auxier, J.A., Ichiban, Technical Information Center, Energy Research and Development Administration, TID-27080, National Technical Information Service, U.S. Dept. of Commerce, Springfield, VA, 1977.
31. Milton, R., and Shohoji, T., Tentative 1965 radiation dose estimation for atomic bomb survivors, Hiroshima and Nagasaki, 1968, ABCC TR 1–68, Hiroshima, Japan, 1968.
32. NRC, National Research Council, An assessment of the new dosimetry for A-bomb survivors, Panel on the reassessment of A-bomb dosimetry, Ellett, W.H. (Ed.), National Academy Press, Washington, D.C., 1987.
33. RERF, Radiation Effects Research Foundation, U.S.-Japan Joint Reassessment of Atomic Bomb Radiation Dosimetry in Hiroshima and Nagasaki – Final Report, Vol 1, Radiation Effects Research Foundation, Hiroshima, Japan, 1987.
34. RERF, Radiation Effects Research Foundation, U.S.-Japan Joint Reassessment of Atomic Bomb Radiation Dosimetry in Hiroshima and Nagasaki – Final Report, Vol 2, Radiation Effects Research Foundation, Hiroshima, Japan, 1988.
35. Bunger, B.M., Cook, J.R., and Barrick, M.K., Life table methodology for evaluating radiation risk: An application based on occupational exposures, Health Phys., Vol 40, p439–455, 1971.
36. NCRP, National Council on Radiation Protection and Measurements, Exposure to population in the US and Canada from natural background radiation, NCRP Report 94, Table 9.3, p142, National Council on Radiation Protection and Measurements, Bethesda, Maryland, 1987.
37. Friedberg, W., Copeland, K., Duke, F., O'Brien, K.O., and Darden, Jr., E.B., Radiation Exposure during air travel: Guidance provided by the Federal Aviation Administration for air carrier crews, Health Phys., Vol. 79, pp591–595, 2000.
38. Barish, R.J., Health physics concerns in commercial aviation, Health Phys., Vol 59, p199–204, 1990.
39. ICRP, International Commission on Radiation Protection, Cost benefit analysis in the optimization of radiation protection, ICRP Publication 37, Ann. ICRP, Vol 10 (2/3), 1983, Pergamon, Elmsford, New York.
40. ICRP, International Commission on Radiation Protection, Optimization and decision making in radiological protection, ICRP Publication 55, Ann. ICRP, Vol 20 (1), 1989, Pergamon, Elmsford, New York.
41. NCRP, National Council on Radiation Protection and Measurements, Implementation of the principle of as low as reasonably achievable (ALARA) for medical and dental personnel, NCRP Report 107, National Council on Radiation Protection and Measurements, Bethesda, Maryland, 1990.
42. NSC, National Safety Council, Accident facts, 1992 ed., National Safety Council, Chicago, Illinois.

Additional Reading

1. Cember, H., Introduction to Health Physics. 3rd ed., McGraw Hill, New York, USA, 1996.
2. Hall, E.J., Radiobiology for the Radiologist (5th Ed.), Lippincott, Williams and Wilkins, Philadelphia, USA, 2000.
3. Kondo, S., Health Effects of Low-level Radiation, Medical Physics Publishing, Madison, Wisconsin, USA, 1993.
4. McCollough, C.H., Schueler, B.A., Calculation of effective dose, Med. Phys., Vol. 27, pp828-837, 2000.

5. Sherer, E., Streffer, C., and Trott, K.R. (Eds.), Radiation Exposure and Occupational Risks, Springer-Verlag, Berlin, Germany, 1990.
6. UNSCEAR, United Nations Scientific Committee on the Effects of Atomic Radiation, Sources, Effects, and Risks of Ionising Radiation, 2001 Report to the U.N. General Assembly, Heriditary Effects of Radiation, United Nations Publications, New York, USA, 2001.
7. UNSCEAR, United Nations Scientific Committee on the Effects of Atomic Radiation, Sources, Effects, and Risks of Ionising Radiation, 2000 Report to the U.N. General Assembly, Vol.1., Sources, and Vol.2., Effects, United Nations Publications, New York, USA, 2001.
8. European Atomic Energy Community, Radiation Protection 125, Low Dose Ionizing Radiation and Cancer Risk, Proceedings of a scientific seminar held in Luxembourg, 9 November 2000, The European Union's Publisher, Luxembourg, 2001.

CHAPTER 19

Radiation Safety in External-Beam Therapy

19.1
Introduction

In Chapter 18, we discussed the harmful effects of radiation and the need to conduct the activities involving radiation so as to keep the radiation dose to workers and the general public within recommended limits. In this chapter, we discuss the major factors that need to be considered in the design and building of any external-beam radiation therapy facility.

The International Commission on Radiological Protection (ICRP) and the National Council on Radiation Protection and Measurements (NCRP) are recognized as authorities on the subject of radiation safety. The 1993 guidelines of the NCRP for limiting the exposure of persons (reviewed in Chapter 18) are adopted for the numerical examples in this chapter. It usually takes a few years before the recommendations of scientific bodies such as the NCRP become assimilated in the binding laws of the regional health-regulatory agencies. At the time of this writing, the 1993 NCRP recommendations had been released a few months earlier.1 There is some ongoing controversy in the scientific community as to whether the dose limits recently recommended by the NCRP and ICRP are based on hypotheses that overestimate the radiation risk and hence are too restrictive [2–5]. Although it is not our purpose in this text to discuss such controversies, it is appropriate to draw attention to the following important facts:

(a) Radiation risk assessments and recommended dose limits have changed with time [6], and they can be expected to change in the future. For example, the NCRP published a report, No. 91, entitled 'Recommendations on Limits for Exposure to Ionizing Radiation,' in 1987 [7]. In 1991, the ICRP revised its past recommendations and published new guidelines for radiation safety based on newer data and analysis [8]. In 1993, the NCRP followed, replacing its 1987 report in its entirety with a new report, No. 116, entitled 'Limitation of Exposure to Ionizing Radiation' [1].
(b) NCRP guidelines are only recommendations and are not legally binding. Although many governments may adopt the NCRP guidelines, there can be variations. Only the rules and regulations formulated by local governments carry the force of law. For purposes of safe design of any facility, the rules and regulations promulgated by the local authorities are binding. Furthermore, any emerging trends or expected changes in the future should be taken into account. Dose limits adopted by a facility should be 'as low as reasonably achievable' (ALARA) [9].

19.2
Time, Distance, and Shielding

Time, *distance*, and *shielding* are the three basic parameters that affect the radiation dose received from a radiation source. A proper mixture of the values of these three parameters is necessary if the exposure of persons involved in the uses of radiation is to be kept at acceptably low levels.

Considering *time*, the shorter the time required for a procedure, the lower will be the dose to which the worker is exposed. That is, if the other two parameters, distance and shielding, remain unchanged, the dose received by a worker will be directly proportional to the time he remains in the radiation field. Thus, it is important for the worker to carry out procedures with dispatch.

The second parameter is the *distance* between the radiation source and the worker. If the physical size of the source is small compared to this distance, the dose to the worker will be inversely proportional to the square of the distance.

The third parameter, *shielding*, refers to the interposition of an attenuating barrier between the source and the worker, with the purpose of reducing the exposure to the worker. Usually, shielding is used in situations where improvement in time and distance alone cannot provide the necessary degree of safety. Sometimes, shielding is added for the purpose of ALARA.

Safe operation of an external-beam therapy machine is possible only when it is installed in a well-shielded treatment room. Several references give detailed presentations of the shielding and design considerations for external-beam therapy facilities [10–14].

19.3
Approach to Shielding Design of a Beam-Therapy Facility

19.3.1
Selection of Acceptable Weekly Equivalent Dose Limits (P)

In order to estimate the shielding to be provided by a protective barrier, one must decide on a maximum weekly dose, P, that is acceptable to the occupants behind the barrier. From Tables 18.7A and B, we extract the following annual and cumulative radiation limits recommended by the NCRP for radiation protection purposes:

(a) A limit of 50 mSv per year for radiation workers, with a cumulative limit of 10 mSv multiplied by the age of the person in years
(b) 1 mSv annually for nonradiation workers and the general public if they are likely to be continuously exposed, and 5 mSv annually if the exposure is infrequent

NCRP Report No. 116 [1], in addition, states the following: 'The 50 mSv annual limit should be utilized only to provide flexibility required for existing facilities and practices. The NCRP recommends that all new facilities and the introduction of all new practices should be designed to limit annual exposures to individuals to a fraction of 10 mSv per year limit implied by the cumulative dose limit by occupation.'

In this chapter, based on (a) and (b) above, we use a limit of 10 mSv per year for areas occupied by radiation workers and of 1 mSv for the other areas where nonradiation workers of the staff, the public, or patients can be present. The high-radiation areas where the radiation workers function are to be controlled to allow only minimum access to nonradiation workers or the public. Such areas are referred to as controlled areas. If we use an organ weighting factor, W_T, of 1.0 (for whole-body irradiation) and a radiation weighting factor, W_R, of 1.0 (for photons), the limits stated above result in approximate P values of 200 μGy/week and 20 μGy/week for the controlled and noncontrolled areas, respectively.

19.3.2
Radiation Components

In the design of the shielding of an external-beam therapy facility, it is important, first, to recognize that (as shown in Figure 19.1) there are three major radiation components, primary photons, scattered photons, and leakage photons, against which the persons have to be protected. The primary component refers to the photons of the direct beam irradiating the patient. The scattered component consists of photons scattered from the patient and the walls of the treatment room. The leakage radiation refers to the photons from the source that emerge by penetrating the source-head shielding. In addition to these, for high-energy machines (above 10 MV), protection against photoneutrons and neutron capture gamma rays should also be taken into account [12, 15].

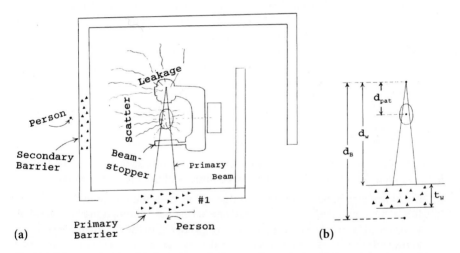

Fig. 19.1. Diagram showing (a) the primary, leakage, and scattered radiation components, primary barrier, secondary barrier, and beam stopper, and (b) the different distances involved in the shielding evaluation

19.3.3
Recommended Leakage Levels

Radiation is emitted from the target within the source head in all directions. The shielding design of the source head should take this fact into account and should be such as to limit the radiation intensity in all directions other than the direction of the useful beam. For accelerators, the leakage ceases when the beam current is turned off. For machines that use radioisotope sources, leakage radiation emerges from the source heads at all times and irradiates the staff even when the source is in the 'OFF' position.

For radiation safety purposes, allowable leakage limits have been given most recently in NCRP Report 102 [16]. For X-ray equipment, NCRP Report 102 divides the source housing assemblies into three categories based upon the energy of the X-rays. The NCRP recommends that the equipment manufacturer construct the source housing to meet the following upper limits for leakage:

(1) For X-ray production at tube potentials from 5 kV to 50 kV, the leakage kerma rate at any position 5 centimeters from the assembly shall not exceed 0.1 cGy in any one hour.
(2) For X-ray production at tube potentials greater than 50 kV and less than 500 kV, the leakage kerma rate measured at a distance of one meter from the source in any direction shall not exceed 1 cGy in any one hour. ... In addition, these assemblies shall limit the kerma rate at a distance of 5 cm from the surface of the assembly to 30 cGy in any one hour.
(3) For X-ray and electron beam equipment operated above 500 kV, the assembly shall be designed so that the following conditions are fulfilled for the regions outside the useful beam.
    (i) The absorbed dose rate due to leakage radiation. ... at any point outside the maximum sized useful beam, but within a circular plane of radius 2 m which is perpendicular to and centered on the central axis of the useful beam at the normal treatment distance, shall not exceed 0.2 percent of the absorbed dose rate to tissue on the central axis at the treatment distance.(The leakage radiation shall be measured with the useful beam blocked by an absorber capable of reducing the useful beam intensity to 0.1 percent of its normal value.)
    (ii) Except for the area defined above, the absorbed dose rate in tissue (excluding that from neutrons) at 1 m from the electron path between the source and the target or the electron window shall not exceed 0.5 percent of the absorbed dose rate in tissue on the central axis of the beam at the normal treatment distance.

For therapy source heads using gamma sealed sources such as ^{60}Co, the leakage limits are stated for both the 'off' and 'on' conditions of the source as follows:

(1) The housing shall be so constructed that at 1 m from the source in the OFF condition, the maximum and average leakage kerma rates through the housing shall not exceed 100 μGy h^{-1} and 20 μGy h^{-1}, respectively. In the design of the housing, consideration should also be given to reducing the surface kerma rate for small diameter housings to less than 2 mGy h^{-1} at 5 cm from surface. (See NCRP Report No. 102 for details as to where measurements are to be made for determining the maximum and average leakage rates.)
(2) The housing shall be so constructed that at 1 m from the source in the ON position the housing leakage kerma rate shall not exceed 0.1 percent of the useful beam kerma rate at one meter. For sources with useful beam kerma rate of less than 10 Gy h^{-1} at 1 m the housing leakage kerma rate shall not exceed 1 cGy h^{-1} at 1 m from the source in the ON position. For both cases the limits apply when the beam is completely intercepted by the collimation or an equivalent barrier. These limits do not apply to housings designed exclusively for whole body irradiations.

19.3.4
Shielding Data

Shielding calculations are meant to give an estimate of acceptable barrier transmissions. A tenth-value thickness (TVT) is the thickness of a barrier that attenuates the radiation to one tenth of its intensity, in the same manner as a half-value thickness (HVT) provides attenuation to one half. TVT and HVT are related as

$$\text{TVT} \approx 3.32\,\text{HVT}$$

A barrier thickness X that can give a barrier transmission B is related to the TVT by

$$10^{-X/\text{TVT}} = B$$

i.e.,

$$X = n(\text{TVT}), \quad \text{where } n = -\log_{10}(B)$$

The value n gives the number of TVTs needed for the barrier. For non-monoenergetic beams, the TVT and HVT can change due to the effect of beam hardening (see Chapter 8, Section 8.6.3). However, after some degree of initial hardening, a steady value called equilibrium TVT (designated TVT_e) is reached.

Scatter and leakage together are referred to as secondary radiations. Unlike the primary beam, the secondaries have no specific direction. Because the primary beam is very intense and is also highly penetrating, the barriers needed for protection against the primary beam are usually very thick. Thus, a wall that is designed to protect against the primary beam is generally also adequate to protect against the secondary radiation. If a wall is exposed only to secondary radiations, a secondary protective barrier will suffice there. By the proper choice of the orientation of the therapy equipment during installation, irradiation of high-occupancy areas by the primary beam can be avoided and the shielding cost reduced. The leaking X-radiation, which has been hardened by the heavy shielding of the source head, is of higher average energy than is the primary. The scattered radiation, on the other hand, is less penetrating than the primary radiation. The energy and penetration of the scattered radiation are a function of the angle of scatter. Here the TVT_e values for primary, scattered, and leakage radiations are designated by $(\text{TVT}_e)_P$, $(\text{TVT}_e)_S$, and $(\text{TVT}_e)_L$, respectively.

Data on the transmission of broad X-ray beams of different energies in various shielding materials have been published. The $(\text{TVT}_e)_P$ values given in Table 19.1 and the $(\text{TVT}_e)_S$ in Table 19.2 will be used for shielding evaluations in this chapter. We also assume that $(\text{TVT}_e)_L \approx (\text{TVT}_e)_P$. Concrete of density 2.35 g cm^{-3} is the most commonly used shielding material for the walls. The density of any proposed shielding material should be ascertained by measurement of a sample. The TVTs for other materials such as earth, sand, brick, or heavy concrete can be derived from the TVT for concrete by density scaling:

$$\text{TVT in material} = \text{TVT in concrete} \times \frac{\text{density of concrete}}{\text{density of material}}$$

Barite (BaSO$_4$) concrete, with a density of 3.0 to 4.5 g cm^{-3}, has been used for reducing the shielding thickness where space is limited. The primary barrier can be

Table 19.1. Tenth-Value Thickness, $(TVT_e)_P$, of Attenuation for Broad Primary Photon Beams of Different Energies and Materials

Beam	Concrete[a] (cm)	Barite[b] (cm)	Steel[c] (cm)	Lead[d] (cm)
0.25-MV X-rays	9	–	–	0.22
0.5-MV X-rays	14	–	–	–
137Cs (0.66-MeV gamma rays)	15.7	–	5.3	2.1
1.0 MV X-rays	20	–	–	3.0
60Co ($\approx$ 1.25-MeV gamma rays)	24	17	7.0	4.0
4 MV X-rays	29	20	8.5	5.3
6 MV X-rays	34	25	10	5.6
10 MV X-rays	39	29	11	5.6
20 MV X-rays	45	34	11	5.6

Note: Values compiled by the authors from references listed in the text.

[a] Density 2.35 g cm^{-3}.
[b] Density 3.2 g cm^{-3}.
[c] Density 7.8 g cm^{-3}.
[d] Density 11.35 g cm^{-3}.

Table 19.2. Tenth-Value Thickness, $(TVT_e)_S$, of Attenuation for Scattered Radiations

Primary Beam	Angle of Scatter	Concrete[a] (cm)	Lead[b] (cm)
137Cs (0.660-MeV gamma rays)	30°	15.7	1.8
	45°	14.6	1.5
	60°	13.3	1.3
	90°	12.3	0.7
	135°	11.3	0.4
60Co ($\approx$ 1.25-MeV gamma rays)	30°	21	3.4
	60°	19	2.5
	90°	16	1.5
4-MV X-rays	90°	17	–
6-MV X-rays	30°	26	–
	60°	21	–
	90°	18	–

Note: Values were compiled by the authors from references listed in the text. Useful for shielding calculations only.

[a] Density 2.35 g cm^{-3}.
[b] Density 11.35 g cm^{-3}.

made partly of steel to save space where necessary. Lead is the material commonly employed in the entrance door. The neutron production at energies above 10 MV requires that the door has hydrogenous material incorporated for protection against these neutrons. Composite roofs involving combinations of concrete, lead, steel, and polyethylene have been studied [17].

19.3.5
Architectural and Equipment Data

NCRP Report No. 49 (page 108) states that, prior to the design of a facility, it is necessary to have the following architectural and equipment information [10]:

(1) Architectural

a) Drawings of radiation rooms and adjacent area, ... including position of radiation source, doors, and windows.
b) Information about occupancy below, above, and adjacent to radiation rooms.
c) Type of proposed, or existing, construction of floors, ceilings, and wall.
d) For megavoltage therapy installations, including cobalt, vertical sections and plot plans.

(2) Equipment

a) Below 150 kV.
   1) Purpose: therapy, radiography, fluoroscopy, etc.
   2) kV and weekly workload, if known.
b) 150 kV and above, including gamma beam apparatus.
   1) kV, or type of gamma source.
   2) mA or R per min (in present usage, rad or cGy per minute) at 1 meter.
   3) Weekly workload, if known, expressed in mA min, or cGy at 1 m.
   4) Restrictions in beam orientations without and with beam interceptor, if any.
c) Possible future increases in workload and radiation energy, and modification in beam orientation.

19.3.6
Workload (W)

Workload (W) is a measure of the degree of use of a particular external-beam therapy machine and is evaluated in terms of the dose delivered by the useful beam at 1 m from the source for 1 week of operation. W is expressed in $Gy\,m^2\,week^{-1}$. For non-pulsed X-ray equipment operating below 1 MV, the workload has also been expressed in terms of milliampere-minutes (mA min) used per week.

EXAMPLE 19.1

It is planned to install an isocentric 4-MV X-ray machine. It is expected that an average time of 7 min for setup and 3 min for irradiation will be needed for each patient treated on the machine. The average daily dose per patient is estimated to be 2.5 cGy at the isocenter of the machine, located at 0.8 m from the source. The clinic expects to work 14 h every day for 5 working days per week. Estimate the workload.

Machine time to be used per patient = 7 min (for setup) + 3 min (for treatment)

$$= 10\,min$$

Patients to be treated per hour = 60 min/10 min = 6 patients/h

Daily patient load in a 14-h working day = 14 h/d × 6 patients/hour = 84 patients/d

2.5 Gy is delivered at 0.8 m treatment distance for every patient. There are 5 working days per week. Total dose delivered by the machine per week

$$= (2.5\,\mathrm{Gy/patient\ at\ 0.8\ m}) \times (84\,\mathrm{patients/day}) \times (5\,\mathrm{day/week})$$
$$= 1050\,\mathrm{Gy\ week}^{-1}\ \mathrm{at\ 0.8\ m}$$

We want to express the workload as normalized at 1 m from the source. This normalization is achieved by multiplication of the above value by $(0.8\,\mathrm{m})^2$. Thus,

$$W = (1050\,\mathrm{Gy/week}) \times (0.8\,\mathrm{m})^2$$
$$= 672\,\mathrm{Gy\ m}^2\ \mathrm{week}^{-1}$$

19.3.7
Use Factor (U)

In general, a radiation therapy machine may have its beam pointed in several directions during its use. The walls, floor, and ceiling to which the beam can be directed are to be designed to shield the primary radiation beam from the source. They are referred to as primary protective barriers. The other walls or barriers, toward which the radiation beam is not directed, are designed to protect against the scatter and leakage radiations. These are called secondary protective barriers. The use factor (U) is a beam direction factor that gives the fraction of the workload W for which the beam has a particular orientation. U for different directions can be based on specific details regarding the anticipated use of the particular equipment that is planned to be installed. Table 19.3 presents the values of U as obtained from the references cited [10, 18–20].

Table 19.3. Use Factors (U) (i. e., Beam Direction Factors) for Primary Protective Barriers for Therapy Installations

Ref.	Floor	Walls	Ceiling[a]
NCRP [10]	1	1/4	1/4
Johns and Cunningham [18]	0.6	0.1	0.3
Farrow [19]	0.625	0.13	0.115
Cobb and Bjarngard [20]	0.48	0.6	0.29

Note: Values given are for use in situations where no specific data for the particular facility are available.

[a] Design features of some radiotherapy equipment may prohibit directing the beam toward the ceiling.

19.3.8
Occupancy Factor (T)

Shielding is designed to protect the possible occupants of an area, rather than to protect the area itself. The purpose for which the protected area is used can be such that it may not be realistic to assume that the area is occupied by any one individual for all of the time that the beam is on. For example, toilets, elevators, hallways, and patients' waiting rooms are occupied only occasionally by any one individual. The occupancy factor (T) is used in the shielding evaluations to take into account such facts. Any area used by a radiation worker should be considered an area with full occupancy, with

Table 19.4. Occupancy Factors

Occupancy	T	Area
Full	1	Work areas, offices, laboratories, shops, nursing station, control panel, occupied spaces in near-by buildings
Partial	1/4	Corridors, restrooms, elevators using operators, unattended parking lots
Occasional	1/16	Waiting rooms, toilets, stairways, unattended elevators, janitors' closets, outside areas used by pedestrians or vehicular traffic

From NCRP Report No. 49 [10], to be used when no data specific to the facility are available.

$T = 1$. Table 19.4 gives the values of T from NCRP Report No. 49, for nonoccupationally exposed persons, in the planning of shielding.10 These values can be used if no other occupancy data specific to the facility are available. Full-occupancy areas ($T = 1$) are work areas such as offices, laboratories, shops, patient wards, and nurses' stations. Areas of partial occupancy ($T = 1/4$) are corridors, rest rooms, unattended parking lots, etc. Areas of occasional occupancy ($T = 1/16$) are waiting rooms, stairways, toilets, janitors' closets, etc. In some jurisdictions, local laws may forbid the use of a value of T less than 1/4.

19.4
Estimating the Allowable Barrier Transmission

19.4.1
Primary Shielding Barrier

Figure 19.1a illustrates a beam from a teletherapy source head directed toward a wall (#1) of the treatment room. This wall should be designed to reduce the exposure of the occupants on its other side to the primary beam. In barrier calculations, the dose reduction due to the inverse-square fall-off should also be allowed for. For this we need to estimate the distance, d_B, from the source to the occupant behind the barrier. The distance d_B is a sum of three distances: the distance, d_W, from the source to the wall, the thickness of the wall, t_W, and a possible distance of clearance between the wall and the occupant, as shown in Figure 19.1b. NCRP Report No. 49 suggests that it can be assumed that there is a 30-cm clearance between any occupant and the wall. Because the purpose in the calculation itself is to determine the value of t_W, assuming that t_W is zero is a possible conservative assumption in the estimation of d_B, unless a first-guess value of t_W is known from past experience. By the definitions of the workload (W), the use factor (U), and the occupancy factor (T), the equivalent dose received in 1 week by a person standing at distance d_B in the absence of any shielding will be

$$\frac{WUT}{(d_B)^2} \tag{19-1}$$

Some therapy heads that are mounted on a gantry for isocentric rotation may have a counterweight that intercepts the beam after it exits the patient, as shown in Figure 19.1a. If there is such a beam interceptor (also called "beam stopper"), the fraction, F_{BS}, of radiation that is transmitted by the beam interceptor should be taken into account in the shielding calculations. NCRP Report No. 102 recommends that a beam interceptor should transmit not more than 0.1% of the useful beam (i. e., $F_{BS} < 0.001$) and cover up to a 30° angle of the central ray [16]. If the equivalent dose to a person behind the wall should not exceed the weekly limit P, the maximum acceptable transmission, B_P, through the primary barrier can be derived from the equation

$$\frac{WUT}{(d_B)^2} F_{BS} \times B_P = P \qquad (19\text{-}2)$$

i. e.,

$$B_P = \frac{P(d_B)^2}{WUT} \frac{1}{F_{BS}} \qquad (19\text{-}3)$$

The width or expanse of the primary barrier should adequately cover the largest field size possible with sufficient margins.

19.4.2
Secondary Protective Barrier

Where there is no primary barrier, a secondary barrier will be needed to provide protection against leakage and scattered radiations.

Leakage Radiation

For any machine, the manufacturers specify the leakage fluence at 1 m from the source as a fraction, F_L, of the useful primary beam fluence at 1 m from the source (see Section 19.3.3). If the distance between a person behind the barrier and the source position is d_B (see Figure 19.1b), the maximum acceptable barrier transmission, B_L, that protects against leakage radiation is obtainable from the relation

$$\frac{WUT}{(d_B)^2} F_L \times B_L = P \qquad (19\text{-}4)$$

i. e.,

$$B_L = \frac{P(d_B)^2}{WUT} \frac{1}{F_L} \qquad (19\text{-}5)$$

Traditionally the use factor U is assigned the value 1 for leakage radiation. However, the newer methods of using intensity-modulated radiotherapy (IMRT) beams can cause the use factor for leakage to be more than 1 for delivery of the same workload W at the patient's position. The use factor for IMRT can be high, in the range of 2-10 depending upon the leaf-sequencing and the degree of inefficient use of the 'beam-on' time [21–24].

Scattered Radiation

The intensity of scattered radiation from the patient that reaches the barrier is related to the primary intensity at the patient position, the cross section of the beam (i. e., the volume irradiated), the angle of deflection of the scattered photons that reach the barrier, and the distance to the barrier. We define a scattering coefficient, α, as the ratio of the scattered dose for a beam of unit cross-sectional area (1 m^2) at a unit distance

Table 19.5. Values of Scatter Coefficient α

Primary Beam	Scattering Angle θ[a]					
	30°	45°	60°	90°	120°	135°
^{137}Cs gamma rays	0.1625	0.125	0.1025	0.07	–	0.0475
^{60}Co gamma rays	0.15	0.09	0.0575	0.0225	–	0.015
4-MV X-rays	–	0.068	–	–	–	–
6-MV X-rays	0.175	0.045	0.0275	0.015	–	0.01

Note: α is the ratio of scattered dose at 1 m from the patient to the primary dose incident on the patient for a beam cross section of 1 m^2. Converted from data in NCRP Report No. 49 [10], which are specific for a beam of cross section of 400 cm^2.

[a] $\theta = 0°$ for forward scatter.

(1 m) away from the scatterer (i. e., the patient) to the primary dose delivered to the scatterer.

Examples of the values of α that can be used for shielding calculations are given in Table 19.5. The value of α changes with the energy of the primary beam and the angle θ of the scatter with respect to the direction of the primary. In general, a machine may have collimators that provide a maximum possible beam cross section of A_{pat} at its normal source-to-patient distance, d_{pat}. Because the workload, W, is specified at a distance of 1 m from the source, the primary dose to the scatterer (i. e., the patient) is $W/(d_{pat})^2$, with d_{pat} measured in meters. Because the values of α are for a beam of 1 m^2 cross section, for a beam of cross section A_{pat} (measured in square meters), the scattered dose at 1 m from the patient is

$$\frac{W}{(d_{pat})^2}(\alpha A_{pat}) \qquad (19\text{-}6)$$

The dose to a person behind the barrier will also be reduced because of the inverse-square fall-off of the scatter fluence over the distance d_B between the person and the scatterer. Hence, in general, the maximum acceptable barrier transmission, B_S, for the scattered radiation is related to P by the expression

$$\frac{WUT}{(d_{pat})^2}F_S B_S = P \qquad (19\text{-}7)$$

where F_S is the scatter factor given by

$$F_S = \frac{\alpha A_{pat}}{(d_B)^2} \qquad (19\text{-}8)$$

Hence,

$$B_S = \frac{P(d_{pat})^2}{WUT}\frac{1}{F_S} \qquad (19\text{-}9)$$

All walls should have enough shielding to protect against 90° side scatter from the patient. The use factor U is 1 for 90° scatter. Sometimes, additional consideration will need to be given to photons scattered in a forward direction (at angles less than 90°) with respect to the incident beam. For example, this happens if the primary barrier of a side wall is designed to be just wide enough to cover the primary beam (as in

Figure 19.1a). If so, the primary barrier may cover a 25° to 30° angle with respect to the central axis of the primary beam. Then the wall beyond the primary barrier should be designed to protect, not only against the leakage through the source housing and 90° scatter, but also against forward scatter from the patient that travels beyond the primary barrier when the beam is directed toward the wall.

Forward-scattered photons are of higher energy than 90° scatter and are more penetrating. Furthermore, the scatter coefficient, α, is greater for forward scatter. When one calculates the barrier thickness for protection against such forward scatter, adoption of a value of U of less than 1.0 can be meaningful. The value of U can be identical to that adopted for the calculation of the thickness of the adjacent primary barrier.

In the above analysis, we addressed scatter and leakage separately, although protection is needed against both simultaneously. To take this into account, the NCRP suggests that, after an independent calculation of the two barrier thicknesses, one should check the difference between them. If the difference exceeds one TVT, using the greater of the two thicknesses will be adequate. Otherwise, one HVT should be added to the greater thickness and adopted as the barrier thickness needed.

19.4.3
Entrance Door Barrier

Most radiotherapy rooms are designed to have a maze entrance. Some plans of maze designs are shown in Figure 19.2. The walls of the entrance path are designed to be such that leakage or scattered radiation from the isocenter cannot reach the door directly without undergoing scatter. A maze of proper design can reduce the lead shielding needed at the door. Multiple reflections through a maze with folds or turns are effective means of reducing both the energy and the fluence of photons reaching the door. Protection against neutrons can also be achieved by making the maze entrance sufficiently long through several turns, if needed.

The kinematics of Compton scattering of high-energy photons (see Section 7.5.3) is such that the maximum energy of photons scattered at 90° is 0.511 MeV. It is possible to show that, for 180° scatter, the scattered photon energy is $0.511/2 = 0.255$ MeV,

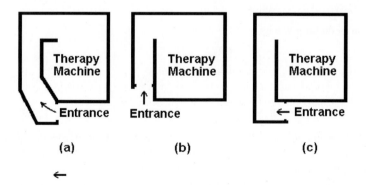

Fig. 19.2. Three different designs of maze entrances to therapy rooms are shown in (a), (b), and (c)

irrespective of the energy of the high-energy primary photon. This is also true when 180° scatter occurs as a consequence of two successive 90° scattering events. Hence, shielding data for 0.25 MeV can be used for shielding against a second scatter. However, for high-energy machines (operating far above the pair-production threshold of 1.02 MeV), there will be a significant number of annihilation photons of 0.511 MeV. Two or three scattering events at smaller angles in a single object can also result in a backscattered photon of energy higher than 0.511 MeV. In such cases, shielding data for 1-MV X-rays can be used.

In a treatment room having a single straight maze entrance (as shown in Figure 19.2b), the walls facing the entrance door to the treatment room can scatter the radiation scattered from the patient and the leakage from the source head toward the door. In principle, any scatterer can have a scatter factor of the form shown in Equation (19-8). If the wall that scatters is at a distance $d_{1,2}$ from the isocenter, the dose at the wall due to scatter from the patient is given by

$$\frac{WUT}{(d_{pat})^2}(F_S)_1$$

where $(F_S)_1$ is the scatter factor for the first scatterer (i. e., the patient), and is given by

$$(F_S)_1 = \frac{\alpha A_{pat}}{(d_{1,2})^2} \tag{19-10}$$

If the wall is treated as a second scatterer having a scatter coefficient α_2 and an area of irradiation A_2, the scatter factor, $(F_S)_2$, for the second scatterer is given by

$$(F_S)_2 = \frac{\alpha_2 A_2}{(d_B)^2} \tag{19-11}$$

where d_B is the distance between the second scatterer (i. e., the wall) and the entrance. Accordingly, we modify Equation (19-7) to obtain the following expression for the dose, $(D_{door})_S$, received by a person at the door due to patient scatter:

$$(D_{door})_S = \frac{WUT}{(d_{pat})^2}(F_S)_1(F_S)_2 \tag{19-12}$$

For this dose to be reduced to the weekly limit P, the door should have shielding that attenuates the scatter by a factor $(B_{door})_S$, given by

$$(B_{door})_S = \frac{P(d_{pat})^2}{WUT}\frac{1}{(F_S)_1}\frac{1}{(F_S)_2} \tag{19-13}$$

The concept of Equations (19-12) and (19-13) can be extended to several successive scatterers. More complex methods of scatter evaluation by Monte Carlo and transport theoretical methods are possible [25–28], but are not discussed here.

The factor $(F_S)_2$ is also applicable to the scattering of the leakage radiation by the wall toward the door. The dose at the door, $(D_{door})_L$, due to the wall scattering of the leakage radiation is

$$(D_{door})_L = WUT\frac{F_L}{(d_{1,2})^2}(F_S)_2 \tag{19-14}$$

For this dose to be reduced to the weekly limit P, the door should have shielding that attenuates this radiation by a factor $(B_{door})_L$, given by

$$(B_{door})_L = \frac{P(d_{1,2})^2}{WUT} \frac{1}{F_L} \frac{1}{(F_S)_2} \tag{19-15}$$

The total dose at the door, D_{door}, is given by the sum of $(D_{door})_S$ and $(D_{door})_L$. The door shielding should be adequate to give protection against both scattered and leakage radiations. After the door shielding is calculated separately for scattered and leakage radiations, the actual door thickness needed to protect against both of them can be arrived at based on the considerations discussed in Section 19.4.2.

19.4.4
Roof Protection and Skyshine

The area above the ceiling of the treatment room may or may not be planned to be an occupied area. If there will be occupancy, the area of the roof struck by the primary beam should have sufficient thickness to function as a primary protective barrier, and the remaining part of the roof should offer protection against leakage and scattered radiation.

Even in situations where there is no occupancy directly above the ceiling, possible irradiation of occupants in upper stories of neighboring buildings should not be overlooked (see Figure 19.3). In addition to the possibility of direct irradiation, the radiation scattered by air, called skyshine or airshine, can pose a problem [11, 17, 29–32]. The skyshine can contribute a significant dose in areas behind the walls of the treatment room, if the ceiling offers only weather protection and no shielding. If a source delivers a dose rate, D_{1m}, at 1 m from it in air, and if the solid angle subtended at the source by the irradiated volume of air is Ω, an estimate of the dose rate from skyshine, $D_{skyshine}$, at a lateral distance, d_p (Figure 19.3), can be obtained from the following equation [11]:

$$D_{skyshine} = \frac{2.5 \times 10^{-2} \times D_{1m} \times \Omega^{1.3}}{(d_p)^2} \tag{19-16}$$

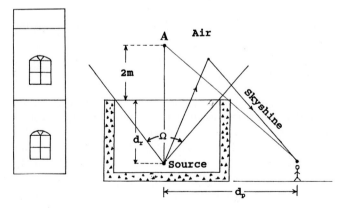

Fig. 19.3. Diagram illustrating air scatter or skyshine. $\pi/2$ is the solid angle subtended at the source by the aperture of the open roof

Fig. 19.4. Solid angle sub-tended by the aperture of a circular roof at the source S. φ is the polar angle subtended by the circular periphery. Points A, B, C, and D on the circumference of the circle form the corners of a rectangular aperture

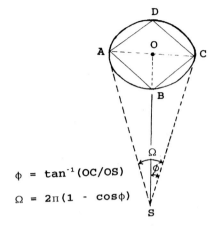

$$\phi = \tan^{-1}(OC/OS)$$

$$\Omega = 2\pi(1 - \cos\phi)$$

For radiotherapy rooms, Ω is the solid angle subtended by the area of the roof irradiated. If a circular roof is irradiated, as shown in Figure 19.4, Ω is given by $2\pi(1 - \cos\phi)$, where ϕ is the polar angle of inclination between the center and the periphery of the roof. In practical situations, the irradiated area of the roof is likely to be close to a square. In such cases, it is possible to find an approximate value of Ω for skyshine calculations by replacing the square or rectangular area by an equivalent circular area. For scatter and leakage radiations, Ω is the value subtended by the entire ceiling. For the primary beam, Ω should be calculated for the largest primary beam cross section provided by the machine. D_{1m} can be substituted by $(WUT F_{BS})$, $(WUT F_L)$, and $(WUT \alpha A_{pat})/(d_{pat})^2$ for primary, leakage, and scatter components, respectively. NCRP Report No. 51 suggests that the acceptable transmission through the roof, $B_{skyshine}$, can be assessed from [11]

$$B_{skyshine} = \frac{P(d_r + 2)^2}{D_{skyshine}} = \frac{P(d_r + 2)^2(d_p)^2}{2.5 \times 10^{-2} \times D_{1m} \times \Omega^{1.3}} \tag{19-17}$$

where d_r is the height of the roof from the source in meters. (The term $(d_r + 2)^2$ is the square of the distance from the source to a point 2 m above the roof, as shown in Figure 19.3.)

Roof shielding of 1 to 2 TVT may often be needed for a therapy facility so that an unacceptable dose from skyshine is prevented.

19.5
High-Energy X-Rays and Neutron Production

19.5.1
Neutron Shielding at the Door

At low photon energies, photoneutron production is absent or negligible. At energies above 10 MV, production of photoneutrons rapidly increases [11, 12, 15, 33]. The photoneutrons result from interaction of photons in materials in the source head, collimators, the patient, and also the materials in the room. From the point of view of dose to the patient, the neutron dose is insignificant compared to the photon dose [15, 34, 35]. For a dose of 1000 cGy delivered by photons, the neutron dose may be in the range of 0.06 to 0.1 cGy. However, for radiation safety of personnel, protection against neutrons cannot be ignored. For understanding the neutron problem, the reader is referred to the references cited above, in particular NCRP Report No. 79 [15].

Neutron fluence is reduced by slowing of neutrons through elastic scattering interactions with nuclei of the shielding material [2, 12, 36, 37]. The slowing-down process is called moderation. In elastic scattering of neutrons with hydrogen nuclides, much energy is transferred to the hydrogen nuclides (which recoil as protons). This large energy transfer happens because the mass of the hydrogen nucleus is almost the same as that of the impinging neutron. Collision of neutrons with heavy nuclides does not cause much loss of energy by the neutrons. Thus, heavy metals are poor neutron shields compared to hydrogenous materials. Water is a good moderator, and so are many plastic materials. The water content of concrete makes it an effective neutron attenuator.

NCRP Report No. 79 [15] presents the following empirical expressions for concrete and polyethylene that relate the tenth-value thickness, TVT_N (in centimeters), for reduction of neutron dose equivalent around medical accelerators to the average neutron energy, E_n (in mega-electron volts):

$$TVT_N = (15.5 + 5.6\,\bar{E}_n) \text{ cm for concrete}$$

and

$$TVT_N = (6.2 + 3.4\,\bar{E}_n) \text{ cm for polyethylene}$$

NCRP Report No. 79 also states that the value of $\bar{E}_N$ would not exceed 1 MeV for medical accelerators. Thus, TVT_N would be less than 21 cm of concrete.

Normally, a therapy room that is shielded with concrete walls can also provide shielding against neutrons. However, neutrons can bounce off the walls and pass through the entrance way to reach the door. The area outside the door is a high-occupancy area. Furthermore, when the equivalent dose from neutrons is evaluated, the radiation weighting factors for neutrons, which are higher than those for X-rays, (see Section 18.3.5) should not be overlooked. Therefore, the door needs to contain a sufficient thickness of a hydrogenous material (like polyethylene) to reduce the neutron dose to the occupants at the entrance. NCRP Report No. 79 states that the average energy of neutrons reaching the door is very low, in the neighborhood of 100 keV, and incorporation of 5 cm ($\approx$ 2 inch) of polyethylene in the door would reduce the fast-neutron component by a factor of 10. Because neutrons that have slowed down considerably (called thermal neutrons) are captured by boron nuclides, polyethylene impregnated with boron offers an advantage.

Approximate methods of estimating the neutron dose equivalent at the entrance to the room are reported in the literature [15, 38, 39]. In one method, which assumes a TVT_N for neutrons of 5 m in air, the equivalent dose, $(D_{door})_N$, from neutrons at the door is derived as

$$(D_{door})_N = \frac{WF_N W_B}{(d_{maze})^2 \, 10^{L/5}} \tag{19-18}$$

where F_N is the neutron dose at 1 m from the isocenter, expressed as a fraction of the dose delivered there by the useful photon beam; W_R is the radiation weighting factor for the neutrons; d_{maze} is the distance (in meters) from the isocenter to the nearend of the maze; and L is the length (in meters) of the central path through the maze from its room end to the entrance door. Equation (19-18) has been ascertained by experimental measurements to err on the safe side [40].

Neutrons can also be produced in the room through photon reactions in objects, including primary barriers of steel [41–44]. The adequacy of protection against neutrons should be confirmed by radiation surveys during the inaugural operation of the therapy machine [15, 45–52]. X-ray dosimeters and survey instruments that may normally be available in a radiotherapy clinic are not adequate for neutron measurements. The neutron survey should be done with neutron-sensitive monitoring devices such as boron trifluoride (BF_3) or ^3He proportional counters or foil activation methods. To react with boron or ^3He, fast neutrons should be slowed down to low (thermal) energies. Hence these detectors are surrounded by plastic spheres which act as moderators. In fact, an array of detectors surrounded by spheres of different diameters can function like a neutron spectrometer [53–55] We discussed neutron activation in Section 5.4. Measurement of the induced activity in indium or gold foils has been used as a method for neutron dosimetry. Neutron dose assessments have also been done by dosimeters based on etching and counting of the damage tracks in plastic materials caused by protons recoiling on neutron hits [56]. One other method depends on counting of the superheated drops formed in gels or soft polymers by neutron interaction. These are called superheated drop detectors (SDDs) or bubble detectors [57–61]. Some of the commercially available neutron measuring devices are called 'rem counters' or 'equivalent-dose counters', as they not only detect the neutrons but also (approximately and inherently) account for neutron-energy-dependent radiation weighting factors (W_R). It is not within the scope of this text to discuss the complex subject of neutron dosimetry.

19.5.2
Neutron Capture Gamma Rays

Neutrons are captured (or absorbed) by many nuclides in reactions that release gamma rays. Such neutron capture gamma rays are emitted from walls, materials in the room, and the door. Capture gamma rays are penetrating. A prominent reaction is neutron capture in hydrogen that releases a 2.2-MeV photon. Capture of a neutron in boron releases a gamma photon of 0.478 MeV. There are other neutron capture reactions in concrete that can release gamma rays having even higher energies, of up to 10 MeV. (Several capture gammas may be emitted from a single neutron capture.) It is usual to design a door with laminations of lead and borated polyethelene. The lead shielding in the door should offer protection against both the scattered photons and the capture gamma rays. The capture gamma rays from hydrogenous material in the entrance door should be absorbed in a lead layer in the outer face of the door. The hydrogenous layers for neutron shielding can be sandwiched between lead sheets to provide structural balance to the door. The overall shielding at the door should offer protection against scattered photons, neutrons, and neutron capture gamma rays [62]. A properly designed maze can reduce all of these components at the door.

19.5.3
Induced Radioactivity

Some of the nuclei resulting from a photoneutron reaction are radioactive [15, 63–67]. Careful studies have shown that such photon-induced activity does not present a safety problem in conventional radiotherapy [63]. This is because the amount of activity induced, although detectable, is minimal and decays rapidly. Some radioactivity is induced in the patient also, resulting in a negligible additional dose to the patient. Some caution has been suggested for the purpose of reducing the dose to staff in situations where a high percentage of patients are treated with IMRT beams with low cGy Mu^{-1} [67].

19.6
An Example of Shielding Calculations for a Facility

19.6.1
Basic Data and Assumptions

In the following sections, we evaluate the shielding requirements for an isocentric rotational 4-MV X-ray therapy machine. Unless specified otherwise, all shielding is provided by concrete of density 2.35 g cm^{-3}. The machine has no primary beam stopper, and patients are treated with the isocenter at 0.8 m from the source. A maximum field size of 40 cm $\times$ 40 cm is obtained at the isocenter. The head leakage is 0.1% of the useful beam. The workload is anticipated to be 672 Gy m^2 week^{-1} (as derived in Example 19.1). The proposed floor layout of the department is shown in Figure 19.5. A corner location has been chosen. The building is a single-storied structure with no occupancy above.

Figure 19.6 shows the layout of the therapy room. The orientation of the gantry of the machine, the plane of rotation of the central axis of the beam, and the width of the beam are also shown. An entrance having a maze is used to ensure that neither primary nor secondary radiations from the machine or patient can directly reach the door. The photon fluence at the door is likely to be mostly due to the radiation scattered by the inside walls that face the door. Radiations scattered two or more times can be weak in both intensity and energy. Hence, the amount of shielding needed at the entrance door can be minimal. In this example, there is no need to be concerned about neutron shielding because no neutrons are produced at 4 MV energy.

In shielding evaluations, some assumptions are inevitable when exact layout details or pertinent data are not available. If, in a particular assumption, one errs on the safe side and overestimates the shielding, this is called a conservative assumption. On the contrary, cost-saving assumptions also can be made. We have tried to be conservative in carrying out the calculations for this facility. For example, where data for 4 MV are not available, we have used values available for either cobalt-60 or 6 MV, depending upon which of these results in a higher shielding estimate. The reader is advised to make a critical appraisal of our assumptions and to repeat these calculations independently.

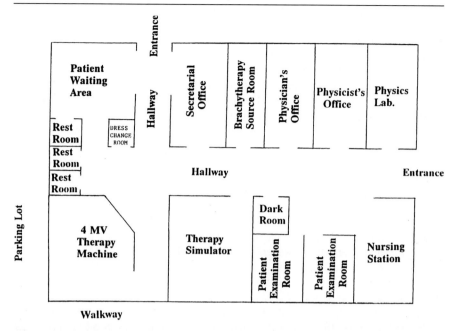

Fig. 19.5. Sample floor plan of a radiotherapy department

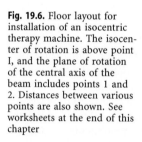

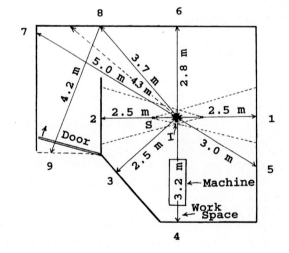

Fig. 19.6. Floor layout for installation of an isocentric therapy machine. The isocenter of rotation is above point I, and the plane of rotation of the central axis of the beam includes points 1 and 2. Distances between various points are also shown. See worksheets at the end of this chapter

19.6.2
Side Walls

Figure 19.6 shows several locations, marked by numbers 1 to 9, where the barrier thicknesses should be estimated for providing adequate safety. A worksheet that can be used for estimating the shielding has been appended at the end of this chapter. The shielding needed at locations 1 to 8 has been calculated on this worksheet. All of the parameters have been assigned appropriate values based on Figure 19.6 and on the data provided in this chapter. The barriers at positions 1 and 2 are primary barriers. At positions 3 to 8, only secondary barriers are needed. For locations 3 and 5, an extra evaluation has been done giving special consideration to 45° forward scatter.

Sometimes a point, such as location 9 in Figure 19.6 that lies just outside the entrance door, may be subjected to different components. (Location 9 receives radiation from the patient that penetrates the wall, the scatter that comes through the maze and the door, and scatter from skyshine.) Although one can consider only one component at a time during the shielding evaluations, it is important to ensure that the sum of the components does not exceed the acceptable dose limit. In such instances, the required safety can usually be achieved by addition of 1 or 2 HVT for the largest of the separately derived thicknesses (as pointed out in Section 19.4.2).

If the beam is obliquely incident on a barrier, the thickness calculated is along a path that is inclined to the wall and aligned with the direction of the beam and is not perpendicular to the wall. However, because scattered photons produced in the wall can travel perpendicular to the wall and have smaller path lengths, this can result in overdosing. This is especially so if the angle of inclination is more than 45°. As a matter of precaution, NCRP Report No. 49 recommends that, if the beam obliquity is taken into account and the perpendicular thickness of the wall is reduced, one HVT be added to the wall thickness to ensure safety. Lines 28 to 31 in the worksheet are meant for adding a safety factor for conditions such as these.

19.6.3
Entrance Door Shield

The door is designed to protect anyone who might be at location 9 of Figure 19.6, which can receive scatter from the walls facing the door. Although the area outside the door is a controlled area, we will use a minimal value of P of only 20 μSv, because of the consideration that the area has already been planned to receive 200 μSv week^{-1} through wall transmission. We will use expressions (19-13) and (19-15) for assessing the shielding requirement for the door for scattered and leakage components separately.

For scattered radiation, we have

$$W = 672 \, \text{Gy m}^2 \, \text{week}^{-1}; \quad U = 1; \quad T = 1;$$
$$d_{\text{pat}} = 0.8 \, \text{m}; \quad A_{\text{pat}} = 0.16 \, \text{m}^2$$

From Table 19.5, for 90° scatter from the patient, for ^{60}Co we obtain $\alpha = 0.0225$. Distance from patient to wall $= d_{1,2} = 4.3$ m. Using Equation (19-10),

$$(F_S)_1 = (0.0225 \times 0.16 \, \text{m}^2)/(4.3 \, \text{m})^2 = 1.947 \times 10^{-4}$$

The wall has a width of 1.5 m and a height of 3.0 m. Thus, the area of the wall contributing to scatter is

$$A_2 = 1.5 \, \text{m} \times 3.0 \, \text{m} = 4.5 \, \text{m}^2$$

For the wall scatter coefficient we will use the value for ^{137}Cs (0.66 MeV) for 90° scatter from Table 19.5. Hence, $\alpha_2 = 0.07$. Distance from wall to door, $d_B = 4.2$ m.

Substituting in Equation (19-11), we obtain

$$(F_S)_2 = (0.07 \times 4.5\,\text{m}^2)/(4.2\,\text{m})^2 = 1.786 \times 10^{-2}$$
$$P = 20\,\mu\text{Gy week}^{-1} \text{ (See Section 19.3.1)}$$

Substituting in Equation (19-13) gives

$$(B_{\text{door}})_S = \frac{20\,\mu\text{Gy week}^{-1}\,(0.8\,\text{m})^2}{672\,\text{Gy week}^{-1}\,\text{m}^2 \times 1.947 \times 10^{-4} \times 1.786 \times 10^{-2}}$$
$$= 5.478 \times 10^{-3}$$

$$\text{TVTs needed} = n = -\log_{10}(B_{\text{door}})_S = 2.26$$

Adopting the (TVT_e) of 0.7 cm of lead for 90° scatter of ^{137}Cs photons from Table 19.2, we obtain

$$\text{Lead shielding needed} = 2.26 \times 0.7\,\text{cm} = 1.6\,\text{cm}$$

For leakage radiation, with $F_L = 0.001$ and $d_{1,2} = 4.3\,\text{m}$ in Equation (19-15), we obtain

$$(B_{\text{door}})_L = \frac{20\,\mu\text{Gy week}^{-1} \times (4.3\,\text{m})^2}{672\,\text{Gy week}^{-1}\,\text{m}^2 \times 0.001 \times 1.786 \times 10^{-2}}$$
$$= 3.08 \times 10^{-2}$$

$$\text{TVTs needed} = n = -\log_{10}(B_{\text{door}})_L = 1.51$$

Adopting the (TVT_e) of 2.1 cm in lead for ^{137}Cs photons of 0.66 MeV, we obtain

$$\text{Lead shielding needed} = 1.51 \times 2.1\,\text{cm} = 3.2\,\text{cm}$$

Overall shielding for the door: we notice that the lead shielding needed for scatter and for leakage is, respectively, 1.6 cm and 3.2 cm. The difference between the two is ≈ 1.6 cm, which is more than the TVT of 0.7 cm that we have used for the scatter component. Hence, we can incorporate a thickness of 3.2 cm of lead in the door.

19.6.4
Skyshine Shielding

There is no occupancy above the roof in this example. However, protection of the surroundings against skyshine is required. We can use the concepts outlined in Section 19.4.4 and Equation (19-17) for the purpose of evaluating the shielding to be provided by the ceiling. First, we will address independently the shielding against (a) the primary beam directed upward, (b) the leakage radiation, and (c) scattered radiation.

(a) Shield against skyshine from primary beam
Let us consider that the primary beam has a maximum rectangular cross section of 0.4 m × 0.4 m at a distance of 0.8 m from the source. The radius of a circle of the same

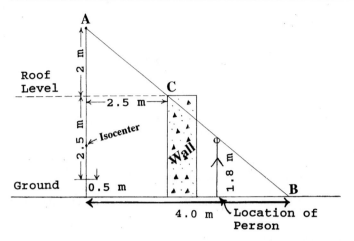

Fig. 19.7. B is the nearest point at which scatter from point A can reach the ground unshielded by the side wall

area is

$$[(0.4\,\text{m} \times 0.4\,\text{m})/\pi]^{1/2} = 0.226\,\text{m}$$

The polar angle subtended by the circle at the source

$$\phi = \tan^{-1}[0.226/0.8] = 15.77°$$
$$\text{Solid angle } \Omega = 2\pi(1 - \cos\phi) = 0.236 \text{ steradian}$$
$$\text{Distance of roof from source, } d_r = 2.5\,\text{m}$$

The machine rotates such that the source is at a height of 0.5 m from ground level when the beam is pointed upward. The diagram in Figure 19.7 connects a point **A** chosen to be at 2 m above the roof on the central axis of the beam, which is pointed upward, and a point **C** on the edge of the ceiling at 2.5 m distance, which is regarded to be the nearest point on the periphery of the roof from the central axis of the beam. We can consider that the points on the ground up to point **B** where line **AC** meets the ground are already protected by the side walls. Only beyond this distance does protection against skyshine have to be achieved by the shielding in the ceiling. Thus, the value of d_p for use in expression (19-17) is ascertained geometrically to be

$$d_p = (2\,\text{m}/2.5\,\text{m}) \times (0.5\,\text{m} + 2.5\,\text{m} + 2.0\,\text{m}) = 4.0\,\text{m}$$

We will further assume that $W = 672\,\text{Gy m}^2\,\text{week}^{-1}$, $F_{BS} = 1$ for no primary-beam stopper, $T = 1$ for full occupancy, $U = 1/2$ for a primary beam pointed upward, $D_{1m} = WUT$, $F_{BS} = 336\,\text{Gy m}^2\,\text{week}^{-1}$, and $P = 20\,\mu\text{Gy week}^{-1}$ for an uncontrolled area. Thus, substituting in Equation (19-17), we obtain

$$B_{skyshine} = \frac{20\,\mu\text{Gy week}^{-1}\,(2.5 + 2)^2 \times (4.0\,\text{m})^2}{2.5 \times 10^{-2} \times 336\,\text{Gy m}^2\,\text{week}^{-1} \times (0.236)^{1.3}}$$
$$= 5.04 \times 10^{-3}$$

The number of TVTs needed is

$$n = -\log_{10}(5.04 \times 10^{-3}) = 2.3$$
$$(TVT_e)_P = 29 \text{ cm (from Table 19.1 for 4 MV)}$$

Shielding needed $= 2.3 \times 29 \text{ cm} = 67 \text{ cm}$. Thus, the part of the ceiling struck by the primary beam should have a thickness of 67 cm.

(b) Shield against skyshine from head-leakage radiation

For leakage radiation, the value of Ω should be based on the entire roof area. We will assume that the roof is approximately a $5 \text{ m} \times 6 \text{ m} = 30 \text{ m}^2$ rectangular area, and that the source is 1 m below the roof. The radius of a circle having the same area is

$$[30 \text{ m}^2/\pi]^{1/2} = 3.1 \text{ m}$$

The polar angle formed by a circle of the above radius at a source 1 m below the roof is

$$\phi = \tan^{-1}[3.1/1] = 72°$$

The solid angle Ω is

$$\Omega = 2\pi(1 - \cos \phi) = 2\pi(1 - 0.309) = 4.34 \text{ steradians}$$

Furthermore,

$$W = 672 \text{ Gy m}^2 \text{ week}^{-1}; \ F_L = 0.001; \ T = 1; \ U = 1;$$

$$D_{1m} = (WUT) \times F_L = 672 \text{ Gy m}^2 \text{ week}^{-1} \times 0.001$$
$$= 0.672 \text{ Gy m}^2 \text{ week}^{-1}$$

$$d_p = 4 \text{ m}; \ d_r = 1 \text{ m}; \ P = 20 \text{ μSv week}^{-1};$$

$$B_{skyshine} = \frac{20 \text{ μSv week}^{-1} \times (1 \text{ m} + 2 \text{ m})^2 \times (4 \text{ m})^2}{2.5 \times 10^{-2} \times 0.672 \text{ Gy cm}^2 \text{ week}^{-1} \times 4.34^{1.3}}$$
$$= 2.54 \times 10^{-2}$$

Number of $(TVT_e)_L$ needed:

$$n = -\log_{10}(2.54 \times 10^{-2}) = 1.6$$

For a $(TVT_e)_L$ of 29 cm, the shielding needed for protection against skyshine from leakage radiation is

$$n \times (TVT_e)_L = 1.6 \times 29 \text{ cm} = 47 \text{ cm}$$

(c) Shield against skyshine from patient scatter

The scattered radiation comes from the patient, who is positioned at the isocenter of treatment. The distance of the isocenter below the roof is

height of roof from ground − height of isocenter $= 3.0 \text{ m} - 1.3 \text{ m} = 1.7 \text{ m}$

Thus, $d_r = 1.7$ m. The radius of a circle having the same area as the roof is 3.1 m (as calculated before). The polar angle subtended by such a circle at a point 1.7 m below it is

$$\tan^{-1}[3.1/1.7] = 61°$$

The solid angle Ω is

$$\Omega = 2\pi(1 - \cos\phi) = 2\pi(1 - 0.481) = 3.26 \text{ steradians}$$

Furthermore,

$$W = 672 \text{ Gy m}^2 \text{ week}^{-1}; \quad U = 1; \quad T = 1;$$
$$\alpha = 0.0225; \quad A_{pat} = 0.16 \text{ m}^2; \quad d_{pat} = 0.8 \text{ m};$$
$$P = 20 \,\mu\text{Sv week}^{-1}; \quad d_p = 4 \text{ m}; \quad d_r = 1.7 \text{ m};$$

$$\begin{aligned}
D_{1m} &= (WUT)(\alpha A_{pat})/(d_{pat})^2 \\
&= (672 \text{ Gy week}^- \text{ m}^2 \times 0.0225 \times 0.16 \text{ m}^2)/(0.8 \text{ m})^2 \\
&= 3.78 \text{ Gy m}^2 \text{ week}^{-1}
\end{aligned}$$

Substituting all of the above values in expression (19-17), we obtain

$$B_{skyshine} = \frac{20 \,\mu\text{Gy week}^{-1} \times (1.7 + 2)^2 \times (4.0 \text{ m})^2}{2.5 \times 10^{-2} \times 3.78 \text{ Gy m}^2 \text{ week}^{-1} \times (3.26)^{1.3}}$$
$$= 9.97 \times 10^{-3}$$

The number of $(TVT_e)_S$ needed is

$$n = -\log_{10}(9.97 \times 10^{-3}) \approx 2.0$$

For $(TVT_e)_S = 17$ cm (from Table 19.2) for the first scattered radiation, the shielding needed for protection against the skyshine from the scattered radiation component is

$$1.9 \times (TVT_e)_S \approx 2.0 \times 17 \text{ cm} = 34 \text{ cm}$$

The difference between the above value and the thickness of 47 cm which we calculated for protection against leakage radiation is less than the $(TVT_e)_S$ of 17 cm. Hence, we will add one $(HVT)_L = 9$ cm to 47 cm and adopt a thickness of 56 cm of concrete for the part of the ceiling that is not struck by the primary beam. Here, it is worthwhile to mention that the skyshine produced by multiple scattering is weaker in energy than the first scattered radiation from the patient, for which the $(HVT)_S$ that we used applies. Thus, the above evaluation is conservative.

Figures 19.8a, b, and c are cross-sectional views of the walls of the treatment room that we just planned.

Fig. 19.8. Sectional diagrams of shielding design of a therapy room. (a) A section parallel to the floor, (b) a section perpendicular to the maze and through the isocenter of the machine, and (c) a section parallel to the maze and through the isocenter

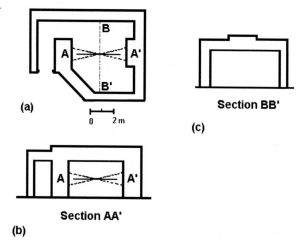

(a)

Section BB'

(c)

Section AA'

(b)

19.7
Ozone Production

Ozone and other noxious gases are produced by the interaction of ionizing radiation with air. Because X-ray beams interact less in air than do electron beams, the problem of ozone production is negligible during the use of X-ray beams. However, electron beam interaction with air can produce a considerable amount of ozone. This is particularly so when total-skin electron treatments are carried out with a large field cross section and a large treatment distance. The ozone should be cleared by provision of adequate ventilation to the room. Ozone is radiomimetic (i. e., mimics radiation) in its adverse effects. The threshold for ozone effects is 0.1 part per million. Nitric oxide and nitrogen dioxide are also produced by ionizing radiation and are harmful, but they have much higher thresholds than does ozone [11]. Kits marketed commercially are available for measurement of the concentration of these gases.

19.8
Miscellaneous Aspects of Planning a Facility

There should be sufficient overlap between the door and the side walls of a treatment room to prevent radiation leakage through gaps. If there is a gap between the door and the floor, radiation can be reflected by the floor and emerge outside the treatment room. Incorporation of layers of lead sheets below the door (i. e., under the floor) can reduce the reflection.

Provision should be made for passing cables into the room for physics measurements to be made on the beam. All of the conduits for wires and cables should preferably be incorporated in the secondary protective barriers. They should follow a slanted or curved course through the barrier to prevent passage of radiation through them to the outside.

There are various other aspects, in addition to the radiation shielding, to which attention should be paid in planning of an external-beam therapy facility [10–12]. Any radiotherapy room should be planned so as to provide a pleasing environment for patients and staff. The access to the room should be such that nonambulatory patients in stretchers can be moved in and out comfortably. In the access planning, one should also consider the need for moving in the therapy equipment during installation. The machine should be installed with sufficient space around it for servicing. The room should also have sufficient space for storage of treatment aids and accessories. There should be good ventilation for removal of the heat generated by the machine, to provide comfort for patients and staff, and to prevent accumulation of ozone. Air conditioners and ducts for ventilation should be located at heights of 8 feet or more. Air conditioners that vent to the outside should be covered by concrete baffles on the outside. Recesses in the walls for placement of localizing lasers can be planned in advance.

The door should be designed in such a way that a patient can open it from the inside of the room in an emergency. The doors are very heavy, especially those for use with high-energy beams. Electromechanical door opening and closing devices, which can also be operated manually in case of power failure, should be installed.

The control console should be placed in close proximity to the access door, so that the operator can readily control who enters the radiation room and when. The facility design should permit two-way oral communications between the patient in the treatment room and the operator at the control console outside.

Provisions for viewing the patient under treatment by the operating staff should be made. A closed-circuit television viewing system can be useful for this purpose. This system may be augmented by a system of viewing that utilizes a lead-glass window in the entrance door as well as a mirror.

Warning signs are a part of the access control system, and they should have a standard format. Unless otherwise specified by law or regulations, the format should include

1)   Words that indicate the degree of hazard
2)   A statement of the type of hazard
3)   The standard radiation warning symbol
4)   A brief statement of instructions for avoiding unwanted exposure

A light should be installed at the entrance to the room to indicate the 'beam on' condition to persons outside the room. An electrical interlock must be installed on the door of the therapy room. The interlock shall be wired into the electrical circuit in such a manner that, when the door is opened for any reason, the generation of the radiation beam will automatically be terminated and irradiation can be resumed only by manual resetting of the controls, after the door is closed.

Radiation alarms that include a flashing light when the beam is 'on' must be installed in the room to warn the staff about the 'beam-on' condition. Systems that give an audible signal that can be heard prior to and during the generation of the beam should also be provided. Emergency switches for turning off the machine should be installed in the treatment room at different points within easy reach of the staff. The staff should be trained to observe the alarm and how to act if the alarm flashes or sounds. Radiation safety measures such as signs and interlocks are the subject of NCRP Report No. 88, entitled 'Radiation Alarms and Access Control Systems' [68]. Machines using radioisotope sources are equipped with manual mechanisms to restore the source to the 'off' position. Staff should be educated about, and made familiar with, the tools and working of the mechanism of the particular machine. An emergency action procedure should be posted for the benefit of the staff.

Some accelerators use klystrons to provide microwave power. Klystrons operate with pulsed electron currents at voltages in the range of 100 to 250 kV and are sources of X-rays themselves. A shielding thickness of 1 to 2 in. of lead is needed for reducing the X-ray leakage from the klystrons to safe levels [11]. After installation, a radiation survey should be conducted around the klystrons. Wrapping films around them can reveal radiation leaking through gaps, if any, in the lead shielding. The film-wrap approach can also be used for checking the machine-head leakage.

The medical physicist on occasion needs to provide a protective-barrier report prior to the construction of a therapy facility. The report typically gives the architect the thicknesses of the protective walls. Most machine vendors may be able to provide a floor and shielding plan for their machines. During the construction phase before the concrete is poured, a careful check should be carried out on the general layout and the distances between the forms that hold the cement while it hardens. Samples of concrete should be obtained and checked for density during the construction phase, so that expensive corrections later on can be avoided. A close consultation between the architect, machine vendor, and a qualified physicist can result in a safe and well-planned facility.

All facilities should be surveyed and certified by a qualified physicist to be safe based on actual radiation levels measured around the installation [48, 69, 70]. In some legal jurisdictions, a copy of the survey may need to be forwarded to the local authorities.

Worksheet for Shielding Calculation

Machine Model: _____; Energy: _____; $W =$ _____ Gy m^2 week^{-1};
Beam Stopper Attenuation $F_{BS} =$ _____; Leakage $F_L =$ _____;

1. Position shielded
2. Controlled area?
3. Limit P (μGy week^{-1})
4. Factor U
5. Factor T
6. d_W (m)*
7. t_W (Anticipated) (m)
8. $d_B = (d_W + t_W + 0.3)$ (m)
9. $B_P = (P\,d_B^2)/(WUT\,F_{BS})$
10. $n = -\log_{10}(B_P)$
11. $(TVT_e)_P$ (cm)
12. $n \times (TVT_e)_P$ (cm)
13. $B_L = (P\,d_B^2)/(WUT\,F_L)$
14. $n = -\log_{10}(B_L)$

Worksheet for Shielding Calculation (Cont.)

15. $(TVT_e)_L$ (cm)	
16. $n \times (TVT_e)_L$ (cm)	
17. d_{pat} (m)	
18. A_{pat} (m^2)	
19. Angle θ	
20. α	
21. $F_S = \alpha A_{pat}/(d_B)^2$	
22. $B_S = P(d_{pat})^2/(WUT\, F_S)$	
23. $n = -\log_{10}(B_S)$	
24. $(TVT_e)_S$ (cm)	
25. $n \times (TVT_e)_S$ (cm)	
26. Larger of 16 or 25	
27. $(HVT)_L$ for leakage (cm)	
28. Do 16 and 25 differ $< 1\ (TVT)_S$?	
29. If 'yes' add 1 $(HVT)_L$	
30. Any thickness added for extra safety	
31. Recommended thickness (cm)	

* For primary-barrier calculations, the value of d_W is the sum of the source-to-isocenter distance and the isocenter-to-wall distance. For scatter and leakage barriers, the value is an average distance represented by the latter.

Worksheet for Shielding Calculation – Example

Machine Model: X-80; Energy: 4 MV; W = 672 Gy m^2 week^{-1};
Beam Stopper Attenuation $F_{BS} = 1.0$; Leakage $F_L = 0.001$;

	1	2	3	4
1. Position shielded	1	2	3	4
2. Controlled area?	No	Yes	Yes	Yes
3. Limit P (μGy week^{-1})	20	200	200	200
4. Factor U	1/4	1/4	1	1
5. Factor T	1/4	1	1	1
6. d_W (m)*	3.3	3.3	2.5	3.2
7. t_W (Anticipated) (m)	1.5	1.5	0.5	0.5
8. $d_B = (d_W + t_W + 0.3)$ (m)	5.1	5.1	3.3	4.0
9. $B_P = (P\, d_B^2)/(WUT\, F_{BS})$	1.24×10^{-5}	3.1×10^{-5}		
10. $n = -\log_{10}(B_P)$	4.91	4.51		

Worksheet for Shielding Calculation – Example (Cont.)

11. $(TVT_e)_P$ (cm)	29	29		
12. $n \times (TVT_e)_P$ (cm)	142	131		
13. $B_L = (P\,d_B^2)/(WUT\,F_L)$			3.24×10^{-3}	4.76×10^{-3}
14. $n = -\log_{10}(B_L)$			2.49	2.32
15. $(TVT_e)_L$ (cm)			29	29
16. $n \times (TVT_e)_L$ (cm)			72	67
17. d_{pat} (m)			0.8	0.8
18. A_{pat} (m^2)			0.16	0.16
19. Angle θ		90°	90°	
20. α		0.0225	0.0225	
21. $F_S = \alpha A_{pat}/(d_B)^2$			3.31×10^{-4}	2.25×10^{-4}
22. $B_S = P(d_{pat})^2/(WUT\,F_S)$			5.76×10^{-4}	8.47×10^{-4}
23. $n = -\log_{10}(B_S)$			3.24	3.07
24. $(TVT_e)_S$ (cm)			17	17
25. $n \times (TVT_e)_S$ (cm)			55	52
26. Larger of 16 or 25			72	67
27. $(HVT)_L$ for leakage (cm)			9	9
28. Do 16 and 25 differ $< 1\ (TVT)_S$?			No	Yes
29. If 'yes' add 1 $(HVT)_L$			–	9
30. Any thickness added for extra safety			–	–
31. Recommended thickness (cm)	142	131	72	76

* For primary-barrier calculations, the value of d_W is the sum of the source-to-isocenter distance and the isocenter-to-wall distance. For scatter and leakage barriers, the value is an average distance represented by the latter.

Worksheet for Shielding Calculation – Example (Cont.)

Machine Model: X-80; Energy: 4 MV; W = 672 Gy m^2 week^{-1};
Beam Stopper Attenuation F_{BS} = 1.0; Leakage F_L = 0.001;

1. Position shielded	5	6	7	8
2. Controlled area?	No	No	Yes	No
3. Limit P (μGy week^{-1})	20	20	200	20
4. Factor U	1	1	1	1
5. Factor T	1/4	1/4	1	1/4
6. d_W (m)*	3.0	2.8	5.0	3.7

Worksheet for Shielding Calculation – Example (Cont.)

7. t_W (Anticipated) (m)	0.5	0.5	0.5	0.5
8. $d_B = (d_W + t_W + 0.3)$ (m)	3.8	3.6	5.8	4.5
9. $B_P = (P\,d_B^2)/(WUT\,F_{BS})$				
10. $n = -\log_{10}(B_P)$				
11. $(TVT_e)_P$ (cm)				
12. $n \times (TVT_e)_P$ (cm)				
13. $B_L = (P\,d_B^2)/(WUT\,F_L)$	1.72×10^{-3}	1.54×10^{-3}	1.0×10^{-2}	2.41×10^{-3}
14. $n = -\log_{10}(B_L)$	2.76	2.81	2.0	2.62
15. $(TVT_e)_L$ (cm)	29	29	29	29
16. $n \times (TVT_e)_L$ (cm)	80	82	58	76
17. d_{pat} (m)	0.8	0.8	0.8	0.8
18. A_{pat} (m^2)	0.16	0.16	0.16	0.16
19. Angle θ	90°	90°	90°	90°
20. α	0.0225	0.0225	0.0225	0.0225
21. $F_S = \alpha A_{pat}/(d_B)^2$	2.49×10^{-4}	2.78×10^{-4}	1.07×10^{-4}	1.78×10^{-4}
22. $B_S = P(d_{pat})^2/(WUT\,F_S)$	3.06×10^{-4}	2.74×10^{-4}	1.78×10^{-3}	4.29×10^{-4}
23. $n = -\log_{10}(B_S)$	3.52	3.56	2.75	3.37
24. $(TVT_e)_S$ (cm)	17	17	17	17
25. $n \times (TVT_e)_S$ (cm)	60	61	47	57
26. Larger of 16 or 25	80	82	58	76
27. $(HVT)_L$ for leakage (cm)	9	9	9	9
28. Do 16 and 25 differ $< 1\ (TVT)_S$?	No	No	Yes	No
29. If 'yes' add 1 $(HVT)_L$	–	–	9	–
30. Any thickness added for extra safety	–	–	–	–
31. Recommended thickness (cm)	80	82	67	76

* For primary-barrier calculations, the value of d_W is the sum of the source-to-isocenter distance and the isocenter-to-wall distance. For scatter and leakage barriers, the value is an average distance represented by the latter.

Worksheet for Shielding Calculation – Example (Cont.)

Machine Model: X-80; Energy: 4 MV; W = 672 Gy m^2 week^{-1};
Beam Stopper Attenuation F_{BS} = 1.0; Leakage F_L = 0.001;

1. Position shielded	3*	5*
2. Controlled area?	Yes	No
3. Limit P (μGy week^{-1})	200	20
4. Factor U	1/4	1/4
5. Factor T	1	1
6. d_W (m)**	2.5	3.0
7. t_W (Anticipated) (m)	0.5	0.5
8. $d_B = (d_W + t_W + 0.3)$ (m)	3.3	3.8
9. $B_P = (P\, d_B^2)/(WUT\, F_{BS})$		
10. $n = -\log_{10}(B_P)$		
11. $(TVT_e)_P$ (cm)		
12. $n \times (TVT_e)_P$ (cm)		
13. $B_L = (P\, d_B^2)/(WUT\, F_L)$	3.24×10^{-3}	1.72×10^{-3}
14. $n = -\log_{10}(B_L)$	2.49	2.76
15. $(TVT_e)_L$ (cm)	29	29
16. $n \times (TVT_e)_L$ (cm)	72	80
17. d_{pat} (m)	0.8	0.8
18. A_{pat} (m^2)	0.16	0.16
19. Angle θ	45°	45°
20. α	0.068	0.068
21. $F_S = \alpha A_{pat}/(d_B)^2$	1.0×10^{-3}	7.42×10^{-4}
22. $B_S = P(d_{pat})^2/(WUT\, F_S)$	7.74×10^{-4}	1.03×10^{-4}
23. $n = -\log_{10}(B_S)$	3.11	3.99
24. $(TVT_e)_S$ (cm)	23	23 (6 MV data from Table 19.2)
25. $n \times (TVT_e)_S$ (cm)	72	92
26. Larger of 16 or 25	72	92
27. $(HVT)_L$ for leakage (cm)	9	9
28. Do 16 and 25 differ < 1 $(TVT)_S$?	Yes	Yes
29. If 'yes' add 1 $(HVT)_L$	9	9
30. Any thickness added for extra safety		
31. Recommended thickness (cm)	81	101

* Repeat calculations for 45° scatter with U = 1/4. U = 1 for leakage.
** For primary-barrier calculations, the value of d_W is the sum of the source-to-isocenter distance and the isocenter-to-wall distance. For scatter and leakage barriers, the value is an average distance represented by the latter.

References

1. National Council on Radiation Protection and Measurements, NCRP Report No. 116, Limitation of Exposure to Ionizing Radiation, National Council on Radiation Protection and Measurements, Bethesda, Maryland, 1987.
2. Dennis, J.A., On the recommendations of ICRP/90/G-01, Radiat. Res., Vol 123, pp349–350, 1990.
3. Dennis, J.A., EURADOS-CENDOS discussion on ICRP draft recommendations, Health Phys., Vol 59, pp936, 1990.
4. Cameron, J.R., Hormesis and high fliers: Radiation risk revisited, Letter, Phys. Today, Vol 45, pp13, 14, and 94, 1992.
5. Yalow, R.S., Is radiation less harmful than BEIR-V reports (letter), Phys. Today, Vol 44, pp13, 14, and 101, 1992.
6. Kocher, D.C., Perspective on historical development of radiation standards, Health Phys., Vol 61, pp519–527, 1991.
7. National Council on Radiation Protection and Measurements, Recommendations on Limits for Exposure to Ionizing Radiation, NCRP Report No. 91, National Council on Radiation Protection and Measurements, Bethesda, Maryland, 1987.
8. International Commission on Radiation Protection, Recommendations of the ICRP, ICRP-60, Ann. ICRP, Vol 21, No. 1–3, Pergamon, Oxford, 1991.
9. National Council on Radiation Protection and Measurements, Implementation of Principles of As Low As Reasonably Achievable for Medical Personnel, NCRP Report No. 107, National Council on Radiation Protection and Measurements, Bethesda, Maryland, 1990.
10. National Council on Radiation Protection and Measurements, Structural Shielding Design and Evaluation for Medical Use of X-rays and Gamma Rays up to 10 MeV, NCRP Report No. 49, National Council on Radiation Protection and Measurements, Bethesda, Maryland, 1976.
11. National Council on Radiation Protection and Measurements, Radiation Protection Design Guidelines for 0.1–100 MeV Particle Accelerator Facilities, NCRP Report No. 51, National Council on Radiation Protection and Measurements, Bethesda, Maryland, 1977.
12. Swanson, W.P., Radiological Safety Aspects of the Operation of Electron Linear Accelerators, IAEA Technical Report Series No. 188, International Atomic Energy Agency, Vienna, 1979.
13. Mckenzie, A.L., Shaw, J.E., Stephenson, S.K., and Turner, P.C.R., Radiation Protection in Radiotherapy, IPSM Report No. 46, The Institute of Physical Sciences in Medicine, London, 1986.
14. International Commission on Radiological Protection, Protection Against Ionizing Radiation from External Sources Used in Medicine, ICRP Publication 33, Pergamon Press, Oxford, 1982.
15. National Council on Radiation Protection and Measurements, Neutron Contamination from Medical Electron Accelerators, NCRP Report No. 79, National Council on Radiation Protection and Measurements, Bethesda, Maryland, 1984.
16. National Council on Radiation Protection and Measurements, Medical X-ray, Electron Beam, and Gamma-ray Protection for Energies up to 50 MeV (Equipment Design, Performance, and Use), NCRP Report No. 102, National Council on Radiation Protection and Measurements, Bethesda, Maryland, 1989.
17. McGinley, P.H., and Butker, E.K., Laminated primary ceiling barriers for medical accelerator rooms, Phys. Med. Biol., Vol. 39, pp1331–1336, 1994.
18. Johns, H.E., and Cunningham, J.R., Physics of Radiology, 4th Edition, p545, Charles C Thomas, Springfield, Illinois, 1983.
19. Farrow, N., The effect of linear accelerator use on primary barrier design, Phys. Med. Biol., Vol 30, pp1151–1153, 1985.
20. Cobb, P.D., and Bjarngard, B.E., Use factors for medical linear accelerators, Health Phys., Vol 31, pp463–465, 1976.
21. Followill, D., Geis, P., Boyer, A., Estimates of whole-body dose equivalent produced by beam intensity conformal therapy, Int. J. Radiat. Oncol. Biol. Phys., Vol. 38, pp667–672, 1997.
22. Verellen, D., and Vanhavere, F., Risk assessment of radiation-induced malignancies based on whole-body equivalent dose estimates for IMRT treatment in the head and neck region, Radiother. Oncol., Vol 53, pp199–203, 1999.
23. Mutic, S., Low, D.A., Klein, E.E., Dempsey, J.F., and Purdy, J.A., Room shielding for intensity modulated radiationtherapy treatment facilities, Int. J. Radiat. Oncol. Biol. Phys., Vol.50, pp239–246, 2001.
24. Rodgers, J.E., Radiation therapy vault shielding calculational methods when IMRT and TBI procedures contribute, J. Appl. Clin. Med. Phys., Vol. 2, pp157-164, 2001.
25. Bigg, P.J., Calculation of shielding door thicknesses for radiation therapy facilities using the ITS Monte Carlo program, Health Phys., Vol 61, pp465–472, 1991.
26. Yuan-Chyuan Lo, Albedos for 4-, 10-, and 18-MV bremsstrahlung X-ray beams on concrete, iron, and lead – normally incident, Med. Phys., Vol 19, pp659–666, 1992.

27. Jaeger, R.G. (Ed. in Chief), Radiation Attenuation Methods, Chapter 3, in Engineering Compendium on Radiation Shielding, Vol 1, Shielding Fundamentals and Methods, Springer-Verlag, Berlin, 1968.
28. McGinley, P.H., Dhaba'an, A.H., and Reft, C.S., Evaluation of the contribution of capture gamma rays, x-ray leakage, and scatter to the photon dose at the maze door for a high energy medical accelerator using a Monte Carlo particle transport code, Med. Phys., Vol. 27, pp225–230, 2000.
29. Clarke, E.T., Photon fields near earth-air interface, p255, in Engineering Compendium on Radiation Shielding, Vol 1, Jaeger, R.G. (Ed. in Chief), Springer-Verlag, New York, 1968.
30. Jenkin, T.M., Accelerator boundary doses and skyshine, Health Phys., Vol 27, pp251–257, 1974.
31. Borak, T.B., A simple approach for calculating gamma ray skyshine for reduced shielding applications, Health Phys., Vol 29, p423–425, 1975.
32. Shultis, J.K., et.al., Approximate beam response functions for gamma-ray and neutron skyshine analysis, EES Report 217, Engineering Experimental Station, Kansas State University, Manhattan, Kansas, 1995
33. Heitler, W., The Quantum Theory of Radiation, 3rd Edition, Oxford University Press, London, 1954.
34. Nath, R., Epp, E.R., Swanson, W.P., and Bond, V., Neutrons from medical accelerators: An estimate of risk to the radiotherapy patient, Med. Phys., Vol 11, pp231–241, 1984.
35. Hoffman, R.J., and Nath, R., On the sources of radiation exposure of technologists in a radiotherapy center with high energy X-ray accelerators, Health Phys., Vol 24, pp525–526, 1973.
36. Jaeger, R.G. (Ed. in Chief), Section 8.2, Attenuation of neutrons, pp497–530, in Engineering Compendium on Radiation Shielding, Vol 1, Springer Verlag, Heidelberg, 1968.
37. National Council on Radiation Protection and Measurements, Protection Against Neutron Radiation, NCRP Report No. 38, National Commission on Radiation Protection and Measurements, Washington, D.C., 1971.
38. Kersey, R.W., Estimation of neutron and gamma radiation doses in the entrance mazes of SL75-20 linear accelerator treatment rooms, Medicamundi, Vol 24, pp151–155, 1979.
39. McCall, R.C., Jenkins, T.M., and Shore, R.A., Transport of accelerator produced neutrons in a concrete room, IEEE Trans. Nucl. Sci., Vol 26, pp1593–1602, 1979.
40. McGinley, P.H., and Butker, E.K., Evaluation of neutron dose equivalent levels at the maze entrance of medical accelerator treatment rooms, Phys. Med. Biol., Vol 18, pp279–282, 1991.
41. McGinley, P.H., Photoneutron production in the primary barriers of medical accelerator rooms, Phys. Med. Biol., Vol 34, pp777–783, 1989.
42. McGinley, P.H., Long, K., and Kaplan, R., Production of photoneutrons in a lead shield by high-energy X-rays, Phys. Med. Biol., Vol 33, pp975–980, 1988.
43. McGinley, P.H., Photoneutron production in the primary barriers of medical accelerator rooms, Health Phys., Vol. 62, pp359–362, 1992.
44. McCall, R.C., McGinley, P.H., and Huffman, K.E., Room scattered neutrons, Med. Phys., Vol. 26, pp206–207, 1999.
45. McGinley, P.H., Wood, M., Mills, M., and Rodriguez, R., Dose levels due to neutrons in the vicinity of high-energy medical accelerators, Med. Phys., Vol 3, pp397–402, 1976.
46. Bading, J.R., Zeitz, L., and Laughlin, J.S., Phosphorus activation neutron dosimetry and its application to an 18 MV radiotherapy accelerator, Med. Phys., Vol 9, pp835–843, 1982.
47. AAPM, American Association of Physicists in Medicine Report #19, "Neutron Measurements Around High Energy X-Ray Radiotherapy Machines," American Institute of Physics, New York, 1986.
48. AAPM Task Group No. 45 Report, (Nath, R., Biggs, P., Bova, F., Ling, C., Purdy, J.A., van de Geijn, J., and Weinhous, M.,) AAPM code of practice for radiotherapy accelerators: Report of AAPM Radiation Therapy Task Group No. 45, Med. Phys., Vol. 21, pp1093–1121, 1994.
49. Tosi, G., Torresin, A., Agosteo, S., Foglio Para, A., Sangiust, V., Zeni, L., and Silari, M., Neutron measurements around medical electron accelerators by active and passive techniques, Med. Phys., Vol 18, pp54–60, 1991.
50. Agosteo, S., Foglio Para, A., and Maggioni, B., Neutron fluxes in radiotherapy rooms, Med. Phys., Vol 20, pp407–414, 1993.
51. Sanchez, F., Madurga, G., and Arrans, R., Neutron measurements around an 18 MV linac, Radiother. Oncol., Vol 15, pp259–265, 1989.
52. Al-Affana, A.M., Estimation of the dose at the maze entrance for x-rays from radiotherapy linear accelerators, Med. Phys., Vol. 27, pp231–238, 2000.
53. Bramblett, R.L., Ewing, R.I., and Bonner, T.W., A new type of neutron spectrometer, Nucl. Instr. Meth., Vol. 9, pp1–12, 1960.
54. Awshalom, M., and Sanna, R.S., Application of Bonner sphere detectors in neutron field dosimetry, Radiat. Prot. Dosim., Vol. 10, pp89–101, 1985.

55. Nakumara, T., Kosako, T., and Iwai, S., Environmental neutron measurements around nuclear facilities with moderated-type neutron detector, Health Phys., Vol. 47, pp729–743, 1984.
56. Bartlett,D.T., J. Booz, J., and K.G. Harrison, K.G., (Eds:), Etched Track Neutron Dosimetry, Proceedings of a Workshop, Harwell, May 1987, Radiat. Prot. Dosim., Vol. 20 Nos. 1–2, 1987.
57. Apfel, R.E. and Yuan Chyuan Lo. "Practical Neutron Dosimetry with Superheated Drop," Health Physics, Vol 56, pp79–83, 1989.
58. Apfel, R.E., Characterisation of new passive superheated drop (bubble) dosemeters." Radiat. Prot. Dosim., Vol. 40, pp343–346, 1992.
59. d'Errico, F. and Curzio, G. Photoneutron Leakage from Medical Accelerators: A Comprehensive Approach to Patient and Personnel Dose Measurement, In: Proc. IRPA8 ISBN 1-55048-657-8, Vol. I, pp833–836 (Montreal: IRPA) 1992.
60. R. Nath, R., A. Meigooni, A., King, C., Smolen, S., and d'Errico, F., Superheated drop detector for determination of neutron dose equivalent to patients undergoing high-energy x-ray and electron radiotherapy, Med. Phys., Vol. 20, pp781–787, 1993.
61. d'Errico, F., Alberts, W.G., and Matzke, M., Advances in Superheated Drop (Bubble) Detector Techniques (In Neutron Dosimetry - Proceedings of the Eighth Symposium, Paris, France, November 13-17, 1995), Radiat. Prot. Dosim. Vol. 70, pp103–108,1997.
62. McCall, R. C., Shielding for thermal neutrons, Med. Phys., Vol. 24, pp135–136, 1997.
63. Glasgow, G.P., Residual radioactivity in radiation therapy treatment aids irradiated on medical linear accelerators, in Radiotherapy Safety, Symposium Proceedings No. 4, American Association of Physicists in Medicine, New York, 1984.
64. McGinley, P.H., Wright, B.A., and Mading, C.J., Dose to radiotherapy technologists from air activation, Med. Phys., Vol. 11, p855–858, 1984.
65. Almen, A., Ahlgren, L., and Mattson, S., Absorbed dose to technicians due to induced activity in linear accelerators for radiation therapy, Phys. Med. Biol., Vol. 36, p815–822, 1991.
66. McGinley, P. H., Miner, M.S., and Mitchum, M.L., A method for calculating the dose due to capture gamma rays in accelerator mazes, Phys. Med. Biol., Vol. 40, p1467–1473, 1995.
67. Rawlinson, J.A., Islam, M.K., and Galbraith, D.M., Dose to radiation therapists from activation of high-energy accelerators used for conventional and intensity-modulated radiation therapy, Vol. 29, p598–608, 2002.
68. National Council on Radiation Protection and Measurements, Radiation Alarms and Access Control Systems, NCRP Report No. 88, National Council on Radiation Protection and Measurements, Bethesda, Maryland, 1986.
69. B'Brien, P., Michaels, H.B., Gillies, B., Aldrich, J.E., and Andrew, J.W., Radiation protection aspects of a new high-energy linear accelerator, Med. Phys., Vol. 12, p101–107, 1985.
70. Powell, N.L., Newing, A., Bullen, M.A., Sims, C., and Leaton, S.F., A radiation safety survey on a clinac-20 linear accelerator, Phys. Med. Biol., Vol. 32, p707–718, 1987.

Additional Reading

1. Chilton, A.B., Shultis, J.K., and Faw, R.E., Principles of Radiation Shielding, Prentice-Hall, Inc., 2nd Ed., Englewood Cliffs., New Jersey, 1996.
2. McGinley, P.H., Shielding Techniques for Radiation Oncology Facilities, 2nd Edition, Medical Physics Publishing, Madison, Wisconsin, 2002.
3. IPEM, Institute of Physics and Engineering in Medicine, The design of Radiotherapy Treatment Room Facilities, IPEM, York, England.
4. McGinley, P.H., and Miner, M. S., A history of radiation shielding of x-ray therapy rooms, Health Phys., Vol. 69, pp759–765, 1995.
5. NCRP, National Council on Radiation Protection and Measurements, Neutron Contamination from Medical Electron Accelerators, NCRP Report No. 79, National Council on Radiation Protection and Measurements, Bethesda, Maryland, 1984.
6. Swanson, W.P., Radiological Safety Aspects of the Operation of Electron Linear Accelerators, IAEA Technical Report Series No. 188, International Atomic Energy Agency, Vienna, 1979.
7. NCRP, National Council on Radiation Protection and Measurements, Structural Shielding Design and Evaluation for Medical Use of X-rays and Gamma Rays up to 10 MeV, NCRP Report No. 49, National Council on Radiation Protection and Measurements, Bethesda, Maryland, 1976.
8. NCRP, National Council on Radiation Protection and Measurements, Radiation Protection Design Guidelines for 0.1–100 MeV Particle Accelerator Facilities, NCRP Report No. 51, National Council on Radiation Protection and Measurements, Bethesda, Maryland, 1977.
9. NCRP, National Council on Radiation Protection and Measurements, Medical X-ray, Electron Beam, and Gamma-Ray Protection for Energies up to 50 MeV (Equipment Design, Performance, and Use), NCRP Report No. 102, National Council on Radiation Protection and Measurements, Bethesda, Maryland, 1989.

10. Deutsches Institut für Normung, DIN-6847-2, "Medizinische Elektronenbeschleuniger-Anlagen – Teil 2: Strahlenschutzregeln für die Errichtung ", (Medical Electron Accelerators, Part 2: Radiation Protection rules for installation,) Deutsches Institut für Normung e. V., Berlin, Germany, 2002.

11. Mills, M.D., Almond, P.R., Boyer, A.L., Ochran, T.G., Madigan, W., Rich, T.A., and Dally, E.B., Shielding considerations for an operating room based intraoperative electron radiotherapy unit, Int. J. Rad. Oncol. Biol. Phys., Vol 18, p1215–1221, 1990.

12. Daves, J.L., and Mills, M.D., Shielding assessment of a mobile electron accelerator for intraoperative radiotherapy, J. Appl. Clin. Med. Phys., Vol. 2, pp165–173, 2001.

13. Maitz, A.H., Dade Lunsford, L., Wu. A., Lindner, G., and Flickinger, J.C., Shielding requirements on-site loading and acceptance testing of the Leksell Gamma Knife, Int. J. Rad. Oncol. Biol. Phys., Vol 18, p469–476, 1990.

CHAPTER 20

Radiation Safety in Brachytherapy

20.1
Introduction

In brachytherapy, small sources that contain radioactive material within a capsule are used. The current methods of brachytherapy can be divided into low-dose-rate (LDR) and high-dose-rate (HDR) techniques [1, 2], which present different hazard control problems. LDR techniques have been practiced since the discovery of radium; HDR techniques have become possible in modern times because of the development and availability of artificially produced radioactive sources of very high specific activities. Whereas LDR brachytherapy is performed with sources of low activity, of the order of a few gigabecquerel, sources having activities of 100 GBq may be employed for HDR brachytherapy. Such high-activity sources used in HDR brachytherapy should be handled only with a remote afterloading device installed in a room specially planned to have sufficient space, distance from the source to personnel, and shielding. The HDR precautions are not unlike those adopted for teletherapy treatments, with remote-control devices, shielding, safety interlocks, and radiation alarms. For an understanding of the safety and quality control problems encountered in HDR remote-loading brachytherapy, the reader is referred to the American Association of Physicists in Medicine (AAPM) Report 41 [3] and other publications [4, 5] cited at the end of this chapter. Our discussion here mainly addresses the conventional LDR techniques, which are the subject of Report No. 40 from the National Council on Radiation Protection and Measurements (NCRP) [6].

It is interesting to compare external-beam therapy with LDR brachytherapy from a radiation safety point of view. In Chapter 19, which deals with external-beam therapy, much emphasis was placed on shielding evaluations, because control of the parameters of time and distance could not provide the needed levels of safety. In LDR brachytherapy, the sources are of much lower strengths than those of the sources used for external-beam therapy. Shielding is necessary for storage and transport of LDR sources. However, during their handling, loading, or removal, a sufficient level of safety can be achieved by use of distance and time. Shielding can be added for the purpose of ALARA (as low as reasonably achievable) at the time of source handling and patient treatment.

Whereas radioisotope sources having activities of the order of 100 TBq are needed for external-beam therapy, LDR brachytherapy sources have activities of the order of only gigabecquerel. Although an external therapy beam is dangerous because it can deliver a lethal dose in a very short time, the external-beam treatment is done with great care in a well-shielded therapy room with engineered safety features, remote 'on' and 'off' mechanisms, safety interlocks, etc. LDR brachytherapy sources can be used without such elaborate built-in safety mechanisms. However, the potential for overexposure from them should not be underestimated. Many incidents of high radiation exposures have resulted because of careless handling of LDR brachytherapy sources. In this chapter, we discuss the radiation hazard control in LDR brachytherapy.

20.2
Role of Time and Afterloading

As a general safety rule, one should work with any radiation source only for the minimum time one needs for its loading or removal. Since the early 1960s, afterloading techniques in brachytherapy have contributed to much reduction in the time spent in the handling of sources and hence in the radiation exposure to personnel [7–10]. This was not so in the first decades of the practice of brachytherapy, when the radioactive sources were loaded into applicators (i. e., source carriers or guide tubes) at the very beginning of the procedure. These applicators were then inserted in the tissues or body cavities of patients. The disadvantage of such a method was that it involved handling of radiation sources even during inserting and positioning of the applicators. The practice of using applicators with sources already loaded has been abandoned. Instead, empty applicators are first inserted and manipulated until they are in the correct configuration in the patient. It is only after ensuring that they have been properly placed with respect to the tumor or anatomic structures in the body that the radioactive sources are loaded into the applicators. Hence, the sources are said to be 'afterloaded,' and the technique is called 'afterloading' technique.

Afterloading methods can be manual or remote. In manual afterloading, the sources are mounted at the tip of a long handle. The sources, which are held by hand at the inactive end of the long handle, are inserted into the applicators. In remote afterloading, a sophisticated remote-handling apparatus steers the sources into and out of the applicators by an electromechanical or pneumatic mechanism which has a timer to control the duration of treatment. Remote-loading techniques have been used for both LDR and HDR treatments.

20.3
Role of Distance

When radioactive sources are handled, it is necessary to maintain a safe distance between the body and the sources. Handling them at too short a distance can result in an unacceptably high dose. As an example, let us compare two possibilities. First, let us say that a worker takes 5 min (300 sec) to pick up and load a brachytherapy source into a catheter by using forceps of 15 cm length. Alternatively, another worker picks up the source with his finger tips and does the loading quickly, in just 1 sec. In the latter instance, the fingers are on the surface of the metallic capsule of the source, and the surface may be only 0.5 mm from the radioactive material in the source. We know that the dose is directly proportional to the time of irradiation, but is inversely proportional to the square of the distance. If we take into account the differences in the times and distances in the two situations, the dose received by the finger tips in the second case will be more than that in the first case by a ratio given by

$$\frac{(15\,\text{cm})^2}{(300\,\text{sec})} \times \frac{1\,\text{sec}}{(0.05\,\text{cm})^2} = 300$$

In other words, it will take as long as 25 h (i. e., 300 × 5 min) for the worker who used the 15-cm forceps to be subjected to the high dose received by the other worker who touched the source capsule. Thus, distance is a very effective parameter for reducing the radiation dose. Especially in brachytherapy, speed of execution cannot substitute for the benefit of distance and inverse-square dose fall-off. At close distances, a very high dose can be received in fractions of seconds.

Sources should never be touched. All source manipulations should be done with forceps or tongs at least 15 cm in length. It is worthwhile for workers to practice the use of forceps or any remote handling procedure with nonradioactive 'dummy' sources, to develop timing efficiency for handling the actual radiation sources.

20.4
Role of Shielding

Shielding is essential for the safe storage and transport of brachytherapy sources. Shielding can be employed, as well, for the purpose of ALARA, to add to the advantages already contributed by control of distance and time. A movable shield placed by the bedside of the patient can reduce the dose levels in the hallways and adjacent rooms.

The physical characteristics and shielding data for several radioisotope sources used in brachytherapy are given in Table 17.1 in Chapter 17. ^{137}Cs and ^{192}Ir have been preferred over ^{226}Ra, ^{60}Co, and ^{182}Ta for temporary implants, because of the more efficient shielding of their radiation by lead. The merits of newer sources such as ^{241}Am, ^{145}Sm, and ^{169}Yb have also been considered for potential use in the future. The very low energy of the photons emitted by these sources (and also by ^{125}I and ^{103}Pd for permanent implants) makes effective shielding possible even by 0.5 mm of lead.

20.5
Monitoring Instruments

Radiation survey meters of the ionization and GM (Geiger-Mueller) counter types should be readily available in the department. The former should be capable of measuring air-kerma rates from $10\,\mu\text{Gy h}^{-1}$ to $1\,\text{Gy h}^{-1}$ (i. e., exposure rates from approximately $1\,\text{mR h}^{-1}$ to $100\,\text{R h}^{-1}$). The latter should have enough sensitivity to measure levels of $0.1\,\mu\text{Gy h}^{-1}$ (i. e., $0.01\,\text{mR h}^{-1}$), comparable to the background. The survey meters should be calibrated periodically by an authorized calibration laboratory providing traceability of the readings to the national and international standards. The meters should be checked often with a test source so that their correct performance is ensured.

20.6
Source Storage and Preparation

Brachytherapy sources must be stored in a safe having 3 to 4 TVL of lead shielding (Figure 20.1). The storage safe may have many drawers with holes or recesses for

Fig. 20.1. A lead safe designed with drawers and slots for placement of encapsulated brachytherapy sources. An L-shaped lead block with a lead glass visor is located in front of the safe

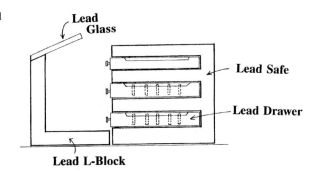

placement of the sources. Each source should have an identification label, engraved mark, or color code that can readily be seen. A fixed magnifying glass should be installed as an aid for reading the identification. Hand-held magnifiers may contribute to unnecessary exposure. Sources can be categorized or grouped in terms of their type, radioisotope content, or strength and stored in separate drawers for quick retrieval for use. The storage safe is to be placed behind an L-shaped block offering 2 to 4 TVL of lead shielding with a lead-glass visor (Figure 20.1). The worker should stand in front of the L-block so that the body is well shielded during retrieval of the sources from the safe and preparation for loading. Forceps and tongs should be provided for ready use. A well-type lead container should be available besides the lead block for temporary storage during the selection and preparation of sources for afterloading. Threading through the eyelet of any source should be done after the source is inserted in a hole in a lead block, so that most of its radioactive length is blocked, with only the eyelet portion protruding outside the shield.

Beta sources, such as ^{90}Sr-^{90}Y, are to be handled behind a shield of a low-Z transparent plastic material such as acrylic. Lead is not a good β-ray shield because the interaction of β radiation with lead produces bremsstrahlung. Beta sources are usually mounted on the tip of a rod (Figure 20.2) that has a plastic shield mounted behind the source. Ophthalmic β applicators may deliver a dose of 100 Gy on their surface in only a few seconds. The source should always be held in such a way that the plastic shield intervenes between the source and the operator. Fingers should not be placed too close to the surface of the source. The source applicator should be stored in a specially designed plastic container having a sufficient thickness of plastic to absorb the β radiation (Figure 20.2b). The applicator should be taken out of its box only for the short time needed for use. All preparation of the patient should be done in advance. The duration of irradiation may be very short, lasting just a few seconds. It is worthwhile to establish a method of timing by using a stopwatch to control the period of treatment exactly. The procedure should be practiced so that it will be accurate and safe when being used on a patient.

The radiation levels in the source storage room should be surveyed frequently to ensure that no source is left outside the storage safe. Survey meters should be readily available in the source room for locating any misplaced, dropped, or lost source. The room where the sources are stored should be locked, and access should be allowed only to authorized personnel.

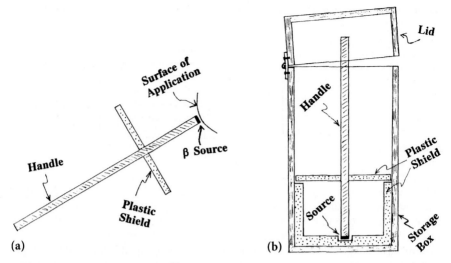

Fig. 20.2. (a) Typical appearance of an ^{90}Sr β-ray eye applicator with the source at the tip of a rod and a plastic shield mounted behind the source. (b) The applicator is stored in a plastic box

20.7
Source Inventory

A record of the brachytherapy sources available in the department and of their actual locations should be maintained. A misplaced or lost brachytherapy source can become a radiation hazard to the public. The removal of any source from storage, its insertion in a patient, its removal from the patient after completion of treatment, and its return to storage should all be recorded in a log book. Records of receipt, storage, use, and return of rental sources should likewise be maintained.

The use of flexible radioactive wires (of ^{192}Ir, ^{182}Ta, or ^{198}Au) can create special problems [11]. A single long wire may be acquired and cut into the desired lengths for use; thus, the total number of sources to be tracked can change. Proper record-keeping of how a particular long wire is used and disposed of is necessary for control of the radiation hazard. Cut pieces of radioactive wires should be traced and accounted for to prevent loss.

20.8
Source Wipe Tests

A basic precaution required with the use of radioactive materials is to prevent any spread of radioactive contamination. The possibility for such a spread is minimal with brachytherapy sources, provided the sources are always handled in such a way as not to threaten the integrity of the encapsulation [12, 13]. Sources should not be heated or subjected to steam for sterilization, because that would damage the capsule. Only chemical sterilization should be used. All brachytherapy sources should be checked periodically for any leakage of radioactivity resulting from cracking or rupture of the capsule. Wiping the surface of a source capsule with cotton swabs and counting the wipes for any radioactive emission by a high-sensitivity counter can reveal any breach in the capsule.

Radium sources are particularly hazardous and should be tested frequently for radon leakage [14]. In radium sources, there is pressure build-up due to both α particles (which are gaseous helium ions) and the radium decay product of radon gas. Leakage of radon from radium sources with defective encapsulation can become a major radiation hazard, because the diffusing radon can contribute to the deposition of its radioactive daughter products on walls, surfaces, and floors throughout a department. Many radium sources used in the past have been phased out and replaced by the safer non-radium substitutes.

The tools used for cutting radioactive wires are likely to become contaminated, albeit with a low probability. Hence it is advisable to keep these tools isolated from others. Wipe tests on them can reveal any contamination, which may require a clean-up.

20.9
Source Transport

Radioactive sources are transported from the source storage facility to the patient room for loading into the patient. A lead-shielded transport container that can be rolled on wheels is useful for this purpose (Figure 20.3). A transport container specifically designed to carry the afterloading inserts for the particular applicators in use at a given clinic can be obtained commercially.

Shipping of radioactive sources to other institutions or receipt or return of sources from or to source vendors should be done in containers that have sufficient shielding. The dose rates on the surface of these containers can be reduced further by the use of internal spacers which increase the distance of the container surface from the sources. In most jurisdictions, there are regulations concerning the transport of radioactive

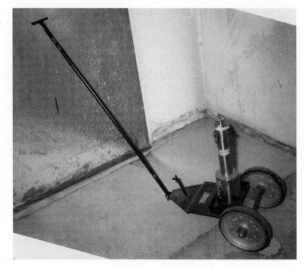

Fig. 20.3. A lead-walled cart for transporting brachytherapy sources between the source storage area and the patient room

materials. These usually require signing of shipping certificates indicating the type of source (needles, wires, sealed, unsealed, etc.), the radioisotope, the amount of activity, and the radiation levels on the surface and at 1 m from the shipping container, and they require labeling of the container with radioactivity warning signs.

20.10
Safety of Nurses and Visitors During Treatment

LDR brachytherapy is a procedure that can extend over several days. Proper care is necessary for avoiding unnecessary irradiation of auxiliary medical staff, particularly nurses, attending the patient, and also exposure of visitors [15]. Preferably, a private room should be made available. This is a regulatory requirement in some jurisdictions. A corner room should be selected where possible, so that traffic is minimal. The location of the patient's bed in the room should be such that irradiation of other patients, staff, and visitors is minimized. After the sources are inserted in the patient, the radiation levels at different points in the room and adjacent areas should be surveyed and noted. Efforts should be made to ensure that the radiation levels in areas to which the public may have access are minimal. Air-kerma rates of less than $2\,\mu Gy\,h^{-1}$ can usually be achieved in the hallways and at the door by proper selection of the position of the bed in the room and the choice of the room itself. Any chair in the room where a visitor may sit can be moved to a location with a low radiation level, preferably less than $2\,mR\,h^{-1}$ (which corresponds approximately to $17\,\mu Gy\,h^{-1}$ air-kerma rate). The visiting time may be restricted to less than an hour.

The dose rate at the bedside and at 1 m from the patient should be recorded. The nursing staff should be advised to keep a distance of at least 2 m from the patient if possible without compromising nursing care. A maximum duration for nursing at the bedside of the patient can be indicated as guidance to the nurses. This can be based on the projected number of radioactive patients whom a nurse may attend in a year during her rotation in the clinic, and on the ALARA policy of the institution. If nursing for an extended period is warranted, the (afterloaded) sources may be removed temporarily and placed in the lead transport container, which may be left in the room until the end of treatment.

Figure 20.4 shows the different warning signs that can be posted. These include a warning sign for the entrance door to the patient's room (Figure 20.4a) indicating the radioisotope and the activity in use. Other signs in Figure 20.4 mark the patient's chart to alert the nurses (Figure 20.4b and c) about either temporary or permanent radioactive implants. Bedside lead shields can be acquired and used for ALARA [16, 17]. The patient should wear a wrist band indicating that he or she is radioactive. Nurses should be educated and informed about radiation safety principles so that they understand how to work with radiation, rather than fearing the radiation [18]. They should be made familiar with the appearance of the sources, applicators, and warning signs.

20.11
Procedure After Treatment

At the end of treatment, all sources should be removed from the patient except in the case of permanent implants (as discussed in Section 20.12). A procedure for safe

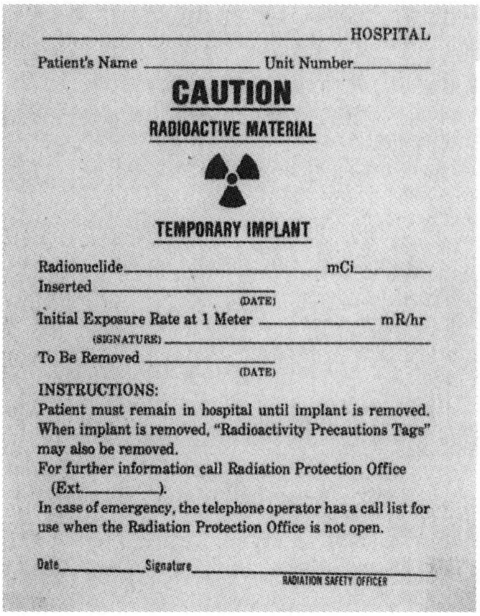

Fig. 20.4. Radiation warning signs (**a**) for labeling the entrance door of the patient treatment room, (**b**) for labeling the patient's treatment chart for a temporary implant, and (**c**) for labeling the patient's treatment chart for a permanent implant

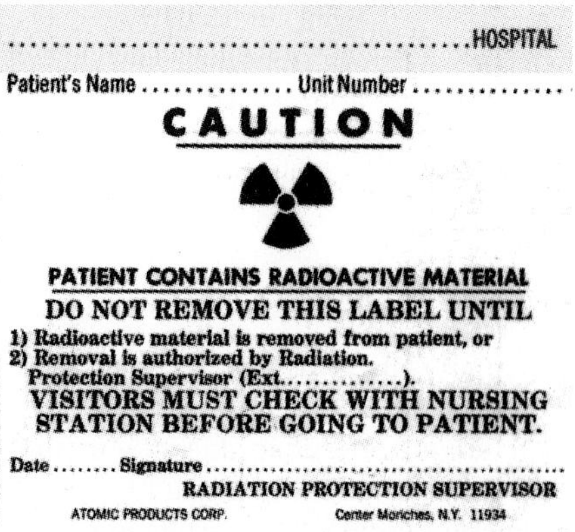

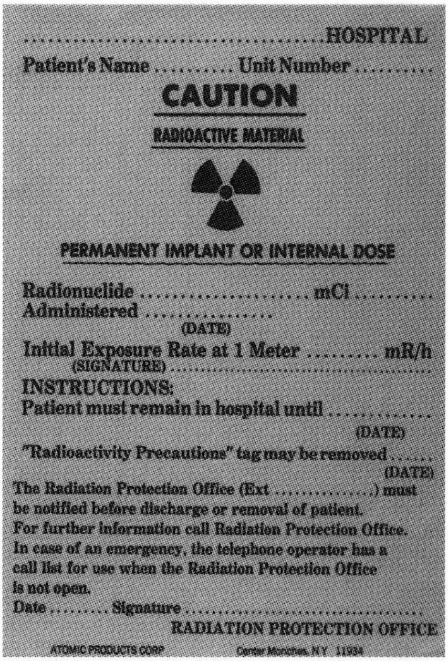

removal of sources should be established in the institution for minimum exposure to personnel. The removal technique should not cause physical damage to the sources. It is also important to have a method that will definitely succeed in removing the sources. There have been instances of afterloaded sources left lodged in patient tissues after an attempt at removal. The patient's body should be surveyed to ensure that all radiation sources have been removed prior to his or her discharge from the hospital. The room should be surveyed for radiation levels so that any left-over or dropped source is detected. All trash from the room should be surveyed for radiation emission prior to disposal. Only after it has been ascertained that all sources have been recovered for return to storage can the safety signs be removed. Without much delay, the removed sources should be taken back for inventory and storage.

20.12
Permanent Implants

Radiation sources of ^{222}Rn, ^{198}Au, ^{125}I, and ^{103}Pd have been used for permanent implants. In the U.S., the use of ^{222}Rn is a thing of the past. ^{125}I, and ^{103}Pd, have lower radiation energies than does ^{198}Au, and hence they are more efficiently shielded by lead. Furthermore, compared to ^{198}Au, they have longer mean lives, giving a longer irradiation period. This results in a lower strength of sources at the time of implantation for the delivery of any desired dose. Even during hospitalization, the patient's self-shielding is greater for ^{125}I and ^{103}Pd than for ^{198}Au [19]. Overall, ^{125}I and ^{103}Pd are preferable to ^{198}Au from the point of view of the radiation safety of hospital personnel.

For permanent implants, the same precautions as for removable implants should be taken while the patient is hospitalized. Local regulations should be observed in deciding on the appropriate time for the discharge of these patients. One guideline requires that the radioactivity in a patient with a permanent implant should reach less than 1.11 Gbq (30 mCi) for the patient to be discharged from the hospital [6]. According to another guideline, the radiation level at 1 m from the patient should be less than $50\,\mu\text{Sv}\,\text{h}^{-1}$ (5 mrem h^{-1}) for discharge [20].

Radioactive seeds may be expelled in urine or other body excretions, especially in the case of permanent prostate implants. The urine should be checked for the presence of radioactive seeds. Any source, if found, should be segregated and taken to the storage room. The source either can be stored for decay over a period of 10 half-lives or can be returned to the source vendor for disposal.

After discharge, a patient with a permanent implant should be advised to follow certain precautions to reduce the irradiation of other members of the household. The patient may be asked to maintain a distance of 1 m from others as much as possible. Particular care should be taken to avoid exposure of pregnant women and persons below the age of 18 years. The patient's relatives should be properly educated and informed and should not be driven to panic. The hazards should not be overrated because, unlike the staff in the hospital, the patient's relatives are not frequently close to patients implanted with radiation sources.

If a patient containing radioactive materials dies in the hospital, the volume of tissue implanted can be excised and isolated to be left to decay. This precaution can also be taken if the body is autopsied.

20.13
Personnel Monitoring

In addition to the use of chest monitors, the use of wrist and finger radiation monitoring badges is helpful and desirable for those who handle brachytherapy sources. The doses recorded by these monitors can alert the radiation safety officer to the possible need to improve the source-handling procedures.

20.14
Conclusion

The use of brachytherapy sources need not be feared if care is exercised. A proper understanding of the role of distance in improving radiation safety is very important. Sources should never be touched for saving time or for obtaining quick results in a panic situation. Preloading techniques should be replaced by afterloading methods.

References

1. Martinez, A.A., Orton, C.G., and Mould, R.F. (Eds.), Brachytherapy HDR and LDR, Proceedings of Remote Afterloading: State of the Art Conference, Nucletron Corporation, Columbia, Maryland, 1990.
2. Joslin, C.A.F., Brachytherapy: A clinical dilemma, Int. J. Radiat. Oncol. Biol. Phys., Vol 19, p801–802, 1990.
3. American Association of Physicists in Medicine, Remote Afterloading Technology, AAPM Report No. 41, American Association of Physicists in Medicine, American Insitute of Physics, New York, 1993.
4. IEC, Particular Requirements for the Safety of Remote Controlled Automatically Driven Gamma-ray Afterloading Equipment, International Standard IEC 601, Medical Electrical Equipment, Part 2, Bureau de la Commission Electrotechnique Internationale, Geneva, 1989.
5. Almond, P.R., Remote Afterloading, p601–619, in AAPM Monograph No. 9, Advances in Radiotherapy Treatment Planning, Wright, A.E., and Boyer, A.L. (Eds.), American Association of Physicists in Medicine, New York, 1983.
6. National Council on Radiation Protection and Measurements, Protection Against Radiation from Brachytherapy Sources, NCRP Report No. 40, National Council on Radiation Protection and Measurements, Washington, D.C., 1972.
7. Paine, C.H., Modern afterloading methods for interstitial radiotherapy, Clin. Radiol., Vol 23, p263–272, 1972.
8. Henschke, U.K., Hilaris, B.S., and Mahan, G.D., Afterloading in interstitial and intracavitary radiation therapy, Am. J. Roentgenol., Vol 90, p386–395, 1963.
9. Suit, H.D., Moore, E.B., Fletcher, G.H., and Worsnop, R., Modification of Fletcher ovoid system for afterloading, using standardized radium tubes (milligram and microgram), Radiology, Vol 81, p126–131, 1963.
10. Horowitz, H., Kereiakes, J.G., Bahr, G.K., Cluxton, S.E., and Barrett, C.M., An afterloading system utilizing cesium-137 for the treatment of carcinoma of the cervix, Am. J. Roentgenol., Vol 91, p176–191, 1964.
11. Arnott, S.J., Law, J., Ash, D. et al., Problems associated with iridium-192 wire implants, Clin. Radiol., Vol 36, p283–285, 1985.
12. International Organisation for Standardisation (ISO), Sealed Radioactive Sources – Leak Test Methods, Technical Report 4862, Geneva, Switzerland, 1979.
13. British Standards Institution, Sealed Radioactive Sources, BS5288, British Standards Institute, London, 1976.
14. Wood, V.A. (Ed.), A collection of radium leak test articles, U.S. Public Health Service Publication, MORP 68-1, U.S. Government Printing Office, Washington, D.C., 1968.
15. National Council on Radiation Protection and Measurements, Precautions in the Management of Patients Who Have Received Therapeutic Amounts of Radionuclides, NCRP Report No. 37, National Council on Radiation Protection and Measurements, Washington, D.C., 1970.
16. Thomadsen, B., van de Geijn, J., Buchler, D., and Paliwal, B., Fortification of existing rooms for brachytherapy patients, Health Phys., Vol 45, p607–615, 1983.
17. Gitterman, M., and Webster, E.W., Shielding hospital rooms for brachytherapy patients: Design, regulatory and cost/benefit factors, Health Phys., Vol 46, p617–625, 1984.
18. Sedham, L.N., and Yanni, M.I., Radiation therapy and nurses' fears of radiation exposure, Cancer Nursing, Vol 8, p129–134, 1985.
19. Dawes, T.J.O.K., and Aird, E.G.A., Preliminary experience with 125I seeds in Newcastle upon Tyne, Clin. Radiol., Vol 36, p359–364, 1985.
20. United States Nuclear Regulatory Commission, Rules and Regulations, Code of Federal Regulation, Energy, Part 10, Paragraph 35.75, p532, Revised Jan 01,1994, U.S. Government Printing Office, Washington, D.C.

Additional Reading

1. International Atomic Energy Agency, Physical Aspects of Radioisotope Brachytherapy, IAEA Technical Report Series No. 75, International Atomic Energy Agency, Vienna, 1967.
2. Institute of Physical Sciences in Medicine, Report 45, Dosimetry and Clinical Uses of Afterloading Systems, Alderson, A.R. (Ed.), Institute of Physical Sciences in Medicine, London, 1986.
3. Institute of Physical Sciences, Report 46, Chapter 3, Brachytherapy, in Radiation Protection in Radiotherapy, Mckenzie, A.L., Shaw, J.E., Stephenson, S.K., and Turner, R.C.R. (Eds.), Institute of Physical Sciences in Medicine, London, 1986.
4. American Association of Physicists in Medicine, Symposium Proceedings No. 4, Radiotherapy Safety, Thomadsen, B. (Ed.), American Institute of Physics, New York, 1982.
5. American Association of Physicists in Medicine, Advances in Radiation Oncology Physics, Dosimetry, Treatment Planning, and Brachytherapy, American Association of Physicists in Medicine Monograph No. 19, American Institute of Physics, New York, 1993.
6. Williamson, J.F., Thomadsen, B.R., Nath, R. (Eds.), Brachytherapy Physics, Lectures presented at 1994 Summer School of American Association of Physicists in Medicine, Medical Physics Publishing, Madison, Wisconsin, 1995.
7. Joslin, C.A.F., Flynn, A., Hall. E.J., (Eds.) Principles and practice of brachytherapy using afterloading systems, Hodder Arnold Publisher, London , 2001.

Appendix A and B

Appendix A

APPENDIX A. Electron Mass Stopping Powers (in MeV cm^2 g^{-1}) for Various Materials

Energy (MeV)	Air (Dry) Collision (S_c/ρ)	Radiative (S_r/ρ)	Total (S/ρ)	Water Collision (S_c/ρ)	Radiative (S_r/ρ)	Total (S/ρ)
0.0100	1.975E+1	3.897E−3	1.976E+1	2.256E+1	3.898E−3	2.257E+1
0.0125	1.663E+1	3.921E−3	1.663E+1	1.897E+1	3.927E−3	1.898E+1
0.0150	1.445E+1	3.937E−3	1.445E+1	1.647E+1	3.944E−3	1.647E+1
0.0175	1.283E+1	3.946E−3	1.283E+1	1.461E+1	3.955E−3	1.461E+1
0.0200	1.157E+1	3.954E−3	1.158E+1	1.317E+1	3.963E−3	1.318E+1
0.0250	9.753E+0	3.966E−3	9.757E+0	1.109E+1	3.974E−3	1.110E+1
0.0300	8.492E+0	3.976E−3	8.496E+0	9.653E+0	3.984E−3	9.657E+0
0.0350	7.563E+0	3.986E−3	7.567E+0	8.592E+0	3.994E−3	8.596E+0
0.0400	6.848E+0	3.998E−3	6.852E+0	7.777E+0	4.005E−3	7.781E+0
0.0450	6.281E+0	4.011E−3	6.285E+0	7.130E+0	4.018E−3	7.134E+0
0.0500	5.819E+0	4.025E−3	5.823E+0	6.603E+0	4.031E−3	6.607E+0
0.0550	5.435E+0	4.040E−3	5.439E+0	6.166E+0	4.046E−3	6.170E+0
0.0600	5.111E+0	4.057E−3	5.115E+0	5.797E+0	4.062E−3	5.801E+0
0.0700	4.593E+0	4.093E−3	4.597E+0	5.207E+0	4.098E−3	5.211E+0
0.0800	4.198E+0	4.133E−3	4.202E+0	4.757E+0	4.138E−3	4.762E+0
0.0900	3.886E+0	4.175E−3	3.890E+0	4.402E+0	4.181E−3	4.407E+0
0.1000	3.633E+0	4.222E−3	3.637E+0	4.115E+0	4.228E−3	4.120E+0
0.1250	3.172E+0	4.348E−3	3.177E+0	3.591E+0	4.355E−3	3.596E+0
0.1500	2.861E+0	4.485E−3	2.865E+0	3.238E+0	4.494E−3	3.242E+0
0.1750	2.637E+0	4.633E−3	2.642E+0	2.984E+0	4.643E−3	2.988E+0
0.2000	2.470E+0	4.789E−3	2.474E+0	2.793E+0	4.801E−3	2.798E+0
0.2500	2.236E+0	5.126E−3	2.242E+0	2.528E+0	5.141E−3	2.533E+0
0.3000	2.084E+0	5.495E−3	2.089E+0	2.355E+0	5.514E−3	2.360E+0
0.3500	1.978E+0	5.890E−3	1.984E+0	2.235E+0	5.913E−3	2.241E+0
0.4000	1.902E+0	6.311E−3	1.908E+0	2.148E+0	6.339E−3	2.154E+0
0.4500	1.845E+0	6.757E−3	1.852E+0	2.083E+0	6.787E−3	2.090E+0
0.5000	1.802E+0	7.223E−3	1.809E+0	2.034E+0	7.257E−3	2.041E+0
0.5500	1.769E+0	7.708E−3	1.776E+0	1.995E+0	7.747E−3	2.003E+0
0.6000	1.743E+0	8.210E−3	1.751E+0	1.963E+0	8.254E−3	1.972E+0
0.7000	1.706E+0	9.258E−3	1.715E+0	1.917E+0	9.312E−3	1.926E+0
0.8000	1.683E+0	1.036E−2	1.694E+0	1.886E+0	1.043E−2	1.896E+0
0.9000	1.669E+0	1.151E−2	1.681E+0	1.864E+0	1.159E−2	1.876E+0
1.0000	1.661E+0	1.271E−2	1.674E+0	1.849E+0	1.280E−2	1.862E+0
1.2500	1.655E+0	1.588E−2	1.671E+0	1.829E+0	1.600E−2	1.845E+0
1.5000	1.661E+0	1.927E−2	1.680E+0	1.822E+0	1.942E−2	1.841E+0
1.7500	1.672E+0	2.284E−2	1.694E+0	1.821E+0	2.303E−2	1.844E+0
2.0000	1.684E+0	2.656E−2	1.711E+0	1.824E+0	2.678E−2	1.850E+0
2.5000	1.712E+0	3.437E−2	1.747E+0	1.834E+0	3.468E−2	1.868E+0
3.0000	1.740E+0	4.260E−2	1.783E+0	1.846E+0	4.299E−2	1.889E+0
3.5000	1.766E+0	5.115E−2	1.817E+0	1.858E+0	5.164E−2	1.910E+0
4.0000	1.790E+0	5.999E−2	1.850E+0	1.870E+0	6.058E−2	1.931E+0
4.5000	1.812E+0	6.908E−2	1.882E+0	1.882E+0	6.976E−2	1.951E+0
5.0000	1.833E+0	7.838E−2	1.911E+0	1.892E+0	7.917E−2	1.971E+0
5.5000	1.852E+0	8.787E−2	1.940E+0	1.902E+0	8.876E−2	1.991E+0
6.0000	1.870E+0	9.754E−2	1.968E+0	1.911E+0	9.854E−2	2.010E+0
7.0000	1.902E+0	1.173E−1	2.020E+0	1.928E+0	1.185E−1	2.047E+0
8.0000	1.931E+0	1.376E−1	2.068E+0	1.943E+0	1.391E−1	2.082E+0
9.0000	1.956E+0	1.584E−1	2.115E+0	1.956E+0	1.601E−1	2.116E+0
10.000	1.979E+0	1.795E−1	2.159E+0	1.968E+0	1.814E−1	2.149E+0
15.000	2.069E+0	2.895E−1	2.359E+0	2.014E+0	2.926E−1	2.306E+0
20.000	2.134E+0	4.042E−1	2.539E+0	2.046E+0	4.086E−1	2.454E+0
25.000	2.185E+0	5.219E−1	2.707E+0	2.070E+0	5.277E−1	2.598E+0

From Attix, F.H., Appendix E, in Introduction to Radiological Physics and Radiation Dosimetry, John Wiley & Sons, New York, 1986. Based on original data of Berger, M.J., and Seltzer, S.M., Stopping Powers and Ranges of Electrons and Positrons, NBSIR 82-2550 A, National Bureau of Standards, Washington, D.C., 1983. With permission.

APPENDIX A. (Contd.). Electron Mass Stopping Powers (in MeV cm^2 g^{-1}) for Various Materials

Energy (MeV)	Adipose Tissue (ICRP)			Cortical Bone (ICRP)		
	Collision (S_c/ρ)	Radiative (S_r/ρ)	Total (S/ρ)	Collision (S_c/ρ)	Radiative (S_r/ρ)	Total (S/ρ)
0.0100	2.347E+1	3.168E−3	2.347E+1	1.971E+1	5.461E−3	1.972E+1
0.0125	1.971E+1	3.184E−3	1.971E+1	1.663E+1	5.579E−3	1.664E+1
0.0150	1.709E+1	3.194E−3	1.709E+1	1.447E+1	5.664E−3	1.447E+1
0.0175	1.515E+1	3.201E−3	1.515E+1	1.286E+1	5.728E−3	1.287E+1
0.0200	1.365E+1	3.207E−3	1.365E+1	1.161E+1	5.778E−3	1.162E+1
0.0250	1.148E+1	3.217E−3	1.149E+1	9.804E+0	5.853E−3	9.810E+0
0.0300	9.984E+0	3.227E−3	9.987E+0	8.546E+0	5.907E−3	8.552E+0
0.0350	8.881E+0	3.238E−3	8.884E+0	7.618E+0	5.951E−3	7.624E+0
0.0400	8.034E+0	3.249E−3	8.037E+0	6.903E+0	5.989E−3	6.909E+0
0.0450	7.362E+0	3.262E−3	7.365E+0	6.335E+0	6.022E−3	6.341E+0
0.0500	6.816E+0	3.275E−3	6.819E+0	5.872E+0	6.054E−3	5.879E+0
0.0550	6.362E+0	3.290E−3	6.365E+0	5.488E+0	6.084E−3	5.494E+0
0.0600	5.979E+0	3.305E−3	5.983E+0	5.163E+0	6.113E−3	5.169E+0
0.0700	5.369E+0	3.338E−3	5.372E+0	4.643E+0	6.171E−3	4.649E+0
0.0800	4.903E+0	3.373E−3	4.906E+0	4.246E+0	6.230E−3	4.252E+0
0.0900	4.535E+0	3.411E−3	4.539E+0	3.932E+0	6.292E−3	3.939E+0
0.1000	4.238E+0	3.452E−3	4.241E+0	3.678E+0	6.356E−3	3.685E+0
0.1250	3.696E+0	3.562E−3	3.700E+0	3.215E+0	6.530E−3	3.221E+0
0.1500	3.330E+0	3.681E−3	3.334E+0	2.901E+0	6.719E−3	2.908E+0
0.1750	3.068E+0	3.808E−3	3.071E+0	2.676E+0	6.923E−3	2.683E+0
0.2000	2.871E+0	3.943E−3	2.875E+0	2.507E+0	7.140E−3	2.514E+0
0.2500	2.597E+0	4.232E−3	2.601E+0	2.272E+0	7.612E−3	2.280E+0
0.3000	2.418E+0	4.547E−3	2.422E+0	2.119E+0	8.129E−3	2.127E+0
0.3500	2.294E+0	4.885E−3	2.299E+0	2.011E+0	8.685E−3	2.020E+0
0.4000	2.204E+0	5.244E−3	2.209E+0	1.931E+0	9.276E−3	1.941E+0
0.4500	2.135E+0	5.623E−3	2.141E+0	1.871E+0	9.901E−3	1.881E+0
0.5000	2.081E+0	6.020E−3	2.087E+0	1.825E+0	1.055E−2	1.836E+0
0.5500	2.039E+0	6.433E−3	2.045E+0	1.789E+0	1.124E−2	1.800E+0
0.6000	2.005E+0	6.860E−3	2.011E+0	1.760E+0	1.194E−2	1.772E+0
0.7000	1.954E+0	7.753E−3	1.962E+0	1.718E+0	1.341E−2	1.732E+0
0.8000	1.921E+0	8.692E−3	1.929E+0	1.690E+0	1.495E−2	1.705E+0
0.9000	1.897E+0	9.674E−3	1.907E+0	1.671E+0	1.657E−2	1.688E+0
1.0000	1.880E+0	1.070E−2	1.891E+0	1.658E+0	1.824E−2	1.677E+0
1.2500	1.858E+0	1.340E−2	1.871E+0	1.642E+0	2.267E−2	1.665E+0
1.5000	1.849E+0	1.629E−2	1.865E+0	1.637E+0	2.740E−2	1.665E+0
1.7500	1.848E+0	1.934E−2	1.867E+0	1.639E+0	3.237E−2	1.671E+0
2.0000	1.850E+0	2.252E−2	1.873E+0	1.643E+0	3.755E−2	1.681E+0
2.5000	1.860E+0	2.921E−2	1.889E+0	1.656E+0	4.840E−2	1.704E+0
3.0000	1.872E+0	3.626E−2	1.908E+0	1.670E+0	5.981E−2	1.730E+0
3.5000	1.885E+0	4.360E−2	1.928E+0	1.684E+0	7.165E−2	1.755E+0
4.0000	1.897E+0	5.120E−2	1.948E+0	1.697E+0	8.386E−2	1.781E+0
4.5000	1.909E+0	5.901E−2	1.968E+0	1.709E+0	9.638E−2	1.805E+0
5.0000	1.920E+0	6.701E−2	1.987E+0	1.720E+0	1.092E−1	1.829E+0
5.5000	1.930E+0	7.518E−2	2.005E+0	1.731E+0	1.222E−1	1.853E+0
6.0000	1.939E+0	8.350E−2	2.023E+0	1.740E+0	1.355E−1	1.876E+0
7.0000	1.956E+0	1.005E−1	2.057E+0	1.758E+0	1.626E−1	1.921E+0
8.0000	1.972E+0	1.181E−1	2.090E+0	1.773E+0	1.904E−1	1.964E+0
9.0000	1.985E+0	1.360E−1	2.121E+0	1.787E+0	2.188E−1	2.006E+0
10.000	1.997E+0	1.542E−1	2.151E+0	1.799E+0	2.476E−1	2.046E+0
15.000	2.042E+0	2.492E−1	2.291E+0	1.844E+0	3.971E−1	2.241E+0
20.000	2.073E+0	3.485E−1	2.421E+0	1.874E+0	5.525E−1	2.427E+0
25.000	2.095E+0	4.505E−1	2.546E+0	1.897E+0	7.117E−1	2.609E+0

APPENDIX A. (Contd.). Electron Mass Stopping Powers (in MeV cm^2 g^{-1}) for Various Materials

Energy (MeV)	Skeletal Muscle (ICRP)			Teflon		
	Collision (S_c/ρ)	Radiative (S_r/ρ)	Total (S/ρ)	Collision (S_c/ρ)	Radiative (S_r/ρ)	Total (S/ρ)
0.0100	2.231E+1	3.835E−3	2.231E+1	1.843E+1	4.211E−3	1.843E+1
0.0125	1.876E+1	3.863E−3	1.877E+1	1.553E+1	4.247E−3	1.554E+1
0.0150	1.628E+1	3.880E−3	1.629E+1	1.351E+1	4.271E−3	1.351E+1
0.0175	1.445E+1	3.892E−3	1.445E+1	1.200E+1	4.287E−3	1.201E+1
0.0200	1.303E+1	3.901E−3	1.303E+1	1.084E+1	4.300E−3	1.084E+1
0.0250	1.097E+1	3.913E−3	1.098E+1	9.141E+0	4.316E−3	9.146E+0
0.0300	9.547E+0	3.924E−3	9.551E+0	7.965E+0	4.329E−3	7.970E+0
0.0350	8.498E+0	3.934E−3	8.502E+0	7.098E+0	4.341E−3	7.102E+0
0.0400	7.692E+0	3.946E−3	7.696E+0	6.430E+0	4.353E−3	6.435E+0
0.0450	7.052E+0	3.959E−3	7.056E+0	5.900E+0	4.366E−3	5.904E+0
0.0500	6.531E+0	3.973E−3	6.535E+0	5.468E+0	4.380E−3	5.472E+0
0.0550	6.099E+0	3.988E−3	6.102E+0	5.109E+0	4.395E−3	5.113E+0
0.0600	5.733E+0	4.004E−3	5.737E+0	4.806E+0	4.410E−3	4.810E+0
0.0700	5.151E+0	4.040E−3	5.155E+0	4.321E+0	4.444E−3	4.325E+0
0.0800	4.706E+0	4.079E−3	4.710E+0	3.951E+0	4.483E−3	3.955E+0
0.0900	4.355E+0	4.122E−3	4.359E+0	3.658E+0	4.525E−3	3.663E+0
0.1000	4.071E+0	4.168E−3	4.075E+0	3.421E+0	4.571E−3	3.426E+0
0.1250	3.552E+0	4.294E−3	3.557E+0	2.989E+0	4.700E−3	2.994E+0
0.1500	3.203E+0	4.431E−3	3.207E+0	2.697E+0	4.844E−3	2.702E+0
0.1750	2.951E+0	4.579E−3	2.956E+0	2.487E+0	5.000E−3	2.492E+0
0.2000	2.763E+0	4.734E−3	2.768E+0	2.330E+0	5.167E−3	2.335E+0
0.2500	2.501E+0	5.070E−3	2.506E+0	2.111E+0	5.530E−3	2.117E+0
0.3000	2.329E+0	5.438E−3	2.335E+0	1.968E+0	5.928E−3	1.974E+0
0.3500	2.211E+0	5.832E−3	2.216E+0	1.869E+0	6.353E−3	1.875E+0
0.4000	2.125E+0	6.252E−3	2.131E+0	1.797E+0	6.805E−3	1.804E+0
0.4500	2.061E+0	6.694E−3	2.068E+0	1.742E+0	7.279E−3	1.749E+0
0.5000	2.012E+0	7.158E−3	2.019E+0	1.699E+0	7.775E−3	1.707E+0
0.5500	1.972E+0	7.642E−3	1.980E+0	1.665E+0	8.291E−3	1.674E+0
0.6000	1.941E+0	8.141E−3	1.949E+0	1.639E+0	8.823E−3	1.647E+0
0.7000	1.895E+0	9.186E−3	1.904E+0	1.600E+0	9.937E−3	1.610E+0
0.8000	1.863E+0	1.028E−2	1.874E+0	1.573E+0	1.111E−2	1.585E+0
0.9000	1.842E+0	1.143E−2	1.853E+0	1.555E+0	1.233E−2	1.568E+0
1.0000	1.827E+0	1.262E−2	1.839E+0	1.543E+0	1.360E−2	1.557E+0
1.2500	1.806E+0	1.578E−2	1.822E+0	1.527E+0	1.697E−2	1.544E+0
1.5000	1.799E+0	1.916E−2	1.818E+0	1.522E+0	2.057E−2	1.542E+0
1.7500	1.799E+0	2.271E−2	1.821E+0	1.522E+0	2.437E−2	1.546E+0
2.0000	1.801E+0	2.642E−2	1.828E+0	1.525E+0	2.834E−2	1.553E+0
2.5000	1.812E+0	3.421E−2	1.846E+0	1.535E+0	3.667E−2	1.572E+0
3.0000	1.824E+0	4.241E−2	1.866E+0	1.546E+0	4.544E−2	1.592E+0
3.5000	1.836E+0	5.095E−2	1.887E+0	1.558E+0	5.456E−2	1.612E+0
4.0000	1.848E+0	5.977E−2	1.908E+0	1.569E+0	6.399E−2	1.633E+0
4.5000	1.860E+0	6.883E−2	1.928E+0	1.579E+0	7.367E−2	1.653E+0
5.0000	1.870E+0	7.811E−2	1.948E+0	1.589E+0	8.357E−2	1.672E+0
5.5000	1.880E+0	8.758E−2	1.968E+0	1.598E+0	9.367E−2	1.692E+0
6.0000	1.889E+0	9.722E−2	1.987E+0	1.606E+0	1.040E−1	1.710E+0
7.0000	1.906E+0	1.170E−1	2.023E+0	1.621E+0	1.250E−1	1.746E+0
8.0000	1.921E+0	1.372E−1	2.058E+0	1.635E+0	1.466E−1	1.781E+0
9.0000	1.934E+0	1.579E−1	2.092E+0	1.646E+0	1.686E−1	1.815E+0
10.000	1.946E+0	1.790E−1	2.125E+0	1.657E+0	1.910E−1	1.848E+0
15.000	1.992E+0	2.887E−1	2.281E+0	1.697E+0	3.071E−1	2.004E+0
20.000	2.023E+0	4.032E−1	2.427E+0	1.724E+0	4.281E−1	2.152E+0
25.000	2.047E+0	5.208E−1	2.568E+0	1.745E+0	5.521E−1	2.297E+0

APPENDIX A. (Contd.). Electron Mass Stopping Powers (in MeV cm^2 g^{-1}) for Various Materials

Energy (MeV)	Polyethylene			Polymethyl Methacrylate		
	Collision (S_c/ρ)	Radiative (S_r/ρ)	Total (S/ρ)	Collision (S_c/ρ)	Radiative (S_r/ρ)	Total (S/ρ)
0.0100	2.441E+1	2.837E−3	2.442E+1	2.198E+1	3.332E−3	2.198E+1
0.0125	2.049E+1	2.847E−3	2.049E+1	1.848E+1	3.349E−3	1.849E+1
0.0150	1.775E+1	2.854E−3	1.776E+1	1.604E+1	3.359E−3	1.604E+1
0.0175	1.573E+1	2.860E−3	1.573E+1	1.423E+1	3.366E−3	1.423E+1
0.0200	1.417E+1	2.864E−3	1.417E+1	1.283E+1	3.372E−3	1.284E+1
0.0250	1.191E+1	2.873E−3	1.192E+1	1.080E+1	3.382E−3	1.081E+1
0.0300	1.035E+1	2.883E−3	1.036E+1	9.400E+0	3.391E−3	9.404E+0
0.0350	9.206E+0	2.894E−3	9.209E+0	8.367E+0	3.401E−3	8.370E+0
0.0400	8.325E+0	2.905E−3	8.328E+0	7.573E+0	3.413E−3	7.576E+0
0.0450	7.627E+0	2.918E−3	7.630E+0	6.942E+0	3.425E−3	6.946E+0
0.0500	7.060E+0	2.931E−3	7.063E+0	6.429E+0	3.438E−3	6.433E+0
0.0550	6.589E+0	2.945E−3	6.592E+0	6.003E+0	3.453E−3	6.007E+0
0.0600	6.191E+0	2.960E−3	6.194E+0	5.644E+0	3.468E−3	5.647E+0
0.0700	5.557E+0	2.992E−3	5.560E+0	5.070E+0	3.502E−3	5.073E+0
0.0800	5.074E+0	3.025E−3	5.077E+0	4.631E+0	3.538E−3	4.635E+0
0.0900	4.692E+0	3.061E−3	4.696E+0	4.286E+0	3.577E−3	4.289E+0
0.1000	4.384E+0	3.099E−3	4.387E+0	4.006E+0	3.619E−3	4.010E+0
0.1250	3.822E+0	3.201E−3	3.825E+0	3.496E+0	3.732E−3	3.500E+0
0.1500	3.443E+0	3.312E−3	3.446E+0	3.152E+0	3.855E−3	3.155E+0
0.1750	3.171E+0	3.429E−3	3.174E+0	2.904E+0	3.987E−3	2.908E+0
0.2000	2.967E+0	3.553E−3	2.970E+0	2.719E+0	4.126E−3	2.723E+0
0.2500	2.683E+0	3.820E−3	2.687E+0	2.461E+0	4.425E−3	2.465E+0
0.3000	2.497E+0	4.110E−3	2.501E+0	2.292E+0	4.751E−3	2.297E+0
0.3500	2.368E+0	4.420E−3	2.373E+0	2.175E+0	5.101E−3	2.180E+0
0.4000	2.272E+0	4.750E−3	2.277E+0	2.090E+0	5.474E−3	2.096E+0
0.4500	2.199E+0	5.098E−3	2.204E+0	2.026E+0	5.867E−3	2.032E+0
0.5000	2.142E+0	5.462E−3	2.147E+0	1.975E+0	6.278E−3	1.981E+0
0.5500	2.097E+0	5.841E−3	2.103E+0	1.935E+0	6.707E−3	1.942E+0
0.6000	2.061E+0	6.233E−3	2.068E+0	1.903E+0	7.149E−3	1.910E+0
0.7000	2.008E+0	7.053E−3	2.016E+0	1.856E+0	8.076E−3	1.864E+0
0.8000	1.972E+0	7.915E−3	1.980E+0	1.825E+0	9.050E−3	1.834E+0
0.9000	1.947E+0	8.816E−3	1.956E+0	1.803E+0	1.007E−2	1.813E+0
1.0000	1.930E+0	9.754E−3	1.940E+0	1.788E+0	1.113E−2	1.799E+0
1.2500	1.905E+0	1.224E−2	1.917E+0	1.767E+0	1.393E−2	1.781E+0
1.5000	1.895E+0	1.490E−2	1.910E+0	1.760E+0	1.693E−2	1.776E+0
1.7500	1.893E+0	1.770E−2	1.911E+0	1.759E+0	2.009E−2	1.779E+0
2.0000	1.895E+0	2.062E−2	1.916E+0	1.762E+0	2.338E−2	1.785E+0
2.5000	1.905E+0	2.678E−2	1.932E+0	1.772E+0	3.031E−2	1.802E+0
3.0000	1.917E+0	3.327E−2	1.950E+0	1.784E+0	3.761E−2	1.822E+0
3.5000	1.930E+0	4.004E−2	1.970E+0	1.797E+0	4.521E−2	1.842E+0
4.0000	1.942E+0	4.704E−2	1.989E+0	1.809E+0	5.307E−2	1.862E+0
4.5000	1.954E+0	5.424E−2	2.008E+0	1.821E+0	6.115E−2	1.882E+0
5.0000	1.965E+0	6.162E−2	2.026E+0	1.832E+0	6.943E−2	1.901E+0
5.5000	1.975E+0	6.916E−2	2.044E+0	1.842E+0	7.788E−2	1.920E+0
6.0000	1.984E+0	7.684E−2	2.061E+0	1.851E+0	8.648E−2	1.938E+0
7.0000	2.002E+0	9.259E−2	2.094E+0	1.868E+0	1.041E−1	1.972E+0
8.0000	2.017E+0	1.088E−1	2.126E+0	1.883E+0	1.222E−1	2.005E+0
9.0000	2.030E+0	1.253E−1	2.156E+0	1.896E+0	1.407E−1	2.037E+0
10.000	2.042E+0	1.422E−1	2.184E+0	1.908E+0	1.596E−1	2.067E+0
15.000	2.087E+0	2.301E−1	2.317E+0	1.952E+0	2.577E−1	2.210E+0
20.000	2.117E+0	3.220E−1	2.439E+0	1.982E+0	3.603E−1	2.342E+0
25.000	2.139E+0	4.166E−1	2.556E+0	2.004E+0	4.656E−1	2.470E+0

APPENDIX A. (Contd.). Electron Mass Stopping Powers (in MeV cm^2 g^{-1}) for Various Materials

Energy (MeV)	Polystyrene			Carbon		
	Collision (S_c/ρ)	Radiative (S_r/ρ)	Total (S/ρ)	Collision (S_c/ρ)	Radiative (S_r/ρ)	Total (S/ρ)
0.0100	2.223E+1	2.982E−3	2.224E+1	2.014E+1	3.150E−3	2.014E+1
0.0125	1.868E+1	2.992E−3	1.869E+1	1.694E+1	3.161E−3	1.695E+1
0.0150	1.621E+1	2.999E−3	1.621E+1	1.471E+1	3.168E−3	1.471E+1
0.0175	1.437E+1	3.004E−3	1.438E+1	1.305E+1	3.172E−3	1.305E+1
0.0200	1.296E+1	3.008E−3	1.296E+1	1.177E+1	3.176E−3	1.177E+1
0.0250	1.091E+1	3.017E−3	1.091E+1	9.913E+0	3.184E−3	9.916E+0
0.0300	9.485E+0	3.027E−3	9.488E+0	8.626E+0	3.194E−3	8.629E+0
0.0350	8.440E+0	3.037E−3	8.443E+0	7.679E+0	3.204E−3	7.682E+0
0.0400	7.637E+0	3.048E−3	7.640E+0	6.950E+0	3.215E−3	6.953E+0
0.0450	7.000E+0	3.061E−3	7.003E+0	6.372E+0	3.228E−3	6.375E+0
0.0500	6.481E+0	3.074E−3	6.484E+0	5.901E+0	3.241E−3	5.904E+0
0.0550	6.051E+0	3.088E−3	6.054E+0	5.510E+0	3.255E−3	5.513E+0
0.0600	5.688E+0	3.103E−3	5.691E+0	5.179E+0	3.270E−3	5.183E+0
0.0700	5.108E+0	3.135E−3	5.111E+0	4.652E+0	3.303E−3	4.655E+0
0.0800	4.666E+0	3.169E−3	4.669E+0	4.249E+0	3.337E−3	4.253E+0
0.0900	4.317E+0	3.206E−3	4.320E+0	3.931E+0	3.375E−3	3.935E+0
0.1000	4.034E+0	3.244E−3	4.038E+0	3.674E+0	3.414E−3	3.677E+0
0.1250	3.520E+0	3.350E−3	3.523E+0	3.204E+0	3.523E−3	3.207E+0
0.1500	3.172E+0	3.463E−3	3.176E+0	2.886E+0	3.640E−3	2.890E+0
0.1750	2.923E+0	3.584E−3	2.926E+0	2.657E+0	3.764E−3	2.661E+0
0.2000	2.735E+0	3.711E−3	2.739E+0	2.485E+0	3.896E−3	2.489E+0
0.2500	2.475E+0	3.985E−3	2.479E+0	2.245E+0	4.179E−3	2.249E+0
0.3000	2.305E+0	4.284E−3	2.309E+0	2.087E+0	4.489E−3	2.092E+0
0.3500	2.187E+0	4.604E−3	2.192E+0	1.977E+0	4.820E−3	1.981E+0
0.4000	2.101E+0	4.945E−3	2.106E+0	1.896E+0	5.173E−3	1.901E+0
0.4500	2.035E+0	5.304E−3	2.040E+0	1.835E+0	5.545E−3	1.841E+0
0.5000	1.984E+0	5.680E−3	1.990E+0	1.788E+0	5.935E−3	1.794E+0
0.5500	1.943E+0	6.071E−3	1.950E+0	1.752E+0	6.340E−3	1.758E+0
0.6000	1.911E+0	6.475E−3	1.918E+0	1.722E+0	6.759E−3	1.729E+0
0.7000	1.864E+0	7.322E−3	1.871E+0	1.679E+0	7.637E−3	1.687E+0
0.8000	1.832E+0	8.212E−3	1.840E+0	1.650E+0	8.559E−3	1.659E+0
0.9000	1.810E+0	9.142E−3	1.819E+0	1.631E+0	9.523E−3	1.640E+0
1.0000	1.794E+0	1.011E−2	1.804E+0	1.617E+0	1.053E−2	1.627E+0
1.2500	1.773E+0	1.267E−2	1.786E+0	1.599E+0	1.318E−2	1.612E+0
1.5000	1.766E+0	1.541E−2	1.781E+0	1.593E+0	1.602E−2	1.609E+0
1.7500	1.765E+0	1.830E−2	1.783E+0	1.594E+0	1.901E−2	1.613E+0
2.0000	1.768E+0	2.132E−2	1.789E+0	1.597E+0	2.213E−2	1.619E+0
2.5000	1.778E+0	2.766E−2	1.806E+0	1.608E+0	2.870E−2	1.637E+0
3.0000	1.791E+0	3.435E−2	1.825E+0	1.621E+0	3.561E−2	1.657E+0
3.5000	1.804E+0	4.132E−2	1.845E+0	1.634E+0	4.281E−2	1.677E+0
4.0000	1.816E+0	4.852E−2	1.865E+0	1.647E+0	5.026E−2	1.697E+0
4.5000	1.828E+0	5.593E−2	1.884E+0	1.658E+0	5.792E−2	1.716E+0
5.0000	1.839E+0	6.353E−2	1.902E+0	1.669E+0	6.576E−2	1.735E+0
5.5000	1.849E+0	7.129E−2	1.920E+0	1.679E+0	7.378E−2	1.753E+0
6.0000	1.859E+0	7.919E−2	1.938E+0	1.689E+0	8.193E−2	1.771E+0
7.0000	1.876E+0	9.539E−2	1.971E+0	1.706E+0	9.865E−2	1.804E+0
8.0000	1.891E+0	1.120E−1	2.003E+0	1.720E+0	1.158E−1	1.836E+0
9.0000	1.904E+0	1.290E−1	2.033E+0	1.733E+0	1.334E−1	1.867E+0
10.000	1.916E+0	1.464E−1	2.062E+0	1.745E+0	1.513E−1	1.896E+0
15.000	1.960E+0	2.367E−1	2.196E+0	1.787E+0	2.444E−1	2.032E+0
20.000	1.989E+0	3.311E−1	2.320E+0	1.816E+0	3.417E−1	2.157E+0
25.000	2.010E+0	4.282E−1	2.439E+0	1.836E+0	4.417E−1	2.278E+0

APPENDIX A. (Contd.). Electron Mass Stopping Powers (in MeV cm^2 g^{-1}) for Various Materials

Energy (MeV)	Aluminum			Silicon		
	Collision (S_c/ρ)	Radiative (S_r/ρ)	Total (S/ρ)	Collision (S_c/ρ)	Radiative (S_r/ρ)	Total (S/ρ)
0.0100	1.649E+1	6.559E−3	1.650E+1	1.689E+1	7.255E−3	1.690E−1
0.0125	1.398E+1	6.700E−3	1.398E+1	1.432E+0	7.431E−3	1.433E−1
0.0150	1.220E+1	6.798E−3	1.221E+1	1.251E+0	7.555E−3	1.252E−1
0.0175	1.088E+1	6.871E−3	1.088E+1	1.115E+0	7.648E−3	1.116E−1
0.0200	9.844E+0	6.926E−3	9.851E+0	1.010E+0	7.720E−3	1.011E−1
0.0250	8.338E+0	7.004E−3	8.345E+0	8.556E+0	7.822E−3	8.564E−1
0.0300	7.287E+0	7.059E−3	7.294E+0	7.480E+0	7.892E−3	7.487E−1
0.0350	6.509E+0	7.100E−3	6.516E+0	6.682E+0	7.946E−3	6.690E−1
0.0400	5.909E+0	7.133E−3	5.916E+0	6.067E+0	7.988E−3	6.075E−1
0.0450	5.430E+0	7.162E−3	5.437E+0	5.576E+0	8.026E−3	5.584E−1
0.0500	5.039E+0	7.191E−3	5.046E+0	5.175E+0	8.061E−3	5.183E−1
0.0550	4.714E+0	7.217E−3	4.721E+0	4.842E+0	8.092E−3	4.850E−1
0.0600	4.439E+0	7.243E−3	4.446E+0	4.559E+0	8.123E−3	4.568E−1
0.0700	3.998E+0	7.295E−3	4.005E+0	4.107E+0	8.185E−3	4.116E−1
0.0800	3.661E+0	7.350E−3	3.668E+0	3.761E+0	8.248E−3	3.769E−1
0.0900	3.394E+0	7.411E−3	3.401E+0	3.487E+0	8.317E−3	3.496E−1
0.1000	3.177E+0	7.476E−3	3.185E+0	3.265E+0	8.389E−3	3.274E−1
0.1250	2.781E+0	7.659E−3	2.789E+0	2.859E+0	8.591E−3	2.867E−1
0.1500	2.513E+0	7.865E−3	2.521E+0	2.583E+0	8.821E−3	2.592E−1
0.1750	2.320E+0	8.096E−3	2.328E+0	2.385E+0	9.076E−3	2.394E−1
0.2000	2.174E+0	8.344E−3	2.183E+0	2.236E+0	9.349E−3	2.245E−1
0.2500	1.972E+0	8.888E−3	1.981E+0	2.028E+0	9.951E−3	2.038E−1
0.3000	1.839E+0	9.487E−3	1.849E+0	1.892E+0	1.062E−2	1.903E−1
0.3500	1.747E+0	1.013E−2	1.757E+0	1.797E+0	1.133E−2	1.809E−1
0.4000	1.680E+0	1.082E−2	1.691E+0	1.729E+0	1.209E−2	1.741E−1
0.4500	1.630E+0	1.154E−2	1.642E+0	1.677E+0	1.290E−2	1.690E−1
0.5000	1.592E+0	1.230E−2	1.604E+0	1.638E=00	1.374E−2	1.652E−1
0.5500	1.563E+0	1.309E−2	1.576E+0	1.608E=00	1.461E−2	1.623E−1
0.6000	1.540E+0	1.390E−2	1.554E+0	1.585E+0	1.551E−2	1.600E−1
0.7000	1.507E+0	1.560E−2	1.522E+0	1.551E+0	1.740E−2	1.568E−1
0.8000	1.486E+0	1.739E−2	1.503E+0	1.529E+0	1.938E−2	1.549E−1
0.9000	1.473E+0	1.925E−2	1.492E+0	1.516E+0	2.145E−2	1.537E−1
1.0000	1.465E+0	2.119E−2	1.486E+0	1.507E+0	2.360E−2	1.531E−1
1.2500	1.457E+0	2.630E−2	1.484E+0	1.500E+0	2.927E−2	1.529E−1
1.5000	1.460E+0	3.177E−2	1.491E+0	1.502E+0	3.533E−2	1.538E−1
1.7500	1.466E+0	3.752E−2	1.504E+0	1.509E+0	4.171E−2	1.551E−1
2.0000	1.475E+0	4.350E−2	1.518E+0	1.518E+0	4.833E−2	1.567E−1
2.5000	1.493E+0	5.605E−2	1.549E+0	1.538E+0	6.223E−2	1.600E−1
3.0000	1.510E+0	6.924E−2	1.580E+0	1.558E+0	7.682E−2	1.634E−1
3.5000	1.526E+0	8.292E−2	1.609E+0	1.575E+0	9.197E−2	1.667E−1
4.0000	1.540E+0	9.702E−2	1.637E+0	1.591E+0	1.076E−1	1.699E−1
4.5000	1.552E+0	1.115E−1	1.664E+0	1.605E+0	1.236E−1	1.729E−1
5.0000	1.564E+0	1.263E−1	1.690E+0	1.618E+0	1.399E−1	1.758E−1
5.5000	1.574E+0	1.413E−1	1.715E+0	1.629E+0	1.566E−1	1.786E−1
6.0000	1.583E+0	1.567E−1	1.739E+0	1.639E+0	1.735E−1	1.813E−1
7.0000	1.599E+0	1.879E−1	1.787E+0	1.657E+0	2.081E−1	1.865E−1
8.0000	1.613E+0	2.200E−1	1.833E+0	1.672E+0	2.435E−1	1.916E−1
9.0000	1.625E+0	2.526E−1	1.877E+0	1.685E+0	2.795E−1	1.965E−1
10.000	1.636E+0	2.858E−1	1.921E+0	1.697E+0	3.161E−1	2.015E−1
15.000	1.676E+0	4.574E−1	2.134E+0	1.740E+0	5.057E−1	2.245E−1
20.000	1.704E+0	6.357E−1	2.340E+0	1.769E+0	7.023E−1	2.472E−1
25.000	1.726E+0	8.180E−1	2.544E+0	1.791E+0	9.035E−1	2.695E−1

APPENDIX A. (Contd.). Electron Mass Stopping Powers (in MeV cm^2 g^{-1}) for Various Materials

Energy (MeV)	Lithium Fluoride (LiF)			Calcium Fluoride		
	Collision (S_c/ρ)	Radiative (S_r/ρ)	Total (S/ρ)	Collision (S_c/ρ)	Radiative (S_r/ρ)	Total (S/ρ)
0.0100	1.796E+1	3.678E−3	1.796E+1	1.666E+1	7.284E−3	1.667E+1
0.0125	1.513E+1	3.712E−3	1.514E+1	1.412E+1	7.499E−3	1.413E+1
0.0150	1.315E+1	3.735E−3	1.316E+1	1.233E+1	7.657E−3	1.233E+1
0.0175	1.168E+1	3.750E−3	1.169E+1	1.099E+1	7.778E−3	1.099E+1
0.0200	1.055E+1	3.762E−3	1.055E+1	9.945E+0	7.874E−3	9.953E+0
0.0250	8.894E+0	3.779E−3	8.898E+0	8.424E+0	8.016E−3	8.432E+0
0.0300	7.748E+0	3.792E−3	7.751E+0	7.363E+0	8.118E−3	7.371E+0
0.0350	6.902E+0	3.804E−3	6.906E+0	6.577E+0	8.197E−3	6.585E+0
0.0400	6.252E+0	3.815E−3	6.256E+0	5.970E+0	8.263E−3	5.979E+0
0.0450	5.736E+0	3.827E−3	5.739E+0	5.487E+0	8.319E−3	5.495E+0
0.0500	5.315E+0	3.840E−3	5.319E+0	5.093E+0	8.370E−3	5.101E+0
0.0550	4.965E+0	3.853E−3	4.969E+0	4.764E+0	8.416E−3	4.773E+0
0.0600	4.670E+0	3.867E−3	4.674E+0	4.486E+0	8.458E−3	4.495E+0
0.0700	4.198E+0	3.898E−3	4.202E+0	4.041E+0	8.541E−3	4.050E+0
0.0800	3.838E+0	3.932E−3	3.842E+0	3.701E+0	8.621E−3	3.709E+0
0.0900	3.553E+0	3.970E−3	3.557E+0	3.432E+0	8.704E−3	3.440E+0
0.1000	3.323E+0	4.011E−3	3.327E+0	3.213E+0	8.788E−3	3.222E+0
0.1250	2.903E+0	4.125E−3	2.907E+0	2.814E+0	9.016E−3	2.823E+0
0.1500	2.619E+0	4.253E−3	2.623E+0	2.544E+0	9.265E−3	2.553E+0
0.1750	2.415E+0	4.392E−3	2.419E+0	2.349E+0	9.534E−3	2.359E+0
0.2000	2.261E+0	4.540E−3	2.266E+0	2.203E+0	9.821E−3	2.213E+0
0.2500	2.048E+0	4.863E−3	2.053E+0	2.000E+0	1.045E−2	2.011E+0
0.3000	1.907E+0	5.215E−3	1.912E+0	1.867E+0	1.113E−2	1.878E+0
0.3500	1.809E+0	5.592E−3	1.814E+0	1.774E+0	1.187E−2	1.786E+0
0.4000	1.737E+0	5.992E−3	1.743E+0	1.706E+0	1.266E−2	1.719E+0
0.4500	1.683E+0	6.412E−3	1.690E+0	1.656E+0	1.348E−2	1.669E+0
0.5000	1.642E+0	6.852E−3	1.649E+0	1.617E+0	1.435E−2	1.631E+0
0.5500	1.609E+0	7.308E−3	1.617E+0	1.587E+0	1.525E−2	1.602E+0
0.6000	1.583E+0	7.779E−3	1.591E+0	1.563E+0	1.618E−2	1.579E+0
0.7000	1.546E+0	8.765E−3	1.555E+0	1.528E+0	1.812E−2	1.547E+0
0.8000	1.521E+0	9.800E−3	1.530E+0	1.506E+0	2.016E−2	1.526E+0
0.9000	1.503E+0	1.088E−2	1.514E+0	1.491E+0	2.229E−2	1.513E+0
1.0000	1.491E+0	1.200E−2	1.504E+0	1.481E+0	2.450E−2	1.505E+0
1.2500	1.476E+0	1.499E−2	1.491E+0	1.470E+0	3.034E−2	1.500E+0
1.5000	1.471E+0	1.818E−2	1.489E+0	1.468E+0	3.658E−2	1.505E+0
1.7500	1.471E+0	2.154E−2	1.493E+0	1.471E+0	4.313E−2	1.515E+0
2.0000	1.474E+0	2.505E−2	1.499E+0	1.477E+0	4.995E−2	1.527E+0
2.5000	1.493E+0	3.244E−2	1.515E+0	1.491E+0	6.423E−2	1.555E+0
3.0000	1.493E+0	4.021E−2	1.533E+0	1.506E+0	7.922E−2	1.585E+0
3.5000	1.503E+0	4.830E−2	1.552E+0	1.520E+0	9.476E−2	1.615E+0
4.0000	1.513E+0	5.666E−2	1.570E+0	1.533E+0	1.108E−1	1.644E+0
4.5000	1.523E+0	6.524E−2	1.588E+0	1.545E+0	1.272E−1	1.673E+0
5.0000	1.531E+0	7.402E−2	1.605E+0	1.557E+0	1.439E−1	1.701E+0
5.5000	1.539E+0	8.298E−2	1.622E+0	1.567E+0	1.610E−1	1.728E+0
6.0000	1.547E+0	9.211E−2	1.639E+0	1.577E+0	1.783E−1	1.755E+0
7.0000	1.560E+0	1.108E−1	1.671E+0	1.594E+0	2.137E−1	1.808E+0
8.0000	1.572E+0	1.299E−1	1.702E+0	1.610E+0	2.499E−1	1.859E+0
9.0000	1.583E+0	1.494E−1	1.732E+0	1.623E+0	2.868E−1	1.910E+0
10.000	1.592E+0	1.693E−1	1.761E+0	1.635E+0	3.243E−1	1.959E+0
15.000	1.629E+0	2.723E−1	1.901E+0	1.679E+0	5.180E−1	2.197E+0
20.000	1.654E+0	3.797E−1	2.034E+0	1.709E+0	7.189E−1	2.428E+0
25.000	1.673E+0	4.896E−1	2.163E+0	1.731E+0	9.243E−1	2.655E+0

APPENDIX A. (Contd.). Electron Mass Stopping Powers (in MeV cm^2 g^{-1}) for Various Materials

Energy (MeV)	Tungsten			Lead		
	Collision (S_c/ρ)	Radiative (S_r/ρ)	Total (S/ρ)	Collision (S_c/ρ)	Radiative (S_r/ρ)	Total (S/ρ)
0.0100	8.974E+0	1.977E−2	8.993E+0	8.428E+0	2.045E−2	8.448E+0
0.0125	7.806E+0	2.165E−2	7.828E+0	7.357E+0	2.251E−2	7.379E+0
0.0150	6.945E+0	2.320E−2	6.968E+0	6.561E+0	2.421E−2	6.585E+0
0.0175	6.281E+0	2.450E−2	6.306E+0	5.946E+0	2.566E−2	5.971E+0
0.0200	5.753E+0	2.563E−2	5.779E+0	5.453E+0	2.693E−2	5.480E+0
0.0250	4.961E+0	2.752E−2	4.989E+0	4.714E+0	2.908E−2	4.743E+0
0.0300	4.394E+0	2.908E−2	4.423E+0	4.182E+0	3.086E−2	4.213E+0
0.0350	3.966E+0	3.042E−2	3.996E+0	3.779E+0	3.240E−2	3.812E+0
0.0400	3.631E+0	3.160E−2	3.662E+0	3.463E+0	3.376E−2	3.497E+0
0.0450	3.360E+0	3.267E−2	3.393E+0	3.208E+0	3.500E−2	3.243E+0
0.0500	3.137E+0	3.364E−2	3.171E+0	2.997E+0	3.613E−2	3.034E+0
0.0550	2.950E+0	3.454E−2	2.985E+0	2.821E+0	3.718E−2	2.858E+0
0.0600	2.791E+0	3.539E−2	2.826E+0	2.670E+0	3.817E−2	2.708E+0
0.0700	2.533E+0	3.694E−2	2.570E+0	2.426E+0	3.998E−2	2.466E+0
0.0800	2.335E+0	3.834E−2	2.373E+0	2.237E+0	4.162E−2	2.279E+0
0.0900	2.176E+0	3.964E−2	2.216E+0	2.087E+0	4.313E−2	2.130E+0
0.1000	2.047E+0	4.084E−2	2.088E+0	1.964E+0	4.454E−2	2.008E+0
0.1250	1.808E+0	4.355E−2	1.852E+0	1.738E+0	4.772E−2	1.785E+0
0.1500	1.646E+0	4.595E−2	1.692E+0	1.583E+0	5.054E−2	1.633E+0
0.1750	1.528E+0	4.814E−2	1.576E+0	1.471E+0	5.312E−2	1.524E+0
0.2000	1.439E+0	5.021E−2	1.490E+0	1.387E+0	5.555E−2	1.442E+0
0.2500	1.315E+0	5.414E−2	1.370E+0	1.269E+0	6.015E−2	1.329E+0
0.3000	1.234E+0	5.797E−2	1.292E+0	1.193E+0	6.460E−2	1.257E+0
0.3500	1.178E+0	6.179E−2	1.240E+0	1.140E+0	6.900E−2	1.209E+0
0.4000	1.138E+0	6.565E−2	1.203E+0	1.102E+0	7.340E−2	1.175E+0
0.4500	1.108E+0	6.956E−2	1.177E+0	1.074E+0	7.781E−2	1.152E+0
0.5000	1.085E+0	7.353E−2	1.159E+0	1.053E+0	8.228E−2	1.135E+0
0.5500	1.068E+0	7.755E−2	1.146E+0	1.037E+0	8.677E−2	1.124E+0
0.6000	1.055E+0	8.162E−2	1.136E+0	1.026E+0	9.132E−2	1.117E+0
0.7000	1.036E+0	8.993E−2	1.126E+0	1.009E+0	1.005E−1	1.110E+0
0.8000	1.025E+0	9.841E−2	1.124E+0	1.000E+0	1.098E−1	1.110E+0
0.9000	1.019E+0	1.071E−1	1.126E+0	9.957E−1	1.193E−1	1.115E+0
1.0000	1.016E+0	1.159E−1	1.132E+0	9.939E−1	1.290E−1	1.123E+0
1.2500	1.016E+0	1.387E−1	1.154E+0	9.966E−1	1.537E−1	1.150E+0
1.5000	1.021E+0	1.624E−1	1.183E+0	1.004E+0	1.792E−1	1.183E+0
1.7500	1.029E+0	1.868E−1	1.215E+0	1.014E+0	2.053E−1	1.219E+0
2.0000	1.037E+0	2.117E−1	1.249E+0	1.024E+0	2.319E−1	1.256E+0
2.5000	1.055E+0	2.630E−1	1.318E+0	1.044E+0	2.866E−1	1.331E+0
3.0000	1.072E+0	3.158E−1	1.388E+0	1.063E+0	3.427E−1	1.406E+0
3.5000	1.087E+0	3.698E−1	1.457E+0	1.080E+0	3.999E−1	1.480E+0
4.0000	1.101E+0	4.248E−1	1.526E+0	1.095E+0	4.582E−1	1.553E+0
4.5000	1.114E+0	4.806E−1	1.595E+0	1.108E+0	5.174E−1	1.626E+0
5.0000	1.126E+0	5.372E−1	1.663E+0	1.120E+0	5.773E−1	1.698E+0
5.5000	1.136E+0	5.945E−1	1.731E+0	1.132E+0	6.379E−1	1.769E+0
6.0000	1.146E+0	6.523E−1	1.798E+0	1.142E+0	6.991E−1	1.841E+0
7.0000	1.163E+0	7.697E−1	1.933E+0	1.160E+0	8.233E−1	1.983E+0
8.0000	1.178E+0	8.890E−1	2.067E+0	1.175E+0	9.495E−1	2.125E+0
9.0000	1.191E+0	1.010E+0	2.201E+0	1.189E+0	1.077E+0	2.266E+0
10.000	1.203E+0	1.132E+0	2.335E+0	1.201E+0	1.206E+0	2.407E+0
15.000	1.247E+0	1.759E+0	3.006E+0	1.246E+0	1.870E+0	3.116E+0
20.000	1.277E+0	2.406E+0	3.682E+0	1.277E+0	2.554E+0	3.830E+0
25.000	1.299E+0	3.065E+0	4.364E+0	1.299E+0	3.252E+0	4.551E+0

Appendix B

APPENDIX B. Mass Attenuation Coefficients, Mass Energy Transfer Coefficients, and Mass Energy Absorption Coefficients (in $cm^2\,g^{-1}$) for Various Materials

Photon Energy E_V (MeV)	Hydrogen			Carbon			Nitrogen		
	μ/ρ	μ_{tr}/ρ	μ_{ab}/ρ	μ/ρ	μ_{tr}/ρ	μ_{ab}/ρ	μ/ρ	μ_{tr}/ρ	μ_{ab}/ρ
0.01	0.385	0.00986	0.00986	2.32	1.97	1.97	3.77	3.38	3.38
0.015	0.376	0.0110	0.0110	0.797	0.536	0.536	1.19	0.908	0.908
0.02	0.369	0.0135	0.0135	0.434	0.208	0.208	0.602	0.362	0.362
0.03	0.357	0.0185	0.0185	0.253	0.0594	0.0594	0.304	0.105	0.105
0.04	0.346	0.0231	0.0231	0.205	0.0306	0.0306	0.229	0.0493	0.0493
0.05	0.335	0.0271	0.0271	0.185	0.0233	0.0233	0.196	0.0319	0.0319
0.06	0.326	0.0306	0.0306	0.174	0.0211	0.0211	0.181	0.0256	0.0256
0.08	0.309	0.0362	0.0362	0.162	0.0205	0.0205	0.164	0.0223	0.0223
0.1	0.294	0.0406	0.0406	0.152	0.0215	0.0215	0.154	0.0224	0.0224
0.15	0.265	0.0481	0.0481	0.135	0.0245	0.0245	0.136	0.0247	0.0247
0.2	0.243	0.0525	0.0525	0.123	0.0265	0.0265	0.124	0.0267	0.0267
0.3	0.211	0.0569	0.0569	0.107	0.0287	0.0287	0.107	0.0287	0.0287
0.4	0.189	0.0586	0.0586	0.0953	0.0295	0.0295	0.0953	0.0295	0.0295
0.5	0.173	0.0593	0.0593	0.0870	0.0297	0.0297	0.0870	0.0297	0.0296
0.6	0.160	0.0587	0.0587	0.0805	0.0296	0.0295	0.0805	0.0296	0.0295
0.8	0.140	0.0574	0.0574	0.0707	0.0289	0.0288	0.0707	0.0289	0.0289
1.0	0.126	0.0555	0.0555	0.0637	0.0279	0.0279	0.0636	0.0280	0.0279
1.5	0.103	0.0507	0.0507	0.0519	0.0256	0.0255	0.0518	0.0256	0.0255
2.0	0.0875	0.0465	0.0464	0.0443	0.0235	0.0234	0.0444	0.0236	0.0234
3.0	0.0691	0.0399	0.0398	0.0356	0.0206	0.0204	0.0357	0.0207	0.0205
4.0	0.0581	0.0353	0.0352	0.0305	0.0187	0.0185	0.0308	0.0189	0.0186
5.0	0.0505	0.0319	0.0317	0.0271	0.0174	0.0171	0.0274	0.0177	0.0173
6.0	0.0450	0.0292	0.0290	0.0247	0.0164	0.0161	0.0251	0.0167	0.0163
8.0	0.0375	0.0253	0.0252	0.0216	0.0151	0.0147	0.0221	0.0156	0.0151
10.0	0.0325	0.0227	0.0225	0.0196	0.0143	0.0138	0.0203	0.0149	0.0143

From Attix, F.H., Appendix D.3, in Introduction to Radiological Physics and Radiation Dosimetry, John Wiley & Sons, New York, 1986; and Evans, R.D.,X and γ ray Interactions, Chapter 3 in Radiation Dosimetry, Vol. 1, (Ed: Attix, F.H. and Roesch, W.C.), Academic Press, New York, 1968, based on original data of Hubbel, J.H. With permission.

APPENDIX B. (Contd.). Mass Attenuation Coefficients, Mass Energy Transfer Coefficients, and Mass Energy Absorption Coefficients (in $cm^2\,g^{-1}$) for Various Materials

Photon Energy E_V (MeV)	Oxygen			Air			Water		
	μ/ρ	μ_{tr}/ρ	μ_{ab}/ρ	μ/ρ	μ_{tr}/ρ	μ_{ab}/ρ	μ/ρ	μ_{tr}/ρ	μ_{ab}/ρ
0.01	5.82	5.39	5.39	5.04	4.61	4.61	5.21	4.79	4.79
0.015	1.75	1.44	1.44	1.56	1.27	1.27	1.60	1.28	1.28
0.02	0.830	0.575	0.575	0.758	0.511	0.511	0.778	0.512	0.512
0.03	0.373	0.165	0.165	0.350	0.148	0.148	0.371	0.149	0.149
0.04	0.257	0.0733	0.0733	0.248	0.0668	0.0668	0.267	0.0677	0.0677
0.05	0.211	0.0437	0.0437	0.206	0.0406	0.0406	0.225	0.0418	0.0418
0.06	0.190	0.0322	0.0322	0.187	0.0305	0.0305	0.205	0.0320	0.0320
0.08	0.168	0.0249	0.0249	0.167	0.0243	0.0243	0.185	0.0262	0.0262
0.1	0.156	0.0237	0.0237	0.155	0.0234	0.0234	0.171	0.0256	0.0256
0.15	0.137	0.0251	0.0251	0.136	0.0250	0.0250	0.151	0.0277	0.0277
0.2	0.124	0.0268	0.0268	0.124	0.0268	0.0268	0.137	0.0297	0.0297
0.3	0.107	0.0288	0.0288	0.107	0.0287	0.0287	0.119	0.0319	0.0319
0.4	0.0957	0.0295	0.0295	0.0954	0.0295	0.0295	0.106	0.0328	0.0328
0.5	0.0871	0.0297	0.0297	0.0868	0.0297	0.0296	0.0966	0.0330	0.0330
0.6	0.0805	0.0296	0.0296	0.0804	0.0296	0.0295	0.0894	0.0329	0.0329
0.8	0.0707	0.0289	0.0289	0.0706	0.0289	0.0289	0.0785	0.0321	0.0321
1.0	0.0637	0.0280	0.0278	0.0635	0.0280	0.0278	0.0706	0.0311	0.0309
1.5	0.0518	0.0256	0.0254	0.0517	0.0256	0.0254	0.0575	0.0284	0.0282
2.0	0.0445	0.0236	0.0234	0.0444	0.0236	0.0234	0.0493	0.0262	0.0260
3.0	0.0359	0.0208	0.0206	0.0358	0.0207	0.0205	0.0396	0.0229	0.0227
4.0	0.0310	0.0191	0.0188	0.0308	0.0189	0.0186	0.0340	0.0209	0.0206
5.0	0.0278	0.0179	0.0175	0.0276	0.0178	0.0174	0.0303	0.0195	0.0191
6.0	0.0255	0.0171	0.0166	0.0252	0.0168	0.0164	0.0277	0.0185	0.0180
8.0	0.0226	0.0160	0.0155	0.0223	0.0157	0.0152	0.0243	0.0170	0.0166
10.0	0.0209	0.0154	0.0148	0.0205	0.0151	0.0145	0.0222	0.0162	0.0157

APPENDIX B. (Contd.). Mass Attenuation Coefficients, Mass Energy Transfer Coefficients, and Mass Energy Absorption Coefficients (in cm^2 g^{-1}) for Various Materials

Photon Energy E_V (MeV)	Striated Muscle (ICRU)			Compact Bone (ICRU)			Methyl Methacrylate (ICRU)		
	μ/ρ	μ_{tr}/ρ	μ_{ab}/ρ	μ/ρ	μ_{tr}/ρ	μ_{ab}/ρ	μ/ρ	μ_{tr}/ρ	μ_{ab}/ρ
0.01	5.30	4.87	4.87	20.3	19.2	19.2	3.31	2.91	2.91
0.015	1.64	1.32	1.32	6.32	5.84	5.84	1.07	0.783	0.783
0.02	0.796	0.533	0.533	2.79	2.46	2.46	0.555	0.310	0.310
0.03	0.375	0.154	0.154	0.962	0.720	0.720	0.300	0.0899	0.0899
0.04	0.267	0.0701	0.0701	0.511	0.304	0.304	0.233	0.0437	0.0437
0.05	0.224	0.0431	0.0431	0.346	0.161	0.161	0.205	0.0301	0.0301
0.06	0.204	0.0328	0.0328	0.273	0.0998	0.0998	0.191	0.0254	0.0254
0.08	0.183	0.0264	0.0264	0.209	0.0537	0.0537	0.176	0.0232	0.0232
0.1	0.170	0.0256	0.0256	0.181	0.0387	0.0387	0.165	0.0238	0.0238
0.15	0.150	0.0275	0.0275	0.150	0.0305	0.0305	0.146	0.0266	0.0266
0.2	0.136	0.0294	0.0294	0.133	0.0301	0.0301	0.133	0.0287	0.0287
0.3	0.118	0.0317	0.0317	0.114	0.0310	0.0310	0.115	0.0310	0.0310
0.4	0.105	0.0325	0.0325	0.102	0.0315	0.0315	0.103	0.0318	0.0318
0.5	0.0958	0.0328	0.0328	0.0926	0.0317	0.0317	0.0939	0.0322	0.0322
0.6	0.0886	0.0326	0.0325	0.0856	0.0315	0.0314	0.0869	0.0319	0.0319
0.8	0.0778	0.0318	0.0318	0.0751	0.0307	0.0306	0.0763	0.0312	0.0311
1.0	0.0699	0.0308	0.0306	0.0675	0.0297	0.0295	0.0686	0.0302	0.0301
1.5	0.0570	0.0282	0.0280	0.0549	0.0272	0.0270	0.0559	0.0276	0.0275
2.0	0.0489	0.0259	0.0257	0.0472	0.0251	0.0249	0.0478	0.0254	0.0253
3.0	0.0392	0.0227	0.0225	0.0382	0.0221	0.0219	0.0383	0.0222	0.0220
4.0	0.0337	0.0207	0.0204	0.0331	0.0204	0.0200	0.0329	0.0202	0.0199
5.0	0.0300	0.0193	0.0189	0.0297	0.0192	0.0187	0.0292	0.0187	0.0184
6.0	0.0274	0.0183	0.0178	0.0274	0.0184	0.0178	0.0266	0.0177	0.0173
8.0	0.0240	0.0169	0.0164	0.0244	0.0173	0.0167	0.0231	0.0162	0.0158
10.0	0.0219	0.0160	0.0155	0.0226	0.0168	0.0159	0.0210	0.0153	0.0148

APPENDIX B. (Contd.). Mass Attenuation Coefficients, Mass Energy Transfer Coefficients, and Mass Energy Absorption Coefficients (in $cm^2\,g^{-1}$) for Various Materials

Photon Energy E_v (MeV)	Polystyrene			Polyethylene			Aluminum		
	μ/ρ	μ_{tr}/ρ	μ_{ab}/ρ	μ/ρ	μ_{tr}/ρ	μ_{ab}/ρ	μ/ρ	μ_{tr}/ρ	μ_{ab}/ρ
0.01	2.17	1.82	1.82	2.04	1.69	1.69	26.2	25.5	25.5
0.015	0.764	0.495	0.495	0.737	0.461	0.461	7.90	7.47	7.47
0.02	0.429	0.193	0.193	0.425	0.180	0.180	3.39	3.06	3.06
0.03	0.261	0.0562	0.0562	0.268	0.0535	0.0535	1.12	0.868	0.868
0.04	0.216	0.0300	0.0300	0.225	0.0295	0.0295	0.565	0.357	0.357
0.05	0.197	0.0236	0.0236	0.207	0.0238	0.0238	0.367	0.184	0.184
0.06	0.186	0.0218	0.0218	0.196	0.0225	0.0225	0.277	0.111	0.111
0.08	0.173	0.0217	0.0217	0.183	0.0228	0.0228	0.201	0.0562	0.0562
0.1	0.164	0.0231	0.0231	0.173	0.0243	0.0243	0.170	0.0386	0.0386
0.15	0.145	0.0263	0.0263	0.154	0.0279	0.0279	0.138	0.0285	0.0285
0.2	0.132	0.0286	0.0286	0.140	0.0303	0.0303	0.122	0.0276	0.0276
0.3	0.115	0.0309	0.0309	0.122	0.0328	0.0328	0.104	0.0282	0.0282
0.4	0.103	0.0318	0.0318	0.109	0.0337	0.0337	0.0926	0.0287	0.0287
0.5	0.0937	0.0321	0.0321	0.0994	0.0340	0.0340	0.0844	0.0287	0.0286
0.6	0.0867	0.0319	0.0318	0.0919	0.0338	0.0337	0.0779	0.0286	0.0286
0.8	0.0761	0.0311	0.0310	0.0807	0.0330	0.0329	0.0682	0.0279	0.0277
1.0	0.0683	0.0300	0.0300	0.0725	0.0319	0.0319	0.0613	0.0270	0.0269
1.5	0.0557	0.0275	0.0275	0.0591	0.0292	0.0291	0.0500	0.0247	0.0245
2.0	0.0476	0.0253	0.0252	0.0505	0.0268	0.0267	0.0431	0.0229	0.0226
3.0	0.0381	0.0221	0.0219	0.0403	0.0234	0.0232	0.0353	0.0206	0.0202
4.0	0.0326	0.0200	0.0198	0.0345	0.0211	0.0209	0.0311	0.0193	0.0188
5.0	0.0289	0.0185	0.0182	0.0305	0.0195	0.0192	0.0284	0.0185	0.0179
6.0	0.0263	0.0174	0.0171	0.0276	0.0182	0.0180	0.0266	0.0181	0.0172
8.0	0.0227	0.0159	0.0155	0.0238	0.0166	0.0162	0.0244	0.0177	0.0168
10.0	0.0206	0.0150	0.0145	0.0215	0.0155	0.0151	0.0232	0.0176	0.0165

APPENDIX B. (Contd.). Mass Attenuation Coefficients, Mass Energy Transfer Coefficients, and Mass Energy Absorption Coefficients (in cm^2 g^{-1}) for Various Materials

Photon Energy E_V (MeV)	Silicon			Calcium			Copper		
	μ/ρ	μ_{tr}/ρ	μ_{ab}/ρ	μ/ρ	μ_{tr}/ρ	μ_{ab}/ρ	μ/ρ	μ_{tr}/ρ	μ_{ab}/ρ
0.01	34.1	33.3	33.3	96.5	91.6	91.6	224.2	160.0	160.0
0.015	10.2	9.75	9.75	30.1	28.6	28.6	74.1	59.4	59.4
0.02	4.36	4.01	4.01	12.9	12.2	12.2	33.7	28.2	28.2
0.03	1.41	1.14	1.14	3.98	3.60	3.60	10.9	9.50	9.50
0.04	0.693	0.472	0.472	1.78	1.50	1.50	4.88	4.24	4.24
0.05	0.435	0.241	0.241	0.994	0.764	0.764	2.61	2.22	2.22
0.06	0.319	0.144	0.144	0.646	0.444	0.444	1.60	1.32	1.32
0.08	0.223	0.0700	0.0700	0.363	0.196	0.196	0.768	0.573	0.573
0.1	0.184	0.0459	0.0459	0.255	0.109	0.109	0.462	0.302	0.302
0.15	0.145	0.0312	0.0312	0.168	0.0497	0.0497	0.223	0.106	0.106
0.2	0.128	0.0292	0.0292	0.138	0.0371	0.0371	0.157	0.0597	0.0597
0.3	0.108	0.0294	0.0294	0.112	0.0318	0.0318	0.112	0.0370	0.0370
0.4	0.0961	0.0298	0.0298	0.098	0.0309	0.0309	0.0942	0.0318	0.0318
0.5	0.0875	0.0298	0.0298	0.0886	0.0304	0.0304	0.0835	0.0298	0.0298
0.6	0.0806	0.0296	0.0295	0.0813	0.0300	0.0299	0.0762	0.0287	0.0286
0.8	0.0708	0.0289	0.0288	0.0712	0.0291	0.0289	0.0659	0.0272	0.0271
1.0	0.0634	0.0279	0.0277	0.0639	0.0280	0.0278	0.0590	0.0261	0.0258
1.5	0.0517	0.0255	0.0253	0.0519	0.0257	0.0254	0.0479	0.0237	0.0233
2.0	0.0447	0.0237	0.0234	0.0452	0.0240	0.0236	0.0419	0.0222	0.0217
3.0	0.0367	0.0214	0.0210	0.0377	0.0220	0.0214	0.0359	0.0211	0.0202
4.0	0.0324	0.0202	0.0196	0.0340	0.0213	0.0205	0.0332	0.0211	0.0200
5.0	0.0297	0.0194	0.0187	0.0317	0.0211	0.0200	0.0318	0.0214	0.0200
6.0	0.0279	0.0191	0.0182	0.0304	0.0211	0.0198	0.0310	0.0220	0.0202
8.0	0.0257	0.0187	0.0177	0.0289	0.0215	0.0198	0.0307	0.0234	0.0209
10.0	0.0246	0.0188	0.0175	0.0284	0.0222	0.0201	0.0310	0.0248	0.0215

APPENDIX B. (Contd.). Mass Attenuation Coefficients, Mass Energy Transfer Coefficients, and Mass Energy Absorption Coefficients (in cm^2 g^{-1}) for Various Materials

Photon Energy E_V (MeV)	Tin			Photon Energy E_V (MeV)	Tin		
	μ/ρ	μ_{tr}/ρ	μ_{ab}/ρ		μ/ρ	μ_{tr}/ρ	μ_{ab}/ρ
0.001	11130	11110	11110	0.10	1.720	1.257	1.250
0.0015	3960	3950	3950	0.15	0.634	0.446	0.442
0.002	1963	1954	1954	0.20	0.333	0.211	0.209
0.003	713	705	705	0.30	0.1649	0.0853	0.0843
				0.40	0.1163	0.0536	0.0530
0.003929 L3 Edge	367	360	360	0.50	0.0948	0.0423	0.0416
0.003929	1118	1067	1067	0.60	0.0811	0.0358	0.0353
				0.80	0.0667	0.0301	0.0294
0.0040	1067	1019	1019	1.0	0.0578	0.0270	0.0264
				1.5	0.0462	0.0233	0.0226
0.004157 L2 Edge	973	930	930	2.0	0.0410	0.0220	0.0210
0.004157	1244	1187	1187	3.0	0.0366	0.0219	0.0205
				4.0	0.0355	0.0232	0.0212
0.004465 L1 Edge	1016	971	971	5.0	0.0353	0.0247	0.0221
0.004465	1264	1207	1207	6.0	0.0357	0.0262	0.0230
0.005	919	880	880	8.0	0.0370	0.0292	0.0245
0.006	561	540	539	10.0	0.0387	0.0319	0.0258
0.008	259	250	249				
0.010	141.6	136.5	136.4				
0.015	45.8	43.7	43.6				
0.0020	21.2	19.83	19.81				
0.029195 K Edge	7.61	6.83	6.82				
0.029195	45.4	16.70	16.69				
0.03	42.1	16.18	16.17				
0.04	18.77	9.97	9.96				
0.05	10.20	6.25	6.24				
0.06	6.34	4.20	4.19				
0.08	3.07	2.19	2.18				

APPENDIX B. (Contd.). Mass Attenuation Coefficients, Mass Energy Transfer Coefficients, and Mass Energy Absorption Coefficients (in cm^2 g^{-1}) for Various Materials

Photon Energy E_V (MeV)	Lead			Photon Energy E_V (MeV)	Lead		
	μ/ρ	μ_{tr}/ρ	μ_{ab}/ρ		μ/ρ	μ_{tr}/ρ	μ_{ab}/ρ
	Ñ	Ñ	Ñ	0.10	5.78	2.28	2.28
M1 Edge				0.15	2.07	1.164	1.154
0.003854	1493	1454	1453	0.20	1.014	0.637	0.629
				0.30	0.406	0.265	0.259
0.004	1333	1298	1297				
0.005	767	747	747	0.40	0.233	0.1474	0.1432
0.006	493	479	479	0.50	0.1614	0.0984	0.0951
0.008	238	230	230	0.60	0.1249	0.0737	0.0710
0.010	136.6	131	130.7	0.80	0.0886	0.0503	0.0481
0.013041	70.1	66.2	66.0	1.0	0.0708	0.0396	0.0377
L3 Edge				1.5	0.0518	0.0288	0.0271
0.013041	165.7	128.8	128.8	2.0	0.0455	0.0259	0.0240
				3.0	0.0417	0.0260	0.0234
0.015	114.7	91.7	91.7				
				4.0	0.0415	0.0281	0.0245
0.015205	112.0	89.6	89.6	5.0	0.0424	0.0306	0.0259
L2 Edge				6.0	0.0436	0.0331	0.0272
0.015205	145.4	113.0	113	8.0	0.0467	0.0378	0.0294
0.015855	129.3	101.7	101.6	10.0	0.0496	0.0419	0.0310
L1 Edge							
0.015855	159.2	123.0	123.0				
0.02	85.5	69.2	69.1				
0.03	29.1	24.6	24.6				
0.04	13.80	11.83	11.78				
0.05	7.71	6.57	6.54				
0.06	4.87	4.11	4.08				
0.08	2.37	1.924	1.908				
0.088005	1.865	1.494	1.481				
K Edge							
0.088005	7.30	2.47	2.47				

Subject Index

AAPM 101, 154, 335, 369
Absolute activity 361, 363–364
Absolute-risk model 432–433
Absorption
  in air 142, 145–146,
  in bone 248–250
  coefficients data 499–505
  of energy
    and dose 137–138, 143–14
    local 76, 84–85
    in Compton scatter 80–81
    in pair production 84
    in photoelectric effect 76
  in medium 137–140
  in microscopic scale 424–425
  in photon interactions 69–88
  of photons 69–88
  in soft-tissue 248–250
  in water 142, 145–146
Acceleration of electrons 95, 100, 107, 118,
    125
Accelerating tube 119
Accelerators 118–132
  betatron 118, 127–129
  clinical 124–126
  cyclotron 118, 129–130
  direct-voltage 103–105
  dual-energy 107, 208, 209
  electrostatic 119–121
  induction 118
  linacs 118, 121–124
  linear 118, 121–124
  magnetic-induction 118, 127–129
  microtron 118, 130–132
  particle 118–132
  resonance 118, 127–132
  standing wave 124
  traveling wave 124
Acceptable weekly equivalent dose limits
    444–445
Access control 445, 467, 468, 484
  (see also Door shielding)
Accredited dosimetry calibration laboratory
    (see ADCL)
Acronyms list 228, 253, 315
Activity units 44, 363

Acute radiation syndrome 422
ADCL 149, 150, 155
Additive-risk projection model 432
Adjacent sites treatment 309–314, 350–351
Afterloading techniques 361, 401, 410, 412, 479,
    487
Air
  -cavity perturbation in electron beams
    342–345
  density of 143
  dose to tissue in 151, 194–195
  electron mass stopping powers 491
  energy absorption 143–145
  energy required produce an ion pair 144
  energy transfer to 144–145
  ionization of secondary charged particles
    142–143
  mass attenuation coefficients 500
  mass energy absorption coefficients 500
  mass energy transfer coefficients 500
Air dose 143–146
Air kerma 142–146
  relationship to dose 143–146
  relationship to exposure 143–146
Air-kerma rate constant 159–162, 358
Air-kerma rate yield 361, 364
Air-kerma strength 162–163, 364
  definition 364
  unit U 163, 364
Air-kerma to water-dose conversion 145–146,
    367
Air-kerma yield of treatment 365–366
  data tables (see dosage tables)
  definition 365
  relation to milligram-hours of radium
    365–366
Air output factor (see Normalized air output
    factor)
Air output rate, calibrated (see Calibrated air
    output rate)
ALARA principle 421, 435, 438, 478
Alarms 468, 478
Alpha decay 31, 33, 34
Alpha particles 3, 31, 34, 56, 130, 168–169
  collision and 59–61
  in particle accelerators 130

radiation weighting factor 426–428
    quality factor for 426–428
Alpha track 59
Alternating current (AC), 100–104, 128
Aluminum
    electron mass stopping powers 496
    filters 105–106, 338–339
    mass attenuation coefficients 496
    mass energy absorption coefficients 502
    mass energy transfer coefficients 502
American Association of Physicists in Medicine
        (see AAPM)
Americium-241 (^{241}Am), 358, 480
Angular distribution, of scattered photons 79
Angular emission of photoelectrons 76
Angular scattering of electrons 323–324,
        327–329
Animal experiments 430
Annihilation
    photons 83–84
    of positron 83–84
Annual maximum dose limits 436–437, 443,
        444–445
Annular zones 271–272, 294
Anode
    rotating 99
    in X-ray tube 95–99
Anthracene crystal 176
Antimatter 24
Antineutrino 21–22, 35
Antiparticles 21–22
Antiprotons 24
Antiquarks 23–24
Apparent activity 361, 364
Appendices 491–505
Applied potential, the role
    in condenser chamber 169–171
    in ionization detector 146, 168–171
    in an X-ray tube 95, 100–104
Arc therapy
    dosimetry 226–227
    by electrons 348–350
    by photons 288, 291–293
Architectural data 449
"As low as reasonably achievable" (see ALARA)
Atomic
    attenuation coefficient 72
    electrons
        binding energies of 13, 38–39, 74
        energy levels of 11–14
        of K-, L-, M- shells 11–14
        orbits of,
Atomic mass 15–16
Atomic mass unit (amu) 16
Atomic number
    Compton cross section 81
    definition 9–11
    effective 87, 241
    pair production 84
    photoelectric interaction 76
    radioactive decay and
        (see Decay schemes)

Atoms
    excitation 14
    formation 8–11
    ionization 14
    physical characteristics 7–9
    physics of, historical background 7
Attenuation coefficient 70–72
    atomic 72
    data 250, 499–505
    electronic 72
    linear 71
    mass 71–72, 75–76, 498–505
    for mixtures and compounds 87
    variation with energy 75–76
Attractive force 21,22, 32
Auger electrons 14–15, 37, 76
Auger electron 10
^{198}Au
    as brachytherapy source 358
    decay scheme 39
    permanent implant 408–409
    water perturbation correction 368
Avogadro's number (N_{Av}) 16

Background radiation 434–435
Back-pointing device 116
Back-scatter factor (see BSF)
Backscattered electrons 226–227
Backscattered photons 80, 198, 339, 454–455
Barite 447–448
Barium contrast medium 296
Baryons 24
Basic dose rate (of implant) 388–389, 408
Batho's method 244–247
Beam (see also calibration)
    collimation 109–110, 126
    for external-beam therapy 93–102
    filtered and unfiltered 105–106, 65–66
    flatness of 239
    geometry (for attenuation,) 88–89
    geometry (of therapy beam,) 189–191,
    hardening of 105–106
    limiting diaphragms 109–110, 126, 261–264,
        324–325,
    penumbra of 111–113, 261–264
    of photons (see photon beam)
    -quality 191
        half-value thickness and 105–106
        peak dose and 193
        peak scatter factors and 200,
        softening 240
    radioisotope, equipment 107–117
"Beam on" indicator 468
Beamlets 316
Beam's-eye projection 308
Beam-stopper 451
Becquerel unit 44
Bedside shields 484
Benzene 181
Beryllium-7 (^{7}Ba) 435
Beta decay 32, 34–37,

Beta energy spectrum 35, 39
Beta eye applicator 172–173,
Beta particles 32–37, 168–169
Beta sources
  for brachytherapy 357–358
  storage and handling 481–482
Betatron 118, 127–129
Binding energy 8, 13, 32, 38–39, 74
BIPM 150
Bilateral arcs 26, 34
Biological damage 422–423, 425
Biological effectiveness 425
Bismuth-210 29
Blocked fields 230–234
Body inhomogeneities,
  in electron beams 342–345
  in photon beams 240–250
Bolusing 280–281, 287
Bonds, types of molecular 17–20
Bone
  attenuation and absorption in 248–250
  as a body inhomogeneity
    in electron beams 342–345
    in high-energy photon beams 248–250
    in low-energy x-ray beams 248–250
  depth-dose profiles through 249
  dose to bone 145–146, 249
  effective atomic number and density 241
  electron mass stopping powers in 492
  electron scattering in 342–344
  mass attenuation coefficients 501
  mass energy absorption coefficients 501
  mass energy transfer coefficients 501
Boron-based shielding 174
Boron tri-fluoride proportional counters 459
Bosons 21–22
Brachytherapy Dosimetry (see Dosimetry and
    Dose calculation)
Brachytherapy, principles 85–139
  afterloading technique 361, 401, 410, 412
  AAPM/ICGW approach 369–371, 376–377
  bronchial 374, 377–379
  cardiovascular 374
  Computer dose evaluation 405–408
  cylindrical mould 383–385
  distribution rules 395–398
  dosage tables (see under same title)
  esophageal 374
  $g(r)$, factor in dosimetry 369–371,
    definition 369
    data for various sources 369
    relation to WPC(r) 369
  gynecologic applications 409–414
  Heyman packing 413
  high-dose-rate (HDR) 361
  interstitial application 359–360
  intracavitary insertions 360, 409–414
  intraluminal 360, 374, 377–379
  line source treatment 374, 377–379
  low-dose-rate (LDR) 361
  multiple source arrays 378–385
  permanent implants 408–409

planar implants
  single plane 378, 383–384, 389, 400–401,406,
    408–409, 486
  two-plane 360, 381–382, 397
  radiographic localization 401–405
  removable implants 360,
  source strength specification 361–364
  surface applications 359, 394–396, 383–385
  systems 384–394
    definition 384–385
    Paris 387–389, 392, 408
    Manchester (Paterson-Parker) 390–398, 400
    Memorial (New York) 389–390
    Quimby 385–387, 392
  temporary implants 360
  uniform and differentially loading 379–385
  vaginal colpostats 410–411
  vaginal cylinder 409–410
  volume implants 360, 383–384, 389, 391–394,
    408–409
Brachytherapy Safety (see Radiation safety and
    shielding)
Brachytherapy sources 358
  as dose building blocks 379
  encapsulated linear source 371–373
  encapsulation 357, 363, 371,
  linear source 371–374
  physical characteristics 358
  point source in water 366–369
  radioactive seeds 369–371, 486
  radioactive wire 374, 377–378, 387, 483
  specification 163, 361–364
  unencapsulated linear source 373–374
Brachytherapy systems 384–394
  definition 384–385
  Paris 387–389, 392, 408
  Manchester (Paterson-Parker) 390–398, 400
  Memorial (New York) 389–390
  pitfalls 394
  Quimby 385–387, 392
Bragg-Gray cavity, 152–154
Bragg ionization curve 62–63
Bragg peak 62–63
Breast irradiation 288
Bremsstrahlung (see also x-rays) 63–64, 85, 324,
    327
  angular distribution 64
  energy distribution 65–66
  loss 85, 144
  production of 63–64, 82
  spectra 65–66
  yield 63–64
Broad-beam geometry 88–89
BSF 198, 200 (see also PSF)
Build-up caps 148–149, 155
Build-up factor 89, 163–164, 368
Build-up, dose (see Dose build-up; Secondary
    electrons)
Build-up zone 271–272
Bureau International des Poids et des Mesures
    (BIPM) 150

Calcium fluoride, electron mass stopping powers 497
Calibrated air output rate (see CAOR)
Calibrated peak output rate (see CPOR)
Calibrated output 206–210
Calibration
  of beams
    in-air output
    in-phantom output
    need for 150–151
    (see also) protocol
  of dosimeter
    need for 150, 174, 183
    NMR 182
    OSL 181
    photographic film 174
    radiochromic film 182–183
    TLD 179–180
  of ion-chamber
    absorbed dose 158
    by ADCL 149–150, 155
    Cobalt-60 exposure 149, 150
Calibration factor
  Absorbed dose 158
  exposure 149–150, 155
Calcium
  in bone 76
  mass attenuation coefficients 503
  mass energy absorption coefficients 503
  mass energy transfer coefficients 503
Calorimetry 157–158
Cancer-risk projection 432–433
CAOR 210–211
  derivation of dose rate 212–214, 232–234, 239–240
Carbon
  electron mass stopping powers 495
  isotopes of 15–16
  mass attenuation coefficients 499
  mass energy absorption coefficients 499
  mass energy transfer coefficients 499
  as standard for amu 15–16
Carbon-14 435
Carcinogenic effect 422–423, 431–433, 436
Covalent bonds 17–18
Cavity chambers 147–148, 169–172
Centerline peripheral dose (CPD) 389
Central-axis dose profile 192–193, 279–280, 282, 284, 327, 329–330, 331, 335, 345
Ceric sulphate 181
Cesium-137 (see ^{137}Cs)
Chamber, walled, in a medium 154–155
Characteristic X-rays 14–15, 37, 74, 76, 105, 85, 357
Charge
  of electrons 8
  of elementary particles 8, 22–23
  relationship to exposure 142–143
Charged-particle equilibrium (see CPE)
Charged particle interactions 59–68
  Bragg peak 62–63
  collision loss 60–63

radiation loss 63–64 (see also bremsstrahlung)
  track 59
Charged particles 20, 23 (see also particles; alpha particles; beta particles)
Chemical bonds
  breaking
  formation 17–20
Chemical dosimeters 180–181, 182
Chernobyl radiation accident 430
Childhood cancers 423
Chromosomal aberrations 425–426
Clinical
  dose prescription 3, 5, 241, 259, 272, 300, 311, 313, 337, 385, 394
  linear accelerator 124–126
  physicist 3–6, 295
Clinical physicist, vii 3–6, 159, 228, 294, 469
Clinical dose prescription 3, 5, 241, 259, 272, 300, 311, 313, 337, 385, 394
  linear accelerator 124–126
  physicist 3–6, 295
  target volume (CTV), 272
Cloud chamber 333
Cobalt-59 53–54
Cobalt-60 source (see ^{60}Co source)
Cobalt-60 beams (see ^{60}Co beams)
Cobalt-61 55
^{60}Co beams
  absorbed dose calibration factor 158–159
  calibration of 151–152
  depth-dose through bone 249
  dose distributions curves for 263, 275, 280–293
  dosimetry of 195, 218–221, 236–237, 245–247, 269–270
  ICFs for 236–247
  on-off mechanisms 110–111
  PDDs for 201–203, 218–219
  penumbra of 111–113, 262–263
  PSFs for 200,
  SARs for 235
  scatter coefficients for 453
  shielding data for 448
  source-head 110
  TARs for 199
  teletherapy machine 108–117
  teletherapy source capsule 111
  typical beam output factors for 211
^{60}Co source 16, 36, 53–55, 108–111, 117, 448,
  air-kerma rate 162–164
  as brachytherapy source 358, 375
  calibration of ion-chamber 149–151
  isodose curves for linear source 375
  scatter coefficients 453
  as teletherapy source 108–111
  values of g(r) 368
  water perturbation correction 368
Cockcroft-Walton voltage multiplier 119–120
Coefficient
  of atomic attenuation 72
  Compton absorption 80–81
  Compton scatter 80–81, 84–86

of electronic attenuation 72
of energy absorption 85, 499–505
of energy transfer 80–81, 85, 499–505
of equivalent thickness (CET) 344
of mass attenuation 71–72, 75, 499–505
of narrow and broad beam attenuation 88–89
of pair production 84–86
photoelectric effect 75–76, 84–86
total attenuation 85–86
Coherent Thompson scattering 69, 72–73
Cold cathode tubes 95–97
Collimators 109–110, 126, 262, 324–325
    assymmetric independent 240
    for intraoperative radiotherapy 347–348
    multi-leaf (see MLC)
Collimator scatter factor 211
Collision loss 60–63, 153
Collision stopping power Data 491–498
Colpostats 410–411
Conformal therapy, 314, 315
Coolidge X-ray tubes 96–97
Compensating filters 287–288
Compounds, attenuation coefficient 87
Compton cross section 77–81
Compton effect (see Compton scattering)
Compton scattering, incoherent 69, 77–81, 85–86, 194–196,
Computed tomography (CT), 260, 295, 306–308, 345, 253
Computer-assisted dosimetry 265, 271, 294, 401, 405–406
Computer planning 294, 308, 405
Concrete shielding materials 447–448, 458
Condenser chamber 169–171
Congenital defects 423
Contour shape, effect of,
    on electron beams 333–335
    on photon beams 267–270, 287
Conservation law
    of electric charge 33
    of lepton number 33
    of mass-energy 8, 35,83
    of momentum 35, 77,83
    of nucleon number 33
Controlled-access areas 445, 467, 468, 484
Copper
    filters 105–106, 338
    mass attenuation coefficients 503
    mass energy absorption coefficients 503
    mass energy transfer coefficients 503
Corpuscular radiation 3
Cosmic radiation 24, 434–435
Coulomb 15
Covalent bonds 17–18
CPE 138–139, 142, 148, 150, 151, 153, 248
CPOR 210–211
    derivation of dose rate 212–214, 232–234
Crookes' tubes 95–96
Cross section (see also coefficint)
    Compton scatter 80–81
    neutron absorption 52

neutron activation 52
pair production 84
photoelectric absorption 77
^{137}Cs
    air-kerma rate constant 161–162
    as brachytherapy source 358, 448
    as fission product 40
    scatter coefficients 453
    shielding data 448
    as teletherapy source 108–109
    values of g(r) 368
    water perturbation correction 369
CT (see Computed tomography)
CT numbers 253
CT scans 253, 306, 308
CT simulation 295, 308
Clinical target volume (CTV) 272
Cumulative effective dose 437, 444
Curie unit 44
Curved surfaces,
    and electron arc therapy 348–350
    and electron beams 333–335
    and photon beams 276–277
Cyclotron 118, 129–130
Cylindrical cavity chamber 148, 151, 171
Cylindrical mould 383–385

Dalton's, Atomic Theory 7
Daughter nuclides 48–52
Daughter product buildup and decay 48–52
Day's method 237, 238
de'Broglie waves 29
DDREF 433–434
Decay (see Radioactive Decay)
Decay chains 48–49
Decay constant 43–46
Decay schemes 34, 36, 38, 39, 40, 48
Deflector 129, 131, see also peeler
Delta rays 59, 67
Densitometer 173
Density
    of body constituents 241
    electron- 61, 240–241, 250,
    ionization 62, 67
    optical 173–175, 148
Depletion layer 178
Depth 196–197
    beam quality and 191–194
    calculation of dose at 195–196, 212–214
    effective 243–247
    treatment 190–191
    water-equivalent 243
Depth-dose data 206, 210, 228, 329–331
    gathering 175
    NAOFs 211
    NPOFs 211
    NPSFs 200, 211
    PDDs 201–205
    PSFs 198, 200, 201–203, 211
    TARs 197, 199
    TMRs 206–209

Depth-dose profile (see central-axis dose profile)
Deterministic radiation effects 422–423, 435, 437
Deuteron
  in nuclear reactions 130
  in particle accelerators 130
Deuterium 9, 130
Diamond crystal detector 178
Diaphragms (see also collimators)
  adjustable 110, 113
  collimating 109–110, 126, 261–264, 325,
  within wave guides 123
Differential SAR (DSAR) 251
Diodes, semiconductor 101–102, 177–178
Dirac's theory of the electron 82–83
Disposal of sources 484–486
Dissipation of heat 97–99, 157–158
Distribution rules (see Manchester System)
Door controls 467
Door shielding 448, 454–456, 462–463
Dosage tables
  cesium-137 sources 376
  linear sources 377
  planar implants 386, 387, 390–393
  volume implant 387, 391, 393
Dose and dose rate effectiveness factor (DDREF) 433–434
Dose build-up (see also Build-up)
  in high-energy photon beams 112, 140–142, 158,
  in oblique beams 270–271
  in electron beams 327, 329
Dose, calculation
  in photon beams
  on central axis 212–214
  at off-axis 238–240
  in blocked fields 230–237
  of non-uniform intensity 251–253
  in IMRT beams 251–253
  in electron beams 336–337
  near point source 159–165, 366–371
  near linear source 371–377
Dose equivalent (H) 425–426
Dose evaluation for radiation protection 423–429
Dose limits, for radiation safety
  adult radiation workers 436–437
  eye, feet, hands 437–439
  fetus 438
  general public 439, 445
  weekly limit for shielding 444–445
  workers under age 18, 438
Dose output (see CAOR; and CPOR)
Dose profile, see also central axis dose profile
  at air-tissue interface 140–142
  off-central axis 112, 191
  through lung and bone 246–248
Dose, radiation 119, 120
  definition 3, 138
  energy transfer 69, 139–140
  evaluation in air 143–146
    in medium 144–146

  in water 152
  to water 157 (see also Dosimetry)
  gathering depth-dose data 175
  kerma profiles and 140–142
  measurement (see dosimetry)
  prescription in radiotherapy 3, 5, 241, 259, 272, 300, 311, 313, 337, 385, 394
  relationship to kerma 139, 140, 141–142, 143–146
  relationship to air kerma and exposure 143–146
  to tissue in air 144, 151, 194–195, 228
  unit of 138
Dose rate constant (Λ) 163–165, 358, 370
Dose-response projection 431–432
Dose to skin (see skin dose)
Dose to tissue-in-air 144, 151, 194–195, 228
Dose-volume histograms (DVH) 301
Dose-volume plots 300–301
Dosimeters
  calorimeter 157–158
  chemical 180–181
  ferrous sulfate 180–181
  for neutrons 459
  Fricke 180–181
  ionization chamber (see under same heading)
  nuclear magnetic resonance (NMR) 182
  optically stimulated luminescence (OSL) 182
  for personnel monitoring 438
  photographic film 173–174
  radiochromic film 182–183
  radiochromic film 182–183
  semiconductor 177–178
  solid-state conductivity 177–178
  thermoluminescent 178–179
  TLD 178–179
Dosimetry (see also Dosimeters)
  in brachytherapy
    AAPM/ICGW empirical approach 369–371, 376–377
    brachytherapy planning 400–401, 405–408
    by computer 405–408
    linear sources 371–377
    permanent implant 408–409
    point source in water 159–165, 366–371
    radioactive seed implants 408–409
  in external beam therapy (see dose calculation)
DRR 295, 315
DSAR 251
Dumb-bell-type loading 409–410
Duration of treatment 210, 214, 365, 385
DVH 301

Effective atomic number (Z_{eff}) 87, 241
Effective depth 243
Effective dose 428–429
Effective field size 243
Effective rectangular field 231–232
Effective SSD,
  for missing-tissue correction 269
  for electron beams 340–341

Electrometer 147, 155, 168, 169, 170, 363
Equivalent squares and circles 214–215
Einstein, Albert 7, 29, 74
Einstein's theory of relativity 7, 29, 77
Electric field 26–28, 83, 118
   in ionization chambers 146–147, 168–169,
   in linear accelerators 118–132
Electricity, and magnetism 27–28
Electromagnetic radiation 3, 14, 26–29
Electromagnetic waves 26–29
Electron angular scattering 59–60
Electron arc therapy 348–350
Electron backscattering 69–70
Electron beam
   adjacent fields 350–351
   agreement of light and radiation fields
      341–342
   angular scattering in 323–324, 327–329
   backscattering in 337–339
   comparison with kilovoltage X-ray beams
      345–346
   delivery port 324–325
   depth-dose curve 329–331, 333–335
      field size and 331
      oblique incidence and 333–335
      shape of 327
   dose distribution 325–335, 350–351
   dose enhancement by shields 337–339
   effective SSD for 340–341
   extrapolated range of 329–330
   factors influencing 326
   field shaping 337, 341–342
   from machine to patient 324–325
   inhomogeneities and 342–344
   intraoperative radiotherapy 347–348
   output factors for 335–351
   pencil beam 324, 333–334
   photographic images of 326
   practical range of 329–330
   selective shielding within 337–339
   surface dose build-up 327–329
   total-skin treatment 346–347, 467
   trimmers 324–325, 340
   water-equivalent depth in 344
Electron capture 37–38
Electron contamination dose 112–113, 141, 193
Electron-density 61
   and collision loss 61
   and Compton effect 81, 249
   and energy absorption 248–250
Electron gun 124–125
Electron, secondary (see Secondary electrons)
Electron Volt (eV) 15
Electronic attenuation coefficient 72
Electronic equilibrium 146 (see also CPE)
Electron-positron annihilation 83–84
Electron scattering 60, 125, 323–325
   electron-electron 323
   electron-nuclear 323
Electron track 59, 67
Electrons 7, 8, 21–22
   Auger (see Auger electrons)

binding energies of 13, 14–15, 39, 74
charge of 8, 15, 82–83
Compton recoil 77–79
contamination and skin dose 112–113,
   138–141, 194–195
free vs. bound 77
from ionization chamber wall 154–155
orbits (see Orbits of electrons)
secondary 14, 112–113, 138–141, 194–195
shells 11–14
tracks of 59, 139–140
Electrostatic accelerators 108–121
Elementary particles 20–24 (see also Charged
   particles)
   forces between 21
   wave-like behavior of 29–30
Elements
   artificially produced 11, 16
   binding energies of atomic orbital electrons
      13
   definition 8
   formation of 8–10
   list of 10
   naturally occurring 11
   periodic table 17–18
   stable, unstable 11
   transuranic 11
Elongation correction factors 398
Embryo exposure limits 438
Emergency action procedure 468
Endocurie therapy 357
Energy 7
   absorption of local 73, 81, 85
   amount absorbed and dose 138
   binding 8, 13, 32
   bremsstrahlung 63–66, 85, 97, 144
   continuous, of beta particles 35, 39
   of dissipation as heat 97, 157–158
   electron volt unit and 15
   law of conservation 8
   needed to produce an ion pair 144–145
   of nucleons 32
   of photons 29
   potential 12–13
   propagation of electromagnetic 26–30
   of quarks 18
   transfer coefficient 85, 499–505
   at rest 3
Energy fluence 136
Energy fluence rate 137
Energy states 7–8
Energy straggling 329
Energy transfer 137
Entrance door shielding 448, 454–456,
   462–463
Entrance maze 454, 455, 458, 459
Epidemiological data 421, 430–431
Equilibrium (see CPE)
Equivalent dose 427–428
"Ether" 28
Excitation 3, 14–15
   and nuclide stability 11

Exclusion principle, Pauli's 11
Exit dose 346
Exit zone 271–272, 294
Exposure 142–145
  concept of 142–143
  measurement of 146–150
  relationship to air kerma 143–145
  relationship to dose 143–145
  unit of 143
Exposure calibration factor 149–150, 155
Extrapolation chamber 172–173
External Beam Therapy Safety (see Radiation
  Safety)
European Atomic Energy Community 421
Eye lens
  opacification 422
  recommended dose limits 437, 438, 439
Eyler's exponential constant 44

Facility design 449, 467–469
Fall-off, inverse-square (see Inverse square
  factor)
Fatal accident risk 436, 437
Feathering adjacent beams 312–313
Ferrous sulfate dosimeter 180–181
Fetus exposure limits 438
Field size
  of beam 190, 191, 196
  effective rectangular 231
  equivalent squares and circles 214–216
  irregularly-shaped, with shields 231–232
Field localizer (see light beam localizer)
Filament tube 96–97
Film
  badges 438, 486
  diagnostic imaging 174–176
  dosimetry by 173–174, 182–183
  high-energy portal 176
  optical density 173
  photographic, silver bromide 173
  radiochromic 182–183
  response curves 174–175
Filters
  Aluminum 105–106
  beam-flattening 125
  Copper 105–106
  Thoreaus 105–106
  Wedge 214, 251, 273–279, 288, 315
  in X-ray tube 96, 99, 104, 105–106
Finger badges 438, 486
Fixed-SAD technique 190, 214, 196–197, 200,
  212–213
Fixed-SSD technique 214, 196–197, 200, 212–213
Flattening filter (see filters)
Fluence 135–136
Fluence rate 136
Fluoroscopy, diagnostic 99–100
Focal spots, X-ray 97–98, 261–264
Foil, electron-scattering 125–126, 323–325
  activation dosimetry 459
Forces, nuclear 32

electro-weak 21
short-range 21
strong and weak 21
Four-field box 284, 286
Four-field-obliques 284, 290
Free electrons 77
Frequency of waves 27–29
Free-air ionization chamber 146–147
Fricke dosimeter 180–181
Full 360 degree rotation 288, 291
Full-wave rectification 102–103

G value 181
Gamma rays 28, 31, 34, 36–40
Gap on skin 309–312, 350–351
Gas-discharge X-ray tube 95–96
Gas multiplication 169
Geiger-Mueller (GM) counter regions 168–169
Genetic effects 423
Geometrical features,
  of single beams 189–191, 260–261
  of penumbra 111–113
Geometric penumbra 111–113
Germanium 177
Given dose 266–267
Glossary of acronyms 228, 253, 315
Gluons 21–22
Gold-198, (see ^{198}Au)
Gravitational field 11–14, 21
Gray unit, definition 137
Grids 81, 175–176
Gross tumor volume, (GTV) 272
Gynecologic applications 409–414

^{3}H 9, 42, 435, 459
H & D curve 174
Hadrons 23–24
Half-life 32, 45–46
Half-value thickness (HVT) 70–71, 106, 191, 441
Half-wave rectification 101–102
Hardening of Beam 105–106, 240
Harmful effects of radiation 422–423
Heat generation,
  by radiation dose 157–158
  in X-ray tubes 97–99
Heel effect 98
Helium, atom 9, 130
  binding energies 9
  in fusion 41–42
  ions in alpha decay 31–34
  isotopes 9
Heyman packing 413
High-dose-rate (HDR) 361, 478–479
High-voltage supply and rectification 100–103,
  108
Hinge angle 277–278
"holes" 82–83, 177–178
Homogeneity index 106
Homogeneity of Beam 106
Hot-cathode tubes 96–97

Hydrogen
  atom 8–9
  deuteron 9
  during fusion 35
  isotopes 9
  mass attenuation coefficients 499
  mass energy absorption coefficients 499
  mass energy transfer coefficients 499
  in molecular bonds of 17, 19–20
  tritium 9, 435
Hydrogen bomb 34
Hydrogen bonds 19–20
Hydrogenous materials 458
Hyperons 23

^{125}I
  characteristics 358, 368, 389, 394
  decay scheme of 38
  permanent implant 47, 389
  value of g(r) for 369
ICF 240–248
  definition 241
  different methods of deriving 245–247
ICRP, safety guidelines 421, 423, 434, 436–439
ICRU 135, 269, 272, 301, 413, 423, 425
ICWG dosimetry approach 369–371, 376–377
Implants (see Brachytherapy principles)
IMRT 252, 314–316, 452
Incoherent Compton scattering 69, 77–81, 85–86, 194–196
Independent collimator 240
Induced nuclear transformations 42
Induced radioactivity 460
Infrared radiation 26, 28
Internal conversion 32, 38–39
Iodine-125 (see ^{125}I)
Iodine-131 36
Ionization 3, 14–15
Ionization chambers
  cavity 147–149, 169–172
  condenser 169–171
  free-air 146–147
  pancake 148–149, 171–172
  parallel plate 148–149, 156, 171–172
  pocket 438
  re-entrant 362–363
  thimble 148, 171
Ionization detectors 168–171
Ionization density 62, 67
In-air output (see CAOR)
Index of harm 423
Infinite limit approximation 344
Inhomogeneities, lung and bone 240–248
Inhomogeneity correction factor (see ICF)
Integral dose 301–302
Intensity Modulated Radiotherapy (IMRT) (see IMRT)
Intensifying screens 148–149
Intensity
  of light 173
  of radiation 65–66, 89, 105

International Atomic Energy Agency 421
International Commission on Radiation Protection (see ICRP)
Interstitial Collaborative Working Group (see ICWG)
International Commission Radiation Units and Measurements (see ICRU)
Intracavitary insertions 360, 374, 377–379, 409–414
Intraluminal therapy 360, 374, 377–379
Intraoperative radiotherapy (IORT), 347–348
Intrauterine irradiation 360, 411–414
Inverse-square factor
  in brachytherapy dosimetry 363–369
  in brachytherapy safety 479–480
  in external beam dosimetry 195, 196, 197, 213, 214
  in radionuclide source dosimetry 159–165
  in shielding evaluation 444, 451–453, 455–456
Iodine-125 (see ^{125}I)
^{192}Ir
  as brachytherapy source 358, 480
  planar implant table 391
  production of 55
  as teletherapy source 108–109
  values of g(r) for
  water perturbation correction 368
  wires in Paris system 387
Iridium-192 (see ^{192}Ir)
Iridium-191 54
Iridium-192 (see ^{192}Ir)
Irradiation parameters 196–197
Isobars 11
Isocentrically mounted system 115, 125, 155
Iso-centric technique 197, 267, 210
Isodose curves and surfaces 259–260
Isodose Distributions
  for adjacent electron beams 350–351
  for adjacent photon beams 309–313
  for a breast implant 406, 407
  derivation of 265–267
  for esophagus treatment 298–299
  for implanted source arrays 378–382,
  in intracavitary applications 410, 411, 414
  for oblique beams 274, 275, 278, 288, 289, 299, 303–305
  for other multiple beams 288–293, 298–299
  for parallel opposed beams 281–283, 285, 288
  for single beams 261, 263, 276, 332
  for wedged beam combinations 274–275, 278–279, 288
Isomeric state 11, 40,
Isomeric transition 11,40,51
Isomers 11, 40
Isotones 11
Isotopes 9–11
  artificially produced 52–55, 130, 357
  of carbon 15–16
  definition 9–11
  of helium 9
  of hydrogen 9

radioactive 11, 52, 107–108, 130, 357–358
   stable 11
   unstable 11

Japanese atomic bomb survivors 150
Joule 15, 97, 157–158

^{40}K, (Potasium-40) 435
K shell 11–14
Kerma
   air- 142–145
   air-kerma rate constant 159–163, 358
   definition 137
   ratio of, to dose at depth 140–142
   relationship to dose 139–140, 143–144
   relationship to exposure 143–145
   water 140–142
Kinetic energy
   of Compton recoil electrons 77–78
   of photoelectrons 74
Klystron 125, 469

L shell 11–14
Lateral electronic equilibrium 248
Laws of conservation (see individual
     conservation laws)
Lead
   for beam collimation 109–110
   collision and radiative loss 64
   electron mass stopping powers 498
   mass attenuation coefficients 505
    in comparison with water 64, 75, 86
    vs. photon energy for 75
   mass energy absorption coefficients 231, 505
   mass energy transfer coefficients 230, 505
   percent of different interactions 86
   types of photon interactions in 75
   shielding
    for brachytherapy sources 480–481, 484
    in electron beams 337–340, 342
    at entrance door 448, 454, 463
    for therapy source 109–110
    for x-ray tube 97
Leakage radiation 2, 4
   from klystrons 469
   protective barrier 452
   skyshine of 465
   from therapy source-head 445–446
Lethal dose 422
Leptons 21–22
LD50/30, 422
LET 67, 424–426,
   and biological effect 424–426
   and microscopic energy deposition 424–426
   and quality factor (QF) 424–426
Light
   transmitted, intensity 173
   velocity of 7, 29
   visible 28

Light beam localizer 110, 115, 125, 325, 341–342
Linear accelerators (linacs) 118, 121–126
Linear-quadratic model 431–432
Linear sources 371–374
Light waves 27–28
Linear attenuation coefficient 71
Linear density of ionization 67
Linear energy transfer (see LET)
Lithium fluoride 17, 19
   dosimeter 178, 180
   mass stopping powers for 497
   molecule 19
   thermoluminescence 178, 180
Loaded wave guides 123
Locally absorbed energy 76, 84–85
Lorentz force 118
Low-dose-rate (LDR) brachytherapy 361,
    478–479
Lung
   as a body inhomogeneity 241–242
   density of 241–242
   depth-dose profiles through 246–247
   dose-volume plots 301
   effective atomic number 241
   lateral electronic equilibrium and 248
   phantom geometry of 242

M shell 11–14, 105
Magnetic field 27–28, 31–32
   in particle accelerators 125–131
Magnetic peeler 127–128
Magnetic resonance Imaging (MRI) 182
Magnetism, and electricity 27–28
Magnetron 125
Manchester system 390, 392, 394–398, 400
   for implants 397–398
    single-plane 397
    two-plane 397
    volume 398
   surface applications 394–397
    circular areas 395
    irregularly shaped areas 396
    rectangular areas 396
Mass
   atomic 8, 15–16
   attenuation coefficient 71–72, 75–76, 86, 250,
    499–505
   of elementary particles 8, 22–24
   of gas in Bragg-Gray cavity 133
   molecular 15–16
   -number (M) 9
Mass attenuation coefficient (see also Energy
    transfer and Energy absorption)
   definition 71–72, 75
   variation with energy 75–76
   for various materials 250, 499–505
Mass-energy relation 7
Mass-equivalent thickness 71–72
Mass unit, atomic 15
Mayneord F factor 217–218
Maze entrance 454, 455, 458, 459

Mean free path 71
Mean life 21–24, 45–47, 409
Medical physics 3
Medical radiation exposures 435
Mental retardation 423
Memorial Hospital system 389–390
Mesons 21–23
Metal oxide field effect transistors (MOSFET) 178
Microscopic energy deposition 67, 424–425
Microtron 118, 130–132
Microwaves 28, 125, 131
Microwave technology 125, 131
Milligram hour of treatment 365–366
Milligram radium equivalent 362–363
Minimum peripheral dose (MPD) 386, 389
Mixtures, attenuation coefficient 87
MLC 230, 252, 315, 316
Molecular bonds 17–20
   covalent bonds 17, 19–20
      Aluminum Oxide 20
      Ammonia 20
      Water 19
   formation of 17–20
   hydrogen bond 19
   ionic bond 17
Molecular mass 15–16
Molybdenum-99 40, 51–52
Momentum
   of Compton recoil electron 77
   Compton scatter photon 77
   conservation law 35, 77
   of free body 7
   of photon 29, 77
Monitor ion chamber 125–126
Monitor unit 210
Monitor units per degree of arc 227
Monitoring (see Radiation Monitoring)
MOSFET 178
MRI dosimetry 182
Multiple source arrays 379–385
Multiplicative-risk projection model 432–433
Muons 21–22
Mutations, radiation induced 425
Muscle
   electron mass stopping powers 493
   mass attenuation coefficients for 250, 501
   mass energy absorption coefficients 501
   mass energy transfer coefficients 501
M value, mass number 9

N value, neutron number 9
^{22}Na 37–38, 435
NAOF 200–211
Narrow-beam geometry 88–89
National Council on Radiation Protection and Measurements (see NCRP)
Natural background radiation 434–435
NCRP 421, 422, 425, 427, 434, 436, 437–438, 446, 458, 468, 478

NCRP, safety guidelines 421, 423, 434, 436, 436–439
Negatron 35
   -positron pair production 37, 82–83
Net minimum dose (NMD) 392–398
Neutrinos
   electron- 21–22
   muon- 21–22
   tau- 21–22
Neutron 8–9, 11
   activation by 52–55
   capture gamma-rays 445, 459
   decay of 35
   detection and dosimetry 459
   induced activity 460
   moderation 458
   from nuclear fission 40–41
   number (N)
   physical characteristics 8–11
   -proton balance 34–35
   -producing reactions 130
   quality factor for 426
   quarks structure within 24
   radiation weighting factor 427–428, 459
   relative biological effectiveness 425
   slowing down of 458
   shielding of 316, 460, 457–459, 460
   and stability of isotopes 11, 34–35
Neutron equivalent dose 458–459
Neutron flux 52–53, 458
Neutron number (N) 9
Neutron-Photon ratio 458
Neutron shielding 457–459
Neutron survey instruments 459
New York (Memorial Hospital) system 389–390
Nitrogen
   in ammonia 19
   isotopes of 11
   mass attenuation coefficients 499
   mass energy absorption coefficients 499
   mass energy transfer coefficients 499
Normalized air output factor (see NAOF)
Normalized peak output factor (see NPOF)
   173–174
   derivation of dose rate 175–177
   effective rectangular field 194–195, 196
   PDD and 184, 186
Normalized peak scatter factor (see NPSF)
NPOF 211
NPSF 200–211
NTP 143
"n-type" semiconductor material 178
Nuclear decay scheme (see Decay schemes)
Nuclear fission 32, 40–41
Nuclear forces 21, 32
Nuclear fusion 41–42
Nuclear reaction 35
Nuclear reactors 52–55, 428, 435
Nuclear transitions 31–42
   induced 42
   isomeric 11, 40, 51
Nucleons 33

Nucleus 8–11, 31–33
Nurse's safety 484

Oblique incidence
  compensation for 287–288
  and depth-dose 269–270, 333–335
  and skin dose 270–271
Occupancy factor (T) 450–451
Occupational effective dose limits 436–437
Oncogenic transformation 425
Optical density 173–174
Optical distance indicator 115
Optical distance indicator (ODI) 114–116
Optically simulated luminescence (OSL) 182, 438
Orbits of electrons 11–14
Organ weighting factors 428–429
Orthogonal radiographic localization 403–406
Oscillator
  microwave 125
  radio frequency 121, 125
OSL dosimeters 182, 438
Outcome 4–5, 317
  examples of treatment
    by beam therapy 4
    by brachytherapy 5
Output factor
  collimator output 211
  in-air output (see CAOR and NAOF)
  peak output (see CPOR and NPOF)
  phantom-scatter 211
  total output 211
Oxalic acid 181
Oxygen
  isotopes of 11
  mass attenuation coefficients 500
  mass energy absorption coefficients 500
  mass energy transfer coefficients 500
  in molecular bonds 17, 19–20,
Ozone 467

Pair production 69, 84–86,
  cross section 84
  negatron-positron 37, 82–83,
  threshold energy 82
  yield 84
Palladium-103, (see ^{103}Pd)
PAR 234–237
Para-cervical triangle 412
Paris system 387–389, 392, 408
Particles (see Charged particles;
    Elementary particles)
  accelerators (see accelerators)
  fluence 135–136
Pancake chamber 148–149, 171–172, 156
Parallel-plate cavity chamber 129, 146
Parallel opposed beams 279–284
  adjacent to single beam 312–313
  at adjacent sites 311–313
  three-field techniques 17, 21

Paterson and Parker system (see Manchester
    system)
Patient positioning 114–116, 189–190, 267, 303
  for electron arc therapy 349
  for total-skin electron treatment 346–347
Patient scatter 445, 452–454
Patient support assembly 114–115
Pauli's, Exclusion principle 11
^{103}Pd
  characteristics 358, 368, 394
  for permanent implant 408, 486
  values of g(r) for 369
  water perturbation correction 368
PDD,
  definition 200, 204
  converting for one SSD to another 217–219
  relationship to TAR and TMR 178, 180
  data 201–205
Peak scatter factor (see PSF)
Peeler (betatron) 127–128
Pencil beam 324, 333–334
Penumbra 111–113, 261–264
  of cobalt-60 beam 111–113, 262
  fall-off of dose in 309
  geometric and transmission 111–113,
    261–264
  for low-energy X-ray 261–262
  for megavoltage X-rays 262–263
  producers 351
  -zone 261, 271–272, 294
Percent depth dose (see PDD) 165–166, 178
  converting for one SSD to another 180–190
  data tables 201–205
  relationship to TAR and TMR 217
Periodic table of elements 17–18
Peripheral dose, minimum (MPD) 386, 389
Permanent implants 408–409, 486
Phantom material 87, 189, 196, 228, 242, 244
  water as 196, 228
Phase stability 122–123, 132
Phosphorus-32 (^{32}P) 358
Photoelectric absorption 69, 75–76, 84–86
Photoelectric cross section 77, 86
Photoelectric effect 73–75
Photoelectric interaction 69, 75–76, 84–86
Photoelectrons 14, 73–75
  angular emission 76,
  kinetic energy 74
Photographic film detector 173–174, 325–326,
    337–340, ,438
Photographic process 173 (see also film)
Photomultiplier 177–179
Photon beam radiation safety (see radiation
    safety)
Photon characteristics,
  emission (see characteristic x-rays and gamma
    rays)
  frequency 29
  momentum 29, 77
  quanta 29
  wavelength 28–29

Photon field 21
Photon flux 70
  diminution of 69–70
Photon-induced activity 460
Photon interactions 69
  relative percentages of different 86
Photons 23–24 (see also Electromagnetic
      radiation, Electromagnetic spectrum,
      and Gamma rays)
  interactions of 69–90
  wavelength of 28–29
Photonuclear reaction 90
Phosphorous-32 130
Physicist
  clinical vii, 3–6, 159, 228, 294
  qualified 469
Physics, historical background of atomic 3–6
Physics, medical 3
Pions 22
Planar implant distribution rules (see
      Distribution rules)
Planar implant dosage table (see Dosage tables)
Planck's constant 29
Planning target volume (PTV) 272
Plasma state of matter 41
Plastic
  in parallel-plate chambers 148–149
  scintillators 177
  use in cavity ionization chambers 148–149
  as water-substitute in dose assessment 157
Pocket ionization chambers 438
Points A and B 412–413
Polonium 31
Polymethyl methacrylate,
  electron mass stopping powers 494
Polyethylene
  electron mass stopping powers in 494
  mass attenuation coefficients 502
  mass energy absorption coefficients 502
  mass energy transfer coefficients 502
  for neutron shielding 458
Polystyrene
  electron mass stopping powers in 495
  mass attenuation coefficients for 502
  mass energy absorption coefficients for
      502
  mass energy transfer coefficients for 502
Port films 176, 294, 307–308
Positioning, of patient 114–115, 189–190,
      267, 303
Positrons 35, 37–38;
  negatron-positron pair production 37,
      82–83
Practical range 329–330
Pregnant women's exposure 438, 486
Preloading,361, 479, 487
Pressure (see also NTP and STP)
  in gas-discharge X-ray tubes 95
  in ion chamber 143, 149–150
Primary-air ratio (see PAR)
Primary and secondary electrons 329
Primary protective barriers 451–452

Proportional counters 168–169, 459
Prostate implants 486
Protocols for beam calibration 150–151,
      157–159,
  using absorbed dose calibration factor
      157–159
  using exposure calibration factor
      150–157
Protons 7–8, 24
  beta-plus decay and 37
  charge of 8,
  collision loss and 61–62
  during electron capture 37–38
  in particle accelerators 130
  physical characteristics 7–8
  quarks structure in 24
Prout's hypothesis 7
PSF
  data, derivation of dose rate 175–176
  definition 198–200
  effective rectangular field 194, 195
  inhomogeneity correction factor 206
  normalized 200–211
  uses of 206, 210–211, 213–214, 232–234,
Public radiation dose limits 439, 445
Pseudo-arc technique 350
"p-type" semiconductor material 178

Quality factor (Q) 425–426
Quanta, and the electromagnetic spectrum
      26–30,
Quantum chromodynamics 21
Quantum electrodynamics 21
Quantum mechanics 11
Quantum numbers 11–13
Quarks 20–24
Quimby system 385–386, 392

^{226}Ra
  alpha decay to radon 34
  as brachytherapy source 357, 358, 480, 483
  decay chain of 48
  equivalent mass of 362–363
  milligram hours of 365–366
  radon leakage hazard 357, 483
  in secular equilibrium with radon 50
  shielding considerations 109, 480
  as teletherapy source 108–109
  water perturbation corrections 368
Radiation alarms 468–478
Radiation chemical yield 181
Radiation components 445
Radiation dose (see Dose)
Radiation dosimetry (see Dosimetry)
Radiation field 135 (see also field size)
Radiation harmful effects 422–423
Radiation leakage (see Leakage radiation)
Radiation monitoring
  badges 438, 486
  of brachytherapy patients 484

instruments for 480
of neutrons 459
of personnel 438, 486
Radiation protection (see Radiation Safety)
Radiation risk assessment 421, 430–434,
    absolute and relative risks 432–433
    ICRP estimate 434
    uncertainties in 430–434
Radiation safety (see also shielding)
    brachytherapy 478–488
        afterloading techniques 479–487
        HDR and LDR 478–479
        handling of sources 478–480
            role of distance 480, 487
            role of shielding 479–480
            role of time 479
        monitoring instruments 480
        nurses and visitors 484
        patient's body survey 485–486
        permanent implants 486
        post-treatment procedures 484–486
        radiation surveys 485–486
        removable implants 480–486
        room survey 484–486
        source inventory 482
        source wipe tests 482–483
        storage and handling 478, 480–482
    dose limits guidelines
        adult radiation workers 436–437
        eye, feet, hands 437–439
        fetus 438
        general public 439, 445
        source-head leakage 445–446
        weekly limit for shielding 444–445
        workers under age 18 438
    external beam therapy 443–477
        (see also Shielding)
        architectural and equipment data 449
        barrier transmission 451–457
        comparison with brachytherapy 195
        effect of distance 451–457
        entrance door barrier 448, 454–456,
            462–463
        facility design and planning 467–469
        neutron capture gamma rays 445–449
        occupancy factor (T) 450–451
        ozone production 467
        patient monitoring 468
        source-head leakage 445–446
        use factor (U) 450
        warning signs and indicators 468
        weekly dose limits 444–445
        workload (W) 449–450
Radiation Safety Committee (RSC) 438
Radiation safety officer (RSO) 438
Radiation safety philosophy 432–436
Radiation safety standards (see Dose limits)
Radiation survey meters 480
Radiation weighting factors 426–427
Radiation worker, dose limits 436–437
Radiation therapy. See Radiotherapy
Radiation units and measurements 135–167

Radiative loss 63–74
Radiative stopping power data , 491–498
Radioactive decay 31–42
    by alpha emission 33
    by beta emission 34–37
    calculations of 43–55
    chains of 48–52
    complete 47, 408
    constant of 46–47
    by electron capture 37
    by fission 40–41
    half-life 45–46
    by internal conversion 38–39
    by isomeric transition 40
    mean life 46–47
    randomness of 43
Radioactive seed implants 378, 383–384, 389,
    400–401, 406, 408–409, 496
Radioactive sources (see Radionuclide
    sources)
Radioactive wires 374, 377–378, 387, 483
Radioactivity, discovery of natural 31
Radioactivity warning signs 484, 485
Radiofrequency (RF) oscillator 121
Radiographic localization of sources
    401–405
Radiography, diagnostic 99, 100, 175–176
Radioisotopes (see Isotopes)
Radiomimetic gas 467
Radionuclide sources,
    for brachytherapy 358
    decay calculations 43–55
    decay modes and schemes 33–42
    for teletherapy 108–109
Radiotherapy simulator (see simulator)
Radio waves 28
Radium 31 (see also Radium-226)
Radium-226 (see ^{226}Ra)
Radium-E 35, 48
Radium-equivalent mass 362–363
Radon, contamination hazard 357–358, 483
Radon-222 34
Range straggling 329
Reactors 40–41, 428, 435
Rectification 101–103
Reentrant ionization chamber 362–363
Relative biological effectiveness (RBE) 425
Relative-risk models 432–433
Relativity, Theory of 7, 29, 77
rem unit 426
Removable implants 360, 480–486
Resonance accelerators 118, 121–132
RF Oscillator 121, 125
Risk assessment (see Radiation risk
    assessment)
Risk-benefit philosophy 435–436
Roentgen equivalent man (see rem)
Roentgen rays 95 (see also X-rays)
Roentgen unit 143
Roof irradiation and protection 456–457,
    463–466
Rotating anode 99

SAD 190–191
Safety standards (see dose limits)
Samarium-145 (^{145}Sm) 358, 369, 480
SAR 234–237
  differential SAR 251
Saturation activity 53–55
S_c 211, 232
Scatter
  in blocked fields 230–231
  coherent Thompson 69, 72–73, 86
  Compton 69, 77–81, 85–86, 194–196
    angular distribution 79
    backscatter 79–80
    forward scatter 79–80
    perpendicular 79–80
  differential scatter 251
  dose to tissue in air 194–195
  electron 60, 125, 323–325,
  use of grid to minimize 81, 175
  from treatment head 232, 195–196
Scatter-air ratio (see SAR and TAR)
Scatter build-up factor 89, 163–164, 368
Scatter-radius integration 235–237
Scattering coefficient (α) 453
Scattering foils 125–126, 324
Sealed sources 357
Secular equilibrium 49–50
Seed implants (see Radioactive seed
      implants)
Semiconductor diodes 177–178
Shipping of sources 483–484
SI system 137
Sievert's integral 373
Silicon 177
  electron mass stopping powers for 496
  mass attenuation coefficients for 503
  mass energy absorption coefficients for
      503
  mass energy transfer coefficients for 503
Simulator,
  general features 294–295
  localization using 303–308, 401, 404, 405
Single-plane implant 359–360, 380–381, 385,
      390, 391
Skin dose,
  at air-tissue interface 140–142
  and bolusing 287
  in electron beams 192–193, 327, 331
  from electron contamination 112, 141
  limits for radiation safety 437–438
  for low-energy X-ray beams 192–193
  in megavoltage X-ray beams 140–142,
      192–193,
  and oblique incidence 271
Sodium-22 38
Skin gap 309–312, 350–351
Skyshine evaluations 456–457, 463–466
Sodium-22 37–38, 435
Somatic effects 423
Source, radionuclide (see Radionuclide
      sources)
Source capsule 111, 371–373

Source-head 109–110, 114 (see also
      treatment-head)
Source disposal 486
Source inventory 482
Source strength 361–364
  specification
    by activity 363–364
    by air-kerma rate 364
    need for 361–362
    by radium-equivalent mass 362–363
    by water-kerma rate 364
  time product 365–366
  traceability 362
Source wipe tests 482–483
Source isotopes,
  for brachytherapy 358
  for teletherapy 108–109
Source on-off mechanism 110–111
Source-to-axis distance (see SAD)
Source-to-skin distance (see SSD)
Space research 24
Special theory of relativity 7, 29, 77
Specific ionization 67
Spectrometer 177
Spherical volume seed implant 383–384
Spin, of elementary particles 21
^{90}Sr beta source 357–358, 481–482
S_p 211, 232
SRT 314, 315
SSD 190–191
St 211, 232
Stability
  of elementary particles 21–23
  of isotopes 11,
  phase 122–124, 131,
Stable isotopes 11
Stable nuclide, definition 32
Standard International System
      (see SI system)
Standing wave 124
Standing wave linear accelerator 124
Stem effect 170–171
Stereotactic Radiotherapy (SRT) 314, 315
Stereo radiography 402–403
Stochastic radiation effects 422
Storage of radioisotope sources 480–482
Stopping power 61–64
  collision- 61–63
  data for many materials 491–498
  linear- 61
  mass- 61
  radiative 61, 63–64
  restricted- 67
  in relation to LET 67
STP 149
Strontium-90 (^{90}Sr) 358, 481–482
Support of patient 114–115
Surface applications 359, 383–385,
      394–397
Surface curvature 267–268
  compensation for 287–288
  and depth-dose 269–270

and dose buildup 270–271
  effect in electron beams 333–335
  effect on skin dose 270–271
Survey instruments 480
  for neutrons 459

Tangentially opposing beams 288
Tantalum-182 (^{182}Ta) 358, 480, 482
TAR
  for cobalt-60 199
  in Day's method 237–238
  definition 197
  derivation of dose rate and 213–214
  in effective rectangular field 231–232
  inhomogeneity correction factor and 243–245
  in relation to TMR 205–206
  in relationship to PDD 217
  in scatter-air ratio correction 234–235
  in scatter-radius integration 235–236
  for zero field size 234
Target (see also Thickness of medium)
  in accelerators 125–126
  and field width and length 265
  localization 296–298
  for nuclear reactions 90
  for planar implants 359–360, 387–389 (see
    also CTV, GTV, PTV)
  volume in radiotherapy 230–231, 259, 264, 265,
    271, 272, 300, 314, 315
  in X-ray tubes 96
Target zone 13–14
Technetium generator 51–52
Technetium-99m 40, 51–52
Teflon, electron mass stopping powers 493
Teletherapy 107–113
Tenth-value thickness (TVT) 447–448,
  for neutrons 458
Temperature pressure correction factor 149
Temporary implants 360, 480–486
Terrestrial radiation 434–435
Thallium-activated sodium iodide 176
Therapy simulator (see simulator)
Thermionic emission 14, 96–97
Thermoluminescence 178
Thermoluminescent dosimeters (TLDs)
  178–180, 438
Thermonuclear bomb 41
Thimble cavity chamber 148, 171
Three Dimensional Conformal Radiotherapy
  (3DCRT), 314, 315
Three-field box 277, 279
Three-field-obliques 288, 289
Three-field techniques, using wedges 277, 278
Thompson scattering 69, 72–73, 86
Thoreaus filter 105–106
Three-phase transformers 103
Threshold energy
  for negatron-positron pair production 82
  for photonuclear reactions 90
Tin
  filters 105–106

mass attenuation coefficients 504
mass energy absorption coefficients 504
mass energy transfer coefficients 504
Tissue
  behavior of water as analogy for 140–142
  dose to 151–152, 194–196,
  effective atomic number and density of 241
  effective atomic number (Z_{eff}) 87
  electron mass stopping powers 492
  mass-energy absorption coefficient 250
  substitute materials 87
Tissue-air ratio (see TAR and SAR)
Tissue-air interface 140
Tissue-compensating filters 287–288
Tissue-equivalent bolus (see bolusing)
Tissue-maximum ratio (see TMR)
Tissue-phantom ratio (TPR) 205–206
Tissue weighting factors 428
TLD reader 179–180
TMR
  data tables 207–209
  definition 205–206
  derivation of dose rate and 213–214
  effective rectangular field and 231–232
  relationship to PDD 217
Tolerance doses 264, 300, 301
Tomotherapy 316
Total-skin electron treatment 346–347, 467
Transformer, Electrical 100, 118
  principle of 100
  three-phase 103
Transient equilibrium 50–51
Transmission penumbra 111–113, 261–264
Transport of sources 483–484
Traveling-wave linear accelerator 124
Treatment duration 210, 214, 365, 385
Treatment (source) head 109–110, 124–126,
  232, 324
Treatment planning (see Isodose distribution)
Treatment planning computer 294, 308, 405
Trimmers, for electron beams 324–325, 340
Triplet production 83
Tube shift radiographic localization 402–403
Tungsten
  electron mass stopping powers in 498
  for shielding and collimation 109
  as target in X-ray tubes 97
Two-plane implants 360, 381–382, 397

Ultraviolet radiation 28
Uncertainties, in radiation risk assessment
  430–434
Units for radiation measurements 135–167
Uranium
  fission 40
  radioactivity of 31
  for source shielding 109
Uranium-235 40
Uranium-238 40
Use factor (U) 450
Uterine applications 360, 411–413

Vaginal colpostats 410–411
Vaginal cylinder 409–410
van de Graff generator 120–121
Voltage
    in ionization detectors 146, 168–171
    in X-ray tube 95–104
Voltage multiplier 119–120
Volume implants 360, 383–384, 389, 391–394,
    408–409

Wall scatter 455, 456, 461–463
Warning signs 468, 484, 485
Water
    collision and radiative loss in 64
    dose buildup at interface 140–142, 193
    dose in 152, 157, 366–369,
    dose to 152, 157, 366–369,
    electron mass stopping powers in 491
    -kerma 140–142, 364,
    kerma rate yield 91
    linear source dosimetry 100–101
    mass attenuation coefficients 500
    mass energy absorption coefficients 250, 500
    mass energy transfer coefficients 500
    molecule 19
    perturbation correction (WPC) 367–368
    as phantom 158, 189, 196, 228
    photon interactions 86
    point source dosimetry 93–97
    significance in radiotherapy dosimetry 157
Water-equivalent depth, effective 243, 344
Water kerma yield 142
Water perturbation correction (WPC),
    definition 367
    in relationship to buildup factor 369
    in relationship to g(r) 369
    for various sources 368
Wave guides 123–124
Wavelength 26–27, 29
    shift in Compton scattering 78–79
Wave propagation 26–28
Waves 27–30
    electromagnetic 27–29
    infrared 26, 28
    matter waves 29
    microwaves 28
    ultra violet 27–28
    visible light 27–28
W/e 144, 157
Wedge angle 273
Wedged beam 276
Wedged oblique pair 17
Wedge filters 2, 14–21
Weekly dose limits (P) 444–445

Weighting factors
    for radiation types 426–427
    for tissue types 428–429
Wipe tests 482–483
Workload (W) 449–450
Worksheet for shielding calculation 469–470
Wrist badges 438, 486

Xenon-131 36
X-ray circuit 104
X-ray machines 95–104, 124–126 (see also
    Accelerators)
X-rays 3, 14, 28 (see also Bremsstrahlung)
    bone and depth-dose profile 209, 211
    characteristic 14–15, 37, 74, 76, 105, 357
    continuous 63
    discovery of 95–96
    in electromagnetic spectrum 28
    historical background 95–96
    kilovoltage 63–64, 105–106,192, 249, 261–262
    megavoltage 95, 124–126, 191–192, 262–264,
        345–346
    spectra and quality of 63, 65–66, 105–106,
        191–192
X-ray beam combinations (see Isodose
    distributions)
X-ray beams (see also photon beams)
    allowable leakage limits 163
    equipment workload 166
    radiation weighting factor 148
    scatter coefficients 170
    shielding back scattering 70, 164
X-ray tube,
    circuit 104
    cold-cathode 95
    constant potential 103
    Coolidge's 96
    Crooke's 95
    full-wave rectified 102
    gas-discharge 95–96,
    half-wave rectified 101
    heat generation in 97
    rotating anode 99
    self-rectified 101

Ytterbium-169 (^{169}Yb) 358, 369, 480

Z value (see Atomic Number)
Z_{eff} value 87, 241
Zinc sulfide 176
Zones, for treatment planning 271–273

Druck: Strauss Offsetdruck, Mörlenbach
Verarbeitung: Schäffer, Grünstadt